CYCLOSPORIN

MODE OF ACTION AND CLINICAL APPLICATIONS

CYCLOSPORIN

Mode of Action and Clinical Applications

Edited by

Angus W. Thomson
BSc(Hons), MSc, PhD, DSc, MRCPath, FIBiol
Reader in Immunology
Department of Pathology
University of Aberdeen
Foresterhill
Aberdeen
Scotland

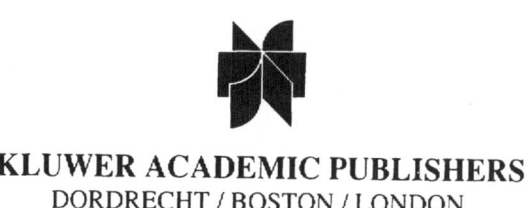

KLUWER ACADEMIC PUBLISHERS
DORDRECHT / BOSTON / LONDON

Distributors

for the United States and Canada: Kluwer Academic Publishers, PO Box 358, Accord Station, Hingham, MA 02018-0358, USA
for all other countries: Kluwer Academic Publishers Group, Distribution Center, PO Box 322, 3300 AA Dordrecht, The Netherlands

British Library Cataloguing in Publication Data

Cyclosporin.
  1. Man. Organs and tissues. Transplantation. Drug therapy. Cyclosporin A
  I. Thomson Angus W.
  615'.7

ISBN-13: 978-94-010-6874-1   e-ISBN-13: 978-94-009-0859-8
DOI: 10.1007/978-94-009-0859-8

Copyright

Kluwer Academic Publishers BV incorporates the publishing programmes of D. Reidel, Martinus Nijhoff, Dr W. Junk and MTP Press.

Typeset by Lasertext, Stretford, Manchester

Contents

List of Contributors

Kerry Atkinson
Department of Haematology
St Vincent's Hospital
Sydney
New South Wales, 2010
Australia

Jean-François Bach
Inserm U 25 CNRS U122
Hôpital Necker
161 Rue de Sèvres 75015
Paris
France

Barbara S. Baker
Department of Dermatology and
    Immunology
St Mary's Hospital
London W2 1NY

M. Danny Burke
Department of Pharmacology
University of Aberdeen
Marischal College
Aberdeen AB9 1AS

D. Cameron
Department of Pharmacology
University of Aberdeen
Marischal College
Aberdeen AB9 1AS

Graeme R. D. Catto
Department of Medicine and Therapeutics
University of Aberdeen
Foresterhill
Aberdeen AB9 2ZD

Janet I. Duncan
Immunopathology Laboratory
Department of Pathology
University of Aberdeen
Aberdeen AB9 2ZD

John V. Forrester
Department of Ophthalmology
University of Aberdeen
Foresterhill
Aberdeen AB9 2ZD

David Friend
Clinical Research
Sandoz Ltd
CH-4002
Basle
Switzerland

Lionel Fry
Department of Dermatology and
    Immunology
St Mary's Hospital
London W2 1NY

Joachim Grevel
Division of Immunology and Organ
    Transplantation
The University of Texas Medical School
6431 Fannin MSB 6.252
Houston
Texas 77030
USA

Allan D. Hess
The Bone Marrow Transplant Unit
Oncology Centre
The Johns Hopkins University
600 N. Wolfe St
Baltimore
Maryland 21205
USA

Michael C. Jones
Department of Medicine and Therapeutics
University of Aberdeen
Foresterhill
Aberdeen AB9 2ZD

Barry D. Kahan
Department of Immunology and Organ
   Transplantation
The University of Texas Medical School
643 Fannin, MSB 6.252
Houston
Texas 77030
USA

John E. Kay
School of Biological Sciences and Centre for
   Medical Research
University of Sussex
Brighton BN1 9QG

Susan M. L. Lim
Department of Surgery
Level 9
Addenbrooke's Hospital
Cambridge CB2 2QQ

Janet Liversidge
Department of Ophthalmology
University of Aberdeen
Foresterhill
Aberdeen AB9 2ZD

Fiona MacIntyre
Department of Pharmacology
University of Aberdeen
Marischal College
Aberdeen AB9 1AS

Iris Motta
Unité d'Immunophysiologie Moléculaire
Institut Pasteur
75724
Paris Cedex 15
France

Anne V. Powles
Department of Dermatology and
   Immunology
St Mary's Hospital
London W2 1NY

Wilfried Schiess
Clinical Research
Sandoz Ltd
CH-4002
Basle
Switzerland

Nicholas Shand
Clinical Research
Sandoz Ltd
CH-4002
Basle
Switzerland

Sathia Thiru
Department of Pathology
Cambridge University
Addenbrooke's Hospital
Cambridge CB2 2QQ

Angus W. Thomson
Immunopathology Laboratory
Department of Pathology
University of Aberdeen
Foresterhill
Aberdeen AB9 2ZD

Pentti Timonen
Clinical Research
Sandoz Ltd
CH-4002
Basle
Switzerland

Hamish M. Towler
Department of Ophthalmology
University of Aberdeen
Foresterhill
Aberdeen AB9 2ZD

Paolo Truffa-Bachi
Unité d'Immunophysiologie Moléculaire
Institut Pasteur
75724
Paris Cedex 15
France

Beat von Graffenried
Clinical Research
Sandoz Ltd
CH-4002
Basle
Switzerland

David J. G. White
Department of Surgery
Level 9
Addenbrooke's Hospital
Cambridge CB2 2QQ

Paul H. Whiting
Department of Clinical Biochemistry
University of Aberdeen
Foresterhill
Aberdeen AB9 2ZD

Foreword

Cyclosporin has had a remarkable effect on clinical organ transplantation. Prior to its introduction, considerable advances had been made in the grafting of vital organs, particularly the kidney, heart and liver. In many developed countries, however, transplantation was not considered worthwhile in terms of gain for the investment of resources. The improved results of kidney grafts following the use of cyclosporin has changed this attitude. For all types of organ transplantation, cyclosporin has resulted in an improvement of functional graft survival and has allowed a reduction in steroid dose and, in some cases, no steroids at all. It has permitted the first successful experimental transplantation of the heart and lungs in primate species by Reitz and colleagues and their results were applied directly to the clinic. It was largely due to the introduction of cyclosporin that the Washington Consensus Meeting on Liver Transplantation came to a favourable recommendation and the result has been the proliferation of units performing liver transplantation, approximately fifty in North America and another fifty in Europe, where previously there had been a handful.

Having been involved in cyclosporin for organ grafting from the beginning, I have been able to witness these developments which have far exceeded my expectations once the nephrotoxicity of cyclosporin was demonstrated in man. It is fitting that Dr. Thomson has put together this important volume of the state of the art of cyclosporin, since he has been one of the leaders in the investigation of its mode of action and side effects. He has brought together a strong team of authors and I am sure that their combined wisdom will be of great use to scientists and clinicians working in transplantation and on autoimmunity. The bibliography will be especially valuable.

It is my pleasure to be associated with this book and to write the Foreword.

Sir Roy Calne FRS
University of Cambridge
May, 1989.

Preface

The advent of a novel immunosuppressive agent with the distinctive anti-T cell properties of cyclosporin came by fortune rather than by design. We still do not comprehend how it exercises its selectivity for helper T cells or how, in precise molecular terms, it suppresses their activation. Since the first descriptions in 1976 of its immunological properties by J. F. Borel and his colleagues in Basel, and since its introduction into clinical use by R. Y. Calne in Cambridge, cyclosporin has been the subject of several thousands of scientific papers. Three major international congresses on cyclosporin (Cambridge, Houston and Washington) have been held, whilst in the clinic, the drug has had a major impact on the nature of, and progress in, clinical organ transplantation.

Cyclosporin has proved a powerful investigative tool for immunologists in the evaluation and dissection of T cell function. Its potential for the treatment of certain autoimmune diseases in which T cells are believed to play a pathogenetic role is presently the subject of extensive investigation. In this book, the mode of action, clinical applications, pharmacology and pathology of cyclosporin are reviewed by expert contributors in Europe, North America and Australia. I am grateful to them all for their roles in this venture.

A. W. Thomson
University of Aberdeen
May, 1989.

1
Inhibitory effects of cyclosporin A on lymphocyte activation

John E. Kay

IMMUNOSUPPRESSION BY CYCLOSPORIN A

Cyclosporin A (CsA) was first identified in the early 1970s by Dr J. F. Borel and colleagues of Sandoz Ltd as a compound in the culture broths of the fungi *Tolypocladium inflatum* and *Cylindrocarpon lucidum* that showed strong *in vivo* immunosuppressive activity in mice, but was otherwise well tolerated. Their influential publication on the properties of CsA in 1976[1] led to successful clinical trials, and the drug is now in routine use in organ transplantation. It also shows promise in the prevention or treatment of some conditions with an autoimmune basis (discussed in subsequent chapters of this volume). It was very quickly apparent that CsA differed in its mechanism of action from pre-existing immunosuppressive drugs, in that at therapeutic concentrations it showed no general inhibition of cell proliferation and was not cytotoxic to lymphocytes.

STRUCTURE AND ANALOGUES

CsA is a strongly hydrophobic cyclic endecapeptide, with a relative molecular mass of 1202. Its structure, first determined in 1976, it shown in Figure 1.1. It contains a 9-carbon amino acid at position 1 that had not previously been discovered, appears to be unique to cyclosporins and is essential for biological activity. Seven of the amino acids are *N*-methylated, and one (at position 8) is in the D configuration. The total synthesis of this molecule has been achieved, and the properties of a large number of natural and synthetic analogues are reviewed in references 2 and 3. None of the analogues so far studied has proved more potently immunosuppressive than CsA, though one natural analogue in which the α-aminoisobutyric acid residue at position 2 is replaced by a norvaline appears to couple similar potency with fewer side-effects[4].

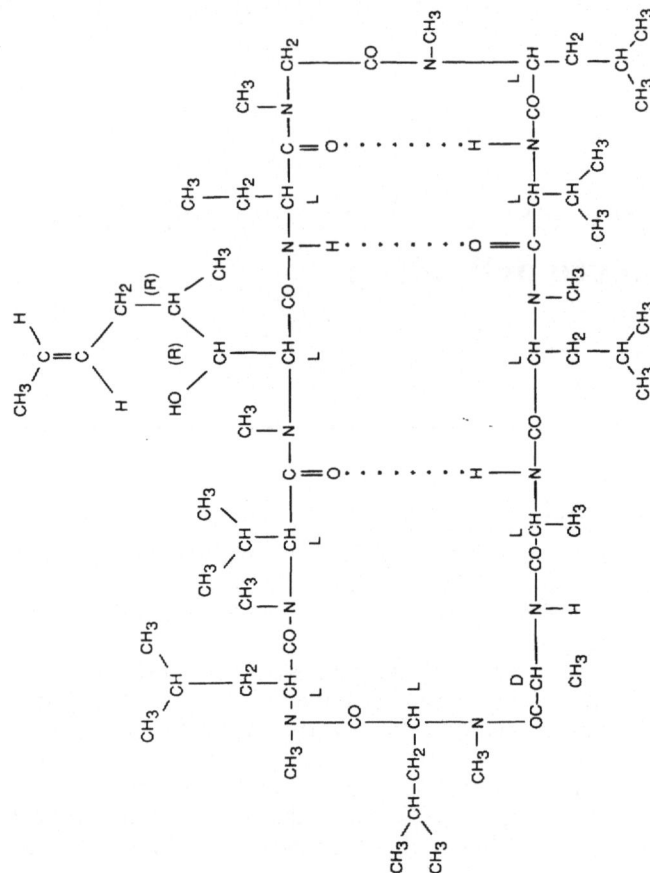

Figure 1.1 The structure of cyclosporin A

TERMINOLOGY

The compound originally named cyclosporin A has now achieved sufficient prominence to attract the attention of several learned international bodies. As a result the molecule shown in Figure 1.1 has been renamed cyclosporine by the United States Adopted Name Council, ciclosporin by the World Health Organization and simply cyclosporin by the British Pharmacopoeia Commission. It is marketed by Sandoz under the trade name Sandimmun, except in North America where it is Sandimmune[5]. It is referred to throughout this chapter as CsA.

INHIBITION OF T AND B LYMPHOCYTE ACTIVATION *IN VITRO*

Although it was found that CsA could suppress both humoral and cell-mediated immunity in the intact animal, the early studies that first showed the drug to inhibit the activation of cultured lymphocytes *in vitro* were interpreted as indicating that it acted primarily by inhibiting an early step in the activation of T lymphocytes[6]. The activation of mouse splenic lymphocytes by the T lymphocyte mitogen concanavalin A (Con A) was much more sensitive to inhibition by CsA than activation by the B lymphocyte mitogen lipopolysaccharide (LPS), so the effects of CsA on humoral immunity *in vivo* were assumed to be secondary to inhibition of T helper cell function.

Subsequent more detailed analysis has shown this conclusion to have been premature. The sensitivity of both T and B lymphocyte activation *in vitro* depends on the specific mitogen used. Thus the activation of T lymphocytes by the lectin Con A is more sensitive to inhibition by CsA than is activation by the lectin phytohaemagglutinin (PHA), while activation by the anti-CD3 monoclonal antibody OKT3 is more sensitive still[7,8]. The mixed lymphocyte reaction, another T lymphocyte response that might be considered more physiological than activation by lectins, also appears to be particularly sensitive to CsA. Similarly the activation of murine B lymphocytes by LPS could be inhibited only by very high concentrations of CsA, but their activation by anti-IgM antibodies was more than two orders of magnitude more sensitive to the drug, and thus as readily inhibited as the most sensitive T lymphocyte responses[9]. Both T lymphocyte-dependent and T-independent immunoglobulin synthesis by human B lymphocytes showed similar sensitivities to CsA[10].

Initially it was thought that these differences in sensitivity could be accounted for by the different mitogens acting on different lymphocyte subpopulations, with only certain T and B lymphocyte subpopulations being sensitive to the action of CsA. Studies on the effects of CsA *in vivo* rather favoured this concept, as treatment of patients or experimental animals with CsA leads to a fall in the ratio of CD4 : CD8 lymphocytes in the peripheral blood[11], and may tip the balance of the response to transplantation from rejections towards tolerance. Although both new cell-mediated and humoral immunological responses are inhibited, priming often occurs much as usual in the presence of CsA[12]. However, it has proved difficult to obtain convincing evidence for CsA-resistant lymphocyte subpopulations *in vitro*, the principal

3

exception being that a number of studies have reported the induction of T suppressor lymphocytes to be relatively resistant to CsA (reviewed in reference 13). The activation by antigen or (most) mitogens of both T helper and T cytotoxic cells or cloned cell lines is inhibited by CsA[14]. It now seems more likely that sensitivity to CsA is a function of the nature of the activating signal delivered to the cell, rather than an immutable property of the cell itself.

The concentrations of CsA needed to inhibit lymphocyte proliferation *in vitro* are in general closely comparable to the serum concentrations that need to be maintained for effective immunosuppression *in vivo*. It has been the common experience that CsA at such concentrations is not cytotoxic to lymphocytes, and that its effects on lymphocyte activation are readily reversible when the drug is removed. The drug has few reported effects on resting lymphocytes. However, CsA and its immunosuppressive analogues have been shown to reduce the membrane potential of both T and B lymphocytes[15,16], and CsA also causes a small but significant inhibition of the rate of protein synthesis in unstimulated lymphocytes[7].

THE ROLE OF ACCESSORY CELLS

The hierarchy of CsA-sensitivity of T lymphocyte activation responses shows a superficial correspondence with their dependence on accessory cells. While all the responses above require such cells to be present in the cultures, activation by anti-CD3 requires higher numbers of accessory cells than activation by Con A, while the accessory cell dependence of the PHA response can only be demonstrated if rigorous depletion procedures are used. Although the addition of an excess of accessory cells does not relieve the inhibition of PHA- or Con A-induced activation by even limiting concentrations of CsA[7], there is evidence that CsA may in at least some circumstances inhibit their functioning.

Two independent studies investigating the mechanism by which CsA inhibited the specific antigen responsiveness of murine T cell lines found that, when irradiated spleen cells were pulsed with antigen in the presence of CsA, their subsequent ability to present antigen to the T cells was impaired[17,18]. Although mixed spleen cell populations rather than purified antigen presenting cells were used in these studies, it is unlikely that the inhibition was mediated by T cells within the spleen cell population, as T cells are not required for the development of antigen presenting capacity.

The work of Knight's laboratory has specifically implicated dendritic cells as a target for CsA action[19-21]. After only brief incubation with CsA, rabbit dendritic cells were blocked in their ability to function as accessory cells in the activation of T lymphocytes by Con A, while murine dendritic cells became unable to provoke a response by allogeneic lymphocytes. In the most recent study[21], *in vivo* administration to mice of CsA concentrations that blocked the development of contact sensitivity was shown to reduce the accumulation of antigen by the dendritic cells that accumulated in the draining lymph node. These dendritic cells from CsA-treated animals were unable to

4

initiate proliferation in syngeneic lymphocytes *in vitro*. Despite the obvious controls being carried out, it is difficult to eliminate the possibility that in the *in vitro* studies the antigen presenting cells might have concentrated CsA and specifically 'presented' it to potentially reponsive T cells along with the antigen. However, the observation that dendritic cells *in vivo* fail to accumulate antigen normally in the presence of CsA cannot be accounted for in this way.

Together these studies present a strong case that CsA may interfere with the process of antigen presentation. However, they do not indicate that this is the only or even the principal action of CsA. Indeed, Varey *et al.*[18] noted that the CsA concentration required to suppress antigen presentation was an order of magnitude higher than that needed to prevent T cell responsiveness to presented antigen. In addition, as noted below, some lymphocyte responses that bypass the requirement for accessory cells are nevertheless sensitive to inhibition by CsA.

THE STAGE IN LYMPHOCYTE ACTIVATION SENSITIVE TO CsA

One early conclusion that has been widely confirmed is that CsA inhibits a relatively early step or steps in lymphocyte proliferation. Studies on the activation of pig lymphocytes by the T lymphocyte mitogens PHA and Con A[22] have shown that sensitivity to CsA is progressively lost over the first 6–8 h. The response of human T lymphocytes to mitogens shows a similar progressive loss of sensitivity to CsA, though over a slightly longer period[8]. The generation of T lymphocyte cytotoxicity in the murine mixed lymphocyte reaction also became progressively less sensitive to CsA over the first 2–3 days of culture[23,24].

CsA does not inhibit T lymphocyte cytotoxicity directly, nor does it inhibit the response of primed T lymphocytes to Il-2[23]. Orosz *et al.*[14] have confirmed that the response of individual clones to mitogen or antigen is CsA-sensitive, while the response of the same clones to IL-2 under identical culture conditions is resistant. The reponse of preactivated B lymphocytes to IL-4 is also not inhibited by CsA, but their response to IL-5 is still sensitive to the drug[25]. With the exception of this anomalous sensitivity to IL-5, the evidence thus suggests that the principal CsA-sensitive step in lymphocyte activation is completed relatively early in the process, well before the initiation of DNA synthesis.

THE CsA-SENSITIVITY OF ACTIVATION CORRELATES WITH Ca^{2+}-DEPENDENCE

There is now strong evidence that the activation of both T and B lymphocytes by antigen or mitogens is initiated by receptor-mediated hydrolysis of phosphatidylinositol bisphosphate to generate two key intracellular mediators, diacylglycerol and inositol-1,4,5-trisphosphate[26,27]. Diacylglycerol is believed to function principally via the activation of protein kinase C, while inositol-1,4,5-trisphosphate elevates the cytoplasmic Ca^{2+} concentration by releasing Ca^{2+} from intracellular stores. The concentration of free Ca^{2+} in the cytoplasm of unstimulated lymphocytes is maintained at about 100 nmol/l, but a wide range of different signals that cause receptor-mediated phosphatidylinositol bisphosphate hydrolysis in T and B lymphocytes or T and B cell lines increase this to 250–500 nmol/l within a few minutes.

This initial increase, caused by the release of Ca^{2+} from intracellular stores, is very transient and is not of itself sufficient to initiate the activation process. However, most successful mitogenic signals result in the initial transient Ca^{2+} signal being followed by a more sustained elevation of the cytoplasmic Ca^{2+} concentration. The Ca^{2+} required for this second phase is taken into the cell from the culture medium, and this key step in activation is blocked if no extracellular Ca^{2+} is available. The intracellular signals mediating this second phase of the Ca^{2+} signal have not yet been clearly established, but there is some evidence to suggest that inositol-1,4,5-trisphosphate and/or other phosphoinositides derived from it, such as inositol-1,3,4,5-tetraphosphate, may be involved[28].

Both the activation of protein kinase C and a sustained elevation of the cytoplasmic Ca^{2+} concentration are thought to be necessary to initiate the chain of events leading to the proliferation of unstimulated lymphocytes, and at least in vitro activation of protein kinase C by exogenous diacylglycerols or phorbol esters together with artificial elevation of the cytoplasmic Ca^{2+} concentration by calcium ionophores are sufficient to initiate the process[29,30]. The scheme presented in Figure 1.2 is thus widely accepted. However, it should be noted that under physiological conditions the two signalling arms may interact, as diacylglycerols activate protein kinase C principally by reducing the Ca^{2+} concentration required for the enzyme's activity. In addition, the activation achieved by naturally formed diacylglycerols is likely to be weaker and more transient than that seen when phorbol esters are added to cultured cells, as the diacylglycerols are rapidly metabolized further, while the phorbol esters are stable under the conditions of culture. It should also be noted that while inositol-1,4,5-trisphosphate can be generated only by the hydrolysis of phosphatidylinositol bisphosphate, diacylglycerol can also be formed by the hydrolysis of other phospholipids. There is evidence to suggest that the induction of lymphocyte proliferation requires protein kinase C activation to be maintained for much longer than the Ca^{2+} signal, and this may well be achieved through the generation of diacylglycerols via alternative receptors, and perhaps by hydrolysis of alternative phospholipids[31].

The enhanced turnover of phosphatidylinositol bisphosphate initiated by addition of anti-Ig to B lymphocytes or of Con A to T lymphocytes is not inhibited by CsA[32,33]. The relatively specific action of CsA as an immunosuppresive drug in vivo could most obviously have been accounted for by some specific action against a receptor required only for immunological responsiveness, but an early report that CsA bound to and blocked the function of the T lymphocyte receptor[34] has received no confirmation, and appears incompatible with more recent research. Certainly CsA can also inhibit the induction of lymphocyte proliferation by agents that bypass the initial antigen receptor, such as combinations of phorbol esters and calcium ionophores (Figure 1.3).

Direct activation of protein kinase C by phorbol esters can, even in the

6

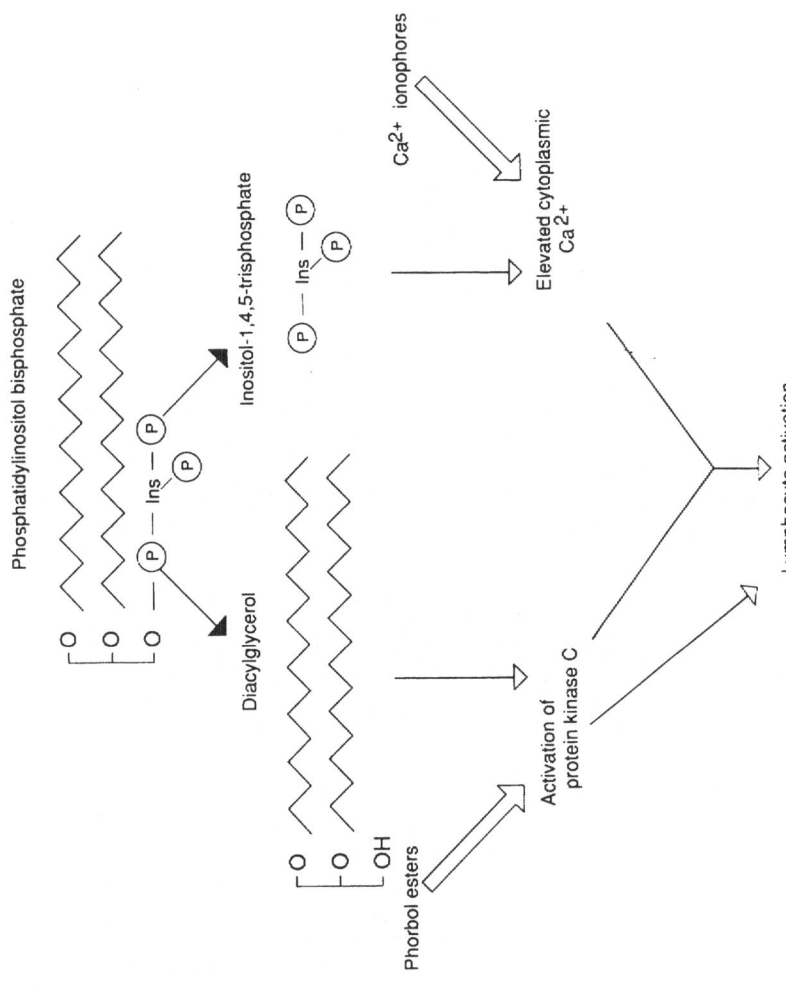

Figure 1.2 Schematic representation of phosphatidylinoitol bisphosphate hydrolysis during lymphocyte activation

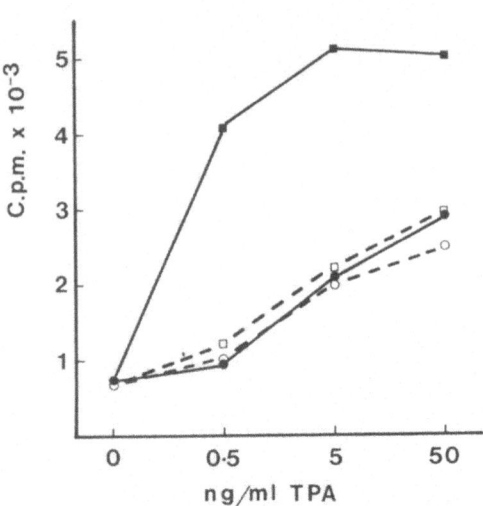

Figure 1.3 Effect of CSA on lymphocyte activation by combination of the phorbol ester TPA with the calcium ionophore A23187. Pig peripheral blood lymphocytes were incubated with TPA alone (●), TPA plus 1 µg/ml CSA (○), TPA plus 100 ng/ml A23187 (■) or TPA plus both 100 ng/ml A23187 and 1 µg/ml CSA (□). Lymphocyte activation was determined by assessment of [³⁵S]methionine incorporation into protein in a pulse given 20–24 h after activation, as little DNA synthesis is seen in cultures stimulated with TPA alone. CSA had little effect on the stimulation of protein synthesis by TPA, but blocked the additional effects of A23187

absence of a Ca^{2+} signal, induce some of the changes characteristic of the early stages of lymphocyte proliferation. Saturating concentrations of phorbol esters can induce such late changes as quite substantial increases in the rate of protein synthesis 24 h after treatment (Figure 1.3), though the increase is smaller than that induced by strongly mitogenic lectins such as PHA or Con A, and there is usually little or no progression of the response to DNA synthesis. These effects that can be induced by activation of protein kinase C alone are not inhibited by CsA[35] (see also Figure 1.3).

Low ionophore concentrations synergize with agents that activate protein kinase C to initiate the early changes characteristic of the induction of lymphocyte proliferation as effectively as the most potent mitogenic lectins[29,30] (see also Figure 1.3). The concentrations of calcium ionophores that synergize effectively in this way have few observable effects when added on their own to unstimulated lymphocytes − not only is there no induction of DNA synthesis, but few if any of the earlier changes associated with lymphocyte activation occur. Higher ionophore concentrations may induce some lymphocyte proliferation, but at these concentrations there appears to be some Ca^{2+}-induced stimulation of phosphatidylinositol bisphosphate turnover and thus indirect activation of protein kinase C, and the intracellular Ca^{2+} may perhaps even rise sufficiently to cause direct activation of protein kinase C in the absence of an activator such as diacylglycerol. Both the synergistic effects of low ionophore concentrations and the mitogenic effects of higher concentra-

8

tions are very sensitive to inhibition by CsA in both B and T lymphocytes[36–38]. This is well illustrated by Figure 1.3, which shows that when lymphocytes are stimulated by a combination of a phorbol ester and a calcium ionophore whatever part of the subsequent activation observed is dependent on the presence of the ionophore is inhibited by CsA, while the stimulation that can be ascribed to the action of the phorbol ester alone remains unaffected. The actual percentage inhibition of the response by CsA varies with the phorbol ester concentration.

The observations presented in Figure 1.3 suggest an explanation for the dependence of CsA-sensitivity on the mitogen used noted above. The hierarchy of sensitivity to CsA would be accounted for if the mitogens all caused an effective Ca^{2+} signal, but varied in their abilities to activate protein kinase C. There is some evidence to support this hypothesis, as the relatively CsA-sensitive response to anti-CD3 monoclonal antibodies is much more strongly augmented by coincubation with phorbol esters than the more CsA-resistant response to the lectin PHA. As those *in vitro* responses that most strongly resemble the physiological induction of lymphocyte proliferation by antigen are all at the more CsA-sensitive end of the spectrum, this hypothesis would suggest that the direct activation of protein kinase C by diacylglycerol generated by antigen–receptor interaction may be physiologically rather weak.

ARE THE STEPS IN ACTIVATION INHIBITED BY CsA THOSE WHICH OCCUR IN RESPONSE TO THE Ca^{2+} SIGNAL?

The rapid and transient increases in the cytoplasmic Ca^{2+} concentration that occur immediately after activation of murine T lymphocytes or thymocytes by Con A[39,33] or of cells of the Jurkat T cell line by the anti-CD3 monoclonal antibody OKT3[40,41] were found not to be inhibited by the simultaneous addition of high concentrations of CsA. Similar results were reported for human lymphocytes stimulated by PHA when CsA or its active analogues were added together with, or up to 15 min before, mitogen[16]. In this latter study the increase in the cytoplasmic Ca^{2+} concentration was greatly reduced when the CsA was added 30 min before the mitogen, although DNA synthesis was depressed to a similar extent whether the cyclosporins were added 10 min or 30 min before mitogen. In one of the reports using mouse thymocytes[33] the increase in cytoplasmic Ca^{2+} concentration was shown to occur normally even when the cells were preincubated for 30 min with a very high cyclosporin concentration (5 μmol/l).

In all four studies above the experimental conditions were such that only the effects of CsA on the initial increase in the cytoplasmic Ca^{2+} concentration caused by the release of Ca^{2+} from intracellular stores were studied. The limitations of the available methodology make it much more difficult to establish whether CsA affects the subsequent uptake of extracellular Ca^{2+} which, as noted above, seems much more closely associated with the Ca^{2+} signal that induces cellular proliferation. However, it seems unlikely that CsA acts primarily by preventing Ca^{2+} uptake, as its effects are not relieved by the addition of Ca^{2+} ionophores such a ionomycin or A23187 – indeed, as also noted above, effects mediated by these ionophores are equally sensitive to inhibition by CsA. It has been confirmed directly that CsA does not affect the enhanced cytoplasmic Ca^{2+} concentration induced by addition of ionomycin[16].

It thus seems that CsA does not act primarily by preventing the elevation of the cytoplasmic Ca^{2+} concentration. However, a possible alternative explanation for the correspondence between CsA-sensitivity and Ca^{2+}-dependence noted above would be that CsA prevents the cells from responding to this signal. It has frequently been observed that when T lymphocytes or T cell lines are exposed to a proliferative stimulus some early changes characteristic of the activation response still occur in the presence of CsA, while others are blocked. The extent to which those that are blocked correlate with those that require a Ca^{2+} signal is discussed below.

The early changes that may still be observed at least in part when T lymphocytes or T cell lines are stimulated in the presence of CsA include translocation of protein kinase C from the cytoplasm to the cell membrane[42], activation of Na^+/H^+ exchange resulting in a rise in cytoplasmic pH[41], accelerated rates of membrane transport of small molecules such as nucleosides[43], induction of transcription- or proliferation-associated genes such as c-fos and c-myc[44,45], expression of the 55 kd Tac chain of the IL-2 receptor[46,47,44,16] and enhanced rates of protein synthesis[7]. These CsA-resistant changes can all also be induced when T cell protein kinase C is activated directly by incubation with phorbol esters.

The extent to which these changes are inhibited by CsA again depends on the nature of the mitogen used, being more marked when cells are activated via the T cell receptor–CD3 complex or with lectins such as Con A than when PHA is used, and least sensitive to CsA when a phorbol ester is used as mitogen or co-mitogen. Thus the rise in intracellular pH following activation of T cell Na^+/H^+ exchange is blocked by CsA when the cells are activated by anti-CD3 monoclonal antibodies, but unaffected when the cells are activated by phorbol esters[41]. Similarly, the induction of c-myc mRNA synthesis by phorbol ester is not inhibited by CsA, but the additional c-myc mRNA induced if a Ca^{2+} signal is also provided is abolished by the drug[45]. Phorbol esters may also enhance the level of some mRNAs constitutively expressed by T cells, such as T cell receptor mRNA. This enhancement is antagonized by a Ca^{2+} signal provided by a calcium ionophore or mitogenic lectin, and here again CsA neutralizes the effect of the Ca^{2+}, increasing the level of the mRNA back to that found when cells are incubated with phorbol ester alone[45]. Failure to recognize the importance of the precise nature of the mitogenic signal used has on occasion led to confusion, and probably contributed to the apparently contradictory results obtained in studies of the effect of CsA on the induction of the IL-2 receptor[16,44,46–51]. In general it seems likely that where CSA inhibits these processes, its action is secondary to the neutralization of an intracellular Ca^{2+} signal responsible for them, rather than a direct effect on the process itself.

Some other early changes have been reported to be strongly inhibited by CsA. Enhanced incorporation of arachidonate and oleate into membrane

10

phosphatidylcholine and phosphatidylethanolamine in rabbit lymphocytes stimulated by the T cell mitogen Con A, the B cell mitogen anti-immunoglobulin or the calcium ionophore A23187 is apparent within the first hour of stimulation, and is strongly inhibited by CSA[37,52]. The enzyme responsible for this incorporation, lysophosphatide acyltransferase, was shown not to be inhibited by CsA directly. Incorporation of these fatty acids into phosphatidylinositol was much less sensitive. CsA has also been reported to inhibit the induction of ornithine decarboxylase, the first enzyme in the pathway leading to polyamine biosynthesis, in the first few hours after mitogen addition[53]. Another early change inhibited was the uptake of amino acids by the Na^+-dependent amino acid transport systems in pig lymphocytes stimulated by A23187[36]. However, in these studies the mitogens used were those most easily inhibited by CsA, and it is not yet clear whether these processes would be similarly CsA-sensitive if a mitogenic signal ensuring strong activation of protein kinase C had been employed.

The action of CsA which has attracted the greatest attention is its effect on lymphokine production. The drug completely abolishes the synthesis by activated T lymphocytes or T cell lines of most lymphokines studied, including IL-2[40,44,47,49,54–58], γ-interferon[59–61,40,44,56,58], IL-3[58,62], IL-4[63] and GM-CSF[55,64] (see also reference 62). Even ongoing synthesis of IL-2 is inhibited. Where studied, inhibition of lymphokine synthesis has invariably been found to be due to an effect at the transcriptional level. Studies of the intracellular signals required for the induction of lymphokine mRNA synthesis in T cells have shown that both protein kinase C activation and a Ca^{2+} signal are absolutely required in normal lymphocytes and in most T lymphocyte-derived cell lines. The CSA-sensitivity of the synthesis of IL-2 and other lymphokines is thus compatible with the hypothesis that the primary target of the drug is the response to the Ca^{2+} signal. The inhibition of the synthesis of these lymphokine mRNAs by CsA is highly selective[44,47,56,57,64], and the suggestion that CsA might directly inhibit RNA polymerase II[65], and thus all lymphocyte mRNA synthesis, can be discounted as the basis for its immunosuppressive action.

In some cell lines derived from neoplastic T cells the control of lymphokine mRNA synthesis is abnormal, and IL-2 may be induced by protein kinase C activation alone. The human leukaemia line HUT 78 produces a low level of IL-2 when incubated with phorbol ester alone, and a much higher level if coincubated with both azacytidine and phorbol ester. There is no increase in the cytoplasmic Ca^{2+} concentration when IL-2 synthesis is induced in this way, and CsA is unable to inhibit this process[42]. However, the mouse thymoma line EL-4 can produce both IL-2 and IL-3 when stimulated with phorbol ester alone, and in this case the synthesis of both lymphokines is strongly inhibited by low concentrations of CsA[56,57,62].

CsA has also been reported to inhibit the production of lymphokines such as IL-1 synthesized by cells of the monocyte/macrophage lineage[51,54,66–68]. In some cases the inhibition may very well be secondary to the inhibition of a T cell-derived signal that induces lymphokine production by the monocytes. However, there has been disagreement between studies using experimental systems from different species as to whether CsA at concentrations that inhibit lymphocyte proliferation also inhibits the lipopolysaccharide-induce synthesis of IL-1[63,66]. Such inhibition would imply a direct action of CsA on the monocytes, and the effects of LPS are not thought to be mediated via a Ca^{2+} signal.

As the induction of IL-2 synthesis is essential for the activation of T lymphocytes to progress to DNA synthesis and proliferation, its prevention could potentially account completely for the inhibition of this process by CsA, and thus the immunosuppressive properties of the drug. However, if inhibition of lymphokine production were the only important effect, then it should be possible to reverse the inhibition caused by CsA by addition of preformed lymphokines. There have been occasional reports of this being achieved – for example Bunjes et al.[54]. In our laboratory we have found that when high phorbol ester concentrations are used to provide maximal activation of protein kinase C, addition of recombinant IL-2 enables the cells to initiate proliferation (Figure 1.4). However, no such synergy is seen with lower phorbol ester concentrations, and we and others have found that when cells are activated via the T cell receptor or with mitogenic lectins in the presence of CsA, neither recombinant IL-2 nor lymphokine-rich culture supernatants gave more than partial restitution of the response[8,16,22,50,69]. Interestingly, the effects of CsA could also be partially counteracted by the addition of insulin[70,71].

Perhaps the clearest evidence about the way in which CsA interferes with lymphocyte activation has come from the study of the factors which are

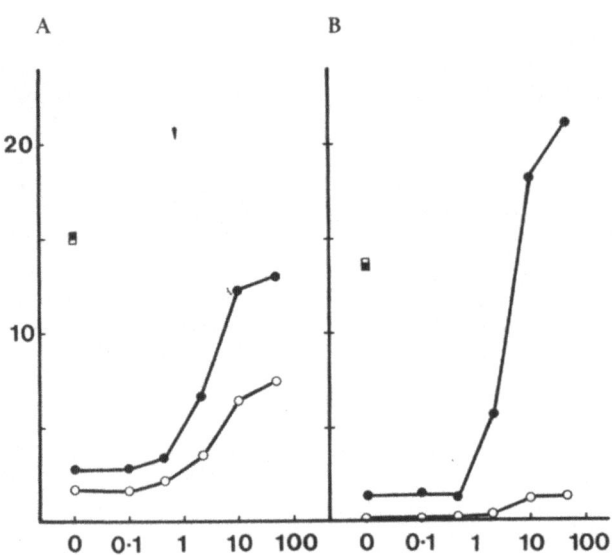

Figure 1.4 High phorbol ester concentrations enable T lymphocytes to proliferate in the presence of recombinant IL-2. Pig peripheral blood lymphocytes were incubated with TPA at the concentration shown, and with (●) or without (○) 100 units/ml recombinant IL-2. Incorporation of [^{35}S]methionine into protein was determined 20–24 h after stimulation (Panel A), and [^{35}H]thymidine into DNA after 44–48 h (Panel B). Incorporation by parallel cultures incubated with PHA and with (■) or without (□) IL-2 is shown for comparison

12

necessary during the first hours after activation for the response to become resistant to CsA. A protocol that we have used is to stimulate cells with PHA for 6–8 h in the presence of a range of inhibitors. The inhibitors are then washed out, and incubation with mitogen continued in the presence of CsA. Normally CsA added at this time would be ineffective, but if the inhibitor used prevents the key CsA-sensitive stage of activation taking place during the preincubation, the response will still be sensitive to CsA added when the inhibitor is washed out[43]. The CsA-sensitive stage of activation is completely dependent on the availability of Ca^{2+} in the culture medium, and on its ability to enter the cell, and it is also inhibited by chlorpromazine (which inhibits both calmodulin and protein kinase C). However, drugs which do not prevent the CsA-sensitive stage of activation being completed include cycloheximide (which inhibits protein synthesis), monensin (which inhibits protein secretion), ouabain (which inhibits Na^+, K^+ ATPase) or colchicine (which inhibits microtubule formation). Unfortunately there is no suitable reversible inhibitor available to study the role of the production of the mRNAs for IL-2 and other lymphokines, which are known to be induced during this initial period. Analogous experiments in which the preincubation phase was carried out with either phorbol esters or calcium ionophores or both showed that neither alone was sufficient to drive the cells through the CsA-sensitive stage, but that both together were able to do so.

HOW DOES CsA BLOCK THE RESPONSE TO THE Ca^{2+} SIGNAL?

CsA binds to a wide range of cells, including B and T lymphocytes of all types. The binding is generally of relatively low affinity, with K_d values for most cells in the range $1–5 \times 10^{-7}$ mol/l. The few cell types reported to show some higher affinity binding include B but not T lymphocytes[72]. As K_d values similar to those for binding to T lymphocytes were found for synthetic phospholipid vesicles, it was initially suspected that the hydrophobic CsA molecule simply partitioned into the membrane and phospholipid bilayer[72] and accumulated in intracytoplasmic lipid droplets[73].

However, in 1984 Handschumacher's laboratory identified and purified cyclophilin, the major CsA-binding protein in the cell[74,75]. Cyclophilin is an abundant basic 18 kd cytoplasmic protein, with a K_d for CsA of 2×10^{-7} mol/l, very similar to that seen in the intact lymphocyte. The binding of a series of cyclosporin analogues to cyclophilin was demonstrated to parallel their immunosuppressive potency[75]. The protein was identified in all mammalian tissues and cell lines examined, with CsA binding activity for most normal and neoplastic cells within the range 0.05–0.3 μg/mg protein, although higher activities were found in a few neoplastic tisues[76]. A minor isoform, less basic but with very similar amino acid composition, was also found in all tissues examined. Similar activities were found in yeast, plants and representatives of several lower eukaryotic phyla, but the activity was not detectable in E. coli[76]. Incubation of T cells with mitogenic lectins, phorbol esters or CsA had little effect on cyclophilin activity[76,77].

The amino acid sequences of the major isoform of bovine[78], human[77] and

13

rat[79] cyclophilins have now been determined. Comparison of the sequences indicates a very high degree of conservation between these mammalian species. Antibodies raised against bovine cyclophilin cross-reacted not only with the human and murine cyclophilins from a variety of tissues, but also with the CsA-binding activity from a marine sponge[78]. Genomic blots of human leukocyte DNA show multiple hybridizing fragments. This strongly suggests that several related genes may exist, although it has not been established how many of these genes are functional[77]. Initial analyses did not reveal any significant homologies between the cyclophilins and other proteins, but it has recently been reported[80] that there is a moderate level of homology between a particularly highly conserved region of cyclophilin and a section of the eukaryotic protein synthesis elongation factor EF-2. The region of homology includes the putative CsA binding site of cyclophilin, and also a sequence that is characteristic of nucleotide binding proteins.

An attractive hypothesis to explain the antagonism of Ca^{2+}-mediated steps in lymphocyte activation by CsA was proposed by Colombani, Robb and Hess in 1985[81]. They presented evidence that CsA bound directly to calmodulin, the protein that mediates many of the effects of Ca^{2+}, and that the binding of CsA to T cells was competitively inhibited by other calmodulin antagonists known to interact at the hydrophobic site on calmodulin exposed by Ca^{2+} binding. They also reported that CsA directly inhibited the activation of bovine brain 3',5'-cyclic nucleotide phosphodiesterase by bovine brain calmodulin, with a significant effect detectable at 10 nmol/l CsA and 50% inhibition with less than 100 nmol/l CsA. In addition they claimed that antibodies to calmodulin showed strong cross-reactivity with cyclophilin and, noting that both proteins had similar molecular weights, suggested that they might be very closely related, if not identical.

While this hypothesis could provide a straightforward explanation for many of the effects of CsA on lymphocyte activation, workers in other laboratories have found it difficult to confirm the evidence on which it is based. Most unambiguously, the subsequent determination of the sequence of cyclophilin has established that it has no homology at all with calmodulin, and it is thus not surprising that Handschumacher's laboratory have failed to observe any immunological cross-reactivity between the two proteins[82]. Purified cyclophilin did not activate calmodulin-dependent enzymes or bind phenathiazine inhibitors of calmodulin. Handschumacher's laboratory found that any binding of CsA to calmodulin was at least two orders of magnitude lower than that to cyclophilin. LeGrue et al.[83] were able to detect some Ca^{2+}-dependent binding of CsA to calmodulin, but only at CsA concentrations two orders of magnitude higher than those necessary to block lymphocyte activation. They also found that two analogues of CsA with much reduced immunosuppressive activity were nevertheless equally effective at binding to calmodulin.

Neither these laboratories nor others including our own have been able to confirm the claim that CsA directly inhibits the activation of 3',5'-cyclic nucleotide phosphodiesterase by calmodulin[82–85,33]. No inhibition was seen even with CsA concentrations as high as 30 μmol/l, more than three orders of magnitude higher than those reported by Colombani et al. to cause

14

detectable inhibition, and two orders of magnitude greater than those they claimed to cause 50% inhibition. The studies have been extended to include the effects of CsA on lymphocyte calmodulin, and the use of alternative calmodulin-dependent enzymes, but in no case has inhibition by CsA been detected, even when great care has been taken to ensure that the amount of calmodulin was limiting, and that the activity of the CsA was not compromised by the assay conditions. In all cases it was confirmed that conventional inhibitors of calmodulin activity were fully effective. This discrepancy is puzzling, as the reagents for the basic experiment are readily available commercially and the experimental protocol is standard and widely used.

Mizushima et al.[33] have also provided direct evidence that CsA does not interfere with calmodulin-dependent changes following the addition of Con A to T lymphocytes. They demonstrated by immunofluorescence microscopy that the rapid patching and capping of Con A receptors on the T lymphocyte surface was calmodulin-dependent and accompanied by the concentration of the actin-linked regulatory proteins calspectin, caldesmon and tropomycin below the caps. This process was prevented by phenathiazine inhibitors of calmodulin, but was unaffected by CsA concentrations as high as 10 μmol/l.

The conclusion to be drawn about the role of calmodulin in immunosuppression by CsA thus remains controversial. In particular it is difficult to see how a compound that acted via such a universal mediator as calmodulin could be so selectively immunosuppressive in vivo – although CsA certainly does have effects on cells other than lymphocytes both in vivo and in vitro, there does not seem to be any obvious correlation in other tissues between events that are calmodulin-dependent and those that are CsA-sensitive. Hess and Colombani, while now accepting that cyclophilin and calmodulin are distinct proteins, have recently presented further circumstantial argument in favour of their hypothesis, and suggested a possible resolution[86]. They noted that the T lymphocytes that bound CsA most strongly contained the same amount of calmodulin, but less cyclophilin, than T lymphocytes that bound less CsA. The cells that bound most CsA were also, paradoxically, more resistant to the action of the drug. They thus proposed that cyclophilin might act as an intracellular buffer for CsA, preventing the inhibition of calmodulin by the drug. The selective immunosuppressive effect of CsA would thus reflect a relative lack of cyclophilin in key lymphoid cells. More detailed studies than those presently published will be required to substantiate this hypothesis, which seems superficially difficult to reconcile with the evidence that it is only the immunosuppressive cyclosporins that bind to cyclophilin, while both immunosuppressive and inactive analogues bind to calmodulin.

As cyclophilin is also a protein that is very widely distributed in nature, it is at present not clear either how it could mediate a selective effect on the proliferation of lymphocytes. The possibility must therefore be considered that the immunosuppressive action of CsA is due to its interaction with some other quantitatively minor but lymphocyte-specific protein or other cellular constituent.

Two receptors found on lymphocytes (but also on other cells) that have been suggested to be blocked by CsA are the receptors for interleukin-1 and prolactin. Inhibition of the binding of immunoadsorbent-purified IL-1 to T lymphocytes by CsA has been reported by Bendtzen and Dinarello[70]. CsA could also cause IL-1 that had already been bound to the cells to be released. However, this cannot be the only mechanism by which CsA inhibits lymphocyte proliferation. As noted above, activation is still sensitive to CsA even when the stimulus used bypasses any requirement for IL-1, such as a combination of a calcium ionophore and a phorbol ester.

CsA has been reported to inhibit prolactin-induced changes in lymphocytes and in some other tissues[87]. In the rat kidney, CsA prevented the normal induction of ornithine decarboxylase by prolactin, but did not affect that induction of the enzyme by growth hormone or insulin. Ornithine decarboxylase is the first enzyme in the pathway leading to the synthesis of the polyamines spermidine and spermine, and its activity is greatly increased early in the cellular response to many stimuli promoting growth or proliferation. The comparatively small increases observed in ornithine decarboxylase activity in thymus and spleen *in vivo* in response to prolactin administration *in vivo* were also abolished by CsA. It is of course difficult to be certain in such experiments that the effects of prolactin were due to a direct action on the spleen and thymus.

However, two laboratories have demonstrated direct and reciprocal interference between the binding of CsA and prolactin to human peripheral blood lymphocytes[87,88]. CsA at sub-immunosuppressive concentrations caused a fourfold increase in the binding of iodinated prolactin to lymphocytes, but binding was then completely inhibited as the CsA concentration was increased into the immunosuppressive range. Cyclosporin analogues without immunosuppressive activity were ineffective. Conversely, prolactin inhibited the binding of tritiated CsA, with 50% inhibition seen at 10^{-11} mol/l prolactin[87]. Generally similar results were obtained with a fluorescent CsA derivative, except that a 100-fold higher prolactin concentration was required to inhibit binding[88]. Prolactin could also displace CsA previously taken up by lymphocytes.

These results appear straightforward, though it is not altogether clear how they are to be reconciled with the evidence above that most cell-associated CsA is bound to cyclophilin in the cytoplasm. It could be proposed that CsA would bind first to the prolactin receptor and then be passed to cyclophilin after endocytosis. The rapid release of CsA on the subsequent addition of prolactin would be anticipated if the CsA–cyclophilin complex were relatively unstable and easily broke down, with the release of CsA from the cell – an explanation in line with the ready reversibility of inhibition of lymphocyte proliferation by CsA if the drug is withdrawn. However, this demands a mechanism for the rapid exit of CsA across the cell membrane, a mechanism that could operate in the outward direction only if this hypothesis were to hold.

Evidence has been presented to indicate that prolactin deprivation may lead to reduced immunological responsiveness *in vivo*, and that increased prolactin release may antagonize immunosuppression by CsA[87,88]. However, there is yet no unambiguous evidence that blockade of the prolactin receptor can account for the inhibition of lymphocyte proliferation *in vitro* by CsA. Hiestand *et al.*[88] have noted that lymphocyte activation by Con A results in increased synthesis of mRNA recognized by probes for both prolactin mRNA and growth hormone mRNA, though of considerably greater size than the authentic mRNA. They suggested that such mRNA might code for autocrine hormone-like factors promoting lymphocyte proliferation.

ACTION OF CsA ON NON-LYMPHOID CELLS

When administered clinically CsA has been found to give rise to side-effects on other tissues, particularly kidney and liver. It is not clear to what extent these reflect effects mediated by the same fundamental biochemical mechanism(s) as the immunosuppression, but at least some actions on other tissues can be distinguished by comparative studies of the effects of different cyclosporin analogues[4]. While a considerable number of effects of CsA *in vivo* and *in vitro* have been described, in only a few cases have the underlying mechanisms been investigated in any detail.

At least one observation of the effects of CsA on lymphocytes has a close parallel in non-lymphoid cells. The addition of vasopressin to cultured rat kidney fibroblasts results in an elevation of the cytoplasmic Ca^{2+} concentration mediated via the hydrolysis of phosphatidylinositol bisphosphate, and this in turn activates Na^+/H^+ exchange and thus leads to a rise in the cytoplasmic pH. This change in cytoplasmic pH is completely inhibited by CsA, while a similar pH change induced by direct activation of protein kinase C with phorbol ester is unaffected by the drug[41]. Similarly, the pH change observed in Swiss 3T3 fibroblasts incubated with platelet-derived growth factor or sodium orthovanadate is strongly inhibited by CsA, while that induced by phorbol ester is not[89].

CsA has also been reported to share with calmodulin inhibitors and Ca^{2+} channel blockers the property of reversing the resistance of both human leukaemia cells and Ehrlich ascites carcinoma cells to vinca alkaloids and anthracycline antibiotics[90]. The mechanism of this effect is unclear, although it has been suggested that it may relate to the inhibition of calmodulin action. The CsA concentrations required are considerably higher than those needed to inhibit the induction of lymphocyte proliferation, and too high to be maintained *in vivo* without unacceptable side-effects.

CsA has also been reported to increase the magnitude and duration of receptor-mediated increases in cytoplasmic Ca^{2+} concentration in hepatocytes stimulated with vasopressin[91] and vascular smooth muscle cells stimulated with angiotensin II[92]. The basal cytoplasmic Ca^{2+} concentration in the absence of stimulus was not affected, but detailed analysis showed that in both cases the underlying cause was a marked increase in the rate of Ca^{2+} influx into the cells caused by CsA. The consequent increase in the amount of Ca^{2+} in the intracellular stores in turn resulted in a larger Ca^{2+} signal in response to a stimulus. Again, high concentrations of Ca^{2+} were required to induce these effects. CsA at concentrations sufficient to inhibit lymphocyte proliferation does not lead to any increase in the Ca^{2+} signal in the lymphocyte cytoplasm after activation, so it seems unlikely that immunosuppression is mediated in this way, but effects of this type may underlie some of the side-effects of the drug.

17

One effect of CsA that can be demonstrated in cell free systems (and at more modest concentrations) is that it can promote the retention of Ca^{2+} by isolated mitochondria[93,94]. Investigation of the mechanism of this effect in isolated heart mitochondria showed that CsA was a potent inhibitor of the operation of a Ca^{2+}- and phosphate-dependent pore in the inner mitochondrial membrane, leading to the suggestion that CsA might interact with the protein conferring Ca^{2+}-sensitivity on the process of pore opening[94].

An entirely different action of CsA is that when administered to mice *in vivo* it inhibits several effects of phorbol esters applied topically to the skin[95]. Some of the phorbol ester effects were very rapid, such as the activation of protein synthesis elongation factor 2, mediated at least in part via the activation of a phosphatase. However, in this case it was shown that both immunosuppressive and inactive cyclosporins were equally effective in antagonizing the phorbol esters, an important control that could advantageously have been included in some of the other studies.

CONCLUSIONS

A great deal of evidence has now accumulated to indicate that the principal mechanism by which CsA inhibits both T and B lymphocyte proliferation is by antagonizing the Ca^{2+} signal that plays a key role in initiating this process. Many, if not yet all, of the effects of CsA on lymphocytes can be accounted for in this way. The balance of the evidence at present suggests that it is the response of the cell to the Ca^{2+} signal that is prevented, rather than the generation of the signal itself. The precise mechanism by which CsA accomplishes this is at present uncertain – none of the hypotheses so far proposed is supported by compelling evidence.

One step in T lymphocyte activation for which the Ca^{2+} signal is essential is the induction of the synthesis of the mRNA for IL-2 and other lymphokines. In some experimental model systems in which very strong protein kinase C activation is provided, usually by addition of phorbol esters, inhibition of IL-2 synthesis appears to be the only step essential for proliferation blocked by CsA, and addition of recombinant IL-2 can largely overcome its effects (see for example Figure 1.4). However, it seems likely that under more physiological conditions the activation of protein kinase C is much less intense, and the Ca^{2+} signal plays a more complex role (probably including the promotion of the activation of protein kinase C itself, which is a Ca^{2+}-dependent enzyme). At least some of these additional effects of the Ca^{2+} signal are also inhibited by CsA. Thus the available evidence would suggest that under physiological conditions, CsA blocks lymphocyte activation at more than one Ca^{2+}-dependent step.

It should be appreciated that while the inhibition of lymphocyte proliferation *in vitro* occurs at CsA concentrations similar to the serum concentrations that must be maintained *in vivo* for immunosuppression, it is still an open question whether this is indeed the sole, or even the principal, explanation for CsA's immunosuppressive action[96,97]. It is possible that the drug has additional effects.

CsA is known to affect cells other than lymphocytes, including antigen-presenting cells. Although it remains uncertain how closely these effects on other cells resemble its effects on lymphocytes, and in at least some cases there seem clear distinctions in its action, a common feature of those systems studied is the involvement of Ca^{2+}. In specific situations CsA has been shown both to enhance and to inhibit the transport of Ca^{2+} across membranes, though it is unclear whether this is a direct effect of CsA on the transport systems affected.

ACKNOWLEDGEMENTS

I thank my colleagues at the University of Sussex, particularly Marianne Gudgeon, Martin Goodier and Robin Benzie, for invaluable discussions and permission to report their unpublished work, and also the MRC and SERC for their support of our work on the action of CsA.

REFERENCES

1. Borel, J. F., Feurer, C., Gubler, H. U. and Stahelin, H. (1976) Biological effects of cyclosporin A: a new antilymphocytic agent. *Agents Actions*, **6**, 468–475
2. Von Wartburg, A. and Traber, R. (1986) Chemistry of the natural cyclosporin metabolites. *Progr. Allergy*, **38**, 28–45
3. Wenger, R. M. (1986) Synthesis of ciclosporin and analogues: structural and conformational requirements for immunosuppressive activity. *Progr. Allergy*, **38**, 46–64
4. Hiestand, P. C., Gunn, H. C., Gales, J. M., Ryffel, B. and Borel, J. F. (1985) Comparison of the pharmacological profiles of cyclosporine, (Nva2)-cyclosporine and (Val2)-dihydrocy-closporine. *Immunology*, **55**, 249–255
5. Borel, J. F. (1986) Ciclosporin and its future. *Progr. Allergy*, **38**, 9–18
6. Wiesinger, D. and Borel, J. F. (1979) Studies on the mechanism of action of cyclosporin A. *Immunobiology*, **156**, 454–463
7. Kay, J. E. and Benzie, C. R. (1983) Effects of cyclosporin A on the metabolism of unstimulated and mitogen-activated lymphocytes. *Immunology*, **49**, 153–160
8. Kay, J. E. and Benzie, C. R. (1986) Lymphocyte activation by OKT3: cyclosporine sensitivity and synergism with phorbol ester. *Immunology*, **57**, 195–199
9. Dongworth, D. W. and Klaus, G. G. B. (1982) Effects of cyclosporin on the immune system of the mouse. I. Evidence for a direct selective effect of cyclosporin A on B cells responding to anti-immunoglobulin antibodies. *Eur. J. Immunol.*, **12**, 1018–1022
10. Paavonen, T. and Hayry, P. (1980) Effect of cyclosporin A on T-dependent and T-independent immunoglobulin synthesis *in vitro*. *Nature (Lond.)*, **287**, 542–544
11. Van Buren, C. T., Kerman, R., Agostino, D., Payne, W., Flechner, S. and Kahan, B. D. (1982) The cellular target of cyclosporin A actions in humans. *Surgery*, **80**, 167–173
12. Lafferty, K. J., Gill, R. and Babcock, S. (1986) Tolerance induction in adult animals. *Progr. Allergy*, **38**, 247–257
13. Hess, A. D. and Colombani, P. M. (1986) Mechanism of action: *in vitro* studies. *Progr. Allergy*, **38**, 198–221
14. Orosz, C. G., Roopenian, D. C., Widmer, M. B. and Bach, F. H. (1983) Analysis of cloned T cell function. II. Differential blockade of various cloned T cell functions by cyclosporine. *Transplantation*, **36**, 706–711
15. Damjanovich, S., Aszalos, A., Mulhern, S., Balazs, M. and Matyus, L. (1986) Cytoplasmic membrane potential of mouse lymphocytes is decreased by cyclosporins. *Mol. Immunol.*, **23**, 175–180
16. Gelfand, E. W., Cheung, R. K. and Mills, G. B. (1987) The cyclosporins inhibit lymphocyte

activation at more than one site. *J. Immunol.*, **138**, 1115–1120

17. Manca, F., Kunkl, A. and Celada, F. (1985) Inhibition of the accessory function of murine macrophages *in vitro* by cyclosporine. *Transplantation*, **39**, 644–649

18. Varey, A.-M., Champion, B. R. and Cooke, A. (1986) Cyclosporine affects the function of antigen-presenting cells. *Immunoloy*, **57**, 111–114

19. Knight, S. C., Balfour, B., O'Brien, J. and Buttifant, L. (1986) Sensitivity of veiled (dendritic) cells to cyclosporine. *Transplantation*, **41**, 96–100

20. Knight, S. C. and Bedford, P. A. (1987) Effects of cyclosporine and retinoic acid on dendritic cell function. *Transplant. Proc.*, **19**, 320–323

21. Knight, S. C., Roberts, M., Macatonia, S. E. and Edwards, A. J. (1988) Blocking of acquisition and presentation of antigen by dendritic cells with cyclosporine. *Transplantation (Suppl)*, **46**, 48S–53S

22. Kay, J. E. and Benzie, C. R. (1984) Rapid loss of sensitivity of mitogen-induced lymphocyte activation to inhibition by cyclosporin A. *Cell. Immunol.*, **87**, 217–224

23. Bunjes, D., Hardt, C., Rollinghoff, M. and Wagner, H. (1981) Cyclosporin A mediates immunosuppression of primary cytotoxic T cell responses by impairing the release of interleukin-1 and interleukin-2. *Eur. J. Immunol.*, **11**, 657–661

24. Wang, B. S., Heacock, E. H., Collins, K. H., Hutchinson, I. F., Tilney, N. L. and Mannick, J. A. (1981) Suppressive effects of cyclosporin A on the induction of alloreactivity *in vitro* and *in vivo*. *J. Immunol.*, **127**, 89–93

25. O'Garra, A., Warren, D. J., Holman, M., Popham, A. M., Sanderson, C. J. and Klaus, G. G. B. (1986) Effects of cyclosporine on responses of murine B cells to T cell-derived lymphokines. *J. Immunol.*, **137**, 2220–2224

26. Isakov, N., Mally, M. I., Scholz, W. and Altman, A. (1987) T lymphocyte activation: the role of protein kinase C and the bifurcating inositol phospholipid signal transduction pathway. *Immunol. Rev.*, **95**, 89–111

27. King, S. (1988) An assessment of phosphoinositide hydrolysis in antigenic signal transduction in lymphocytes. *Immunology*, **65**, 1–7

28. Zilberman, Y., Howe, L. R., Moore, J. P., Hesketh, T. R. and Metcalfe, J. C. (1987) Calcium regulates inositol 1,3,4,5-tetrakisphophate production in lysed thymocytes and in intact cells stimulated with concanavalin A. *EMBO J.*, **6**, 957–962

29. Truneh, A., Albert, F., Golstein, P. and Schmitt-Verhulst, A.-M. (1985) Early steps of lymphocyte activation bypassed by synergy between calcium ionophores and phorbol ester. *Nature (Lond.)*, **313**, 318–320

30. Kaibuchi, K., Takai, T. and Nishizuka, Y. (1985) Protein kinase C and calcium ion in mitogenic response of macrophage-depleted human peripheral lymphocytes. *J. Biol. Chem.*, **260**, 1366–1369

31. Rosoff, P. M., Savage, N. and Dinarello, C. A. (1988) Interleukin-1 stimulates diacylglycerol production in T lymphocytes by a novel mechanism. *Cell*, **54**, 73–81

32. Bijsterbosch, M. K. and Klaus, G. G. B. (1985) Cyclosporine does not inhibit mitogen-induced inositol phospholipid degradation in mouse lymphocytes. *Immunology*, **56**, 435–440

33. Mizushima, Y., Kosaka, H., Sakuma, S., Kanda, K., Itoh, K., Osugi, T., Mizushima, A., Hamaoka, T., Yoshida, H., Sobue, K. and Fujiwara, H. (1987) Cyclosporin A inhibits late steps of T lymphocyte activation after transmembrane signalling. *J. Biochem.*, **102**, 1193–1201

34. Palacios, R. (1982) Concanavalin A triggers T lymphocytes by directly interacting with their receptors for activation. *J. Immunol.*, **128**, 337–342

35. Kay, J. E., Meehan, R. T. and Benzie, C. R. (1983) Activation of T lymphocytes by 12-O-tetradecanoylphorbol-13-acetate is resistant to inhibition by cyclosporin A. *Immunol. Lett.*, **7**, 151–156

36. Kay, J. E., Benzie, C. R. and Borghetti, A. F. (1983) Effect of cyclosporin A on lymphocyte activation by the calcium ionophore A23187. *Immunology*, **50**, 441–46

37. Szamel, M., Martin, A. and Resch, K. (1985) Inhibition of lymphocyte activation by cyclosporin A: interference with the early activation of the membrane phospholipid metabolism in rabbit lymphocytes stimulated with concanavalin A, anti-rabbit immunoglobulin or the Ca^{2-} ionophore A23187. *Cell. Immunol.*, **93**, 239–249

38. Klaus, G. G. B. (1987) Cyclosporin as a probe for different modes of lymphocyte activation. *Ann. Inst. Pasteur/Immunol.*, **138**, 626–628

39. Metcalfe, S. M. (1984) Cyclosporine does not prevent cytoplasmic calcium changes associated with lymphocyte activation. *Transplantation*, **38**, 161–164
40. Wiskocil, R., Weiss, A., Imboden, J., Kamin-Lewis, R. and Stobo, J. (1985) Activation of a human T cell line: a two stimulus requirement in the pre-translational events involved in the coordinate expression of interleukin-2 and gamma interferon genes. *J. Immunol.*, **134**, 1599–1603
41. Rosoff, P. M. and Terres, G. (1986) Cyclosporin A inhibits Ca^{2+} dependent stimulation of the Na^+/H^+ antiport in human T cells. *J. Cell Biol.*, **103**, 457–463
42. Manger, B., Hardy, K. J., Weiss, A. and Stobo, J. D. (1986) Differential effect of cyclosporin A on activation signalling in human T cell lines. *J. Clin. Invest.*, **77**, 1501–1506
43. Kay, J. E., Benzie, C. R. and Gudgeon, M. C. Unpublished data.
44. Granelli-Piperno, A., Andrus, L. and Steinman, R. M. (1986) Lymphokine and non-lymphokine mRNA levels in stimulated human T cells. *J. Exp. Med.*, **163**, 922-937
45. Goodier, M. R. and Kay, J. E. Unpublished data.
46. Miyawaki, T., Yachie, A., Ohzeki, S., Nagaoki, T. and Taniguchi, N. (1983) Cyclosporin A does not prevent expression of Tac antigen, a probable TCGF receptor molecule, on mitogen-stimulated human T cells. *J. Immunol.*, **130**, 2737–2742
47. Kronke, M., Leonard, W. J., Depper, J. M. Arya, S. K., Wong-Staal, F., Gallo, R. C., Waldmann, T. A. and Greene, W. C. (1984) Cyclosporin A inhibits T-cell growth factor gene expression at the level of mRNA transcription. *Proc. Natl. Acad. Sci. USA*, **81**, 5214–5218
48. Larsson, E-L. (1980) Cyclosporin A and dexamethasone suppress T cell responses by selectively acting at distinct sites of the triggering process. *J. Immunol.*, **124**, 2828–2833
49. Lillehoj, H. S., Malek, T. R. and Shevach, E. M. (1984) Differential effect of cyclosporin A on the expression of T and B lymphocyte activation antigens. *J. Immunol.*, **133**, 244–250
50. Reed, J. C., Abidi, A. H., Alpers, J. D., Hoover, R. G., Robb, R. J. and Nowell, P. C. (1986) Effect of cyclosporin A and dexamethasone on interleukin 2 receptor gene expression. *J. Immunol.*, **137**, 150–154
51. Aiello, F. B., Maggiano, N., Larocca, L. M., Piantelli, M. and Musiani, P. (1986) Inhibitory effect of cyclosporin A on the OKT3-induced peripheral blood lymphocyte proliferation. *Cell. Immunol.*, **97**, 131–139
52. Szamel, M., Berger, P. and Resch, K. (1986) Inhibition of T lymphocyte activation by cyclosporin A: interference with the early activation of plasma membrane phospholipid metabolism. *J. Immunol.*, **136**, 264–269
53. Fidelius, R. K., Laughter, A. H., Twomey, J. J., Taffet, S. M. and Haddox, M. K. (1984) The effect of cyclosporine on ornithine decarboxylase induction with mitogens, antigens and lymphokines. *Transplantation*, **37**, 383–389
54. Bunjes, D., Hardt, C., Rollinghoff, M. and Wagner, H. (1981) Cyclosporin A mediates immunosuppression of primary cytotoxic T cell responses by impairing the release of interleukin 1 and interleukin 2. *Eur. J. Immunol.*, **11**, 657–661
55. Kaufmann, Y., Chang, A. E., Robb, R. J. and Rosenberg, S. A. (1984) Mechanism of action of cyclosporin A: inhibition of lymphokine secretion studied with antigen-stimulated T cell hybridomas. *J. Immunol.*, **133**, 3107–3111
56. Granelli-Piperno, A., Inaba, K. and Steinman, R. (1984) Stimulation of lymphokine release from T lymphoblasts. Requirement for mRNA synthesis and inhibition by cyclosporin A. *J. Exp. Med.*, **160**, 1792–1802
57. Elliott, J. F., Lin, Y., Mizel, S. B., Bleackley, R. C., Harnish, D. G. and Paetkau, V. (1984) Induction of interleukin 2 mRNA inhibited by cyclosporin A. *Science*, **226**, 1439–1442
58. Herold, K. C., Lancki, D. W., Moldwin, R. L. and Fitch, F. W. (1986) Immunosuppressive effects of cyclosporin A on cloned T cells. *J. Immunol.*, **136**, 1315–1321
59. Kalman, V. K. and Klimpel, G. R. (1983) Cyclosporin A inhibits the production of gamma interferon but does not inhibit production of virus-induced interferon alpha and beta. *Cell. Immunol.*, **78**, 122–129
60. Palacios, R., Martinez-Maza, O. and De Ley, M. (1983) Production of human immune interferon studied at the single cell level. Origin, evidence of spontaneous secretion and effect of cyclosporin A. *Eur. J. Immunol.*, **13**, 221–225
61. Reem, G. H., Cook, L. A. and Vilcek, J. (1983) Gamma interferon synthesis by human thymocytes and T lymphocytes inhibited by cyclosporin A. *Science*, **221**, 63–65

21

62. Bickel, M., Tsuda, H., Amstad, P., Evequoz, V., Mergenhagen, S. E., Wahl, S.M. and Pluznik, D. H. (1987) Differential regulation of colony stimulating factors and interleukin 2 production by cyclosporin A. *Proc. Natl. Acad. Sci. USA*, **84**, 3274–3277

63. Granelli-Piperno, A. (1988) Effects of cyclosporin A on T lymphocytes and accessory cells from human blood. *Abstr. 9th European Immunology Congress (Rome)*, p. 230

64. Shaw, J., Meerovitch, K., Elliott, J. F., Bleackley, R. C. and Paetkau, V. (1987) Induction, suppression and superinduction of lymphokine mRNA in T lymphocytes. *Mol. Immunol.*, **24**, 409–419

65. Brack, C., Mattaj, I. W., Gautschi, J. and Cammisuli, S. (1984) Cyclosporin A is a differential inhibitor of eukaryotic RNA polymerases. *Exp. Cell Res.*, **151**, 314–321

66. Andrus, L. and Lafferty, K. J. (1982) Inhibition of T cell activity by cyclosporin A. *Scand. J. Immunol.*, **15**, 449–458

67. Thomson, A. W., Moon, D. K., Geczy, C. L. and Nelson, D. S. (1983) Cyclosporin A inhibits lymphokine production, but not responses of macrophages to lymphokines. *Immunology*, **48**, 291–299

68. Helin, H. J. and Edgington, T. S. (1984) Cyclosporin A regulates monocyte/macrophage effector functions by affecting instructor T cells. Inhibition of monocyte procoagulant response to allogeneic stimulation. *J. Immunol.*, **132**, 1074–1076

69. Havele, C. and Paetkau, V. (1988) Cyclosporine blocks the activation of antigen-dependent cytotoxic T lymphocytes directly by an IL-2-independent mechanism. *J. Immunol.*, **140**, 3303–3308

70. Bendtzen, K. and Dinarello, C. A. (1984) Mechanism of action of cyclosporin A. Effect on T-cell-binding of interleukin 1 and antagonizing effect of insulin. *Scand. J. Immunol.*, **20**, 43–51

71. Galatowicz, G., Benzie, C. R., Kay, J. E. and Soos, M. (1986) The role of insulin in lymphocyte activation. *Biochem. Soc. Trans.*, **14**, 326

72. LeGrue, S. J., Friedman, A. W. and Kahan, B. D. (1983) Binding of cyclosporine by human lymphocytes and phospholipid vesicles. *J. Immunol.*, **131**, 712-718

73. Koponen, M. and Loor, F. (1983) Cytoplasmic lipid droplets as the possible eventual cellular fate of active forms of cyclosporin. *Exp. Cell Res.*, **149**, 499–512

74. Merker, M. M. and Handschumacher, R. E. (1984) Uptake and nature of the intracellular binding of cyclosporin A in a murine thymoma cell line, BW5147. *J. Immunol.*, **132**, 3064–3070

75. Handschumacher, R. E., Harding, M. W., Rice, J., Drugge, R. J. and Speicher, D. W. (1984) Cyclophilin: a specific cytosolic binding protein for cyclosporin A. *Science*, **226**, 544–547

76. Koletsky, A. J., Harding, M. W. and Handschumacher, R. E. (1986) Cyclophilin: distribution and variant properties in normal and neoplastic tissues. *J. Immunol.*, **137**, 1054–1059

77. Haendler, B., Hofer-Warbinek, R. and Hofer, E. (1987) Complementary DNA for human T-cell cyclophilin. *EMBO J.*, **6**, 947–950

78. Harding, M. W., Handschumacher, R. E. and Speicher, D. W. (1986) Isolation and amino acid sequence of cyclophilin. *J. Biol. Chem.*, **261**, 8547–8555

79. Danielson, P. E., Forss-Petter, S., Brow, M. A., Calavetta, L., Douglass, J., Milner, R. J. and Sutcliffe, J. G. (1988) p1B15: a cDNA clone of the rat mRNA encoding cyclophilin. *DNA*, **7**, 261–267

80. Gschwendt, M., Kittstein, W. and Marks, F. (1988) Sequence homology between cyclophilin and elongation factor 2. *Biochem. J.*, **256**, 1061

81. Colombani, P. M., Robb, A. and Hess, A. D. (1985) Cyclosporin binding to calmodulin: a possible site of action on T lymphocytes. *Science*, **228**, 337–339

82. Hait, W. N., Harding, M. W. and Handschumacher, R. E. (1986) Calmodulin, cyclophilin and cyclosporin A. *Science*, **233**, 987–988

83. LeGrue, S. J., Turner, R., Weisbrodt, N. and Dedman, J. R. (1986) Does the binding of cyclosporine to calmodulin result in immunosuppression? *Science*, **234**, 68–71

84. Gudgeon, M. C., Benzie, C. R. and Kay, J. E. (1986) Role of Ca^{2+} and calmodulin in the inhibition of lymphocyte activation by cyclosporine. *Biochem. Soc. Trans.*, **14**, 1050–1051

85. Gudgeon, M. C. (1986) Studies on the mechanism of action of cyclosporin A. D.Phil. thesis, University of Sussex, pp. 136–149

86. Hess, A. D. and Colombani, P. N. (1987) Cyclosporin-resistant and -sensitive T lymphocyte subsets. *Ann. Inst. Pasteur/Immunol.*, **138**, 606–611 & 648–650

87. Larson, D. F. (1986) Mechanism of action: antagonism of the prolactin receptor. *Progr. Allergy*, **38**, 222–238

88. Hiestand, P. C., Mekler, P., Nordmann, R., Grieder, A. and Permmongkol, C. (1986) Prolactin as a modulator of lymphocyte responsiveness provides a possible mechanism of action for cyclosporine. *Proc. Natl. Acad. Sci. USA*, **83**, 2599–2603

89. Daniel, T. C and Ives, H. E. (1987) Cyclosporin A inhibits kinase C-independent activation of the Na^+/H^+ exchange by platelet-derived growth factor and vanadate. *Biochem. Biophys. Res. Commun.*, **145**, 111–117

90. Slater, L. M., Sweet, P., Stupecky, M. and Gupta, S. (1986) Cyclosporin A reverses vincristine and daunorubicin resistance in acute lymphatic leukaemia *in vitro*. *J. Clin. Invest.*, **77**, 1405–1408

91. Nicchitta, C. V., Kamoun, M. and Williamson, J. R. (1985) Cyclosporine augments receptor-mediated cellular Ca^{2+} fluxes in isolated hepatocytes. *J. Biol. Chem.*, **260**, 13613–13618

92. Pfeilschifter, J. and Ruegg, U. T. (1987) Cyclosporin A augments angiotensin II-stimulated rise in intracellular free calcium in vascular smooth muscle cells. *Biochem. J.*, **248**, 883–887

93. Fournier, N., Ducet, G. and Crevat, A. (1987) Action of cyclosporine on mitochondrial calcium fluxes. *J. Bioenerg. Biomembr.*, **19**, 297–303

94. Crompton, M., Ellinger, H. and Costi, A. (1988) Inhibition by cyclosporin A of a Ca^{2+}-dependent pore in heart mitochondria activated by inorganic phosphate and oxidative stress. *Biochem. J.*, **255**, 357–360

95. Gschwendt, M., Kittstein, W. and Marks, F. (1988) Effect of tumor promoting phorbol ester TPA on epidermal protein synthesis: stimulation of an elongation factor 2 phosphatase activity by TPA *in vivo*. *Biochem. Biophys. Res. Commun.*, **153**, 1129–1135

96. Chisholm, P. M., Drayson, M. T., Cox, J. H. and Ford, W. L. (1985) The effects of cyclosporin on lymphocyte activation in a systemic graft-vs.-host reaction. *Eur. J. Immunol.*, **15**, 1054–1059

97. Klaus, G. G. B. and Chisholm, P. M. (1986) Does cyclosporine act *in vivo* as it does *in vitro*? *Immunol. Today*, **7**, 101–103

2
Effect of cyclosporin A on the immune response: pivotal role of the interleukin-2/ interleukin-2 receptor autocrine pathway

Allan D. Hess

INTRODUCTION

In 1976 Borel first described the potent immunosuppressive activity of cyclosporin A (CsA) and its apparent selective action on T lymphocyte-dependent, cell-mediated immune responses[1,2]. Within a decade of these initial observations CsA has become the front-line immunosuppressive agent to prevent solid organ graft rejection and graft-versus-host disease in clinical transplantation[3]. Its usefulness is currently being evaluated in a wide variety of autoimmune disorders with some remarkable successes[4,5]. Despite the wide empiric application of CsA, the precise mechanism of action of this drug remains elusive. Nevertheless, many studies have provided some insight into the action of this unique immunosuppressive drug on the cells of the immune system which mediate the events of graft rejection. It has become increasingly apparent that one of the primary actions of CsA is on the interleukin-2 (IL-2)/interleukin-2 receptor autocrine pathway. This chapter will attempt to summarize the salient features of the effects of CsA on the complex cellular events necessary for a competent immune response with a particular focus on the IL-2/IL-2 receptor pathway.

EFFECT OF CsA ON CELLS OF THE IMMUNE SYSTEM

Initial studies by several investigators attempted to define the effect of CsA on the *in vitro* lymphocyte proliferative response to mitogen and alloantigen stimulation and these have recently been reviewed[6]. Several important features of CsA-mediated suppression of lymphocyte responses were determined in these early descriptive studies. First, CsA primarily suppressed in a dose-dependent fashion the lymphocyte proliferative response to mitogen and/or

24

alloantigen stimulation with an apparent selectivity for T cells. Secondary responses were more resistant to CsA than were primary immune responses. The second important feature was that CsA was not lymphotoxic since cells were capable of responding after culture with CsA provided that this drug was removed. The third, and perhaps most important, observation was the narrow time frame for CsA to effectively inhibit T lymphocyte responses requiring that CsA be added within the first few hours of culture. Thereafter, the effect of CsA on lymphoproliferation was significantly reduced. These data suggest that this unique drug interfered with the early events of T cell activation prior to DNA synthesis and cell division.

These initial studies clearly indicated that CsA effectively inhibited the proliferative response of T lymphocytes. However, they offered no insight into the action of CsA in preventing graft rejection, and could not account for the ability of CsA to facilitate the induction of transplantation tolerance or for the prolonged survival of allogafts after discontinuation of CsA treatment or reduction of dose[7]. Similarly, inhibition of lymphocyte proliferation was only a simple measure of the efficacy of this immunosuppressive agent. Furthermore, these studies offered no insight into the effect of CsA on the requisite cell-to-cell collaboration and cellular and subcellular communication necessary for a competent allograft response.

The immune response to an allograft is a complex immune process requiring communication and interaction of a variety of cell populations. An *in vitro* model of this process is the mixed lymphocyte reaction with the generation of antigen-specific cytotoxic T lymphocytes (CTL) and the production of cytokines which participate in delayed-type hypersensitivity responses. Simplistically, this *in vitro* model of the allograft response requires several important steps in addition to antigen recognition:

1. presentation of antigen by macrophages with the subsequent production and release of interleukin 1 (IL-1);
2. activation of the precursor CTL with the acquisition of a receptor for IL-2;
3. activation of T helper lymphocytes with production and release of IL-2 (the production of IL-2 is accentuated by IL-1);
4. clonal amplication of activated CTL by IL-2;
5. activation of suppressor T lymphocytes, which down-regulate or control this response.

One of the critical elements that appears to be rate-limiting in this response is the IL-2/IL-2 receptor autocrine pathway. The primary effect of this pathway is the amplification of effector mechanisms, particularly the clonal expansion of antigen-specific CTL. It is generally thought that this *in vitro* model accurately reflects some of the events that occur in graft rejection and in graft-versus-host disease. The effect of CsA has been studied on several components of this model and the results have revealed informative data regarding our understanding of the mechanism of action of CsA at the cellular level.

To summarize a series of investigations (reviewed in references 6 and 8) and as schematically illustrated in Figure 2.1:

25

1. CsA inhibits the activation of cytotoxic T lymphocytes but permits the activation and amplification of suppressor T lymphocytes. This imbalance results in the induction of specific immunologic unresponsiveness to the stimulating alloantigen *in vitro*.
2. CsA inhibits the production of IL-2 and other lymphokine mRNA transcription, presumably by ablating the activation signal.
3. CsA does not inhibit the clonal expansion of activated cells expressing the IL-2 receptor in response to exogenous IL-2.
4. CsA inhibits the precursor CTL from acquiring functional responsiveness to IL-2, which may be mediated via inhibition of IL-2 receptor formation.
5 CsA appears to inhibit monocyte/macrophage function by inhibiting antigen presentation, but only at much higher concentrations than is necessary for inhibition of lymphocyte proliferation.

It is extremely important to note that the effects of CsA on the various components of this model are extremely dependent on the dose of drug utilized as summarized in Table 2.1. Examination of the 50% inhibitory concentration (IC_{50}) for each function assessed reveals that the IL-2/IL-2 receptor autocrine pathway is the lymphocyte function/response most sensitive to the effects of CsA. From these data it appears that CsA primarily mediates its immunosuppressive effect on the rate-limiting step for the clonal amplification of the immune response.

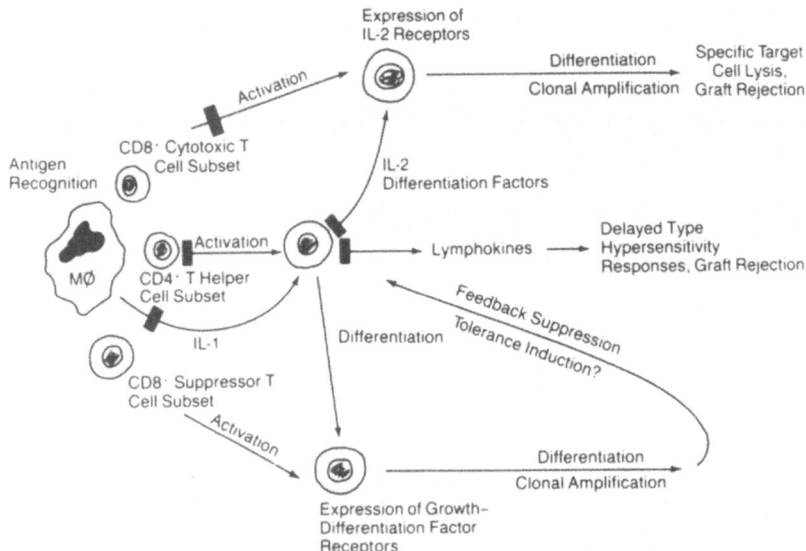

Figure 2.1 Schematic representation of an allograft response and the primary effect of cyclosporin (■ = CsA blockade)

26

Table 2.1 CsA-sensitive and resistant lymphocyte functions

Lymphocyte function	50% Inhibitory concentration (ng/ml
CsA-sensitive	
Proliferation	20–50
IL-2 production	10–20
CTL induction	
(without exogenous IL-2)	20–50
CTL induction	
(with exogenous IL-2)	100–150
IL-2 receptor formation	
MLR	100–200
Con A	200–500
PHA	500–1000
CsA-resistant	
IL-2 dependent proliferation	> 1000
Suppressor cell activation	> 1000
Cell-mediated lympholysis	> 1000

EFFECT OF CsA ON THE IL-2/IL-2 RECEPTOR AUTOCRINE PATHWAY

Inhibition of IL-2 production

Production of IL-2 occurs after antigenic stimulation of T helper lymphocytes and is essential for the amplification of the immune reponse including the clonal expansion of cytotoxic T lymphocytes. Initial studies by Bunjes et al.[9] and by Hess et al.[10] showed that CsA effectively inhibited the production of IL-2 after alloantigen stimulation of lymphocytes in MLR. Since these first reports, several studies have now indicated that the production of this lymphokine after stimulation of lymphocytes with a variety of agents (specific antigen, mitogens, anti-T cell receptor antibodies), is exquisitely sensitive to the immunomodulatory effects of CsA[11–13]. Effective inhibition (50%) of IL-2 production requires minimal concentration of CsA, usually around 10–20 ng/ml with complete suppression of IL-2 production occurring at levels of 50 ng/ml.

One possible explanation to account for the inhibition of IL-2 production by CsA was the absence of IL-1, a monocyte-derived cytokine which promotes the production of IL-2 by the T helper cell. Recent studies have suggested that even addition of exogenous IL-1 to the in vitro test systems (i.e. MLR, mitogen stimulated cultures) will not overcome the inhibitory effects of CsA on IL-2 production, suggesting that CsA renders the T helper cell refractive to the effects of IL-1[9,14,15]. Apparently, CsA mediates the down-regulation of the receptor for IL-1 on this T lymphocyte subset. Although CsA was found to effectively inhibit IL-2 production upon primary stimulation of resting lymphocytes with alloantigens or mitogens, more recent studies have indicated that CsA will inhibit the production of IL-2 by sensitized lymphocytes after antigen-specific restimulation[16,17] and even down-regulate IL-2 production of actively secreting cells. These data indicate that CsA may be useful in suppressing the response of sensitized individuals (i.e. sensitized against

27

antigens of the allograft donor) or may affect ongoing immune responses (i.e. active graft rejection or autoimmunity).

More recently, the application of molecular biological approaches to study the effect of CsA has yielded some insight into how this novel immunosuppressive drug inhibits IL-2 production. Elliott et al. first[18] reported that CsA inhibited the induction of IL-2 messenger RNA (mRNA). In their studies, human and murine cell lines were cultured under conditions in which these cells normally secrete high levels of IL-2 (in the presence of phorbol-12-myristyl-13 acetate). Addition of CsA blocked production of IL-2 and was found to be associated with an absence of IL-2 mRNA accumulation. More recently, studies by Granelli-Piperno et al.[19,20] have confirmed and extended these findings. They used as a model system, 3-day-old Con A-induced lymphoblasts. Mitogen and/or phorbol ester restimulation of these blast cells resulted in the synthesis of IL-2, interferon, B cell stimulating factor, and a cytotoxic differentiation factor. Addition of CsA to this system strongly inhibited production of these lymphokines, and similar observations were recently demonstrated at a clonal level using in situ hybridization techniques. In contrast, mRNA transcripts for constitutive components (actin) and the IL-2 receptor were not affected by CsA. These authors demonstrated that the effect of CsA was to block the induction or production of active lymphokine mRNA. Even though lymphokine production and lymphokine mRNA were inhibited in these studies, total protein synthesis and proliferation were not affected by CsA, suggesting that CsA can selectively inhibit certain cellular biochemical processes. Based on these studies, several possibilities were postulated to account for this effect and included: (1) specific inhibition of lymphokine mRNA formation (via inhibition of a specific enzyme); (2) binding of CsA and an intracellular receptor to a promoter region on the IL-2 gene; and (3) a specific destabilization of lymphokine mRNA[19,21]. However, from recent studies it appears likely that the mechanism accounting for down-regulation of lymphokine and/or IL-2 mRNA transcription is ablation of a calcium-dependent, intracellular signal transmitted from the cell membrane after interaction of the T cell receptor with its ligand (antigen)[22,23]. This intracellular activation signal appears to be required for continued lymphokine production, and CsA blocks the delivery of this antigen-dependent signal. Of interest are the findings of Citterio and Kahan[24], which demonstrate that CsA not only blocks the production of a cytoplasmic factor which activates resting nuclei but also inhibits the action of this cytoplasmic signal. In addition, recent studies by June et al.[25] have identified an activation cascade with subsequent IL-2 gene expression that is resistant to the effects of CsA. Stimulation of resting T lymphocytes via the CD 28 cell surface determinant (a cell surface glycoprotein on T cells) in conjunction with phorbol ester resulted in IL-2 gene transcription and IL-2 production that was insensitive to the effects of CsA. Similarly, a CsA-resistant and CsA-sensitive activation pathway leading to differential gene expression was also reported by Reed et al.[26] for the c-myc and p 53 proto-oncogenes.

Taken together, these data clearly suggest that the inhibitory effect of CsA on IL-2 production is not a direct effect on the transcription process, but rather, the ablation of a calcium dependent cytoplasmic activation signal that occurs distal to the interaction of the T cell receptor with its specific antigen and leads to lymphokine gene activation.

Induction of IL-2 receptors and the development of cytotoxic T lymphocytes

For a complete CTL response two independent steps are required: first, the antigen-activated precursor CTL must mature and acquire a receptor for IL-2; secondly, it must undergo clonal amplification in the presence of IL-2 which mediates the growth signal. This response can be inhibited either by prevention of CTL maturation, by inhibition of IL-2-dependent clonal amplification or by inhibiting IL-2 production. Although one of the major effects of CsA is to inhibit the production of IL-2, subsequently limiting the clonal expansion of CTL, CsA also appears to directly affect the activation of pCTL. This inhibition of CTL activation appears to be associated with a failure to acquire responsiveness to IL-2 and the absence of IL-2 receptor generation. However, the effect of CsA on IL-2 receptor generation has been controversial.

Initial studies by Larsson[27] in a lectin-dependent system showed that CsA inhibited the acquisition of responsiveness to IL-2, leading to the postulation that the CsA inhibits the pCTL from acquiring receptors to this growth factor. The results from Hess et al.[10] using the human MLR treated with CsA at levels greater than 500 ng/ml did not result in significant CTL activity. However, after IL-2 stimulation of primed lymphocytes harvested from MLR treated with these levels of CsA, the CTL did not develop the ability to respond to IL-2, but did acquire responsiveness at lower doses of this agent. However, in all instances a proliferative response of the primed lymphocytes from MLR could be demonstrated upon culture with IL-2, indicating that a proportion of cells activated by alloantigen do acquire the ability to respond to IL-2. Recent studies by Wagner[28], in a limiting dilution assay system (in the presence of exogenous IL-2), indicated that CsA will prevent naive pCTL activation and the subsequent development of IL-2 responsiveness. Further studies by Hess[11] also provided evidence on the ability of CsA to prevent the development of functional IL-2 responsiveness of the CTL by CsA in the human MLR system. Addition of exogenous IL-2 to MLR containing graded doses of CsA restored the proliferative response to alloantigen challenge *in vitro* almost to normal levels. In contrast, the effect of exogenous IL-2 on the induction of CTL in primary MLR in the presence of CsA was completely dependent on the dose of CsA. At the highest doses of CsA (0.5−2.5 μg/ml), no cytotoxic T cell activity could be detected regardless of the presence of exogenous IL-2. However, at a lower dose of CsA (0.1 μg/ml), which routinely resulted in the total inhibition of detectable CTL activity, addition of exogenous IL-2 resulted in significant levels of CTL activity. These results suggested that at this dose of CsA the pCTL was activated but not clonally amplified due to an absence of IL-2. This effect of CsA on the induction of functional IL-2 responsiveness by the pCTL was critically dose-dependent. The studies by Hess[11] also examined the effect of timed sequential addition of CsA or CsA plus exogenous IL-2 to probe the acquisition of functional responsiveness to IL-2 by the pCTL. The results demonstrated that, in the absence of adequate levels of CsA, the pCTL acquires functional IL-2 responsiveness within the first 18 h of culture after alloantigen stimulation, leading to the hypothesis that adequate levels of CsA must be achieved early *in vivo* to prevent sensitization of the pCTL. This is especially important, since CsA will not inhibit the proliferative response to IL-2 of lymphocytes which have developed the ability to respond to this lymphokine, findings which have been established in a variety of studies[9–11,23]. The triggering of IL-2 production by environmental antigens at lower maintenance doses of CsA in clinical transplantation may lead to clonal amplification of sensitized CTL, and to the initiation of graft rejection, since CsA does not block the action of these effector cells[29].

Recent studies show that the influence of CsA on the maturation and amplification of CTL appears to be much more complex than just an inhibitory effect of CsA on the IL-2/IL-2 receptor autocrine pathway. Heeg *et al.*[30] have shown that maturation of CTL in the presence of CsA required the presence of both IL-2 and IL-4. It is thought that IL-4 is a maturation factor for the activated pCTL in this setting. Wagner *et al.*[31] demonstrated that a cytotoxic differentiation factor was required for the maturation of the CTL. Lytic function could be achieved only in the presence of this factor. Clearly, these studies demonstrate that a combination of T lymphocyte-derived cytokines are required for the generation of a competent CTL response, and not just a function of the IL-2/IL-2 receptor autocrine pathway.

The recent development of a monoclonal antibody capable of detecting the IL-2 receptor (TAC) has allowed for the determination of the effect of CsA on IL-2 receptor formation rather than acquisition of functional responsiveness. Recent studies by Miyawaki *et al.*[32] demonstrated that CsA did not inhibit TAC expression on phytohaemagglutinin A- or concanavalin A (Con A)-stimulated human lymphocytes. However, other activation antigens expressed on T lymphocytes, such as class II major histocompatibility antigens or those antigens detected by the OKT9 and OKT10 monoclonal antibodies, were reduced in the presence of CsA. Comparable observations with no effect of CsA on TAC expression on mitogen-stimulated human lymphocytes were reported by Ryffel *et al.*[33]. Even though TAC expression was not reduced in cultures with CsA, proliferation was abolished in a dose-dependent manner. In contrast, the expression of TAC antigen and class II major histocompatibility antigen was reduced in CsA-treated human MLR cultures[11,34]. Similarly, Lillehoj *et al.*[35] demonstrated that CsA inhibited IL-2 receptor formation in mitogen-stimulated murine lymphocytes when tested after 3 days of culture. However, no effect on IL-2 receptor expression was observed when the cells were tested after 24 h of culture. The cells from these cultures were not responsive to IL-2, a surprising finding, since various studies have indicated that CsA does not inhibit primed cells from responding to this soluble factor[9–11]. Taken together, these studies indicate that the effect of CsA on IL-2 responsiveness and IL-2 receptor formation may be much more complex than originally thought.

The discrepant results with regard to the effect of CsA on IL-2 receptor expression on mitogen and alloantigen-stimulated cells remain unclear at present but appear to be related to type of stimulus and certainly to be dose-dependent. It may be that much higher doses of CsA must be used to prevent TAC expression on mitogen-stimulated T lymphocytes as compared to alloantigen-stimulated lymphocytes. It may also be that activation of lymphocytes by alloantigen (especially the CTL) requires an intricate set of signals and cell-to-cell collaboration, whereas mitogen stimulation may bypass some of the necessary events required for alloantigen stimulation. Thus, CsA may allow the discrimination of signalling events between mitogen and alloantigen stimulation. This dichotomy in stimulus is especially important with regard to the stimulation of lymphocytes with phorbol esters which strongly promote IL-2 receptor generation that is exceptionally resistant to CsA. Phorbol esters directly stimulate protein kinase C and bypass many sequential steps in the activation cascade of T lymphocytes.

SYNTHESIS AND CONCLUSIONS

The available data strongly suggest that CsA has a sparing effect on the activation and establishment of suppressor regulatory mechanisms while inhibiting cytotoxic T lymphocyte generation in response to transplantation antigens. The inhibition of the CTL response is due primarily to the inhibitory effect of CsA on the IL-2/IL-2 receptor autocrine pathway as assessed *in vitro*. The production of IL-2 is most sensitive to the effects of CsA. It appears that CsA results in the ablation of a cytoplasmic activation signal that is necessary for promotion of IL-2 mRNA transcription and subsequent IL-2 production. This intracellular signal is apparently transmitted from the interaction of the T cell receptor with a foreign MHC antigen. Because of the exquisite sensitivity of IL-2 and other lymphokine production including IL-2 to the effects of CsA ($IC_{50} = 10-20$ ng/ml), many investigators have suggested that this is the primary mechanism by which CsA prevents graft rejection. In this regard little attention has been paid to the effects of CsA on the pCTL, apart from limiting clonal expansion due to an absence of IL-2. However, the inhibitory effects of CsA on the activation and maturation of this cell may be critical in preventing graft acceptance and prevention of graft rejection. It is of interest that maintenance doses of CsA attempt to produce serum trough levels of 100–200 ng/ml, and the area under the curve for 24 h of levels approximating 500 ng/ml – levels (see Table 2.1) that would inhibit both IL-2 production and pCTL activation[36]. Levels of less than 100 ng/ml (but adequate enough to inhibit IL-2 production) are associated with rejection crises. These data would suggest that prevention of CTL sensitization, as reflected by the failure to develop functional responsiveness to the IL-2 autocrine growth signal, is a very critical component of immunosuppression with CsA.

ACKNOWLEDGEMENTS

This work was supported in part by grants from the US Department of Health and Human Services (CA 15396), and the American Cancer Society (IM 398), and a gift from the Harley W. Howell Foundation.

REFERENCES

1. Borel, J. F. (1976) Comparative study of *in vitro* and *in vivo* drug effects on cell-mediated cytotoxicity. *Immunology*, **31**, 631
2. Borel, J. F., Feurer, C., Gubler, H. U. and Stahelin, H. (1976) Biological effects of cyclosporin \: a new antilymphocytic agent. *Agents Actions*, **6**, 468
3. Morris, P. J. (1981) Cyclosporin A. *Transplantation*, **32**, 349
4. Schindler, R. (ed.) (1985) *Ciclosporin in Autoimmune Diseases* (Berlin: Springer-Verlag)
5. Stiller, C. R., Durpe, J., Gent, M., Jenner, M. R., Keown, P. A., Laupacis, A., Martell, R., Rodger, N. W., von Graffenreid, B. and Wolfe, B. M. J. (1984) Effects of cyclosporine immunosuppression in insulin-dependent diabetes mellitus of recent onset. *Science*, **223**, 1362
6. Hess, A. D., Colombani, P. M. and Esa, A. H. (1986) Cyclosporine and the immune response: basic aspects. *Crit. Rev. Immunol.*, **6**, 123
7. Green, C. L. and Allison, A. C. (1978) Extensive prolongation of rabbit kidney allograft survival after short-term Cyclosporin A treatment. *Lancet*, **1**, 1182
8. Hess, A. D., Esa, A. H. and Colombani, P. M. (1985) Mechanisms of action of cyclosporine: Effect on cells of the immune system and on subcellular events in T cell activation. *Trans. Proc.*, **20** (Suppl. 2), 29
9. Bunjes, D., Hardt, C., Rollinghoff, M. and Wagner, H. (1981) Cyclosporin A mediates immunosuppession of primary cytotoxic T cell responses by impairing the release of interleukin 1 and interleukin 2. *Eur. J. Immunol.*, **8**, 657
10. Hess, A. D., Tutschka, P. J., Pu, Z. and Santos, G. W. (1982) Effect of cyclosporine A on human lymphocyte responses *in vitro*. IV. Production of stimulatory growth factor in CsA treated primary MLR cultures. *J. Immunol.*, **128**, 360
11. Hess, A. D. (1985) Effect of interleukin 2 on the immunosuppressive action of cyclosporine. *Transplantation*, **39**, 62
12. Thomson, A. W., Moon, D. K. and Nelson, D. S. (1983) Suppression of delayed type hypersensitivity reactions and lymphokine production by cyclosporin A in the mouse. *Clin. Exp. Immunol.*, **52**, 599
13. Wang, G. S., Zheng, C., Heacock, E. H., Tilney, N. L., Strom, T. B. and Mannick, J. A. (1983) Inhibition of the production of a soluble helper mediator by cyclosporin A results in the failure to generate alloreactive cytolytic cells in mixed-lymphocyte culture. *Clin. Immunol. Immunopathol.*, **27**, 160
14. Hess, A. D., Tutschka, P. J. and Santos, G. W. (1983) Effect of cyclosporine on the induction of cytotoxic T lymphocytes: Role of interleukin 1 and interleukin 2. *Transplant. Proc.*, **15**, 2248
15. Palacios, R. and Moller, G. (1981) Cyclosporin A blocks receptors for HLA-DR antigens on T cells. *Nature*, **290**, 792
16. Andrus, L. and Lafferty, K. J. (1981) Inhibition of T-cell activity by cyclosporin A. *Scand. J. Immunol.*, **15**, 449
17. Hess, A. D., Tutschka, P. J. and Santos, G. W. (1982) Effect of cyclosporin on human lymphocyte response *in vitro*. III. CS inhibits the production of T lymphocyte growth factors in secondary mixed lymphocyte responses but does not inhibit the response of primed lymphocytes to TCGF. *J. Immunol.*, **128**, 355
18. Elliott, J. F., Lin, Y., Mizel, S. B., Bleackley, R. C., Harnish, D. G. and Paetkau, V. (1984) Induction of interleukin 2 messenger RNA inhibited by cyclosporin A. *Science*, **226**, 1439
19. Granelli-Piperno, A., Inaba, K. and Steinman, R. (1984) Stimulation of lymphokine release from T lymphoblasts. Requirement for mRNA synthesis and inhibition by cyclosporin A. *J. Exp. Med.*, **160**, 1792
20. Granelli-Piperno, A. (1988) In situ hybridization for interleukin 2 and interleukin 2 receptor mRNA in T cells activated in the presence and absence of CsA. *J. Exp. Med.*, **168**, 1649
21. Borel, J. F. and Ryffel, B. (1986) The mechanism of action of cyclosporin: a continuing puzzle. In Schindler, R. (ed.), *Ciclosporin in Autoimmune Diseases*, (Berlin: Springer-Verlag), pp. 24–32
22. Weissm, A. and Imboden, J. (1987) Cell surface molecules and early events in T lymphocyte activation. *Adv. Immunol.*, **41**, 1
23. Hodgkin, P. D., Hapel, A. J., Johnson, R. M., Young, I. G. and Lafferty, K. J. (1987)

Blocking of the delivery of the antigen-mediated signal to the nucleus of T cells by Cyclosporine. *Transplantation*, **43**, 685

24. Citterio, F. and Kahan, B. P. (1988) Effects of cyclosporine on nuclear function. *Trans. Proc.*, **20** (Suppl. 2), 75

25. June, C. H Ledbetter, J. A., Gellespie, M. M., Lindtsen, T. and Thompson, C. B. (1987) T cell proliferation involving the CD 28 pathway is associated with cyclosporine-resistant interleukin 2 gene expression. *Molec. Cell. Biol.*, **7**, 4472

26. Reed, J. C., Prystowsky, M. B. and Nowell, P. C. (1988) Regulation of gene expression in lectin-stimulated or lymphokine-stimulated T lymphocytes. Transplantation, **26** (Suppl.), 85

27. Larsson, E. L. (1980) Cyclosporin A and dexmethansone suppress T cell responses by selectively acting at distinct sites of the triggering process. *J. Immunol.*, **124**, 2828

28. Wagner, H. (1983) Cyclosporine A: mechanism of action. *Transplant. Proc.*, **15**, 523

29. Hess, A. D. and Tutschka, P. J. (1980) Effects of cyclosporine A on human lymphocyte responses *in vitro*. 1. CsA allows for the expression of alloantigen-activated suppressor cells whilep referentially inhibiting the induction of cytolytic effector lymphocytes in MLR. *J. Immunol.*, **124**, 2601

30. Heeg, K., Gillis, S. and Wagner, N. (1988) IL-4 bypassed the immune suppressive effect of Cyclosporin A during the *in vitro* induction of immune cytotoxic T lymphocytes. *J. Immunol.*, **141**, 2330

31. Wagner, H., Hardt, C., Rouse, B., Rollinghoff, M., Scheurich, P. and Pfizermaier, F. (1982) Dissection of the proliferative and differentiative signals controlling murine cytotoxic T lymphocyte responses. *J. Exp. Med.*, **155**, 1876

32. Miyawaki, T., Yachie, A., Ohzeki, S., Nagoaki, T. and Taniguchi, N. (1983) Cyclosporin A does not prevent expression of TAC antigen, a probable TCGF receptor molecule on mitogen stimulated human T cells. *J. Immunol.*, **130**, 2737

33. Ryffel, B., Tammi, K., Greider, A. and Hess, A. D. (1985) Effects of cyclosporine on human T cell activation. *Transplant. Proc.*, **17**, 1268

34. Hess, A. D., Donnenberg, A. D., Tutschka, P. J. and Santos, G. W. (1983) Effect of cyclosporin A on human lymphocyte responses *in vitro*. V. Analysis of responding T lymphocytes subpopulation in primary MLR with monoclonal antibodies. *J. Immunol.*, **130**, 717

35. Lillehoj, H. S., Malek, T. R. and Shevach, E. M. (1984) Differential effect of cyclosporin A on the expression of T and B lymphocyte activation antigens. *J. Immunol.*, **133**, 244

36. White, D. J. G. (1982) Pharmacology of cyclosporin A. *Drugs*, **24**, 322

3

Influence of CsA on humoral immunity and on B lymphocyte activation

Iris Motta and Paolo Truffa-Bachi

INTRODUCTION

CsA is a hydrophobic cyclic undecapeptide of fungal origin with potent specific immunosuppressive effects *in vivo* and *in vitro*. Since its discovery by Borel and his group in 1976[1], CsA has proved an effective and valuable agent for suppression of allograft rejection in animals and has found widespread clinical acceptance[2,3]. CsA is highly specific for lymphocytes and this property suggested that these cells possess some unique features of growth control which might be unravelled through an understanding of the CsA mode of action. Consequently, many laboratories have investigated the effect of this drug on lymphocyte stimulation by antigens or by polyclonal mitogenic or non-mitogenic B cell activators.

One of the most important features of CsA is that it exerts reversible non-cytotoxic inhibitory effects on the activation of quiescent lymphocytes by antigens or other polyclonal activators. The reports of Borel *et al.*[1,4] in 1976–77 demonstrated that administration of CsA to mice concomitantly with antigen inhibited the production of antibodies. CsA was first thought to act exclusively on T lymphocytes, and the lack of a humoral response was considered to be secondary to the effect of this molecule on the T lymphocyte population. However, subsequent analyses have revealed that the specificity of CsA for T cells was less stringent than first thought, and that B cells were also affected[5]. CsA seems to block some as yet unidentified early event(s), following the binding of antigen to the surface Ig receptors or the binding of polyclonal activators to discrete structures on the lymphocyte membrane. CsA may also influence later phases of B lymphocyte growth and maturation controlled by T lymphocyte-derived cytokines (reviewed in reference 6).

Space limitations prevent discussion of all the topics covering the effects of CsA on the B lymphocyte population. We have focused our attention on some of the experiments pertaining to the influence of CsA on the humoral immune response and polyclonal B cell activation.

34

CsA EFFECTS ON THE HUMORAL IMMUNE RESPONSE

Thymus-dependent humoral responses

Primary response

In their early reports Borel et al.[1,4] described the inhibitory effect of CsA on the immune response of rats and mice to the thymus-dependent (TD) antigen sheep red blood cells (SRBC). CsA was given orally at a dose of 900 mg/kg. Later, it was found that lower doses (50–100 mg/kg) were as efficient as higher doses, and CsA is now often given to mice, subcutaneously dissolved in olive oil. In humans CsA is given either orally or by intravenous injection. In early clinical trials CsA was given at doses similar to the one utilized in mice; however, the human immune system is extremely sensitive to CsA inhibition and the doses which are actually utilized, of the order of 5 mg/kg, efficiently block the immune response.

The primary response to TD antigens depends on the production by activated T lymphocytes of lymphokines essential for the proliferation and the differentiation of B lymphocytes into antibody-secreting cellls[7,8]. The effect of CsA on TD antigen responses might be explained by the blockade by CsA of the production of these T lymphocyte-derived factors. This concept was supported by the studies of Kunkl and Klaus in the mouse[5]. These authors have shown that if the primary response to a TD antigen (trinitrophenylated Keyhole limpet haemocyanin, TNP-KLH) was blocked by CsA, the secondary response to this antigen was unaffected by this drug. This finding prompted Kunkl and Klaus to measure the effect of CsA on the primary response to TNP-KLH in mice previously primed with the carrier (KLH). They found that the primary response to TNP in these animals was not inhibited by CsA. Thus, the inhibition of the primary anti-TNP response by CsA was due to its effect(s) on the virgin KLH-specific T cells. They concluded that hapten-specific naive B lymphocytes responding to TD antigens are CsA-resistant[5].

If the suppression of TD responses is due to the inhibitory effect of CsA on T lymphocytes, it would be expected that some of the lymphokines produced by activated T cells could overcome the drug effect. In this regard, Xue et al.[9] have examined the capacity of T cell-derived supernatants and of recombinant interleukin 2 (IL-2) to overcome *in vivo* the suppressive effect of CsA on antibody production to TNP-KLH. These authors found that injection of crude supernatants but not IL-2 (250 U/mouse) had restorative effects. Although a role of IL-2 in B cell responses has been debated, it now appears that this cytokine stimulates B cell proliferation and differentiation[10]. Xue et al.[9] thus postulated a direct effect of CsA on B cells, although they did not exclude the fact that the inability of IL-2 to reverse CsA inhibition may reflect the need for other lymphokines. We have found that addition of T cell replacing factors (as defined by Schimpl and Wecker[11]) to B cell cultures in the presence of CsA (1 μg/ml) did not reverse the inhibitory effect of this molecule on a TD response (anti-SRBC) suggesting a direct effect of CsA on B cells (Motta, I. and Truffa-Bachi, P., unpublished results). The observations of both Xue et al. and ourselves challenge the report by Kunkl and Klaus that naive B cells responding to TD antigens are CsA-resistant. B cell sensitivity or resistance to CsA seems to depend on the model utilized: *in vitro* the B

35

cell response is CsA-sensitive, *in vivo* their response is mainly unaffected by this drug.

Conflicting data exist with respect to the effect of CsA on *in vivo* humoral responses of CsA-treated patients. In one report[12], bone marrow transplant recip ents were treated with 6.25 mg/kg CsA and in the other, patients suffe ing from chronic uveitis[13], were treated with 8.9 mg/kg. Bone marrow transplant recipients had received CsA for approximately 5 months[12], and none of them developed an antibody response following KLH immunization but all responded normally to TI antigen, DNP-Ficoll. The authors concluded that CsA acts, as it does in mice, on T-dependent but not T-independent responses[12]. In contrast, when patients with autoimmune uveitis were treated with CsA the T lymphocyte proliferative response and IgM antibody response to KLH were not affected[13]. It is possible that the different disease states contributed to the different results observed in these studies.

The effect of CsA administration on the immune response to TD antigens was also examined in other species. The response of rabbits to A-positive red cells was inhibited by CsA[14]. Depending on the time of CsA administration, CsA suppressed, or had no effect on, the primary and secondary antibody response of guinea pigs to DNP-BGG. No effect of CsA was seen when given 3 days prior to, or on the day of, immunization, whereas CsA given 3 days after immunization suppressed the response[15]. CsA administration to chickens appears to result in a decreased immune response to different antigens (SRBC, human gamma globulin and *Brucella abortus*). However, a clear conclusion could not be reached since a high variation in individual response was observed[16].

Secondary humoral response
The primary and secondary responses to TD antigens differ in their cellular and soluble factor prerequisites[17], and CsA has highlighted some of the differences involved. It was initially reported by Borel *et al.*[1] that the secondary response to TD antigens was inhibited by CsA. However, in later studies it became clear that the secondary response is insensitive to CsA. The difference in dose and regimen explains the apparent discrepancy between these findings.

The secondary humoral response to TNP coupled to KLH was analysed in detail by Kunkl and Klaus in mice, and was found much less CsA-sensitive than the primary response, indicating that, like naive B lymphocytes responding to TD antigens, B-memory cells are insensitive to CsA[5]. In addition, these results show that the effector functions of T-memory cells are insensitive to this drug. It can be hypothesized that activation and/or proliferation of T-memory cells is not susceptible to CsA. Alternatively, T-memory cells do not need to proliferate in order to perform their effector functions, a hypothesis consistent with the well-established finding that the activity of these cells is resistant to X-ray irradiation.

In contrast to the CsA resistance of murine T-memory cells, human T cell populations are susceptible to CsA. Using peripheral blood lymphocytes (PBL) obtained from human volunteers previously immunized with KLH or tetanus toxoid (TT), Harley and Fauci[18] showed that PBL from human volunteers treated with CsA did not produce IgM and IgG antibodies when

36

cultured with either KLH or TT. CsA blocked the response even when added 3 days after the onset of the culture, suggesting that functional T lymphocytes are required during this period. These authors reported that T lymphocytes were more sensitive to the CsA effect than B cells, as T cells treated with CsA for 4 h ir culture were unable to reconstitute a B lymphocyte response, whereas CsA-pulsed B cells mixed with normal T cells gave a response to 60% of control cultures. These studies also demonstrated large differences in the sensitivity of different individuals to CsA. PBL from some donors were inhibited by low concentrations of Csa (0.1 ng/ml), while antibody production by PBL from other donors was relatively resistant (1000 ng/ml). The different sensitivity of patients to CsA is of great importance in the clinical use of this drug.

Thymus-independent humoral responses

Primary response

Many reports have established that B lymphocytes are heterogeneous in their susceptibility to activation by thymus-dependent (TD) and thymus-independent (TI) antigens (for a review see reference 19). Furthermore, murine B cell susceptibility to activation by various antigens is progressively acquired. The response to LPS appears earlier in ontogeny than the response to Ficoll. A more precise delineation of B lymphocyte responsiveness to B cell antigens was derived from studies of CBA/N mice which carry an X-linked genetic defect (*Xid*) in B cell maturation[20]. B cells fom CBA/N mice respond to LPS or *Brucella abortus*, classified as TI class 1 antigens (TI-1) but not to Ficoll or dextran derivatives, termed TI class 2 antigens (TI-2). Such studies suggest that TI-1 and TI-2 antigens stimulate different B lymphocyte subsets and that TI-1 sensitive B lymphocytes appear earlier in ontogeny than do the TI-2-sensitive B lymphocytes.

Kunkl and Klaus[5] established that CsA also affected the immune response of a murine B cell subpopulation. Administration of 50 mg/kg of CsA, which inhibits the primary TD response, did not suppress the response of a TI-1 antigen, TNP-LPS, but did suppress by more than 90% the response to a TI-2 antigen, DNP-Ficoll. The regimen and the timing of CsA administration were found to be very important. The greatest inhibition of the response to DNP-Ficoll was observed when CsA was given on days -1, 0 and +1, with respect to antigen administration. However, even a single injection of 50 mg/kg of CsA at day -1 or 0 or +1 was sufficient to suppress the anti-DNP-Ficoll response by more than 80%. CsA acts early during B lymphocyte activation, and once the cells have been triggered the drug no longer has any inhibitory effects. For instance, CsA given 2 days after antigenic challenge did not affect the humoral response and actually augments by 2–5-fold the response to TNP-LPS.

The general findings of Kunkl and Klaus[5] were confirmed by many other laboratories including our own[6]. Higham and collaborators[21], using an *in vitro* system, also showed that CsA could increase the B cell response to TNP-LPS. This enhanced response, which can be of the order of 8-fold, could not

37

be accounted for by a shift in the kinetics of the response nor by the inactivation by CsA of T-suppressor activities. As B lymphocyte proliferation can occur without differentiation to antibody production[22], it can be hypothesized that CsA inhibits early differentiation, but not mitogen-induced B cell proliferation. Thus the number of antigen-specific cells will increase, and if these cells escape CsA inhibition the result will be a high antibody production.

Susceptibility or resistance to CsA could be explained by difference in B lymphocyte activation pathways stimulated by the two classes of TI antigens. One of the major features distinguishing TI-1 from TI-2 antigens is the mitogenic properties of the former. However, a non-mitogenic derivative of TNP-LPS, TNP-LPS-polymyxin B, can induce antibody synthesis in the presence of CsA[23], confirming the conclusion of Kunkl and Klaus that CsA sensitivity versus resistance is a marker defining two distinct B lymphocyte subsets[5].

Kunkl and Klaus clearly established that sensitivity to CsA distinguishes two subpopulations of B lymphocytes which had been suggested by other criteria[19]. The suppression of B cell responses to TI-2 but not to TI-1 antigens by CsA differs from the suppression of B cell function induced by cyclophosphamide or 6-thioguanine, which block the B cell response to both TI-1 and TI-2 antigens[5].

The effect of CsA on the humoral response to particulates such as viruses, as opposed to soluble antigens, has also been studied. The humoral response of mice to vesicular stomatitis virus (VSV) is composed of an early TI IgM response and a later IgG TD response[24]; Zinkernagel and his group[25] have shown that CsA had no effect on the TI IgM response to VSV, but abolished the primary IgG response. The secondary response to VSV, as well as to influenza virus[26], was unaffected by CsA, supporting the view that secondary T helper cells are CsA-resistant.

The immune response of human bone marrow transplant recipients undergoing CsA therapy to DNP-Ficoll revealed no differences from controls[14]. These results seem at first sight to contradict those reported for mice; however, it should be kept in mind that the dichotomy in B lymphocyte subsets responding to TI-1 or to TI-2 antigens has been established in the mouse, and that in the humans a similar classification has not been reported.

Secondary response

The simultaneous utilization of TI antigens and CsA has been particularly rewarding in studying memory cell generation. We have found that CsA does not interfere with the generation of B-memory cells by TI-antigens including those of class 2 TI antigens such as TNP-Ficoll[27]. This is so despite the fact that CsA has dramatic suppressive effects on the primary response to this antigen. Our interpretation of these findings is that memory cell precursors proliferate in the presence of CsA, and are derived from a cell lineage distinct from that of the antibody-secreting cell precursors. Since CsA acts preferentially on more mature B-lymphocytes it can also be hypothesized that memory cells are generated from the less mature, CsA-resistant B cell subset[27].

Whether or not TI-1 antigens generate different subpopulations of memory cells was approached by determining the effects of CsA on B-memory cells induced by TNP-LPS. Our data show that CsA blocks the expression of these TNP-specific memory B cells when the challenge is given with TNP-Ficoll. However, Cs A does not block the response to TNP-LPS, suggesting that two distinct subsets of memory B lymphocytes are generated by TNP-LPS priming: one sensitive and the other insensitive to CsA suppression[27].

CsA EFFECTS ON POLYCLONAL B CELL ACTIVATION

B cell proliferation and differentiation

The interaction of antigen with the surface membrane immunoglobulin of B lymphocytes, or the crosslinking of the Ig receptor by anti-Ig initiates a complex process in resting B lymphocytes leading to activation, proliferation and differentiation into an Ig-secreting cell. Mitogens, which activate lymphocytes of a variety of antigen specificities, have helped to define some of the stages involved in the biochemical pathways of lymphocyte activation. A growing body of data obtained with B cell and T cell activation suggests that these cells require two distinct signals for commitment to DNA synthesis[28,29]. Signal 1 drives the cell from a resting G_0 to a G_1 stage, and signal 2 from G_1 to S. In attempts to delineate the signals required for activation (for a review see reference 30), proliferation and differentiation of B lymphocytes, the analysis of the mechanisms whereby CsA inhibits cell proliferation and/or differentiation has been of great importance.

Murine B lymphocytes
It was recognized early that the humoral response, as well as the B lymphocyte proliferation induced by LPS, was CsA-resistant[1]. These observations led to the conclusion that B cells are resistant to CsA. Since the report in 1980 by Kunkl and Klaus[5] that TI-2 responses are highly susceptible to CsA, the effect of this drug on B lymphocyte proliferation induced by different polyclonal B cell activators has been reinvestigated.

Anti-μ antibodies are able to induce the proliferation of B lymphocytes[31]; however, this stimulation differs from that induced by LPS as anti-μ stimulates B lymphocytes appearing late in ontogeny that are absent in CBA/N mice[22,32]. In addition, anti-μ induces only DNA synthesis while the differentiation to Ig-secreting cells requires T cell-derived factors[31,30].

The B lymphocyte proliferation induced by $F(ab'_2)$ anti-μ antibodies was found to be particularly sensitive to CsA inhibition[33]. Dongworth and Klaus established that a concentration of CsA as low a 10 ng/ml inhibited cellular proliferation. In contrast, CsA at concentrations below 2000 ng/ml has no effect on murine or human (see below) B lymphocyte proliferation induced by LPS. However, pig lymphocyte activation by anti-immunoglobulins was reported to be insensitive to CsA inhibition[34].

Resting (G_0) B lymphocytes can also be driven to enter the G_1 phase of the cell cycle by tumour-promoting phorbol esters such as phorbol miristic acetate (PMA)[35]. Using the two-step culture system devised by De Franco *et al.*[36,37], Klaus and Hawrylowicz[38] have shown that the activation signal provided by PMA is CsA-resistant and thus distinct from that given by anti-μ antibodies. These data suggest that B cells can receive two biochemically dist'nct forms of signal 1: one given by anti-μ is CsA-sensitive; the other giv:n by PMA or LPS is CsA-resistant. Klaus and Hawrylowicz hypothesized that anti-Ig binding to B lymphocyte receptors initiates a biochemical cascade, one of the early steps of which is blocked by CsA. The CsA resistance of PMA and LPS activation indicates that, along this cascade of biochemical events leading to cell activation, these molecules operate at some later stage of cell activation than anti-μ[38].

As mentioned above, anti-μ-induced B lymphocyte proliferation is extremely sensitive to CsA. In contrast, T lymphocyte responses to Con A are less susceptible: the amount of CsA required for 50% inhibition is much lower for anti-μ than for Con A activation[33]. Furthermore, activation by anti-μ remains CsA-sensitive for a long period (24–48 h), whereas activation by Con A is sensitive to CsA for only a short time. While there is presently no explanation for the persisting CsA sensitivity of B cell activation by anti-μ, these results suggest that the mechanisms of CsA-mediated inhibition of B and T lymphocytes could be different.

Much evidence has been presented that the triggering of B lymphocyte division and differentiation towards antibody secretion is influenced by various T cell-derived lymphokines[8]. O'Garra *et al.*[39] have studied the effect of CsA on the responses of murine B cells to B cell-stimulatory factor I (BSF-I)[40], and to eosinophil differentiation factor/B cell growth factor II (EDF/BCGF II)[41–43]. Activation of B lymphocytes by BSF-I results in the increased expression of cell surface Ia antigens which is not affected by CsA. This suggests that BSF-I acts on resting B lymphocyte through a signalling pathway distinct from that employed by anti-μ. Perhaps relevant to this finding is the fact that, unlike anti-μ, BSF-1 does not cause an elevation in inositol phospholipid metabolism or in intracellular free Ca^{2+} concentration[44] (see below).

EDF/BCGF II stimulates preactivated B cells to proliferate and differentiate into Ig-secreting cells[41–43]. Addition of CsA to large (presumably activated) B cells has a marked inhibitory effect on these factor-dependent responses. This contrasts with studies reported by Muraguchi *et al.*[45], who found that anti-μ-induced responsiveness to B cell growth factor (BCGF) of human tonsillar B lymphocytes is CsA-resistant (see below). This distinction may reflect a fundamental difference between the properties of human and murine cell growth and differentiation factors. The susceptibility of the EDG/BCGF II-induced response of murine B cells is difficult to reconcile with the fact that, once activated, these cells are resistant to CsA.

Tumour cell lines have also been used to study the mode of action of CsA. The lymphoma cells tested by Gorelick *et al.*[46] produce autoantibodies and appear to have arisen from a restricted subset of B lymphocytes, since they share specificity, idiotype and cell surface markers. The growth of these cells was sensitive to addition of CsA. CsA-susceptibility seems to be a general phenomenon of malignant murine B cell lines. In contrast, human transformed EBV cell lines are resistant to CsA (see below).

Human B lymphocytes

Human B lymphocyte polyclonal activation can be achieved by either T-independent or T-dependent means. T-independent activation of small resting human tonsillar B lymphocytes can be obtained with anti-μ antibodies or *Staphylococcus aureus* Cowan I (SAC). Like murine B lymphocytes, human B lymphocytes show several sequential progressions in cell cycle following anti-μ activation. Cells first increase in size within 36 h and then acquire responsiveness to the proliferative signals delivered by BCGF[47]. Using a low concentration of anti-μ in conjunction with BCGF, Muraguchi and colleagues[45] found that 5−500 ng/ml of CsA blocked B cell proliferative response, increase in size and mRNA production. The inhibitory action of CsA on the anti-μ-induced synthesis of mRNA was observed only when the drug was added within 24 h of the onset of cultures. After this time, and once B lymphocytes were activated, CsA no longer had any effect on the subsequent cell differentiation and proliferation stimulated by the addition of BCGF. Thus, CsA selectively suppresses an early step of the human B lymphocyte activation without inhibiting the effect of subsequent T cell factor-dependent proliferation and differentiation. This conclusion stands in marked contrast with O'Garra *et al.*'s recent report[39] that EDF/BCGF II-induced DNA synthesis and differentiation of preactivated murine B lymphocytes is CsA-sensitive. This indicates that CsA can inhibit not only activation, but also the proliferative and differentiative steps of B lymphocyte stimulation.

The proliferative response to SAC results from the interaction of staphylococcal Protein A with the Fab region of B lymphocyte surface Ig[48], and is thus similar to the target of anti-μ action. Thus it provides a valid model for antigen interaction with surface Ig on B lymphocytes. Muraguchi *et al.*[45] have also shown that the proliferative response of B cell induced by SAC can be inhibited by CsA. However, 50 to 100-fold more CsA was required to inhibit the B lymphocyte response to SAC than to anti-μ. One interpretation which can be drawn by these experiments is that there are two distinct B cell subsets: one responding to anti-μ which is sensitive to CsA, the other responding to SAC in humans or LPS in mouse which is more resistant to CsA. However, the possibility that the activation pathways utilized by the two mitogens are different, one being CsA-sensitive and the other CsA-resistant, cannot be ruled out.

There is ample evidence that pokeweed mitogen (PWM)-induced stimulation of human B lymphocytes, which relies on T lymphocytes and macrophages[49,50], is blocked by CsA[51−53]. T cell products such as IL-2, BCGF, B cell differentiation factor (BCDF) as well as interferon-γ (IFN-γ), have been reported to be directly involved in B cell differentiation[8]. Since the synthesis by T lymphocytes of IL-2, BCGF and IFN-γ, but not of BCDF, is blocked by CsA, it is uncertain whether B lymphocytes are the target of the suppressive effect of CsA on PWM-induced activation. Different investigators have reported contradictory results.

Berger *et al.*[45] have analysed the effect of adding T cell helper-factor(s)-containing supernatant to cultures of human PBL stimulated by PWM. Under these conditions, when the necessary T lymphocyte help was provided, B lymphocyte proliferation induced by PWM was inhibited by CsA, suggesting a direct effect of CsA on this cell lineage[54]. Similar conclusions were reached by Hannan-Harris et al.[55], who reported that neither IL-1 (1 U/ml), recombinant IL-2 (6–12 U/ml) nor BCGF, individually or in combination, reversed the inhibition by CsA of PWM-induced proliferation of human tonsillar B lymphocytes.

Nakagawa et al.[56] have assessed the capacity of exogenous IL-2, IFN-γ and BCGF to counteract the CsA-mediated suppression of PWM-driven differentiation of human PBL into Ig secretors. In contrast to the studies cited earlier, Nakagawa et al.[56] showed that 10–50 U/ml of recombinant IL-2 reconstituted Ig production in CsA-treated, PWM-stimulated PBL cultures. Neither IFN-γ nor BCGF, alone or with IL-2, had an effect. These data are consistent with T cells being the primary targets of CsA, B lymphocytes being insensitive to CsA-induced suppression. Moreover, they demonstrate a crucial role for IL-2 in this system as IL-2 is required during the whole process of PWM-induced stimulation leading from B lymphocyte activation to B lymphocyte differentiation.

A difference worth noting in these studies is that the responses to PWM were measured either by proliferation or by Ig secretion. The contradictory data reported may reflect different factor requirements for PWM-induced B cell proliferation and PWM-induced differentiation of B cells into Ig-secreting cells.

The high concentration of CsA used in the early clinical trials generated a high incidence of lymphoblastomas and a general tendency for increased anti-Epstein-Barr virus (EBV) titre in CsA-treated patients. In contrast to PWM-induced B cell proliferation, which requires the presence of T cells, the B cell transformation by EBV occurs in the absence of T lymphocytes and monocytes[51]. If EBV transforms B lymphocytes into lymphoblastoid cell lines the proliferation induced by the virus is kept under control by T lymphocytes which prevent outgrowth of lymphoblastomas. Bird and colleagues[49] reported in 1981 that the response of human B lymphocytes to EBV was not affected by CsA, and that this drug promoted the early and complete in vitro outgrowth of EBV lymphoblastomas from EBV immune donors in the absence of experimental infection. However, the effect of CsA on EBV-induced proliferation and Ig production depends on many parameters, i.e. the source of the donor lymphocyte and the dose of virus[57]. It has been reported that CsA inhibits[58], enhances[59,60], or has no effect[50] on the EBV-induced Ig response. The apparent inconsistencies in the literature are probably due to the multiple effect of CsA on this system. While the B cell response to EBV is resistant to CsA, it is likely that regulatory T lymphocytes are also the target of CsA action[61] and the T cell blockade will allow the EBV-induced B cell proliferation.

Modulation of B cell receptors

We have reported above that, in mice and humans, CsA inhibits anti-μ-induced B lymphocyte activation. Capping of membrane immunoglobulin alters the interactions of the plasma membrane with the cytoskeleton and the properties of the membrane, leading to depolarization, altered flux of ions through the membrane and metabolism of phophatidylinositol (see below).

A study of the CsA effect on capping by anti-Ig was undertaken by Loor and his colleagues[62,63]. These authors found that CsA at a dose of 500 ng/ml increased the initial rate of immunoglobulin capping. The acceleration induced by CsA is apparent within the first 2 min but not at later times. The physicochemical changes in the membrane last for a few minutes and the CsA-induced acceleration of capping may result in an insufficient signal 1 delivery, and thus in the inhibition of the B cell response.

Transferrin receptors are found on activated T and B cells and their expression precedes cell growth. Lillehoj et al.[64] have analysed the effect of CsA on the expression of IL-2 and transferrin receptors on B lymphocytes by LPS. CsA has no effect on LPS-induced B cell proliferation and does not affect IL-2 receptor expression at a concentration which interferes with IL-2 receptor induction on T lymphocytes. CsA blocks transferrin receptor induction on T lymphocytes, but does not interfere with LPS-induced transferrin receptor expression on B cells[64]. Whether CsA also inhibits the synthesis of these activation antigens in B cells stimulated with anti-μ is not known at present. Since LPS-induced B cell proliferation is resistant to CsA, it can be concluded that the cellular programmes leading to the expression of various genes such as for IL-2 and transferrin receptors are not *per se* sensitive to CsA, but that some as yet unidentified pathway is the target of this drug.

Prolactin receptors may have a physiological role in the regulation of the humoral and cell-mediated immune responses[65]. CsA can interfere with prolactin binding. At 10^{-9} mol/l, CsA elevated specific prolactin binding to B cells 2-fold, and at concentrations of $10^{-7}/10^{-6}$ CsA totally blocked prolactin binding. The effect of CsA on prolactin receptor on T cells was investigated by Hiestand et al.[66], who confirmed and extended the findings of Russel et al.[65]. Although a specific receptor for CsA had not been found on the membrane of B or T lymphocytes, the non-specific blockade of prolactin receptors may play a role in the CsA-induced suppression by displacing pituitary prolactin.

EFFECTS OF CsA ON THE ACTIVATION OF BIOCHEMICAL PATHWAYS

Binding of an antigen to the immunoglobulin receptor on B and T lymphocytes induces an increase in free Ca^{2+} concentration and activation of protein kinase C. These two intracellular signals are the consequence of receptor-induced hydrolysis of inositol phospholipids (phosphatidylinositol biphosphate, PIP_2) in the plasma membrane which give rise to two second messengers, inositol 1,4,5-triphosphate (IP_3) and diacylglycerol (DAG). These two molecules participate in the early stages of cell activation: (a) IP_3 causes Ca^{2+} mobilization from intracellular stores; and (b) DAG induces the protein kinase C translocation from the cytosol to the membrane, and its activation will lead to protein phosphorylation (reviewed in reference 67).

The selectivity of CsA for certain B cell activators prompted a search for the biochemical lesion caused by this drug in the activation cascade. For this reason, differences in lipid metabolism and Ca^{2+} mobilization induced by these activators in the presence of CsA, were analysed.

As already mentioned, activation of B cells by anti-μ or by ionophores is ex.remely sensitive to CsA. Crosslinking of immunoglobulin receptors by anti-μ antibodies leads to cell proliferation but not differentiation; at the biochemical level, anti-μ binding induces PIP_2 degradation and thus Ca^{2+} mobilization[68]. Calcium ionophores (ionomycin and A23187), which in the mouse are non-mitogenic polyclonal activators, cause the expression of Ia antigens but do not induce PIP_2 breakdown or RNA synthesis in B cells[69]. CsA does not interfere with the anti-μ-stimulated PIP_2 breakdown but efficiently blocks the increase in Ia antigens induced by ionophores[70].

In contrast with the above findings, activation of B cells by LPS or PMA is insensitive to CsA inhibition. The effects of these activators on B cells are, however, different since LPS drives B cells into proliferation and differentiation, whereas PMA induces an increased expression of Ia antigens but neither DNA synthesis nor cell proliferation[38]. Interestingly, activation by LPS or PMA products does not cause IP_3 liberation or Ca^{2+} mobilization and/or uptake[68], indicating that these two second messengers are not involved in cell triggering by LPS or PMA. Whether LPS and PMA follow an entirely different biochemical pathway, or whether they bypass the requirement for IP_3 and Ca^{2+}, activating a later step in the pathway initiated by these two second messengers, is still unknown. Since LPS and PMA polyclonal activation are insensitive to CsA inhibition, whereas anti-μ and ionophore are sensitive, it has been suggested that CsA acts on a Ca^{2+}-dependent event or sequence of events occurring early during cell activation[71].

This hypothesis is consistent with the data reported by Bijsterbosch and Klaus on the effects of CsA on the B cell response to Con A[72]. This lectin has been utilized for a long time as a model mitogen that exclusively activates T lymphocytes. Nevertheless, although Con A is incapable of inducing B cell proliferation, it drives B lymphocyte from G_0 to a transitional activation state close to but different from G_1, and there is evidence that at this stage the B cell becomes responsive to proliferative signals produced by T lymphocytes[73]. This stage is characterized by increased Ia expression and increased intracellular Ca^{2+} concentration in B lymphocytes. CsA blocks Ia expression and Ca^{2+} flux induced by Con A in B cells[72]. One exception to the generalization of the concept that CsA acts on a Ca-dependent event is the data reported by the Klaus group[39] that the response to EDF/BCGF II, which, as previously mentioned, does not involve Ca^{2+} mobilization, is sensitive to CsA inhibition.

CONCLUSION

The investigations made during the past 10 years on the effect of CsA on the immune system have shed some light on the site of CsA action. The supposed specificity of this drug for T lymphocytes is not as stringent as was first thought. Indeed, the activation of B cells can be blocked by this drug. Furthermore, the secondary humoral response is, at least in the mouse, much less sensitive to inhibition, pointing to a different sensitivity of virgin and primed T cells. Finally, the inhibition of B cell activation depends on the activator and/or on the B cell subpopulation responding to the polyclonal stimulus. This last point has sparked many controversies; the data in the literature suggest two possible explanations for the mechanism of CsA action: (a) the existence of two B cell compartments, one sensitive and the other insensitive to the drug; (b) a single B cell compartment which can be activated by distinct biochemical pathways which differ in their susceptibility to CsA inhibition. The first interpretation fits well with the existence of different B cell populations[20] and the data on the induction of B memory cells by TI antigens[27,6]. However, the recent studies of Klaus and his group have shown that CsA has selectivity for certain modes of lymphocyte activation, and that its efficiency depends thus on the biochemical pathway induced by the polyclonal activator (reviewed in reference 71). From these and other investigations of T cell activation it can be hypothesized that the activation pathways which requires Ca^{2+} mobilization and/or influx are CsA-sensitive, whereas pathways bypassing these steps are CsA-resistant. This implies that CsA interferes with a Ca^{2+}-dependent event or sequence of events which occur relatively early in the antigen-induced activation cascade[71].

Our ignorance of the molecular target of CsA action makes it difficult to choose between the two above-mentioned hypotheses. The definition of the target of CsA action in B lymphocytes which is undertaken in many laboratories will hopefully clarify this dilemma. In addition to this issue, other prominent questions on CsA mode of action remain unanswered. While there is a large body of evidence which favours the concept that CsA acts on a Ca^{2+}-dependent early event in cell activation, various data obtained *in vivo* are not readily explained by this model[74]. First, there is compelling evidence that B and T lymphocytes can proliferate either in mice treated with immunosuppressive doses of CsA or in spleen cell cultures containing CsA[78]. These data are difficult to reconcile with the conclusion that CsA acts on a very early step of cell activation preceding DNA synthesis. Furthermore, the *in vitro* analyses point to a general sensitivity of B cells to CsA, whereas the *in vivo* studies suggest that these cells are insensitive to CsA inhibition.

The pursuit of the analysis on the mode of action of CsA, both at the cellular and at the molecular level, will allow a better understanding of the process involved in lymphocyte activation and the optimization of the therapeutic application of CsA.

ACKNOWLEDGEMENTS

We are indebted to Drs M. E. Weksler, J-H. Colle, I. Saint Girons and E. Abraham for competent advice, helpful discussions and critical reading of the manuscript. The work from the authors' laboratory was financed by CNRS, the Institut Pasteur and ARC.

REFERENCES

1. Borel, J. F., Feurer, C., Gubler, H. U. and Stahelin, H. (1976) Biological effects of cyclosporin A: a new antilymphocytic agent. *Agents Actions*, 6(4), 468–475

2. Shevach, E. M. (1985) The effects of cyclosporin A on the immune system. *Ann. Rev. Immunol.*, **3**, 397–423

3. Hess, A. D., Colombani, P. M. and Esa, A. H. (1986) Cyclosporin and the immune response: basic aspects. *Crit. Rev. Immunol.*, **6**, 123–149

4. Borel, J.-F., Feurer, C., Magnee, C. and Stahelin, H. (1977) Effects of the new antilymphocytic ;·eptide cyclosporin A in animals. *Immunology*, **32**, 1017–1025

5. Kunkl, A. and Klaus, G. G. B. (1980) Selective effects of cyclosporin A on functional B cell subsets in the mouse. *J. Immunol.*, **125**, 2526–2531

6. Truffa-Bachi, P. (1987) Mode of action of CsA. *Ann. Inst. Pasteur (Immunol.)*, **138**, 161–217

7. Kishimoto, T. and Hirano, T. (1988) Molecular regulation of B lymphocyte response. *Ann. Rev. Immunol.*, **6**, 485–512

8. O'Garra, A., Umland, S., De France, T and Chistiansen, J. (1988) 'B-cell factors' are pleiotropic. *Immunol. Today*, **9**, 45–54

9. Xue, B., Dersarkissian, R. M., Baer, R. L., Thorbecke, G. J. and Belsito, D. V. (1986) Reversal by lymphokines of the effect of cyclosporine A on the contact sensitivity and antibody production in mice. *J. Immunol.*, **136**, 4128–4133

10. Miedema, F. and Melief, C. J. M. (1986) T-cell regulation of human B-cells. *Immunol. Today*, **6**, 258–259

11. Schimpl, A. and Wecker, E. (1972) Replacement of T-cell function by a T-cell product. *Nature*, **237**, 15–17

12. Amlot, P. L., Hayes, A. E., Gray, D., Gordon-Smith, E. C. and Humphrey, J. H. (1986) Human immune responses *in vivo* to protein (KLH) and polysaccharide (DNP-Ficoll) neoantigens: normal subjects compared with bone marrow transplant patients on cyclosporine. *Clin. Exp. Immunol.*, **64**, 125–135

13. Palestine, A. G., Roberge, F., Charous, B. L., Lane, H. C., Fauci, A. S. and Nussenblatt, R. B. (1985) The effect of cyclosporine on immunization with tetanus and keyhole limpet hemocyanin (KLH) in humans. *J. Clin. Immunol.*, **5**, 115–121

14. Smith, G. N. (1982) The effect of cyclosporin A on the primary immune response to allogeneic red cells in rabbits. *Immunology*, **45**, 163–167

15. Parker, D., Drossler, K. and Turk, J. L. (1984) Kinetics of the effect of a single dose of cyclosporin-A on antibody and cell mediated immune responses in the guinea pig. *Int. J. Immunopharmacol.*, **6**(1), 67–74

16. Nowak, J. S., Kai, O., Peck, R. and Franklin, R. M. (1982) The effect of cyclosporin A on the chicken immune system. *Eur. J. Immunol.*, **12**, 867–876

17. Singer, A. and Hodes, R. J. (1983) Mechanisms of T cell–B cell interaction. *Ann. Rev. Immunol.*, **1**, 211–241

18. Harley, J. B. and Fauci, A. S. (1983) Cyclosporine modulates the human in vitro T-dependent antigen-induced synthesis of specific antibody. *Transplant. Proc.*, **15**, 2315–2320

19. Mosier, D. E. and Subbarao, B. (1982) Thymus-independent antigens: complexity of B-lymphocyte activation revealed. *Immunol. Today*, **3**, 217–222

20. Scher, I. (1982) CBA/N immune defective mice: evidence for the failure of a B cell subpopulation to be expressed. *Immunol. Rev.*, **64**, 17–136

21. Higham, A. D., Sells, R. A. and Marshall-Clarke, S. (1986) Cyclosporin A has differential effects on the responses of murine B cells to T1 antigens and B-cell mitogens. *Immunology*, **59**, 203–207

22. Parker, D. C., Fothergill, J. J. and Wadsworth, D. C. (1979) B lymphocyte activation by insoluble anti-immunoglobulin: induction of immunoglobulin secretion by T cell-dependent soluble factor. *J. Immunol.*, **123**, 931–941

23. Shidani, B., Motta, I. and Truffa-Bachi, P. (1985) Mitogenic signal(s) are not required to circumvent the cyclosporin-induced inhibition of TNP-specific B memory cell expression. *Ann. Immunol. (Inst. Pasteur)*, **136C**, 313–321

24. Burns, W. H., Billups, L. C. and Notkins, A. L. (1975) Thymus dependence of viral antigens. *Nature*, **248**, 657–661

25. Charan, S., Huegin, A. W., Cerny, V., Hengartner, H. and Zinkernagel, R. M. (1986) Effects of cyclosporin A on humoral immune response and resistance against vesicular stomatitis virus in mice. *J. Virol.*, **57**, 1139–1144

26. Schiltknecht, E. and Ada, G. L. (1985) Influenza virus-specific T cells fail to reduce lung

virus titers in cyclosporin-treated infected mice. *Scand. J. Immunol.*, **22**, 99–103

27. Shidani, B., Colle, J. H., Motta, I. and Truffa-Bachi, P. (1983) Effect of cyclosporin A on the induction and activation of B memory cells by thymus-independent antigens in mice. *Eur. J. Immunol.*, **13**, 359–363

28. Andersson, J., Lernhardt, W. and Melchers, F. (1979) The purified protein derivative of tuberculin, a B-cell mitogen that distinguishes in its action resting, small B-cells from activated B cell blasts. *J. Exp. Med.*, **150**, 1339–1350

29. Andersson, J., Schreier, M. H. and Melchers, F. (1980) T-cell dependent B-cell stimulation is H-2 restricted and antigen dependent only at the resting B-cell level. *Proc. Natl. Acad. Sci. USA*, **77**, 1612–1616

30. Howard, M. and Paul, W. E. (1983) Regulation of B-cell growth and differentiation by soluble factors. *Ann. Rev. Immunol.*, **1**, 307–333

31. Parker, D. C. (1980) Induction and suppression of polyclonal antibody responses by anti-Ig reagents and antigen-non-specific help factors: a comparison of the effects of anti-Fab, anti-IgM and anti-IgD on murine B cells. *Immunol. Rev.*, **52**, 115–139

32. Sieckmann, D. G., Scher, I., Asofsky, R., Mosier, D. E. and Paul, W. E. (1978) Activation of mouse lymphocytes by anti-immunoglobulin. II. A thymus-independent response by a mature subset of B lymphocytes. *J. Exp. Med.*, **148**, 1628–1643

33. Dongworth, D. W. and Klaus, G. G. B. (1982) Effects of CSA on the immune system of the mouse. I. Evidence for a direct selective effect of CSA on B cells responding to anti-Ig antibodies. *Eur. J. Immunol.*, **12**, 1018–1022

34. White, D. J. G., Plumb, A. M., Pawelec, G. and Brons, G. (1979) Cyclosporin A: an immunosuppressive agent preferentially active against proliferating T cells. *Transplantation*, **27**, 55–58

35. Hawrylowicz, C., Keeler, K. D. and Klaus, G. G. B. (1984) Activation and proliferation signals in mouse B cells. I. A comparison of the capacity of anti-Ig antibodies or phorbol myristic acetate to activate B cells from CBA/N or normal mice into G1. *Eur. J. Immunol.*, **14**, 244–250

36. DeFranco, A. L., Kung, J. T. and Paul, W. E. (1982) Regulation of growth and proliferation in B cell subpopulations. *Immunol. Rev.*, **64**, 161–182

37. DeFranco, A. L., Raveche, E. S., Asofsky, R. and Paul, W. E. (1982) Frequency of B lymphocytes responsive to anti-immunolobulin. *J. Exp. Med.*, **155**, 1523–1536

38. Klaus, G. G. B. and Hawrylowicz, C. M. (1984) Activation and proliferation signals in mouse B cells. II. Evidence for activation (G_0 to G_1) signals differing in sensitivity to cyclosporine. *Eur. J. Immunol.*, **14**, 250–254

39. O'Garra, A., Warren, D. J., Holman, M., Popham, A. M., Sanderson, C. J. and Klaus, G. G. B. (1986) Effects of cyclosporine on responses of murine B cells to T cell-derived lymphokines. *J. Immunol.*, **137**, 2220–2224

40. Rohem, N. W., Leibson, H. J., Zlotik, A., Kappler, J., Marrack, P. and Cambier, J. C. (1984) Interleukin-induced increase in Ia expression by normal mouse cells. *J. Exp. Med.*, **160**, 679–694

41. Swain, S. L. and Dutton, R. W. (1982) Production of a B cell growth-promoting activity, (DL) BCGF, from a cloned T cell line and its assay on the BCL1 B cell tumor. *J. Exp. Med.*, **156**, 1821–1834

42. Warren, D. J. and Sanderson, C. J. (1985) Production of a T-cell hybrid producing a lymphokine stimulating eosinophil differentiation. *Immunology*, **54**, 615–623

43. Sanderson, C., O'Garra, A. J., Warren, D. J. and Klaus, G. G. B. (1986) Eosinophil differentiation factor also has B cell growth factor activity. Proposed name interleukin-4. *Proc. Natl. Acad. Sci. USA*, **83**, 437–440

44. Mizuguchi, J., Beaven, M. A., Ohara, J. and Paul, W. E. (1986) BSF-1 action on resting B cells does not require elevation of inositol phopholipid metabolism or increased $(Ca^{2+})i$. *J. Immunol.*, **137**, 2215–2219

45. Muraguchi, A., Butler, J. L., Kehrl, J. H., Falkoff, J. M. and Fauci, A. S. (1983) Selective suppression of an early step in human B lymphocytes by cyclosporin A. *J. Exp. Med.*, **158**, 690–702

46. Gorelick, M. H., Bishop, G. A., Haughton, G. and Pisetsky, D. S. (1987) Cyclosporine inhibition of CH series murine B-cell lymphomas. *Cell Immunol.*, **107**, 219–226

47. Muraguchi, A., Butler, J. L., Kehrl, J. H. and Fauci, A. S. (1983) Different sensitivity of human B cell subsets to activation signal delivered by anti-μ antibody and proliferative

47

signals delivered by monoclonal B cell growth factor. *J. Exp. Med.*, **157**, 530–546
48. Romagnani, S., Giudizi, M. G., Biagiotti, R., Almerigogna, F., Maggi, E., Del Prete, G. and Ricci, M. (1981) Surface immunoglobulins are involved in the interaction of protein A with human B cells and in the triggering of B cell proliferation induced by protein A-containing *Staphylococcus aureus. J. Immunol.*, **127**, 1307–1313
49. 3ird, A. G. and Britton, S. (1979) A live human B-cell activator operating in isolation of other cellular influences. *Scand. J. Immunol.*, **9**, 507–510
50. Janossy, G., Gomez de la Concha, E., Waxadal, M. J. and Platts-Mills, T. (1976) The effects of purified mitogenic proteins (Pa-1 and Pa-2) from pokeweed on human T and B lymphocytes *in vitro. Clin. Exp. Immunol.*, **26**, 108–117
51. Bird, A. G., McLachlan, S. M. and Britton, S. (1981) Cyclosporin A promotes spontaneous outgrowth *in vitro* of Epstein–Barr virus-induced B-cell lines. *Nature*, **289**, 300–301
52. Tosato, G., Pike, S. E., Koshi, I. R. and Blease, R. M. (1982) Selective inhibition of immunoregulatory cell functions by Cyclosporin A. *J. Immunol.*, **128**, 1986–1991
53. Paavonen, T. and Häyry, P. (1980) Effect of cyclosporin A on T-dependent and T-independent immunolobulin synthesis *in vitro. Nature*, **287**, 542–544
54. Berger, R., Meingassner, J. G. and Knapp, W. (1983) *In vitro* effects of cyclosporin A on human B-cell responses. *Scand. J. Immunol.*, **17**, 241-249
55. Hannam-Harris, A. C., Taylor, D. S. and Nowell, P. C. (1985) Cyclosporin A directly inhibits human B-cell proliferation by more than a single mechanism. *J. Leuk. Biol.*, **38**, 231–239
56. Nakagawa, N., Nakagawa, T., Volkman, D. J., Ambrus, J. L. Jr. and Fauci, A. S. (1987) The role of interleukin-2 in inducing Ig production in a pokeweed mitogen-stimulated mononuclear cell system. *J. Immunol.*, **138**, 795–801
57. Irving, W. L., Lockwood, D. and Lydyard, P. M. (1986) The effects of cyclosporin A on the early responses of B and T cells to Epstein–Barr virus infection. *Immunol. Lett.*, **13**, 173–178
58. Britton, S. and Palacios, R. (1982) Cyclosporin A: usefulness? Risk and mechanisms of action. *Immunol. Rev.*, **65**, 5–22
59. Mayus, J. L., Semper, K. F. and Pisetsky, D. S. (1985) Inhibition of *in vitro* anti-DNA B-cell responses by cyclosporine. *Cell. Immunol.*, **94**, 195–204
60. Pereira, R. S., Gear, A. J., Dore, C. J. and Webster, D. B. (1983) Effects of cyclosporin A on immunoglobulin production by EB virus stimulated lymphocytes. *Clin. Exp. Immunol.*, **53**, 115–121
61. Rickinson, A. B., Rowe, M., Hart, I. J., Yao, Q. Y., Henderson, L. E., Rabin, H. and Epstein, M. A. (1984) T-cell-mediated regression of spontaneous and of Epstein–Barr virus-induced B-cell transformation *in vitro*: studies with cyclosporin A. *Cell. Immunol.*, **87**, 646–658
62. Mosbach-Ozmen, L., Humez, S., Koponen, M., Fonteneau, P. and Loor, F. (1986) Cyclosporine facilitates B-cell membrane immunoglobulin capping. *Immunology*, **57**, 573–577
63. Mosbach-Ozmen, L., Humez, S., Koponen, M., Fonteneau, P. and Loor, F. (1986) Increased membrane immunoglobulin capping of B-cells from C57Bl/6 lpr/lpr and C57Bl/6 nu/nu mice. *Cell. Immunol.*, **98**, 517–524
64. Lillehoj, H. S., Malek, T. R. and Shevach, E. M. (1984) Differential effect of cyclosporin A on the expression of T and B lymphocyte activation antigens. *J. Immunol.*, **133**, 244–250
65. Russel, D. H., Kibler, R., Matrisian, L., Larson, D. F., Poulos, B. and Magun, B. E. (1985) Prolactin receptors on human T and B lymphocytes: antagonism of prolactin binding by cyclosporine. *J. Immunol.*, **5**, 3027–3031
66. Hiestand, P. C., Mekler, P., Nordmann, R., Grieder, A. and Permmongkol, C. (1986) Prolactin as a modulator of lymphocytes responsiveness provides possible mechanism of action for cyclosporine. *Proc. Natl. Acad. Sci. USA*, **83**, 2599–2603
67. Cambier, J. C. and Ransom, J. T. (1987) Molecular mechanisms of transmembrane signalling in B lymphocytes. *Ann. Rev. Immunol.*, **5**, 175–199
68. Bijsterbosch, M. K., Meade, C. M., Turner, G. A. and Klaus, G. G. B. (1985) B lymphocyte receptors and polyphophoinositide degradation. *Cell*, **41**, 999–1006
69. Klaus, G. G. B., Bijsterbosch, M. K. and Holman, M. (1985) Activation and proliferation signals in mouse B cells. VII. Calcium ionophores are non-mitogenic polyclonal activators. *Immunology*, **56**, 321–327

70. Bijsterbosch, M. K. and Klaus, G. G. B. (1985) Cyclosporine does not inhibit mitogen-induced inositol phospholipid degradation in mouse lymphocytes. *Immunology*, **56**, 435–440

71. Klaus, G. G. B. (1987) Cyclosporin as a probe for different modes of lymphocyte activation. *Ann. Inst. Pasteur (Immunol.)*, **138**, 626–628

72. Bijsterbos.h, M. K. and Klaus, G. G. B. (1986) Concanavalin A induces Ca^{2+} mobilization, but only minimal inositol phospholipid breakdown in mouse B cells. *J. Immunol.*, **137**, 1294–1299

73. Hawrylowicz, C. M. and Klaus, G. G. B. (1984) Activation and proliferation signals in mouse B cells. IV. Concanavalin A stimulates B cells to leave G_0 but not to proliferate. *Immunology*, **53**, 703–711

74. Klaus, G. G. B. and Chisholm, P. M. (1986) Does cyclosporine act *in vivo* as it does *in vitro*? *Immunol. Today*, **7**, 101–103

75. Milon, G., Truffa-Bachi, P., Shidani, B. and Marchal, G. (1984) Cyclosporin A inhibits the delayed type hypersensitivity effector function of T lymphocytes without affecting their clonal expansion. *Ann. Immunol. (Inst. Pasteur)*, **135D**, 237–245

76. Klaus, G. G. B. and Kunkl, A. (1983) Dissociation of T helper-cell function and helper-cell priming by cyclosporine. *Transplant. Proc.*, **15**, 2321–2322

77. Thomson, A. W., Moon, D. K., Inoue, Y., Geczy, C. L. and Nelson, D. S. (1983) Modification of delayed-type hypersensitivity reaction to ovalbumin in cyclosporin A-treated guinea pigs. *Immunology*, **48**, 301–308

78. Shidani, B., Motta, I. and Truffa-Bachi, P. (1987) Cyclosporin A does not affect the in vitro induction of antigen-specific delayed-type hypersensitivity-mediating T cells. *Eur. J. Immunol.*, **17**, 291–294

4

The influence of cyclosporin A on T cell activation, cytokine gene expression and cell-mediated immunity

Angus W. Thomson and Janet I. Duncan

INTRODUCTION

The potential of cyclosporin A (CsA) for the immunotherapy of allograft rejection and certain autoimmune disorders was evident in the first account by Borel et al. (1976) of the immunosuppressive properties of the drug. It was clear from such early publications that CsA exerted a powerful and selective inhibitory action against T lymphocytes. Whilst the capacity of CsA to abrogate the activation of CD4$^+$ (T helper/inducer) lymphocytes and the secretion of interleukin-2 (IL-2) and other cytokines in vitro is now well recognized, the molecular basis of this remarkably sophisticated selectivity remains to be elucidated. Although the generation of specific cytotoxic T cells is impaired by CsA, the activity of natural cytotoxic cells (NK cells) appears unaffected.

In this chapter we do not intend to review all aspects of the influence of CsA on cell-mediated immunity. We wish, rather, to focus on aspects of the mode of action of CsA which have generated most interest and controversy. Thus, initially we shall discuss the cell surface binding and intracellular fate of CsA, molecular interactions which determine the inhibition of very early processes in lymphocyte activation. A further, important consideration, is whether CsA interferes directly (and if so, how) with the role of antigen presenting cells (APC) in the initiation of the T cell-mediated response. Whilst the capacity of CsA to inhibit IL-2 production is not in dispute, its influence, if any, on the expression of IL-2 receptors – a very early event in T cell activation, remains the subject of considerable controversy. It is possible that not all T helper (T$_H$) cell clones or production of all interleukins by these cells are equally susceptible to CsA. Moreover, in culture conditions and in certain organ allograft models, CsA spares the generation of antigen-specific suppressor cells – a phenomenon which is most likely to be cytokine-

50

regulated. Examination of the influence of CsA on the expression of major histocompatibility complex (MHC) antigens on potential cellular targets of cytotoxic T cells *in vivo* is currently receiving increased attention.

There is now a substantial body of evidence, contradictory to *in vitro* studies, which indicates that, *in vivo*, CsA may allow T cell priming and even clonal expression of alloactivated T lymphocytes, although not the expression of their effector functions. This clearly raises important issues regarding lymphokine-mediated control of these events and the intermittent clinical use of CsA in cell-mediated autoimmune disorders. In addition to these topics we shall also briefly discuss the documented interactions between CsA and other anti-lymphocytic agents and the search for synergistic immunosuppressive effects which could permit considerable curtailment of CsA dosage. The extent to which the immunosuppressive action of CsA might be mediated by drug metabolites is also considered in this review.

BINDING, INTRACELLULAR FATE AND MOLECULAR ACTION OF CsA

It is now well documented that CsA prevents the activation of naive lymphocytes of the $CD4^+$ T helper/inducer series by preventing their production of the T cell growth factor, IL-2. Currently there is a consensus of opinion that CsA may exert its action at either of two subcellular locations. It is thought that the drug may mediate its immunosuppressive effect by perturbation of a cell membrane event essential for cell activation or, alternatively, that it may interfere with cytosolic proteins which regulate the activity of enzymes involved in the transcription of lymphokine mRNA.

If CsA mediates its action at a membrane level, then binding of the drug to a membrane 'receptor' may be a prerequisite for its specific action against T cells. Ryffel et al.[1] reported a specific membrane receptor for CsA on human lymphocytes after measuring the binding affinity of [^{3}H]CsC, a dihydrocyclosporin. This observation however, was subsequently disputed and described instead as the existence of low-affinity 'acceptor sites' using [^{3}H]CsA[2].

Although another CsA 'receptor' was reported as the OKT3 (CD3) recognition site, which is closely associated with the T cell antigen receptor[3], this finding has also been contended. The use of a fluorescent, dansylated derivative of CsA (dans-CsA) and flow cytometric analysis, which allowed measurements at a single cell level, showed that only CsA competed directly for its 'own' binding site, and that the OKT3 antibody did not interfere with CsA binding[4]. This CsA-binding site may be the prolactin receptor, as CsA has been shown to compete with prolactin, an inducer of ornithine decarboxylase for binding to this receptor[5,6]. Most recently, Hess and Colombani have revealed rather paradoxical results for the binding affinities of dans-CsA with functionally defined T cell subsets[7]. They found that, instead of displaying more binding, cells expressing the markers of helper and precursor cytotoxic T cells stained only weakly, while intense fluorescence was expressed on suppressor lymphocytes. In order to eliminate the possibility that the dimly staining subset may have represented quenched cells from the bright fraction, cells from each fraction were incubated separately with [³H]CsA. Uptake of radiolabel was up to eight times greater in the brightly staining population than in the weakly staining fraction, therefore eliminating this possibility. On the basis of these findings it was proposed that cells with fewer receptors required less CsA to inhibit their proliferative response and vice-versa.

While the actual molecular identity of the 'receptor' remains elusive, it is worth speculating that the previously mentioned membrane-bound CsA might represent non-specific integration of molecules into the plasma membrane. Indeed, this possibility has been alluded to by LeGrue et al., who have suggested that the homeostatic control of membrane function is disturbed when the hydrophobic CsA molecule partitions into the membrane lipid bilayer[2].

This view has also been explored by Rossaro et al.[8], utilizing magnetic resonance techniques to investigate liposome membrane lipid dynamics following CsA incorporation. They found that, in a concentration-dependent fashion, CsA decreased lipid motion of the inner leaflet lipids. From this they inferred that CsA, by increasing membrane viscosity, could affect certain membane-bound enzyme systems. Evidence that membrane phospholipid metabolism is sensitive to CsA has been shown, although not through a fluidity effect. CsA inhibited the activation of the membrane-located enzyme, lysolecithin acyltransferase, which catalyses the transfer of long-chain fatty acids into plasma membrane phospholipids in Con A-stimulated but not unstimulated thymocytes[9]. In view of results from Foxwell et al.[10], however, on the cellular localization of CsA in erythrocytes, it is quite possible that the hitherto described membrane-bound CsA in lymphocytes might be a secondary feature to its binding in the cytosol. CsA was found to diffuse passively into erythrocytes (transport was unaffected by metabolic inhibitors) and cytoplasmic accumulation of the drug was due to high-affinity binding to a 16 Kd protein resembling cyclophilin (see below). Moreover, following saturation of the cytosolic pool, large-scale unsaturable binding of CsA occurred in the membrane, which was concluded to be the drug partitioning into the hydrophobic environment of the membrane as no membrane-binding protein was identified. It is the binding of CsA to cytosolic regulatory proteins, such as cyclophilin, which is proposed as the alternative effector mechanism in inhibiting the activation process.

The lymphocyte activation process involves antigen or mitogen binding to the T cell receptor which mediates a cascade of intracellular events culminating in the synthesis of interleukins, expression of growth factor receptors and, finally, proliferation of the cell. Upon transduction of the antigen signal, membane-associated phosphatidylinositol 4,5-biphosphate (PIP_2) is hydrolysed and two second messenger molecules form. These are: (a) inositol, 1,4,5-triphosphate (IP_3), which is released into the cytoplasm where it mobilizes calcium (Ca^{2+}) from internal stores and, in the presence of extracellular derived Ca^{2+}, results in an overall increase in cytoplasmic Ca^{2+}; and (b) diacylglycerol, which operates within the membrane to activate protein kinase C (PKC). Activation of PKC, calmodulin-dependent protein kinases by Ca^{2+} and cyclic AMP-dependent protein kinases, leads to the induction of nuclear ornithine decarboxylase and polyamine synthesis essential for gene activation[11,12].

CsA does not interfere with mitogen-induced PIP_2 hydrolysis[13] or with the translocation of PKC in cell lines following its direct activation by phorbol esters[13,14]. Some effect of this drug, however, has been demonstrated in certain studies on the expression of IL-2 receptors (see below), a PKC-mediated event[15]. Although some reports suggest that CsA does not affect IL-2 receptor (IL-2R) expression[16,17], this has been disputed on the basis of the diversity of cells studied and the time at which measurements were made after incubation with CsA[18-20]. Not in dispute is the finding that IL-2 production is inhibited by CsA through the prevention of mRNA transcription[12,21,22]. This suppression, however, is selective, since expression of the gene for the T cell receptor β chain is not abolished by CsA following PKC activation[23]. On examination of the Ca^{2+} arm of the activation cascade, it has been found that CsA has no influence on the intracellular rise in Ca^{2+} following activation[20,24,25], but it appears that it exerts its effect on a subsequent Ca^{2+}-dependent step, necessary for the transcription of mRNA for IL-2 and other cytokines[12-14].

This effect may be due to saturation by CsA of the Ca^{2+}-binding 19 kd acid protein, calmodulin, which is known to regulate certain enzyme systems involved in cell activation[26]. Doubt remains, however, as to whether calmodulin is the direct target of CsA. The less immunosuppressive isomers of CsA (CsD and CsH) exhibit equivalent binding to calmodulin[27] and similar suppression of calmodulin-dependent processes[27,28]. In contrast, cyclophilin, a 17 kd basic protein which also binds CsA and appears to have some protein kinase activity[29,30], does demonstrate good corelation between binding affinity and the immunosuppressive action of CsA and its analogues[29,31]. Recent studies conducted to elucidate the nature of the cyclophilin binding site on CsA have shown that the surface residues on CsA associated with the immunosuppressive activity of the molecule were the only moieties recognized specifically by cyclophilin[32]. In addition, binding of cylophilin was highly specific for the peptide-ring conformation of CsA itself, rather than for the configurations of different derivatives (e.g. CsH). Quesniaux et al.[32] have suggested that CsA could be concentrated by cyclophilin, which binds to the 'active site' on the drug and, by inducing a steric effect on cyclophilin, could result in the complex being recognized by specific receptor molecules involved in T cell activation. This theory, however, does not account for the selective nature of CsA action. In contrast, Hess and Colombani[33] explain the selectivity of CsA on the premise that cyclophilin acts as a cytosolic 'sink' by binding CsA, and thus preventing the drug interfering with calmodulin-dependent processes. This hypothesis was based on their findings that cyclophilin concentrations were much higher in the T lymphocyte suppressor subset and would confer greater resistance to the drug effects, compared to the helper/cytotoxic series, which had lower cyclophilin levels. As yet, neither calmodulin nor cyclophilin has been identified as the sole site of CsA action and, as other proteins have been shown to have CsA-binding properties[34], the enigma of its precise subcellular site of action persists.

53

INFLUENCE OF CsA ON INDUCTION OF CYTOKINE mRNA AND CYTOKINE PRODUCTION

Early evidence indicated that the capacity of murine antigen-presenting cells or human macrophage cell line cells to produce IL-1 was inhibited by CsA[35,36]. Additional studies, however, showed that T-cell-independent induction of macrophage IL-1 production by lipopolysaccharide (LPS) was not affected by CsA[37]. Recent investigations, by Granelli-Piperno and her colleagues[38] on the responses of cultured human blood monocytes to either Con A and phorbol myristate acetate (PMA) or LPS have reinforced the view that the induction of mRNA for IL-1 (α and β) is insensitive to CsA. In contrast to these observations concerning mononuclear phagocytes, there is overwhelming evidence that CsA blocks lymphokine release at the level of the T cell, and that this blockade is effected at the level of lymphokine mRNA transcription (Table 4.1). While the production of IL-2, certain B cell stimulatory factors, various lymphokines affecting macrophage activities and interferon gamma (IFN-γ) is inhibited by CsA, there is little evidence that the concomitant induction of other T cell genes (e.g. the IL-2 receptor, heat shock protein or c-fos genes) in response to the same stimuli are affected[38]. Thus, CsA selectively inhibits the de-repression of T cell lymphokine genes. This potent inhibitory effect on lymphokine gene expression is not found using poorly immunosuppressive cyclosporin analogues, such as CsF or CsH[38,39].

There is general agreement that CsA inhibits *de novo* synthesis of IL-2 in

Table 4.1 Influence of CsA on induction of cytokine mRNAs and/or cytokine production

Cytokine	Effect of CsA	Authors and reference
IL-1	Inhibited Not inhibited	Bunjes *et al.*, 1981[35]; Andrus and Lafferty, 1982[36] Wagner, 1983[37]; Granelli-Piperno *et al.*, 1988[38]
IL-2	Inhibited	Hess *et al.*., 1982[40] Granelli-Piperno *et al.*, 1984[21]; Elliot *et al.*, 1984[48]; Reed *et al.*, 1988[49]
IL-3	Inhibited	Orosz *et al.*, 1983[50]; Palacios, 1985[51]
IL-4	Inhibited	Granelli-Piperno *et al.*, 1988[38]; Sideras *et al.*, 1988[54]
IL-5 (TRF/BCGF II)	Inhibited	Granelli-Piperno *et al.*, 1984[21]
IFN-α/β	Not inhibited	Kalman and Klimpel, 1983[58]; Palacios *et al.*, 1983[59]; Wiskocil *et al.*, 1985[25]
IFN-γ	Inhibited	Reem *et al.*, 1983[60]; Granelli-Piperno *et al.*, 1986[39]; Herold *et al.*, 1986[61]
GM-CSF	Inhibited Not inhibited	Shaw *et al.*, 1987[53] Bickel *et al.*, 1987[52]
TNF	Inhibited Not inhibited	Espevik *et al.*, 1987[64] (TNF α/β) Granelli-Piperno *et al.*, 1988[38]
MIF, MCF	Inhibited	Thomson *et al.*, 1983[66,67]
PIF	Inhibited	Thomson *et al.*, 1983[66,67] Helin and Edgington, 1984[68]

IL = interleukin; TRF, T cell replacement factor; BCGF, B cell growth factor; IFN, interferon; GM-CSF, granulocyte/macrophage colony stimulating factor; TNF, tumour necrosis factor; MIF, migration inhibition factor; MCF, macrophage chemotactic factor; PIF, procoagulant inducing factor.

activated T cells. Impairment of IL-2 production by CsA has been demonstrated in human[40], murine[35,41] and guinea pig[42] mixed lymphocyte cultures (MLC) and with respect to antigen, mitogen or PMA-stimulated human T cells[36,38] or human T cell hybridoma[43]. CsA also inhibits the IL-2-dependent growth of alloantigen-activated cloned human T cells[44] and IL-2 secretion by cloned human[45] and murine T_H cells[46]. Significantly, Heeg et al.[47] found that only murine helper, and not cytotoxic T cell clones, was sensitive to inhibition of IL-2-driven proliferation by CsA. It is also noteworthy, however, that IL-2 production by constitutively producing tumour cell lines is unaffected by CsA[22].

Two sets of observations indicate that CsA blocks T cell proliferation primarily at the level of IL-2 production rather than IL-2 responsiveness. First, several studies have now shown that CsA inhibits IL-2 gene expression at the level of mRNA transcription[21,48,49], and second, exogenous IL-2 at least partially restores proliferative responses of T cells to mitogens, such as Con A and anti-CD3 monoclonal antibody[38].

CsA has also been shown[50,51] to inhibit antigen and lectin-induced, but not constitutive, production of IL-3, a haemopoietic stem cell differentiation factor. On the other hand, evidence concerning the influence of CsA on production of GM-CSF is at present conflicting[52,53]. Thus, in CsA-treated patients, in whom haemopoietic stem cell development and differentiation is normal, either the production of GM-CSF and other non-T cell-derived factors is normal, or cells other than T cells can produce IL-3 in a CsA-insensitive fashion.

Recent experiments indicate that CsA-treated cells do not produce the multifunctional lymphokine as evidenced by in situ hybridization of mouse thymic cells with IL-4-specific probes[54] or the induction of IL-4 mRNA in stimulated human T cells[38]. Since there is now evidence that IL-4 is a potent co-stimulator of resting T cells[55], and that it mediates autocrine growth of T_H cells after antigen stimulation[56], inhibition of its production by CsA could be an important contributory factor to the impairment of T cell proliferation.

Although the corresponding studies to those performed using specific probes for IL-2 and IL-4 mRNAs have not yet been reported with respect to IL-5, there is evidence, including the inhibition by CsA of T-dependent eosinophilia in the rat, that the production of this growth factor is also inhibited by CsA[21,57].

CsA exerts differential effects on production of the different classes of IFN. Whilst it has been shown that the drug does not affect IFN-α/β production[25,58,59], CsA inhibits induction of IFN-γ mRNA[39] and its secretion[39,60,61] by T cells. These findings have important implications as regards resistance to viral infection and the induction of MHC antigen expression in CsA-treated hosts. The down-regulatory effect on IFN-γ production probably underlies the low expression of MHC class II antigens observed as a consequence of CsA treatment. CsA does not, however, block the induction of HLA-DR on human or animal APC in response to exogenous IFN-γ or lymphokine-rich lymphocyte culture supernatants[39,62]. Recently, Halloran et al.[63] have suggested, on the basis of observations on LPS-induced MHC expression in mice, that there may be a T-cell independent pathway for IFN-γ release (and induction of MHC gene expression) which is sensitive to CsA. The capacity of CsA also to inhibit tumour necrosis factor (TNF) production[64] could further interfere with the induction of MHC expression which has been shown to be positively affected by TNF[65].

CsA also markedly affects the production of lymphokines influencing the behaviour of macrophages. Thus, as shown by Thomson et al.[66,67], CsA inhibits secretion of migration inhibition factor, chemotactic factor and procoagulant-inducing factor (PIF) by antigen- or mitogen-stimulated rodent T cells. Impairment of production of PIF by alloactivated human T cells has also been demonstrated[68]. It has also been observed that the responses of macrophages to preformed lymphokines, like those of T cells to exogenous IL-2, are largely unimpaired by CsA[40,66] (Figure 4.1). Clearly, these inhibitory effects of CsA on production of a wide spectrum of T cell-derived cytokines, with diverse immunoregulatory properties, underlie its potent immunosuppressive activity.

CsA AND IL-2 RECEPTOR EXPRESSION

The influence, if any, of CsA on expression of the IL-2 receptor (IL-2R) remains the most controversial issue concerning the mode of action of the drug on the immune system. Using a variety of cellular models, several groups have reported that inhibition of IL-2 production by CsA is not accompanied by modification of IL-2R (CD25) expression[17,39,42,45,69–72] (see also Figure 4.2) or that IL-2R expression is at least partially inhibited[3,18,20,73,74]. Shaw et al.[53] recently found that, while CsA totally prevented the induction of IL-2 mRNA in human peripheral blood mononuclear (PBM) cells, it only partially inhibited the induction of CD25 mRNA in these cells. Similarly, Reed et al.[75] reported that expression of the human IL-2R gene was reduced by about 50% in CsA-treated cultures of peripheral blood lymphocytes. Apart from the diversity of methods of analysis used, these obserations are difficult to interpret and reconcile, since it is recognized that IL-2 up-regulates the expression of its own receptor[76,77].

The expression of high-affinity IL-2R is critical for the proliferation and differentiation of most T cells[77]. Expression of the functional, high-affinity receptor complex is wholly dependent on the association of the 55 kd IL-2R gene product with a newly defined 75 kd converter polypeptide[78] which may only be expressed on T cells. It is possible that CsA could interfere at the post-transcriptional level, with the combination of surface molecules essential for the formation of high-affinity IL-2R. This hypothesis could help explain some of the apparent discrepancies concerning the expression of IL-2R as defined by monoclonal antibodies. It is also conceivable that the mechanism which operates to inhibit high-affinity IL-2R expression on T cells may also be effective against the expression of similar receptors on activated B lymphocytes.

SENSITIVITY OF ACCESSORY CELL FUNCTIONS TO CsA

Accessory cells are essential for the presentation of antigen to T cells in association with MHC gene products, and as a source of incompletely defined

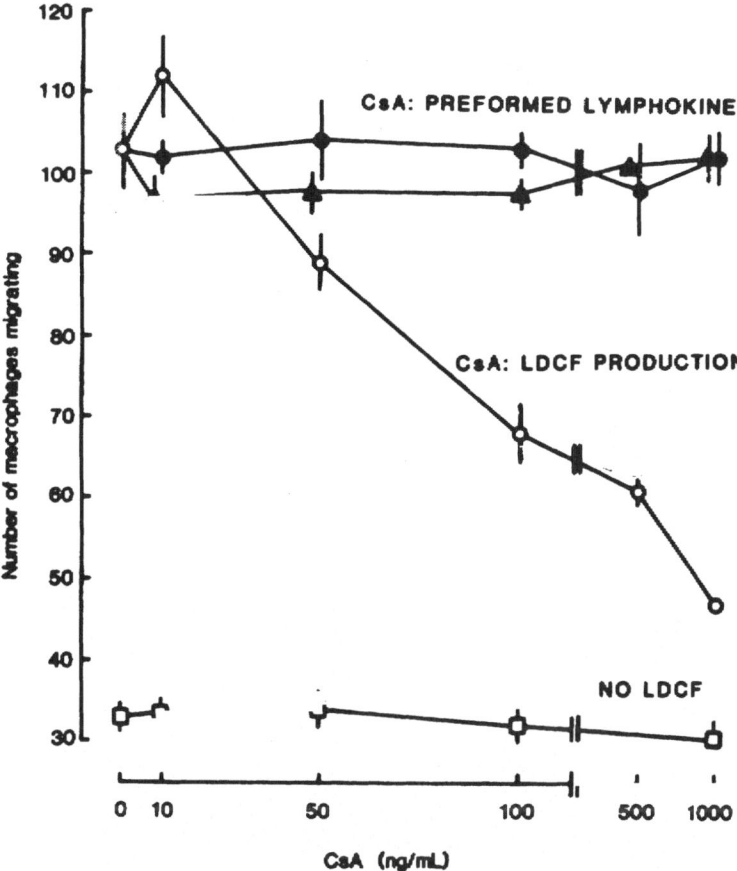

Figure 4.1 Inhibitory effect of CsA on production of the lymphokine lymphocyte-derived macrophage chemotactic factor (LDCF) by mouse splenic T cells. Symbols show the mean numbers of macrophages migrating in response to LDCF produced in the presence of various CsA concentrations (○) or in the absence of lymphokine (□). The failure of CsA to affect the response of macrophages to preformed lymphokine when the drug was added either to the upper (●) or lower (■) wells of the chemotaxis chamber is also shown

'signals' (such as IL-1) which induce T cell activation and lymphokine production. CsA inhibits T cell proliferation only when added in the early stage of accessory cell–T cell interaction. An alternative hypothesis to the view that CsA exerts its immunosuppressive effects by a direct inhibitory action on T cell lymphokine gene expression, is that the drug interferes with the signal normally transmitted to T cells by these antigen-presenting cells (APC).

Early work which examined macrophage functions other than antigen presentation, such as migratory[79] or phagocytic activity[80] and LPS-induced IL-1 production[35,81] suggested that these were insensitive to CsA. More recent studies, conducted by several groups, however, have shown (Table 4.2) that

57

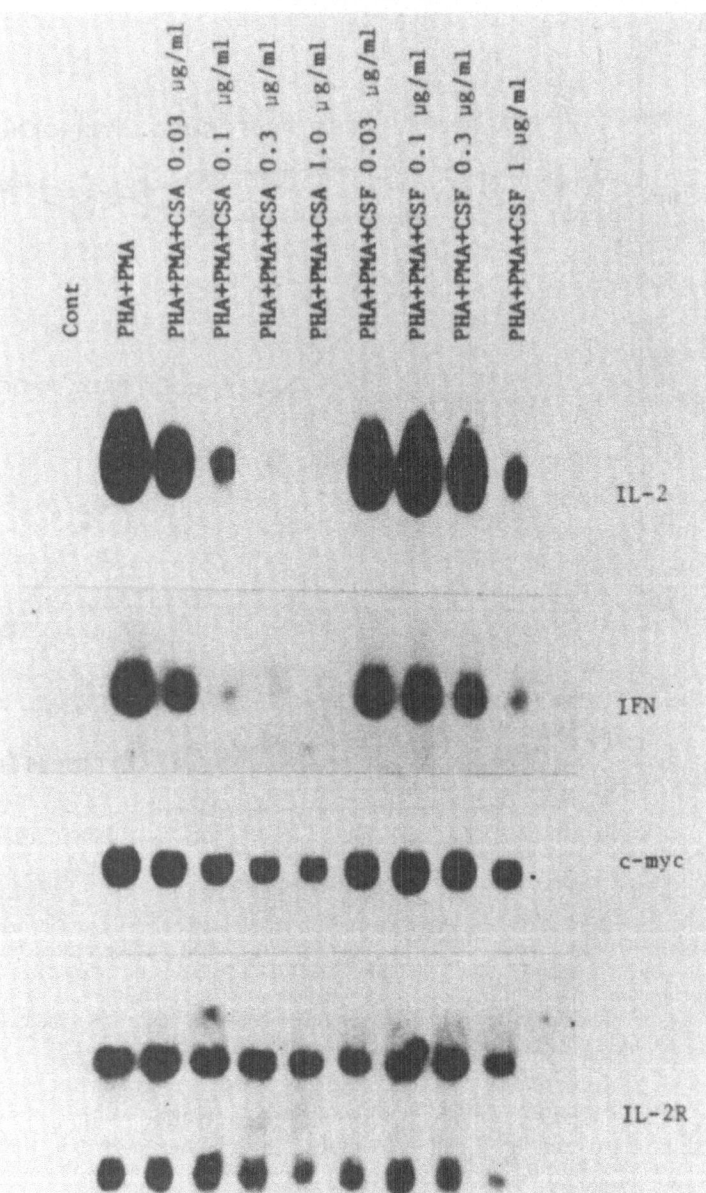

Figure 4.2 The differential effect of CsA on the induction of several human T cell mRNAs. Blood mononuclear cells were cultured in the presence of PHA and PMA and various concentrations of CsA or the less potent immunosuppressant, CsF. After 12 h, total RNA was extracted, fractionated on agarose gels and 20 μg hybridized with the appropriate ^{32}P-labelled cDNA probes. Whilst CsA inhibited production of the lymphokines IL-2 and IFN-γ in a dose-dependent manner, there was no corresponding effect on induction of IL-2R or c-myc mRNAs. Reproduced with permission from Granelli-Piperno et al.[38]

Table 4.2 Evidence that CsA may interfere with accessory cell function

APC	Function	Authors and reference
Murine macrophages	MHC restricted antigen presentation to T cells	Manca et al., 1985[82]; Varey et al., 1986[84]; Paley et al., 1986[83]
Murine Langerhar s cells	Antigen presentation to T cell clones	Furue and Katz, 1988[94]
Rabbit veiled cells	Accessory role in mitogen responses	Knight and Bedford, 1987[93]
Human blood monocytes	Antigen presentation; stimulation of MLR	Whisler et al., 1985[84]; Esa et al., 1988[91]; Snyder et al., 1987[86]
Murine/human macrophages	IL-1 production	Bunjes et al., 1981[55] Andrus and Lafferty, 1982[36]

APC = antigen presenting cell
For further information and discussion, see text

CsA can interfere with the antigen-presenting role of accessory cells[82–86]. Thus, Varey et al.[84] reported that CsA impaired the ability of irradiated mouse spleen cells to present pre-processed antigen (thyroglobulin, PPD) to T cell lines. Similar results were obtained by Manca et al.[82] with respect to β-galactosidase. These observations were supported by Paley et al.[83], who proposed that CsA prevented the complexing of antigen (heat-killed bacteria) and MHC class II gene products, thus causing selective inhibition of antigen presentation, whilst leaving intact non-specific macrophage activities, such as phagocytosis and responsiveness to lymphokines. In human systems, CsA impairs the antigen (PPD)-presenting role of blood monocytes[87] and the ability of monocytes to stimulate autologous and allogeneic mixed lymphocyte reactions[88]. In contrast, Granelli-Piperno et al.[38] reported that CsA did not impair monocyte accessory function for secondary T cell proliferation or primary MLR. These findings with antigen-specific systems are corroborated by data obtained using oxidation and mitogen-driven models[89,90]. Very recently, Esa et al.[91] have further suggested that, with respect to human blood monocytes, there may exist two subpopulations, one efficient at antigen-presentation to T_H cells and which is CsA-sensitive, and a second population, preferentially inducing suppression, which is relatively insensitive to the drug.

Knight and her colleagues[92] have shown that pulsing of rabbit veiled cells (the dendritic cells of afferent lymph) with as little as 5 ng/ml CsA blocks their accessory function in mitogen stimulation of syngeneic blood lymphocytes. In addition, pulsing of mouse dendritic cells with CsA was found to inhibit their capacity to initiate a mixed leukocyte reaction in allogeneic lymphocytes[93]. CsA has also been reported to inhibit accessory and Ag-presenting functions of murine epidermal Langerhans cells[94].

Muller et al.[95], however, have recently pointed out the difficulties in interpreting results of experiments concerning the influence of CsA on antigen presentation, where the nature of the antigen and antigen-handling mechanisms may be quite distinct and where there may be possible carryover of drug to the responder T cell population. In their own experiments, in which the possibility of carryover was minimized, they found that CsA did not interfere specifically with antigen presentation by either murine spleen cells or a B lymphoma cell line to hen egg lysozyme-specific hybridomas. Furthermore, Manca et al.[87] have shown that while CsA inhibits MHC-restricted solution antigen uptake and presentation to T cells, it fails to impair antigen presentation consequent upon receptor-mediated endocytosis of immune complexes.

EFFECTS OF CsA ON MHC GENE EXPRESSION

MHC product induction facilitates both antigen presentation and the interaction of effector T cells with their cellular targets. It has been argued that the inhibition of MHC gene expression by CsA may be important in its suppressive action on T cell responses. The results of recent studies which have addressed this issue are summarized in Table 4.3. Whistler et al.[88] suggested that CsA inhibited autologous and allogeneic MLR stimulated by human blood monocytes by blocking monocyte HLA-DR expression, at least in part by prostaglandin (PG) synthesis. In contrast, Paley et al.[83] found that the inhibitory effect of CsA on murine macrophage antigen presentation was by a mechanism independent of MHC (Ia) antigen expression. This latter observation was corroborated by Snyder et al.[86], who found that CsA inhibited neither basal nor γ-IFN-stimulated human monocyte HLA-DR expression. Both Paley et al.[83] and Snyder et al.[86] found that the inhibitory effect of CsA on the antigen-presenting role of monocytes/macrophages was also independent of IL-1 production and PG secretion. Using Northern blotting analysis Granelli-Piperno et al.[38] have reported that the induction of mRNAs for MHC class II gene products (HLA-DR) in Con A/PMA stimulated human blood monocytes is not inhibited by CsA. Thus the balance of experimental in vitro evidence is clearly in favour of the failure of CsA to interfere with monocyte MHC antigen expression.

Table 4.3 Inhibition of MHC gene expression by CsA

Cell	Response	Authors and reference
Not affected		
Human monocyte	Mitogen-induced HLA-DR mRNA expression	Granelli-Piperno et al., 1988[38]
Human monocyte	Basal/γ-IFN-induced HLA-Dr expression	Snyder et al., 1987[86]
Rat lymphocytes	Ia expression on graft infiltrating cells	Cox and Chisholm, 1987[96]
Murine macrophage	Ia antigen expression	Paley et al., 1986[83]
Retinal pigment epithelial cells*	Ia antigen expression	Liversidge et al., 1988[62]
Inhibited		
Human monocyte	HLA-DR expression in MLR	Whisler et al., 1985[88]
Murine renal epithelium	Basal and GVHD/γ-IFN-induced Ia expression	Halloran et al., 1986[97]; 1988[63]
Vascular endothelium (canine kidney	MHC class II expression	Buurman et al., 1985[98]; Groenevegen et al., 1985[99]

*Postulated antigen-presenting cells in autoimmune uveitis.
For further information and discussion see text

In vivo, the induction of MHC expression in response to strong antigenic stimuli, such as allogeneic cells, is T cell-dependent and presumed to be mediated by γ-IFN, the production of which is inhibited by CsA. Cox and Chisholm[96], however, found that CsA did not affect Ia antigen expression on cells infiltrating rat cardiac allografts. On the other hand, Halloran et al.[97] have shown that CsA treatment of mice with acute graft-versus-host disease (GVHD) diminishes MHC antigen expression on renal proximal tubular epithelial cells, in a dose-dependent manner. The same authors also observed some inhibition by CsA of renal Ia expression in normal mice. Moreover, they found that, *in vitro*, CsA could partially inhibit the induction of MHC products on cultured murine kidney cells in response to γ-IFN. Inhibitory effects of CsA on MHC expression on vascular endothelium *in vivo*[98] and *in vitro*[99] have also been reported. It thus appears that indirect (via inhibition of γ-IFN release) or possibly direct inhibition of MHC antigen expression on target cells may play a key role in the down-regulation of T cell responses by CsA in immunopathological processes, including allograft rejection, GVHD and cell-mediated disease.

In more recent studies, Halloran et al.[63] have reported that the *in vivo* hyperexpression of MHC products induced by LPS administration (and attributable to γ-IFN) in normal or T-cell deficient mice is inhibited by CsA. This finding has raised the possibility that there may also be a T-cell independent pathway for γ-IFN release and, consequently, MHC induction, which is sensitive to CsA.

DIFFERENTIAL SENSITIVITY OF T CELL FUNCTIONS TO CsA: *IN VITRO* STUDIES

Not only are the inhibitory effects of CsA on T cell functions, such as lymphoproliferation, highly dependent both on drug dosage and the temporal relationship between its administration and that of antigen/mitogen, but the various responses of T cell populations exhibit differential sensitivity to CsA. By far the most CsA sensitive function is the *de novo* synthesis, by CD4+ cells, of IL-2 and other lymphokines (Table 4.4). CsA concentrations as low a 10–20 ng/ml are sufficient to cause substantial reductions in lymphokine production; at similar concentrations (20–50 ng/ml) the drug is also extremely effective in inhibiting the clonal amplification and functional differentiation of CD8+ cytotoxic T cells, mediated possibly by the failure of these cells to acquire IL-2R in the absence of IL-2. In general, CsA is believed to exert little direct effect on proliferation or acquisition of cytolytic activity by cytotoxic T cells, although recent investigations using limiting dilution analysis suggest that the drug may directly inhibit human alloantigen-specific cytolytic T cells and their precursors, independent of T_H cell dysfunction[100]. In contrast, CsA (at doses up to 1000 ng/ml) permits the activation, differentiation and clonal expansion of CD8+ suppressor T cells (see Table 4.4). The resulting imbalance in immunoregulatory T cell populations leads to the induction of specific immunological unresponsiveness to the stimulating alloantigen *in vitro* and to allograft specific tolerance in some animal model systems[101,102] (see also

61

Table 4.4 Differential sensitivity of T cell functions to CsA *in vitro*

Function	50% inhibitory concentration (ng/ml)
CsA-sensitive	
Expression of IL-2 receptors	
MLR	100–200
Phytomitogens (PHA, Con A)	200–1000
Production of IL-2 and other lymphokines	10–20
Induction of cytotoxic T cells	
No exogenous IL-2	20–50
With exogenous IL-2	100–150
Proliferation (no exogenous IL-2)	20–50
CsA-resistant	
Proliferation (with exogenous IL-2)	> 1000
Activation of suppressor cells	> 1000
Cell-mediated lympholysis	> 1000

Modified after Hess *et al.* (1988) *Trans. Proc.*, **20**(2), Suppl. 2

Lim and White, Chapter 5 in this volume). The mechanism(s) by which suppressor T cells are resistant to CsA remains to be defined.

Although production of IL-2 is exquisitely sensitive to CsA, the drug (at doses up to 100 ng/ml) does not inhibit the clonal expansion of activated T cells expressing the IL-2R in response to exogenous IL-2. Moreover, the effector arm of cellular immunity, T-cell mediated lympholysis, is insensitive to CsA. Whilst the influence of CsA on acquisition of IL-2R remains controversial, there is evidence that phytomitogen-induced IL-2R expression may be less sensitive to the drug than receptor expression in response to alloantigens.

EFFECTS OF CsA ON T CELL POPULATIONS IN ANIMALS

CsA exerts a wide range of well-documented effects on T cell responses *in vivo* which are consistent with its immunosuppressive properties (Table 4.5). In laboratory rodents, CsA induces rapid ablation of the thymic medulla[103–107], associated with loss of medullary but not cortical epithelium. Accompanying the medullary atrophy are decreases in numbers of mature medullary

Table 4.5 Effects of CsA on T cells *in vivo* consistent with its immunosuppressive properties

Interference with thymocyte maturation
Reductions in T-dependent areas of spleen
Reductions in CD4 : CD8 ratio
Reduction in expression of T cell activation markers
Generation of suppressor cells
Reduced lymphoproliferative and lymphokine-secreting capacity
Inhibition of cytotoxic T cell generation
Capacity to adoptively transfer transplantation tolerance (rat)
Interference with cell migration

See text for further information and references

thymocytes, as defined by the mutually exclusive expression of CD4 or CD8 antigens, and in the amount of MHC class II antigen expression evident within the medulla, especially the Hassall's corpuscles[107]. In contrast, the cortical thymocytes show no apparent alterations in thymocyte or MHC class II antigen expression. Following CsA withdrawal in young adult rats there is full recovery of medullary components within 3 weeks. These observations have important implications with regard to the influence of CsA on cell-mediated immunity. In specific terms, they indicate that there is temporary loss of thymic hormones and self MHC class II antigens necessary for the generation of T_H and antigen recognition.

Marked reductions in T lymphocytes within periarteriolar sheaths and marginal zones of the spleen, whilst the splenic red pulp and thymic cortex remained relatively unaffected, have been observed in normal rodents given high doses of CsA[104] and in cardiac allografted rats with lower doses of the immunosuppressant[108]. This selective depletion of T_H and T_c areas lends credence to the view that CsA spares the $T_{c/s}$ compartment *in vivo* and, indeed, flow cytometric analysis of spleen cells of CsA-treated rats reveals significant reductions in absolute numbers of CD8$^+$ cells and the CD4$^+$: CD8$^+$ ratio (Table 4.6). The dose-related reductions in overall bone marrow cellularity induced by CsA in rats[103,104] are consistent with 'subclinical marrow depression' encountered in human immunotherapy with CsA[109].

SELECTIVE EFFECTS OF CsA ON REGULATORY T CELL POPULATIONS *IN VIVO*

Considerable research effort has been focused on the cellular mechanisms underlying the capacity of short courses of CsA to induce long-term donor-specific transplantation tolerance in some (rat and rabbit) but not all (e.g. dog, monkey) non-human species. Extensive work performed in the rat cardiac allograft model has shown that the adaptive transfer of thymic or splenic

Table 4.6 Effects of CsA on T cell subsets in the spleen

Treatment	CD 4$^+$ W3/25$^+$	CD 8$^+$ OX8$^+$	B OX12$^-$	CD 4$^+$ /CD8$^+$
Vehicle				
Percentage positive cells	22.6 ± 5.3	13.2 ± 3.4	54.3 ± 7.0	1.7 ± .3
Positive cells per spleen (× 10^7)	12.7 ± 4.4	7.5 ± 2.9	30.4 ± 6.3	—
CsA				
Percentage positive cells	27.9 ± 4.9	23.2 ± 4.2***	61.1 ± 7.2	1.2 ± 0.2**
Positive cells per spleen (× 10^7)	14.3 ± 7.3	12.1 ± 5.4*	32.1 ± 14.0	—

Results are means ± 1 SD
*$p < 0.05$; **$p < 0.01$; ***$p < 0.001$ compared to vehicle controls.
Normal rats were immunized with SRBC and treated with either CsA (25 mg/kg) or drug vehicle for 7 days. Numbers of T and B cells in spleen were estimated by flow cytometry (EPICS C) after indirect immunofluorescence staining. CsA caused a decrease in relative and absolute numbers of CD8$^+$ cells and significantly reduced the CD4$^-$: CD8$^+$ ratio, but had no effect on B lymphocytes

lymphocytes from CsA-treated allografted donors into untreated syngeneic recipients leads to prolongation of donor strain but not third-party heart graft survival[110]. Use of monoclonal antibodies and cell separation procedures revealed that the $CD8^+$ $T_{c/s}$ cell population was responsible for mediating the CsA effect[111] whilst abrogation of suppressor cells was found to provoke acute rejection in CsA-treated heart graft recipients[112]. The effectiveness of CsA in prevention of bone marrow transplant rejection and GVHD has also been ascribed to the accelerated appearance of suppressor cells[113]. Studies on the migration of adoptively transferred radiolabelled lymphocytes in rat cardiac transplantation have also indicated that CsA may interfere with allograft recognition by lymphocyte surface receptors[114].

EFFECTS OF CsA ON LYMPHOID CELLS IN PATIENTS

There have been clinical reports that transplant or autoimmune disease patients show reductions in the CD4:CD8 T cell ratio within the first few weeks of CsA treatment[115–118] and that CsA therapy inhibits the *in vivo* expression of activation markers on the surfaces of lymphoid cells, including MHC class II antigens on peripheral blood lymphocytes[119]. Other workers, however, examining absolute lymphocyte counts and T lymphocyte subset distribution in the blood of transplant recipients treated with CsA as the only immunosuppressant, have reported no effect of the drug on these parameters[120–123] or on the *in vitro* proliferative responses of T cells from CsA-treated patients[123]. As in animals, alterations in lymphoproliferative responses and the capacity of lymphocytes from CsA-treated transplant recipients to produce lymphokines, including both IL-2 and γ-IFN, have, however, been reported[124–126]. Moreover, the inhibition of *in vivo* cytotoxic T cell generation, as well as the non-specific generation of suppressor cells, has been observed in CsA-treated allograft recipients[118,127,128]. In autoimmune disease, Assan *et al.*[117] have reported decreased IL-2 production in type 1 diabetics given CsA, whilst in rheumatoid arthritis, CsA treatment leading to significant clinical improvement was associated with a decrease in IL-2 production by synovial lymphocytes[129].

INFLUENCE OF CsA ON DELAYED-TYPE HYPERSENSITIVITY REACTIONS

The capacity of systemic CsA to inhibit classical cutaneous delayed-type hypersensitivity (DTH) reactions to tuberculin or contact sensitizing agents (oxazalone or dinitrochlorobenzene) in rodents was among the first-described effects of the drug on cell-mediated immunity[130]. In these initial studies the immunosuppressive properties of CsA were evident when the drug was administered during either the sensitization or effector phases of the response. Inhibitory effects of CsA on DTH to a variety of antigens have subsequently been demonstrated by other workers[131–135], who have shown that CsA-induced immunosuppression is linked to the impairment of phytomitogen-induced or antigen-dependent lymphokine production[66,67,81,131]. Moreover, the reversal by either lymphokines or a synthetic cytokine inducer of the effect of CsA on DTH has been demonstrated in mice[136,137]. Study of delayed cutaneous hypersensitivity in renal transplant patients receiving CsA as the only immunosuppressant has revealed decreased responses to DNCB immunizatior but normal recall responses to microbial antigens[123].

As with cytotoxic immunosuppressive agents, such as cyclophosphamide, cycloheximide or methotrexate, CsA can exert diverse effects on DTH in different experimental models. Thus, Thomson et al.[131] first showed that in guinea pigs, short (5-day) courses of CsA given from the time of immunization (with ovalbumin) could result in significant augmentation of DTH reactions elicited 2 weeks later (at day 14). In addition, pretreatment of guinea pigs with a high dose of CsA, 2–3 days before immunization, has been shown to augment DTH responses[138], whilst similar treatment of mice can prevent high-dose antigen-induced unresponsiveness to sheep erythrocytes[139,140] (see Figure 4.3). These paradoxical observations are clearly dependent on a variety of factors, including the temporal relationship between drug and antigen

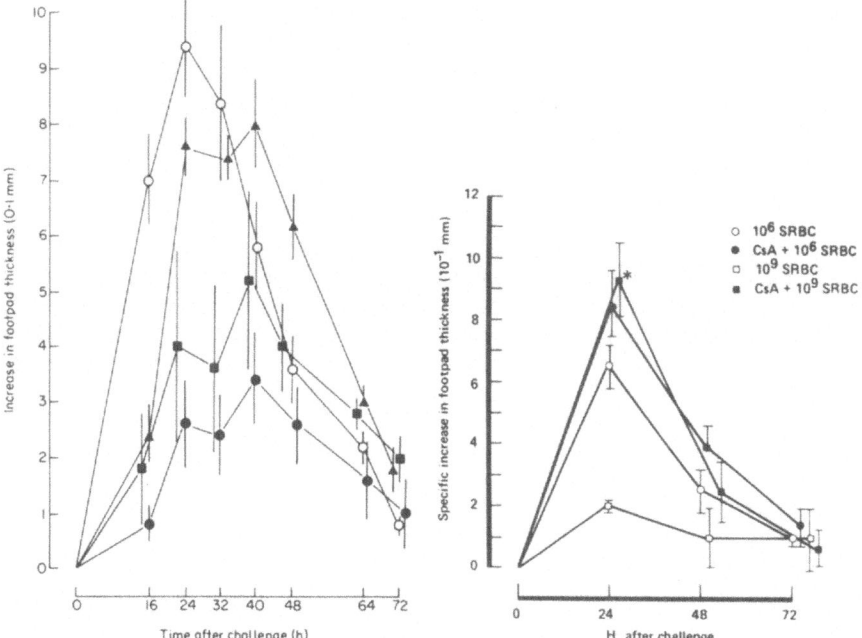

Figure 4.3 The effect of CsA on delayed-type hypersensitivity to SRBC in mice is dependent on antigen and drug dosage and on the temporal relationship between antigen and drug administration. *Left*, dose-dependent immunosuppressive effect of CsA administered 24 and 48 h after immunization (with 10^6 SRBC) on DTH responses elicited on day 4. Note also the delay in the peak of the immune response. (○), Drug vehicle-treated controls; (▲), 50 mg/kg; (■), 75 mg/kg; (●), 100 mg/kg. *Right*, prevention by CsA (200 mg/kg) administered 48 h before immunization (with 10^9 SRBC), of high-dose antigen-induced tolerance. DTH responses in animals immunized with 10^6 SRBC were not significantly affected by CsA pretreatment. Similar results were obtained with animals pretreated with doses of CsA a low as 10 mg/kg. For further details see Thomson et al.[67] and Webster and Thomson[39]

65

administration, the choice and quantity of antigen and the concentration of CsA[141,142]. It has, however, been suggested that augmentation of DTH or inhibition of tolerance induction by CsA is attributable to failure of induction or functional activity of (T) suppressor cells[131,138,142-144].

In guinea pigs, CsA markedly suppressed DTH reactions in animals pre-treated with cyclophosphamide, indicating that in this species, Cy-sensitive suppressor cells (thought to be B cells) are not essential for the immunosuppressive action of CsA. The influence of topical CsA on DTH reactions is of particular relevance to the prospective clinical applications of CsA in the treatment of T cell-mediated cutaneous inflammatory disorders. Topical CsA has been shown to inhibit contact sensitivity reactions to DNFB in guinea pigs[145] and to nickel in a proportion of patients with proven nickel contact sensitivity[146]. Immunohistochemical analyses of skin biopsies in both animal and human studies revealed that clinical responses were accompanied by marked reductions in T cell infiltration. No differential effect on CD4$^+$ or CD8$^+$ cells, however, was observed in the human biopsies, whilst in guinea pigs a possible differential effect on immunoregulatory lymphoid cell populations was suggested, though basophil numbers were unaffected[147].

In a recent study of the immunosuppressive action of CsA in contact sensitivity to DNFB in mice, Knight et al.[148] found that although CsA did not affect the increase in dendritic cells within draining lymph nodes following skin painting, it markedly reduced the level of antigen expression on these cells, and their stimulatory activity in primary syngeneic lymphoproliferative responses. Thus, in contact sensitivity, CsA may prevent antigen acquisition and presentation, in addition to any direct effects on T cells.

Under normal circumstances, T cell-mediated immunity is not accompanied by eosinophilia. There is evidence, however, that eosinophilia in response to parasite antigens is T cell-dependent. Moreover, in rats, the depletion of T cell precursors by high-dose cyclophosphamide followed by immunization with a soluble T-dependent antigen (ovalbumin) can induce pronounced eosinophilia, which is abrogated by CsA[57,149]. The most plausible explanation of this finding is that CsA inhibits production by T_H cells of eosinophil differentiation factor ($=$ interleukin 5). CsA has also been shown, in rats, to reduce numbers of mucosal mast cells elevated in response to helminth infection or GVHD[150].

CONTRADICTORY EFFECTS ON T CELLS IN VIVO

Despite the relatively clear-cut nature of the foregoing proposed model for the action of CsA on T cell proliferation in vitro, doubts have been raised about the validity of extrapolating these mechanisms to interpretation of the drug's mode of action in vivo[151,152]. These reservations are based largely on a number of observations made by various authors using different experimental animal models of T cell-mediated immunity (Table 4.7). Thus, lymphocytic infiltration is a consistent feature of surviving allografts in CsA-treated animals and patients[153] and recipients of renal allografts often undergo rejection crises, despite CsA treatment[154]. Moreover, augmented immune reactivity has been

Table 4.7 Contradictory effects of CsA on T cells *in vivo*

Species	Observation	Authors and reference
Guinea pig; rat	Augmented DTH following drug withdrawal	Thomson et al., 1981[131]; Kaibara et al., 1983[155]
Rat (lethally irradiated, reconstituted)	Syngeneic GVHD	Glazier et al., 1983[114]; Sorokin et al., 1985[156]
Rat, mouse	Failure to block T cell activation	Chisholm et al., 1985[157]; Kroczek et al., 1987[159]; Chisholm and Bevan, 1988[158]
Mouse	Clonal expansion of T cells	Milon et al., 1984[160]; Schildknecht and Ada, 1985[161]
Mouse	Prevention of high-dose antigen-induced tolerance	Webster and Thomson, 1987[139]; 1988[140]
Mouse	Inhibition of T suppressor cells	Altmann and Blyth, 1985[143]; Braida and Knop, 1986[144]
Man	Rejection crises; lymphocytic infiltrate of surviving allografts; exacerbation of autoimmune disease activity following drug withdrawal	Morris 1981[153]; Land et al., 1986[154]

For further information and discussion see text

reported in DTH[131,155] and autoimmune disease models following drug withdrawal[114,156]. Data obtained by Chisholm and her colleagues[157,158] in experimental rat allograft models indicate that, although CsA blocks T effector cell maturation/function, it does not inhibit the earliest stages of T cell activation (IL-2R and MHC class II antigen expression and the co-expression of CD4 and CD8 markers). Similar results, concerning the failure of CsA to inhibit T cell activation in response to alloantigens in the mouse, have been reported by Kroczek et al.[159]. In other experimental systems clonal expansion of T cells, including those involved in DTH reactions[160] or in cytotoxicity against influenza virus[161], has been reported, despite inhibition of their effector function by CsA. In an effort to reconcile these apparent discrepancies between the sites of CsA action *in vitro* and *in vivo*, it has been suggested that there may be an IL-2-dependent pathway(s) of T cell growth *in vivo* which is regulated by CsA-insensitive lymphokine/growth factor production[158,159]. The existence of an IL-2-independent T-cell stimulatory pathway has recently been suggested[55,162,163]. Indeed, the existence of a CsA-resistant pathway for induction of antigen-specific CD8$^+$ murine cytotoxic T cells *in vitro* has recently been demonstrated. Thus the authors have postulated that the capacity of IL-4 to induce cytotoxic T cell differentiation may be CsA-resistant[164] and that systemic CsA may be unable to suppress the local synergistic effects of combined IL-2 and IL-4 on development of cytolytic activity. These observations, together with data indicating that, in certain experimental models of DTH, CsA can inhibit the activity of T suppressor cells, have important cautionary implications with regard to the possible covert priming of patients' T cells during intermittent use of the drug and the possibility of exacerbated immune reactivity following CsA withdrawal.

Notably, Freed et al.[165] have shown that, although CsA suppresses proliferation in the primary human MLC, T cells are nevertheless primed to respond as soon as the drug is removed.

A poorly understood phenomenon is CsA-induced syngeneic GVHD (or 'CsA-induced autoimmunity'), first described in rats by Glazier et al.[114]. This special, severe type of GVHD which appears to be mediated by CD8$^+$ CD4$^-$ cytotoxic T cells, occurs as early as 2 weeks after discontinuation of CsA in lethally irradiated animals, reconstituted with syngeneic bone marow[166]. Lethal disease can be adoptively transferred using relatively small numbers of CD4$^+$ spleen and lymph node cells into irradiated syngeneic recipients[156], but can be overcome by co-transfer of a large excess of lymphocytes from normal donors. Two hypotheses have been offered as possible explanations of CsA-induced syngeneic GVHD. First, as suggested by Lafferty et al.[167], lymphokine-dependent natural suppressor cells arising in irradiated animals during haemopoietic reconstitution may delete anti-self T cells – a process which could be negated by CsA, resulting in abrogation of self-tolerance. Second, as suggested by Beschorner et al.[168], destruction of the thymic medullary microenvironment by CsA[103,106,169] could lead to immature thymocytes entering the circulation and potential target tissues where, under the influence of MHC class II antigen expression, they may develop into anti-self helper-type T cells.

EFFECTS OF CsA ON NK CELL ACTIVITY

Natural killer (NK) cells are lymphoid cells found within the large granular lymphocyte (LGL) population in humans, mice and rats, and are believed to play an important role in host resistance to malignancy and viral infections. They may also have a role in the regulation of haematopoiesis. In humans the cytotoxic activity of NK cells is augmented by IL-2 or all classes of interferons. With respect to CsA, Xi-En et al.[170] found only mild impairment of NK activity in cells from renal transplant patients treated with CsA, compared to the activity of mononuclear cells from those receiving conventional immunosuppressive therapy. Similar results on basal NK cell activity have recently been obtained by Versluis et al.[171], who have also shown that conversion from CsA to azathioprine therapy leads to reduction in basal NK activity and with the numbers of cells expressing the Leu-11a antigen.

In vitro it has been reported that CsA has no direct effect on human basal NK cell-mediated cytotoxicity[172] or on γ-IFN-induced augmentation of target cell killing[171]. Concentrations of CsA much in excess of those used in vivo have, however, been shown to impair NK cell activity, without evidence of direct interference with target cell lysis[173]. Maintenance of basal NK cell activity during CsA administration may explain the reported reduced incidence of viral infections in patients receiving the drug[174], despite interference with IL-2 and γ-IFN production. On the basis of their findings, however, Cauda et al.[175] have argued that CsA may reduce NK cell activity against virally (CMV and HSV)-infected cell targets in renal allograft recipients compared with normal subjects.

68

In an experimental rat model recently described by Stewart *et al.*[176], CsA failed to affect the generation of large granular lymphocytes or the augmented NK cell activity which followed cyclophosphamide administration and systemic immunization (Figure 4.4). In this and a recent report of murine cytotoxic T cell induction[164], it has been suggested that CsA-resistant, cytokine-dependent pathways for induction of NK cells or cytotoxic T cells, respectively, may exist *in vivo*.

SYNERGY BETWEEN CsA AND OTHER AGENTS

Since the administration of CsA is associated with nephrotoxicity and certain other side-effects (see other chapters in this volume), additional immunosuppressive agents for use in combination with reduced doses of CsA are currently being sought.

ANTI-IL-2R

CsA inhibits production of IL-2 by activated T lymphocytes but allows the expression of IL-2R. An attractive approach to combination therapy envisages

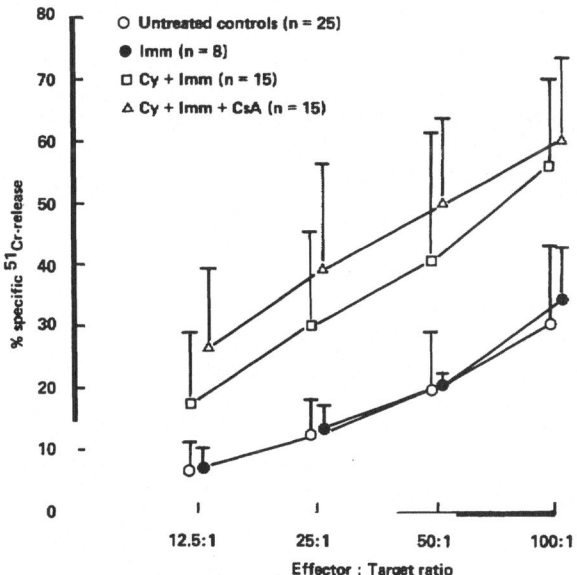

Figure 4.4 Failure of CsA to inhibit NK cell activity. Treatment of rats with 25 mg kg⁻¹ day⁻¹ CsA for 14 days did not impair splenic NK cell activity (against YAC-1 tumour targets). NK cell activity was determined in untreated normal rats and in animals pretreated with high-dose cyclophosphamide (Cy) 48 h before immunization (imm) with a T-dependent antigen — a procedure which significantly increases splenic NK cell activity. For further details see Stewart *et al.*[176]

use of anti-IL-2R monoclonal antibodies together with low-dose CsA. In recent studies Tellides *et al.*[177] have shown that a combination of subtherapeutic doses of CsA (1.5 mg kg^{-1} day^{-1}) and NDS-61 (300 μg kg^{-1} day^{-1}), a mouse IgG1 monoclonal antibody which inhibits rIL-2-induced rat T cell proliferation, has a striking synergistic inhibitory effect on rat (Lew-DA) renal allograft rejection. The same subtherapeutic dose of CsA has been found to potentiate the effect of a suboptimal dose of another anti-IL-2R monoclonal antibody (ART-18) on rat cardiac allograft survival[178], whilst a combination of low doses of both these agents prolonged rat pancreatic islet allograft or skin allograft survival[178,179] in the same species. Kupiec-Weglinski *et al.*[178] have also reported that CsA facilitates the beneficial effect of ART-18 therapy against T cell-mediated β cell destruction in the spontaneously diabetic BB rat. CsA in a dose also ineffectual on its own also potentiates the inhibitory action of ART-18 in suppression of local graft-versus-host reactivity in rats[178]. The potential of CsA and anti-IL-2R in combination immunosuppressive therapy is further emphasized by the capacity of either agent to spare and/or stimulate CD8$^+$ T$_s$ cells[180–182].

FK-506

FK-506 is a recently discovered macrolide antibiotic, isolated from the fermentation broth of a soil fungus, *Streptomyces tsukubaensis*. It shares many of the properties of CsA, including interference with production of IL-2 and other lymphokines, absence of myelotoxicity and tolerance induction following short courses in allografted rats. FK-506, however, is considerably more potent than CsA (reviewed recently by Thomson[183]. There is also evidence that CsA and FK-506 may act synergistically with CsA both *in vivo* and *in vitro*[184,185]. The potential of this new immunosuppressive agent which, on its own, has severe side-effects in dogs and baboons, although not in rats[186], will depend on further toxicology evaluation.

IMMUNOSUPPRESSIVE AND ANTI-INFLAMMATORY AGENTS

There have been reported synergistic effects between CsA and cytotoxic immunosuppressive drugs, including methotrexate[187] and in particular, azathioprine[188–192] in experimental allograft rejection models. Thus, subtherapeutic daily doses of azathioprine, with either daily or alternate-day CsA, prolonged rat cardiac allograft survival far beyond that achieved with either agent alone[192]. The capacity of anti-thymocyte globulin and CsA to act synergistically in the inhibition of one-way human mixed lymphocyte reactions has also been demonstrated[193]. With respect to steroids, synergistic effects of CsA and dexamethasone on the response of human lymphocytes to phytomitogens have been reported[194]. Freed *et al.*[195], however, later observed that whilst both CsA and methylprednisolone were potent inhibitors of human IL-2 production and T cell proliferation, and exhibited additive effects, they were not synergistic. In studies of the interaction between CsA and the anti-rheumatic drugs, bromocriptine and chloroquine[196], only an additive inhibitory effect with bromocriptine on pokeweed mitogen-induced lymphocyte proliferation was observed, but an apparent synergistic effect with chloroquine was reported. The lack of effect of the cyclo-oxygenase blocker indomethacin on CsA-induced immune suppression[83] is consistent with the view that prostaglandir.s do not play a significant role in its antilymphocytic activity.

Another (immunosuppressive) agent which has been examined in experimental combination therapy with CsA is thalidomide. Vogelsang et al.[197] have recently demonstrated the effectiveness of combination low-dose thalidomide and CsA in prophylaxis of acute GVHD in rats.

CALCIUM CHANNEL-BLOCKING AGENTS

Calcium channel-blocking agents, such as verapamil and nicardipine, have recently been advocated to prevent and treat CsA-induced hypertension and/or nephrotoxicity. These drugs, which inhibit calcium uptake from the extracellular fluid, suppress T cell proliferation and function. Recent data indicate that verapamil enhances the inhibitory effects of CsA on murine[198] or human T cell proliferation and the generation of cytotoxic cells[199]. Whilst nicardipine[200] enhances the action of CsA on human T cell proliferation, it does not further depress IL-2 production, indicating that the two agents do not share the same site of action.

CsA METABOLITES

CsA is metabolized primarily in the liver by hydroxylation and N-demethylation through the mono-oxygenase cytochrome P-450 system. The metabolites are excreted into the bile and eliminated through the intestinal tract. The isolation of CsA metabolites from the bile of liver transplant recipients has been described, and the antilymphocytic activity of several bile-derived metabolites has been demonstrated in vitro using PHA and Con A-induced proliferation assays and MLR culture[201,202]. Certain metabolites have also been shown to inhibit IL-2 production in MLC and the generation of cytotoxic T cells[201]. Freed et al.[202] and Zeevi et al.[203] have shown that, in particular, metabolite M17 followed by M1 (each with single hydroxylations of amino acids in positions 1 and 9, respectively), are the most active CsA metabolites with effects approaching that of CsA. In Con A and primary MLR assays the most active metabolite, M17, was found to be about 100 times less inhibitory than CsA[203,204]. Metabolites M8 (hydroxylated at both amino acids 1 and 9) and M21 (N-methylated amino acid at position 4) showed even more reduced activity in relation to the parent compound[202-204].

Recently, Zeevi et al.[203,204] have reported that bile-derived CsA metabolites (M17, M1, M21) are significantly (approximately 10-fold) more active in the inhibition of secondary proliferation of cloned alloactivated human T cells isolated from human heart and liver transplant biopsies. Moreover, differential sensitivity of alloreactive T cells derived from individual patients' biopsies at various times post-transplant could be demonstrated[203,204] in response to either CsA or M17. It appears from these observations that CsA metabolites

71

may exert greater inhibitory activity on primed alloreactive T cells than on unprimed cells. In addition, synergistic inhibition of T cell proliferation was shown by combination of CsA and M17 *in vitro*. Conceivably, low levels of CsA together with active metabolite(s) may effect adequate immunosuppressive activity when concentrations of either alone might be inadequate. The relative concentrations of CsA and metabolites thus appear to be important in mediating immunosuppression.

CONCLUSION

The mechanisms by which CsA exerts its potent suppressive effects on cell-mediated immune responses are not understood. A great deal remains to be learned about the intracellular molecular effects and the influence of this agent on antigen presentation, cytokine–cytokine receptor autocrine pathways, sensitivity of regulatory T cell populations and MHC gene expression *in vivo*. Further understanding of the mode of action of CsA, and of the consequences of its effects on immunoregulatory mechanisms, are essential before more widespread clinical use of the drug can be contemplated.

ACKNOWLEDGEMENTS

The work of the author's laboratory is supported by grants from the Medical Research Council, the Cancer Research Campaign and Grampian Health Board. We also thank Sandoz Pharmaceuticals for supporting our clinical research investigations on cyclosporin and cell-mediated immunity. The manuscript was typed by Mrs I. M. Watson.

REFERENCES

1. Ryffel, B., Götz, U. and Heuberger, B. (1982) Cyclosporin receptors on human lymphocytes. *J. Immunol.*, **129**, 1978
2. LeGrue, S. J., Friedman, A. W. and Kahan, B. D. (1983) Binding of cyclosporine by human lymphocytes and phospholipid vesicles. *J. Immunol.*, **131**, 712
3. Palacios, R. (1982) Mechanisms of T cell activation: role and functional relationship of HLA-DR antigens and interleukins. *Immunol. Rev.*, **63**, 73
4. Ryffel, B., Willard-Gallo, K. E., Tammi, K. and Loken, M. R. (1984) Quantitative fluorescence analysis of cyclosporine binding to human leukocytes. *Transplantation*, **37**, 276
5. Russel, D. H., Kibler, D. H., Matrison, L., Larson, D. P., Poulos, B. and Magun, B. E. (1985) Prolactin receptors on human T and B lymphocytes: antagonism of prolactin binding of cyclosporin. *J. Immunol.*, **134**, 3027
6. Heistand, P. C., Mekler, P., Nordmann, R., Grieder, A. and Permmongkol, C. (1986) Prolactin as a modulator of lymphocyte responsiveness provides a possible mechanism of action of CsA. *Proc. Natl. Acad. Sci. USA*, **83**, 2599
7. Hess, A. D. and Colombani, P. N. (1988) Inverse correlation of cyclosprine binding with sensitivity and resistance. *Transplantation*, **46** (Suppl.), 61S
8. Rossaro, L., Dowd, S. R., Ho, C. and Van Thiel, D. H. (1988) ^{19}F Nuclear magnetic resonance studies of cyclosporine and model unilamellar veiscles: where does the drug sit within the membrane? *Transplant. Proc.*, **20** (Suppl. 2), 41
9. Szamel, M., Berger, P. and Resch, K. (1986) Inhibition of T lymphocyte activation by cyclosporin A: interference with the early activation of plasma membrane phospholipid metabolism. *J. Immunol.*, **136**, 264
10. Foxwell, B. M. J., Frazer, G., Winters, M., Heistand, P., Wenger, R. and Ryffel, B. (1988) Identification of cyclophilin as the erythrocyte ciclosporin-binding protein. *Biochim. Biophys. Acta*, **938**, 447

72

11. King, S. L. (1988) An assessment of phosphoinositide hydrolysis in antigenic signal transduction in lymphocytes. *Immunology*, **65**, 1
12. Hess, A. D., Esa, A. and Colombani, P. M. (1988) Mechanisms of action of cyclosporine: effects on cells of the immune system and on subcellular events in T cell activation. *Transplant. Proc.*, **20** (Suppl. 2), 29
13. Isakov, N., Scholz, W. and Altman, A. (1987) Effect of cyclosporine A on early stages of T cell activation. *Transplant. Proc.*, **14**, 1186
14. Manger, B., Hardy, K. J., Weiss, A. and Stobo, J. D. (1986) Differential effect of cyclosporin A on activation signalling in human T cell lines. *J. Clin. Invest.*, **77**, 1501
15. Isakov, N. and Altman, A. (1987) Human T lymphocyte activation by tumor promoters: role of protein kinase C. *J. Immunol.*, **138**, 3100
16. Gelfand, E. W., Cheung, R. K. and Mills, G. B. (1987) The cyclosporins inhibit lymphocyte activation at more than one site. *J. Immunol.*, **138**, 1115
17. Ryffel, B., Müller, S. and Foxwell, B. (1987) CsA allows the expression of high affinity IL-2 binding sites on anti-T cell antibody activated human T lymphocytes. *Transplant. Proc.*, **19**, 1199
18. Lillehoj, H. S., Malek, T. R. and Shevach, E. M. (1984) Differential effect of CsA on the expression of T and B lymphocyte activation antigens. *J. Immunol.*, **133**, 244
19. Prince, H. E. and John, J. K. (1986) Cyclosporin inhibits the expression of receptors for IL-2 and transferrin on mitogen-activated human T lymphocytes. *Immunol. Invest.*, **15**, 463
20. Redelman, D. (1988) Cyclosporin A does not inhibit the PHA-stimulated increase in intracellular Ca^{2+} concentration but inhibits the increase in E-rosette receptor (CD2) expression and appearance of interleukin-2 receptors (CD25). *Cytometry*, **9**, 156
21. Granelli-Piperno, A., Inaba, K. and Steinman, R. (1984) Stimulation of lymphokine release from T lymphoblasts-requirement for mRNA synthesis and inhibition by CsA. *J. Exp. Med.*, **160**, 1792
22. Hodgkin, P. D., Hapel, A. J. Johnson, R. M., Young, I. G. and Lafferty, K. J. (1987) Blocking of delivery of the antigen-mediated signal to the nucleus of T cells by cyclosporin. *Transplantation*, **43**, 685
23. Noonan, D. J., Isakov, N., Theofilopoulos, A. N., Dixon, F. J. and Altman, A. (1987) Protein kinase C-activating phorbol esters augment expression of T cell receptor genes. *Eur. J. Immunol.*, **17**, 803
24. Metcalfe, S. (1984) Cyclosporin does not prevent cytoplasmic calcium changes associated with lymphocyte activation. *Transplantation*, **38**, 161
25. Wiskovil, R., Weiss, A., Imboden, J., Kamin-Lewis, R. and Stobo, J. (1985) Activation of a human T cell line: A two-stimulus requirement in the pretranslational events involved in the coordinate expression of interleukin 2 and γ-interferon genes. *J. Immunol.*, **134**, 1599
26. Colombani, P. M., Robb, A. and Hess, A. D. (1985) CsA binding to calmodulin: a possible site of action on T lymphocytes. *Science*, **228**, 338
27. LeGrue, S. J., Turner, R., Weisbrodt, N. and Redman, J. R. (1986) Does the binding of cyclosporin to calmodulin result in immunosuppression? *Science*, **234**, 68
28. Gschwendt, M., Kittstein, W. and Marks, F. (1988) The weak immunosuppressant cyclosporine D as well as the immunologically inactive cyclosporine H are potent inhibitors *in vivo* of phorbol ester TPA-induced biological effects in mouse skin and of Ca^2/calmodulin dependent EF-2 phosphorylation *in vitro*. *Biochem. Biophys. Res. Commun.*, **150**, 545
29. Handschumacher, R. E., Harding, M. W., Rice, J. and Drugge, R. J. (1984) Cyclophilin: a specific cytosolic binding protein for cyclosporin A. *Science*, **226**, 544
30. Harding, M. W. and Handschumacher, R. E. (1988) Cyclophilin, a primary molecular target for cyclosporine. *Transplantation*, **46** (Suppl.), 29S
31. Durette, P. L., Boger, J., Dumont, F., Firestone, R., Frankshun, R. A., Koprak, S. L., Lin, C. S., Melino, M. R., Pessolano, A. A., Pisano, J., Schmidt, J. A., Sigal, N. H., Staruch, M. J. and Witzel, B. E. (1988) A study of the correlation between cyclophilin binding on *in vitro* immunosuppressive activity of cyclosporine A and analogues. *Transplant. Proc.*, **20** (Suppl. 2), 51
32. Quesniaux, V. F. J. and Schreier, M. H., Wenger, R. M., Hiestand, P. C., Harding, M. W. and Van Regenmortel, M. H. V. (1988) Molecular characteristics of cyclophilin-cyclosporin interaction. *Transplantation*, **46** (Suppl.), 23S

33. Hess, A. D. and Colombani, P. M. (1987) Mechanisms of action of cyclosporine: role of calmodulin, cyclophilin and other cyclosporin-binding proteins. *Transplant. Proc.,* **18** (Suppl. 5), 219

34. Foxwell, B. M. J., Hiestand, P. C., Wenger, R. and Ryffel, B. (1988) A comparison of cyclosporine binding by cyclosporin-binding proteins. *Transplant. Proc.,* **18** (Suppl.), 35S

35. Bunjes, D., Hardt, C., Röllinghoff, M. and Wagner, H. (1981) CsA mediates immunosuppression of primary cytotoxic T cell responses by impairing the release of IL-1 and IL-2. *Eur. J. Immunol.,* **11**, 657

36. Andrus, L. and Lafferty, K. J. (1982) Inhibition of T cell activity by CsA. *Scand. J. Immunol.,* **15**, 449

37. Wagner, H. (1983) CsA: mechanism of action. *Transplant. Proc.,* **15**, 523

38. Granelli-Piperno, A., Keane, M. and Steinman, R. M. (1988) Evidence that cyclosporine inhibits cell-mediated immunity primarily at the level of the T lymphocyte rather than the accessory cell. *Transplantation,* **46**, Suppl. 53S

39. Granelli-Piperno, A., Andrus, L. and Steinman, R. M. (1986) Lymphokine and non-lymphokine mRNA levels in stimulated human T cells. Kinetics, mitogen requirements and effects of CsA. *J. Exp. Med.,* **163**, 922

40. Hess, A. D., Tutschka, P. J. and Santos, G. W. (1982) Effect of CsA on human lymphocyte responses *in vitro.* III. CsA inhibits production of T cell growth factor in secondary MLC but does not inhibit response of primed lymphocytes to T cell growth factor. *J. Immunol.,* **128**, 355

41. Wang, B. S., Zheng, C., Heacock, G. H., Tilney, N. L., Strom, T. B. and Mannick, J. A. (1983) Inhibition of the production of a soluble helper mediator by CsA results in the failure to generate alloreactive cytolytic cells in MLC. *Clin. Immunol. Immunopathol.,* **27**, 160

42. Dos Reiss, G. A. and Shevach, E. M. (1982) Effect of CsA on T cell function *in vitro:* the mechanism of suppression of T cell proliferation depends on the nature of the T cell stimulus as well as the differentiation state of the responding T cell. *J. Immunol.,* **129**, 2360

43. Kaufmann, Y., Chang, A. E., Robb, R. T. and Rosenberg, S. A. (1984) Mechanism of action of CsA: inhibition of lymphokine secretion studied with antigen-stimulated T cell hybridomas. *J. Immunol.,* **133**, 3107

44. Pawelec, G. and Wernet, P. (1983) CsA inhibits IL-2-dependent growth of alloactivated cloned human T cells. *Int. J. Immunopharmacol.,* **5**, 315

45. Ferrini, S., Moretta, A., Biassoni, R., Nicolin, A. and Moetta, I. (1986) CsA inhibits IL-2 production by all human T cell clones having this function, independent of the T4/T8 phenotype or the co-expression of cytolytic activity. *Clin. Immunol. Immunopathol.,* **38**, 79

46. Weiss, J., Schwinzer, B., Kirchner, H., Gemsa, D. and Resch, K. (1986) Effects of CsA on functions of specific murine T_H cell clones: inhibition of proliferation, lymphokine secretion and cytotoxicity. *Immunobiology,* **171**, 234

47. Heeg, K., Deusch, K., Solbach, W., Bunjes, D. and Wagner, H. (1984) Frequency analysis of cyclosporin-sensitive cytotoxic T lymphocyte precursors. *Transplantation,* **38**, 532

48. Elliot, J. F., Lin, Y., Mizel, S. B., Bleackley, R. C., Harnish, D. G. and Paetkau, V. (1984) Induction of IL-2 mRNA inhibited by CsA. *Science,* **226**, 1439

49. Reed, J. C., Prystowsky, M. B. and Nowell, P. C. (1988) Regulation of gene expression in lectin-stimulated or lymphokine-stimulated T lymphocytes. *Transplantation,* **46** (Suppl.), 75S

50. Orosz, C. G., Roopenian, D. C., Widmer, M. B. and Back, F. H. (1983) Analysis of cloned T cell function. II. Differential blockade of various cloned T cell functions by cyclosporin. *Transplantation,* **36**, 706

51. Palacios, R. (1985) CsA inhibits antigen and lectin-induced but not constitutive production of IL-3. *Eur. J. Immunol.,* **15**, 204

52. Bickel, M., Tsuda, H., Amstad, P. *et al.* (1987) Differential regulation of colony-stimulating factors and interleukin 2 production by cyclosporin A. *Proc. Natl. Acad. Sci. USA,* **84**, 3276

53. Shaw, J., Meerovitch, K., Elliot, J. F., Bleackley, R. C. and Paetkau, V. (1987) Induction, suppression and superinduction of lymphokine mRNA in T lymphocytes. *Mol. Immunol.,* **24**, 409

54. Sideras, P., Funa, K., Zalcberg-Quintana, I., Xanthopoulos, K. G., Kisielow, P. and Palacios, R. (1988) Analysis by *in situ* hybridization of cells expressing mRNA for IL-4 in the developing thymus and in peripheral lymphocytes from mice. *Proc. Natl. Acad. Sci. USA,* **85**, 218

55. Hu-Li, J., Shevach, E., Mizuguchi, J., Ohara, J., Mosmann, T. and Paul, W. (1987) B cell stimulatory factor 1 (interleukin 4) is a potent costimulant for normal resting T lymphocytes. *J. Exp. Med.,* **165**, 157

56. Gernandez-Botran, R., Krammer, P., Diamantstein, T., Uht, J. and Vitetta, E. (1986) B cell-stimulatory factor 1 (BSF-1) promotes growth of helper T cell lines. *J. Exp. Med.,* **164**, 580

57. Mathie, I. H., Sewell, H. F. and Thomson, A. W. (1987) Generation of large granular lymphocytes and subset changes linked with cyclophosphamide-induced eosinophilia in rats and the effects of ciclosporin. *Scand. J. Immunol.,* **26**, 417

58. Kalman, V. K. and Klimpel, G. R. (1983) CsA inhibits the production of gamma interferon (INFγ) but does not inhibit production of virus-induced IFNα/β. *Cell Immunol.,* **78**, 122

59. Palacios, R., Martinez-Maza, O. and DeLey, M. (1983) Production of human gamma IFN studied at the single cell level: origin, evidence for spontaneous secretion and effects of CsA. *Eur. J. Immunol.,* **13**, 221

60. Reem, G. H., Cook, L. A. and Vilcek, J. (1983) Gamma IFN synthesis by human thymocytes and T lymphocytes inhibited by CsA. *Science,* **221**, 63

61. Herold, K. C., Lancki, D. W., Moldwin, R. L. and Fitch, F. W. (1986) Immunosuppressive effects of CsA on cloned T cells. *J. Immunol.,* **136**, 1315

62. Liversidge, J., Sewell, H. F., Thomson, A. W. and Forrester, J. V. (1988) Lymphokine induced expression of MHC class II antigen expression on cultured retinal pigment epithelial cells and the influence of cyclosporin A. *Immunology,* **63**, 313

63. Halloran, P. F., Urmson, J., Farkas, S., Phillips, R. A., Fulop, G., Cockfield, S. and Autenried, P. (1988) Effects of cyclosporine on systemic MHC expression. Evidence that non-T cells produce interferon-gamma *in vivo* and are inhibitable by cyclosporine. *Transplantation,* **46** (Suppl.), 68S

64. Espevik, T., Figari, I. S., Shalaby, M. F., Lackides, G. A., Lewis, G. D., Shepard, H. M. and Palladino, M. A. (1987) Inhibition of cytokine production by cyclosporin A and transforming growth factor β. *J. Exp. Med.,* **166**, 571

65. Scheurich, P., Kronke, M., Schluter, C., Ucer, U. and Pfizenmaier, K. (1986) Noncytocidal mechanisms of action of tumour necrosis factor-α on human tumour cells: enhancement of HLA gene expression synergistic with interferon-γ. *Immunobiology,* **172**, 291

66. Thomson, A. W., Moon, D. K., Geczy, C. L. and Nelson, D. S. (1983) CsA inhibits lymphokine production but not the response of macrophages to lymphokines. *Immunology,* **48**, 291

67. Thomson, A. W., Moon, D. K. and Nelson, D. S. (1983) Suppression of delayed type hypersensitivity reactions and lymphokine production by CsA in the mouse. *Clin. Exp. Immunol.,* **52**, 599

68. Helin, H. and Edgington, T. S. (1984) CsA regulates monocyte/macrophage effector functions by affecting instructor T cells: inhibition of monocyte procoagulant response to allogeneic stimulation. *J. Immunol.,* **132**, 1074

69. Larson, E-L. (1980) CsA and dexamethasone suppresses T cell responses by selectively acting at distinct sites of the triggering process. *J. Immunol.,* **124**, 2828

70. Miyawaki, T., Yachie, A., Ohzeki, S., Nagaoki, T. and Taniguchi, N. (1983) CsA does not prevent expression of Tac antigen, a probable T cell growth factor receptor molecule on mitogen-stimulated human T cells. *J. Immunol.,* **130**, 2737

71. Kronke, M., Leonard, W. J., Depper, J. M., Arya, S. K., Wong-Stall, F., Gallo, R. C., Waldmann, T. A. and Greene, W. C. (1984) CsA inhibits T cell growth factor gene expression at the level of mRNA transcription. *Proc. Natl. Acad. Sci. USA,* **81**, 5124

72. Bloemena, E., van Oers, M. H. J., Weinreich, S., Yong, S-L. and Schellekens, P. T. A. (1988) Cyclosporine A does not prevent expression of biologically active IL-2 receptors *in vitro. Transplant. Proc.,* **20**(2), Suppl. 2, 131

73. Aiello, F. B., Maggiano, N., Larocca, L. M., Piantelli, M. and Musiani, P. (1986). Inhibitory effect of CsA on the OKT3-induced PBL proliferation. *Cell Immunol.,* **97**, 131

74. Gauchat, J.-F., Khandjian, E. W., Nabholz, M. and Weil, R. (1986) Cyclosporin A 'seems' to exert its immunosuppressive action primarily by preventing the activation of a set(s)

of T lymphocyte-specific genes. *Proc. Natl. Acad. Sci. USA*, **83**, 6430

75. Reed, J. C., Abidi, A. H., Alpers, J. D., Hoover, R. G., Robb, R. J. and Nowell, P. C. (1986) Effect of cyclosporin A and dexamethasone on interleukin-2 receptor gene expression. *J. Immunol.*, **137**, 150

76. Smith, K. A. and Cantrell, D. A. (1985). Interleukin-2 regulates its own receptors. *Proc. Natl. Acad. Sci. USA*, **82**, 864

77. Harel-Bellan, A., Bertoglio, J., Quillet, A., Marchiol, C., Wakasugi, H., Mishall, Z. and Fradelizi, D. (1986) Interleukin 2 (IL-2) up-regulates its own receptor on a subset of human unprimed peripheral blood lymphocytes and triggers their proliferation. *J. Immunol.*, **136**, 2463

78. Kondo, S., Shimizu, A., Saito, Y., Kinoshita, M. and Honjo, T. (1986) Molecular basis for two different affinity states of the interleukin 2 receptor: affinity conversion model. *Proc. Natl. Acad. Sci. USA*, **83**, 9026

79. White, D. J. G., Plumb, A. M., Pawelec, G. and Brons, G. (1979) Cyclosporin A: an immunosuppressive agent preferentially active against proliferating T cells. *Transplantation*, **27**, 55

80. McIntosh, L. C. and Thomson, A. W. (1980) Activity of mononuclear phagocytes in CsA-treated mice. *Transplantation*, **30**, 384

81. Alberti, S., Boeraschi, D., Luini, W. and Tagliabue, A. (1981) Effects of *in vivo* treatments with CsA on mouse cell-mediated immune responses. *Int. J. Immunopharmacol.*, **3**, 357

82. Manca, F., Kunkl, A. and Celada, F. (1985) Inhibition of the accessory function of murine macrophages *in vitro* by cyclosporine. *Transplantation*, **39**, 644

83. Paley, D. A., Cluff, C. W., Wentworth, P. A. and Ziegler, H. K. (1986) CsA inhibits macrophage-mediated antigen presentation. *J. Immunol.*, **136**, 4348

84. Varey, A., Champion, B. R. and Cooke, A. (1986) Cyclosporine affects the function of APC. *Immunology*, **57**, 111

85. Esa, A. H., Converse, P. J. and Hess, A. D. (1987) Cyclosporine inhibits soluble antigen and alloantigen presentation by human monocytes *in vitro*. *Int. J. Immunopharmacol.*, **9**, 893

86. Snyder, D. S., Wright, C. L. and Ting, C. (1987) Inhibition of human monocyte antigen presentation, but not HLA-DR expression, by cyclosporine. *Transplantation*, **44**, 407

87. Manca, F., Fenoglio, D., Kunkl, A., Caltabellotta, M. and Celada, F. (1988) Effect of cyclosporine on the antigen-presenting function of human and murine accessory cells. *Transplantation*, **46** (Suppl.), 40S

88. Whisler, R. L., Lindsey, J. A., Proctor, K. V. W., Newhouse, Y. G. and Cornwell, D. G. (1985) The impaired ability of human monocytes to stimulate autologous and allogeneic MLC after exposure to cyclosporine. *Transplantation*, **40**, 57

89. Uyemura, K., Dixon, J. F. P. and Parker, J. W. (1983) Inhibitory effect of cyclosporine on adherent cells in oxidation-induced lymphocyte proliferation. *Transplant. Proc.*, **15**, 2376

90. Uyemura, K., Dixon, J. F. P. and Parker, J. W. (1985) Cyclosporine inhibits macrophage accessory cell function in mitogen-induced lymphocyte proliferation. *Transplant. Proc.*, **17**, 1374

91. Esa, A. H., Paxman, D. G., Noga, S. J. and Hess, A. D. (1988) Sensitivity of monocyte subpopulations to cyclosporine arachidonate metabolism and *in vitro* antigen presentation. *Transplant. Soc.*, **20** (Suppl. 2), 80

92. Knight, S. C., Balfour, B. M., O'Brien, J. and Buttifant, L. (1987) Sensitivity of veiled (dendritic) cells to cyclosporine. *Transplantation*, **41**, 96

93. Knight, S. C. and Bedford, P. A. (1987) Effect of cyclosporine and retinoic acid on dendritic cell function. *Transplant Proc.*, **19**, 320

94. Furue, M. and Katz, S. I. (1988) Cyclosporine A inhibits accessory cell and antigen-presenting cell functions of epidermal Langerhans cells. *Transplant. Proc.*, **20** (Suppl. 2), 87

95. Muller, S., Adorini, L., Appella, E. and Nagy, Z. A. (1988) Lack of influence of cyclosporine on antigen presentation to lysozyme-specific T cell hybridomas. *Transplantation*, **46** (Suppl.), 44S

96. Cox, J. H. and Chisholm, P. M. (1987) Mechanism of action of cyclosporin in preventing cardiac allograft rejection. I. Rate of entry of lymphocytes from the blood, fibrin deposition and expression of Ia antigens on infiltrating cells. *Transplantation*, **43**, 338

97. Halloran, P. F., Wadgymar, A. and Autenried, P. (1986) Inhibition of MHC product

induction may contribute to the immunosuppressive action of ciclosporin. *Progr. Allergy,* **38**, 258

98. Groenewegen, W. A., Buurman, W. A. and Jeunhomme, G. M. A. A. (1985) Class II expression of endothelial cells is affected by cyclosporine. *Transplant Proc.,* **17**, 1417

99. Groenewegen, G., Buurman, W. A., Jeunhomme, G. M. A. A. and Linden, G. J. van der (1985) Effect of cyclosporin on MHC class II antigen expression on arterial and venous endothelium *in vitro. Transplantation,* **40**, 21

100. Orosz, C. G., Adams, P. W. and Ferguson, R. M. (1988) Frequency of human alloantigen-reactive T lymphocytes. III. Evidence that cyclosporine has an inhibitory effect on human CTL and CTL precursors, independent of CsA-mediated helper T cell dysfunction. *Transplantation,* **46** (Suppl.), 73S

101. Shevach, E. M. (1985) The effects of CsA on the immune system. *Ann. Rev. Immunol.,* **3**, 397

102. Hess, A. D. and Colombani, P. M. (1986) Mechanisms of action: *in vitro* studies. *Progr. Allergy,* **38**, 198

103. Thomson, A. W., Whiting, P. H., Blair, J. T., Davidson, R. J. L. and Simpson, J. G. (1981) Pathological changes developing in the rat during a three week course of high dose cyclosporin A and their reversal following drug withdrawal. *Transplantation,* **32**, 271

104. Blair, J. T., Thomson, A. W., Whiting, P. H., Davidson, R. J. L. and Simpson, J. G. (1982) Toxicity of the immune suppressant cyclosporin A in the rat. *J. Pathol.,* **138**, 163

105. Demitris, A. J., Nalesnik, M. A., Kunz, H. W., Gill, T. J. and Shinozuka, H. (1984). Sequential analysis of the development of lymphoproliferative disorders in rats receiving cyclosporine. *Transplantation,* **38**, 239

106. Beschorner, W. E., Di Gennaro, K. A., Hess, A. D. and Santos, G. W. (1987) Cyclosporine and the thymus: influence of irradiation and age on thymic immunopathology and recovery. *Cell Immunol.,* **110**, 350

107. Beschorner, W. E., Namnoum, J. D. and Hess, A. D. (1987) Immunopathology of rat thymus after cyclosporin A. *Transplant. Proc.,* **19**, 1230

108. Baldwin, W. M., Hutchison, I. F., Maijer, C. J. L. M. and Tilney, N. L. (1981) Immune responses to organ allografts. III. Marked decrease in medullary thymocytes and splenic T lymphocytes after cyclosporin A treatment. *Transplantation,* **31**, 117

109. Calne, R. Y., White, D. J. G., Evans, D. B., Thiru, S., Henderson, R. G., Hamilton, D. V., Rolles, K., McMaster, R., Duffy, T. J., MacDougall, B. R. D. and Williams, R. (1981) Cyclosporin A in cadaveric organ transplantation. *Br. Med. J.,* **282**, 934

110. Hutchison, I. F., Shadur, C. A., Duarte, J. S. A., Strom, T. B. and Tilney, N. L. (1981) Cyclosporin A spares selectively lymphocytes with donor-specific suppressor characteristics. *Transplantation,* **32**, 210

111. Bordes-Aznar, J., Kupiec-Weglinski, J. W., Duarte, A. J. S. (1983) Function and migration of suppressor lymphocytes from cyclosporin-treated heterograft recipients. *Transplantation,* **35**, 185

112. Kupiec-Weglinski, J. W., Lear, P. A., Bordes-Aznar, J., Tilney, N. L. and Strom, T. B. (1983) Acute rejection in cyclosporin A-treated graft recipients occurs following abrogation of suppressor cells. *Transplant. Proc.,* **15**, 531

113. Kuromoto, N., Iga, C., Fawwaz, R., Nowygrod, R., Reemstma, K. and Hardy, M. A. (1983) Effect of cyclosporin on lymphocyte migration in rat cardiac transplantation. *Transplant. Proc.,* **15**, 2973

114. Glazier, A., Tutchka, P. J., Farmer, E. R. and Santos, G. W. (1983) Graft-versus-host disease in cyclosporin A-treated rats after syngeneic and autologous bone marrow reconstitution. *J. Exp. Med.,* **158**, 1

115. Sweny, P. and Tidman, N. (1982) The effect of cyclosporin A on peripheral blood T cell subpopulations in renal allografts. *Clin. Exp. Immunol.,* **47**, 445

116. Nussenblatt, R. B., Hoak, A. H., Wacker, W. B., Palestine, A. G., Schir, I. and Gery, I. (1983) Treatment of intraocular inflammatory disease with cyclosporin A. *Lancet,* **2**, 235

117. Assan, R., Derray-Sachs, M., Laboie, C., Chatenoud, L., Feutren, G., Quiniou-Debrie, M. C., Thomas, B. and Bach, J. F. (1985) Metabolic and immunological effects of cyclosporin in recently diagnosed type 1 diabetes mellitus. *Lancet,* **1**, 67

118. Kerman, R. H., Flechner, S. M., van Buren, C. T., Lorber, M. I. and Kahan, B. D. (1987) Role of suppressor cells in cyclosporin-treated allograft recipients. *Transplant. Proc.,* **19**, 1580

119. Henny, R. L., Weening, J. L., Baldwin, W. M., Olsans, P. J., Tanke, H. J., Vanes, L. A. and Paul, L. C. (1986) Expression of HLA-DR antigens on peripheral blood T lymphocytes and renal graft tubular epithelial cells in association with rejection. *Transplantation,* **42,** 479

120. Morris, P. J., Carter, N. P., Cullen, P. R., Thompson, J. F. and Wood, R. F. M. (1982) Role of T-cell-subset monitoring in renal allograft recipients. *N. Engl. J. Med.,* **306,** 1110

121. Daniel, U., Opelz, G. and Dreihorn, K. (1985) Lymphocyte subpopulations in kidney transplant patients with different types of immunosuppression. *Transplant. Proc.,* **17,** 2554

122. Birkeland, S. A. (1985) Immunological monitoring of renal transplant patients treated with prednisolone/azathioprine or cyclosporine A. *Transplant. Proc.,* **17,** 2543

123. Van der Heyden, A. A. P. A. M., van Oers, M. H. J., Cornelissen, P., Yong, S-L., Wilmink, J. M. and Schellekens, P. T. A. (1988) The influence of cyclosporin A treatment on immune responsiveness *in vitro* and *in vivo* in kidney transplant recipients. *Transplant. Proc.,* **20** (Suppl. 2), 190

124. DuPont, E., Huygen, K., Schandene, L., Vandercruys, M., Palfliet, K. and Wybran, J. (1985) Influence of *in vivo* immunosuppressive drugs on production of lymphokines. *Transplantation,* **39,** 143

125. Yoshimura, N., Oka, T., Ohmori, Y., Aikawa, I., Fukuda, M. and Kahan, B. D. (1987) Influence of *in vivo* cyclosporin on interleukin production in kidney transplant recipients. *Transplant. Proc.,* **19,** 1193

126. Abbud-filho, M. (1984) Unpublished data; cited by Kupiec-Weglinski, J. W. *et al.*[180]. *Transplantation,* **133,** 2582

127. Flechner, S. M., Kerman, R. H., Van Buren, G. T., Epps, L. and Kahan, B. D. (1984) The use of cyclosporine in living-related renal transplantation. Donor specific hyporesponsiveness and steroid withdrawal. *Transplantation,* **38,** 685

128. Keown, P. A., Essery-Rice, G., Hellstrom, A., Sinclair, N. R. and Stiller, C. R. (1985) Inhibition of human *in vivo* cytotoxic T lymphocyte generation by cyclosporine following organ transplantation. *Transplantation,* **40,** 45

129. Kerman, R. H. (1988) Effects of cyclosporine immunosuppression in humans. *Transplant. Proc.,* **20** (Suppl. 2), 143

130. Borel, J. F., Feurer, C., Magnee, C. and Stahelin, H. (1977) Effects of the new antilymphocytic peptide CsA in animals. *Immunology,* **32,** 1017

131. Thomson, A. W. and Aldridge, R. D. (1984) Absence of dependence on cyclophosphamide-sensitive suppressor cells in suppression of cell-mediated immunity by CsA in the guinea pig. *Transplantation,* **38,** 76

133. Dunn, C. J. and Miller, S. K. (1986) The effects of CsA on leukocyte infilration and procoagulant activity in the mouse DTH response *in vivo. Int. J. Immunopharmacol.,* **8,** 635

134. Shidani, B., Milon, G., Marchal, G. and Truffa-Bachi, P. (1984) CsA inhibits the DTH reaction: impaired production of early pro-inflammatory mediators. *Eur. J. Immunol.,* **14,** 314

135. Mottram, P. L., Mirisklavos, A., Dumble, L. J. and Clunie, G. J. A. (1986) Effects of CsA, antilymphocyte serum, and donor-specific transfusions on murine DTH and skin graft survival. *Int. Arch. Allergy Appl. Immunol.,* **79,** 296

136. Xue, B., Dersarkissian, R. M., Baer, R. L., Thorbecke, G. J. and Belsito, D. V. (1986) Reversal by lymphokines of the effect of cyclosporin A on contact sensitivity and antibody production in mice. *J. Immunol.,* **11,** 4128

137. Woo, J. and Thomson, A. W. (1989) Alleviation of cyclosporin-induced immune suppression by the cytokine inducer ADA-202-718. *Immunopharmacology* (In press)

138. Webster, L. M. and Thomson, A. W. (1987) Cyclosporin A prevents suppression of delayed-type hypersensitivity in mice immunized with high dose sheep erythrocytes. *Immunology,* **60,** 409

140. Webster, L. M. and Thomson, A. W. (1988) Augmentation of delayed-type hypersensitivity to high dose sheep erythrocytes by cyclosporin A in the mouse: influence of drug dosage and route of administration and analysis of spleen cell populations. *Clin. Exp. Immunol.,* **71,** 149

141. Aldridge, R. D. and Thomson, A. W. (1986) Paradoxical augmentation of tuberculin-like hypersensitivity but not Jones-Mote or contact sensitivity in CsA-treated guinea pigs. *Int. Arch. Allergy Appl. Immunol.,* **79,** 225

142. Aldridge, R. D. and Thomson, A. W. (1986) Factors influencing the enhancement of DTH to ovalbumin by CsA in the guinea pig: possible role of suppressor cells. *Int. Arch. Allergy Appl. Immunol.*, **81**, 17

143. Altmann, D. M. and Blyth, W. A. (1985) The effects of CsA on the induction, expression and regulation of the immune response to Herpes Simplex virus. *Clin. Exp. Immunol.*, **59**, 17

144. Braida, M. and Knop, J. (1986) Effect of CsA on the T effector and T suppressor cell response in contact sensitivity. *Immunology,* **59**, 503

145. Aldridge, R. D., Thomson, A. W., Rankin, R., Whiting, P. H., Cunningham, C. and Simpson, J. G. (1985) Inhibition of contact sensitivity reactions to DNFB by topical cyclosporin application in the guinea pig. *Clin. Exp. Immunol.*, **59**, 23

146. Aldridge, R. D., Sewell, H. F., King, G. and Thomson, A. W. (1986) Topical cyclosporin A in nickel contact hypersensitivity: results of a preliminary clinical and immunohistochemical investigation. *Clin. Exp. Immunol.*, **66**, 582

147. Payne, S. N. L. and Thomson, A. W. (1989) Immunohistochemical analysis of contact sensitivity reactions in the guinea pig using novel monoclonal antibodies: the influence of topical cyclosporin A. *Clin. Exp. Immunol.* (In press)

148. Knight, S. C., Roberts, M., Macatonia, S. E. and Edwards, A. J. (1988) Blocking of acquisition and presentation of antigen by dendritic cells with cyclosporine. Studies with fluorescein isothiocyanate. *Transplantation,* **46** (Suppl.), 48S

149. Thomson, A. W., Milton, J. I., Aldridge, R. D., Davidson, R. J. L. and Simpson, J. G. (1986) Inhibition of drug-induced eosinophilia by cyclosporin A. *Scand. J. Immunol.*, **24**, 163

150. Cummins, A. G., Munro, G. H. and Ferguson, A. (1988) Effect of cyclosporin A on rat mucosal mast cells and the associated protease MCPII. *Clin. Exp. Immunol.*, **72**, 136

151. Klaus, G. G. B. and Chisholm, P. M. (1986) Does cyclosporine act *in vivo* as it does *in vitro*? *Immunol. Today*, **7**, 101

152. Thomson, A. W. (1987) Immunobiology of cyclosporin A, with particular reference to its effects on delayed hypersensitivity and regulatory T-cell functions. *Ann. Inst. Pasteur/Immunol.*, **138**, 639

153. Morris, P. J. (1981) Cyclosporin A. *Transplantation,* **32**, 349

154. Land, W., Castro, L. A., White, D. J. G., Hillebrand, G., Hammer, C., Klare, B. and Fornara, P. (1986) Ciclosporin in renal transplantation. *Progr. Allergy,* **38**, 293

155. Kaibara, N., Hotokebuchi, T., Takagishi, K. and Katsuki, I. (1983) Paradoxical effects of cyclosporin A on collagen arthritis in rats. *J. Exp. Med.,* **158**, 2007

156. Sorokin, R., Kimura, H., Schroder, K., Wilson, D. H. and Wilson, D. B. (1986) Cyclosporin-induced autoimmunity: conditions for expressing disease, requirements for intact thymus and potency estimates of autoimmune lymphocytes in drug-treated rats. *J. Exp. Med.,* **164**, 1615

157. Chisholm, P. M., Drayson, M. T., Cox, J. H. and Ford, W. L. (1985) the effects of cyclosporin on lymphocyte activation in a systemic graft-versus-host reaction. *Eur. J. Immunol.*, **15**, 1054

158. Chisholm, P. M. and Bevan, D. J. (1988) T cell activation in the presence of cyclosporine in three *in vivo* allograft models. *Transplantation,* **46** (Suppl.), 80S

159. Kroczek, R. A., Black, C. D. V., Barbet, J. and Schevach, E. M. (1987) Mechanism of action of cyclosporin A *in vivo*. I. Cyclosporin A fails to inhibit T lymphocyte activation in response to alloantigens. *J. Immunol.*, **139**, 3597

160. Milon, G., Truffa-Bachi, P., Shidani, B. and Marchal, G. (1984) CsA inhibits the DTH effector function of T lymphocytes without affecting their clonal expansion. *Ann. Inst. Pasteur, Immunol.*, **135D**, 237

161. Schiltknecht, E. and Ada, G. L. (1985) The generation of effector T cells in influenza-infected, cyclosporin A-treated mice. *Cell Immunol.*, **95**, 340

162. Severinson, E., Naito, T., Tokumoto, H., Fukushima, D., Hirano, A., Hama, K. and Honjo, T. (1987) Interleukin 4 (IgG1 induction factor): a multifunctional lymphokine acting also on T cells. *Eur. J. Immunol.*, **17**, 67

163. Widmer, M. M. and Grabstein, K. H. (1987) Regulation of cytolytic T-lymphocyte generation by B-cell stimulatory factor. *Nature*, **326**, 795

164. Heeg, K., Gillis, S. and Wagner, H. (1988) IL-4 bypasses the immune suppressive effect of cyclosporin A during the *in vitro* induction of murine cytotoxic T lymphocytes. *J. Immunol.*, **141**, 2330

165. Freed, B. M., Stevens, C., Zhang, G., Rosano, T. F. and Lempert, N. (1988) A comparison of the effects of cyclosporine and steroids on human T lymphocyte responses. *Transplant. Proc.*, **20** (Suppl. 2), 233
166. Hess, A. D., Horwitz, L., Beschorner, W. E. and Santos, G. W. (1985) Development of graft-vs-host disease-like syndrome in cyclosporine-treated rats after syngeneic bone marrow transplantation. *J. Exp. Med.*, **161**, 718
167. Lafferty, K. J., Gill, R. and Babcock, S. (1986) Tolerance induction in adult animals. The cicloporin anomaly. *Progr. Allergy*, **38**, 247
168. Beschorner, W. E., Shinn, C. A., Fischer, A. C., Santos, G. W. and Hess, A. D. (1988) Cyclosporine-induced pseudo-graft-versus-host disease in the early post cyclosporine period. *Transplantation*, **46** (Suppl.), 112S
169. Ryffel, B., Deyssenroth, H. and Borel, J. F. (1981) Cyclosporin A: effects on the mouse thymus. *Agents Actions*, **11**, 373
170. Xi-En, G. U. I., Rinaldo, C. R. and Monto, H. O. (1983) NK cell activity in renal transplant recipients receiving cyclosporin. *Infect. Immun.*, **41**, 965
171. Versluis, D. J., Metselaar, H. J., Bijma, A. M., Vaessen, L. M. B., Wenting, G. J. and Weimar, W. (1988) The effect of long-term cyclosporine therapy on natural killer cell activity. *Transplant. Proc.*, **20** (Suppl. 2), 179
172. Shao-Hsien, C., Lang, I., Gunn, H. and Lydyard, P. (1983) Effect of *in vitro* CsA treatment on human natural and antibody-dependent cell-mediated cytotoxicity. *Transplantation*, **35**, 127
173. Introna, M., Allavena, P., Spreafico, F. and Mantovani, A. (1981) Inhibition of human NK activity by CsA. *Transplantation*, **31**, 113
174. Peterson, P. K., Rynasiewicz, J. J., Simmons, R. L. *et al.* (1983) Decreased incidence of overt cytomegalovirus disease in renal allografted recipients receiving cyclosporin A. *Transplant. Proc.*, **15**, 457
175. Cauda, R., Citierio, F., Tamborrini, E., Pozzetio, U., Tumbarello, M., Castagneto, M. and Ortona, L. (1988) Natural killer activity against targets in cyclosporine-treated renal allograft recipients. *Transplant. Proc.*, **20** (Suppl. 2), 186
176. Stewart, L. S., Sewell, H. F. and Thomson, A. W. (1989) Failure of cyclosporine A to affect generation of large granular lymphocytes (OX-8$^+$, OX-19$^-$) and natural killer cell activity following systemic cyclophosphamide administration and immunization in the rat. *Transplant. Proc.* (In press).
177. Tellides, G., Dallman, M. J. and Morris, P. J. (1988) Synergistic interaction of cyclosporine A with interleukin 2 receptor monoclonal antibody therapy. *Transplant. Proc.*, **20** (Suppl. 2), 202
178. Kupiec-Weglinski, J. W., Hahn, H. J., Kirkman, R. L., Volk, H. D., Mouzaki, A., Di Stefano, R., Tellides, G., Dallman, M., Morris, P. J., Strom, T. B., Tilney, N. L. and Diamantstein, T. (1988) Cyclosporine potentiates the immunosuppressive effects of anti-interleukin 2 receptor monoclonal antibody therapy. *Transplant. Proc.*, **20** (Suppl. 2), 207
179. Hahn, H. J., Kuttler, B., Dunger, A., Klöting, I., Lucke, S., Volk, H. D., Baehr, R. V. and Diamantstein, T. (1987) Prolongation of rat pancreatic islet allograft survival by treatment of recipient rats with monoclonal anti-interleukin-2 receptor antibody and cyclosporin. *Diabetologia*, **30**, 44
180. Kupiec-Weglinski, J. W., Filho, M. A., Strom, T. B. and Tilney, N. L. (1984) Sparing of suppressor cells: a critical action of cyclosporine. *Transplantation*, **38**, 97
181. Kupiec-Weglinski, J. W., Diamantstein, T., Tilney, N. L. *et al.* (1986) Therapy with monoclonal antibody to interleukin 2 receptor spares suppressor T cells and prevents or reverses acute allograft rejection in rats. *Proc. Natl. Acad. Sci. USA*, **83**, 2624
182. Kupiec-Weglinski, J. W., Padberg, W., Uhteg, L. C., Ma, L., Lord, R. H., Araneda, D., Strom, T. B., Diamantstein, T. and Tilney, N. L. (1987) Selective immunosuppression with anti-interleukin 2 receptor-targeted therapy: helper and suppressor cell activity in rat recipients of cardiac allografts. *Eur. J. Immunol.*, **17**, 313
183. Thomson, A. W. (1989) FK-506. How much potential? *Immunol. Today*, **10**, 6
184. Zeevi, A., Duquesnoy, R., Eiras, G., Rabinwich, H., Todo, S., Makowka, L. and Starzl, T. E. (1987) Immunosuppressive effect of FK-506 on *in vitro* lymphocyte alloactivation: synergism with cyclosporine A. *Transplant. Proc.*, **19** (Suppl. 6), 40
185. Murase, N., Todo, S., Lee, P-H. *et al.* (1987) Heterotopic heart transplantation in the rat receiving FK-506 alone or with cyclosporine. *Transplant. Proc.*, **19** (Suppl. 6), 71

80

186. Stephen, M. E., Woo, J., Hasan, N. U., Whiting, P. H. and Thomson, A. W. (1989) Immunosuppressive activity, lymphocyte subset analysis and acute toxicity of FK-506 in the rat: a comparative and combination study with cyclosporine. *Transplantation*, **47**, 60
187. Storb, R., Deeg, H. J., Whitehead, J., Appelbaum, F., Beatty, P., Besinger, W., Buckner, C. D., Cl ft, R., Doney, K., Farewell, V., Hansen, J., Hill, R., Witherspoon, R., Yee, G., Thomas, ⁚. D. (1986) Methotrexate and cyclosporine compared with cyclosporine alone for prophylaxis of acute graft versus host disease after marrow transplantation for leukemia. *N. Engl. J. Med.*, **314**, 729
188. Rynasiewicz, J. J., Sutherland, D. E. R., Ferguson, R. M., Squifflet, J. A., Morrow, C. E., Goetz, F. C. and Najarian, J. S. (1988) Cyclosporin A for immunosuppression: observations in rat heart, pancreas and islet allograft models and in human renal and pancreas transplantation. *Diabetes*, **31** (Suppl. 4), 92
189. Squifflet, J. P., Sutherland, D. E. R., Rynasiewicz, J. J., Field, J., Heil, J. and Najarian, J. S. (1989) Combined immunosuppressive therapy with cyclosporin A and azathioprine. A synergistic effect in three of four experimental models. *Transplantation*, **34**, 315
190. Aeder, M. I., Lewis, W. I., Sutherland, D. E. R. *et al.* (1985) Combination immunotherapy for prolongation of renal allograft survival. *Transplant. Proc.*, **17**, 2675
191. Collier, D. St. J., Thick, M., Curtins, M. D., White, D. J. G., Calne, R. Y.,, Jamieson, N. V., Barroso, E. and Thiru, S. (1986) Alternate-day immunosuppression. *Lancet*, **1**, 267
192. Yen, C. Y., Greenstein, S. M., Lipkowitz, G. S., Hong, J. H., Nitta, K., Friedman, E. A. and Butt, K. M. H. (1987) Daily and alternate day cyclosporine immunosuppressive regimens and synergism with azathioprine. *Transplant. Proc.*, **19**, 1272
193. Brady, H. R., Peters, P. and Cardella, C. J. (1988) Synergistic effects of cyclosporine and rabbit antilymphocyte sera on suppression of the one-way allogeneic mixed lymphocyte response. *Transplant. Proc.*, **20** (Suppl. 2), 229
194. Gordon, D. and Nouri, A. M. E. (1981) Comparison of the inhibition by glucocorticosteroids and cyclosporin A of mitogen-stimulated human lymphocyte proliferation. *Clin. Exp. Immunol.*, **44**, 287
195. Freed, B. M., Stevens, C., Zhang, G., Rosano, T. G. and Lempert, N. (1988) A comparison of the effects of cyclosporine and steroids on human T lymphocyte responses. *Transplant. Proc.*, **20** (Suppl. 2), 253
197. Vogelsang, G. B., Wells, M. C., Santos, G. W., Chen, T. L. and Hess, A. D. (1988) Combination low dose thalidomide and cyclosporine prophylaxis for acute graft-versus-host disease in a rat mismatched model. *Transplant. Proc.*, **20** (Suppl. 2), 226
198. McMillen, M. A., Tesi, R. J., Baumgarten, W. B., Jaffe, B. M. and Wait, R. B. (1985) Potentiation of cyclosporine by varapamil *in vitro*. *Transplantation*, **40**, 444
199. Weir, M. R., Peppler, R., Gomolka, D. and Handwerger, B. S. (1988) Additive effect of cyclosporine and verapamil on the inhibition of activation and function of human peripheral blood mononuclear cells. *Transplant. Proc.*, **20** (Suppl. 2), 240
200. van Eendenburg, J. P., Brisson, E., Klatzmann, D. and Gluckman, J-C. (1988) Nicardipine enhances the effect of cyclosporine A on T lymphocyte activation *in vitro*. *Transplant. Proc.*, **20** (Suppl. 2), 245
201. Rosano, T. G., Freed, B. M., Cerilli, J. and Lempert, N. (1986) Immunosuppressive metabolites of cyclosporine in the blood of renal allograft recipients. *Transplantation*, **42**, 262
202. Freed, B. M., Rosano, T. G. and Lempert, N. (1987) *In vitro* immunosuppressive properties of cyclosporin metabolites. *Transplantation*, **43**, 123
203. Zeevi, A., Eiras, G., Burckart, G., Makowka, L., Venkataramanan, R., Wang, C. P., Van Thiel, D. H., Murase, N., Starzl, T. E. and Duquesnoy, R. (1988) Immunosuppressive effect of cyclosporine metabolites from human bile on alloreactive T cells. *Transplant. Proc.*, **20** (Suppl. 2), 115
204. Zeevi, A., Venkataramanan, R., Burckart, G., Wang, C. P., Nurase, N., Van Thiel, D. H., Starzl, T. E., Makowka, L. and Duquesnoy, R. J. (1988) Sensitivity of activated human lymphocytes to cyclosporine and its metabolites. *Human Immunol.*, **21**, 143

5
Cyclosporin A and tolerance induction in experimental animals

Susan M. L. Lim and David J. G. White

INTRODUCTION

Since the discovery of the immunosuppressive properties of cyclosporin A (CsA) in 1972[1], and its introduction into transplantation research in 1977[2,3], there have been numerous publications reporting the successful induction, by CsA, of 'tolerance' to a wide range of organ allografts in a broad spectrum of animal models. Heterotopic heart grafts between fully incompatible inbred strains of rats were the first organ allografts to be used as a model for tolerance induction with CsA[2]. This model has been tested and confirmed by others using different strain combinations[4-6]. Tolerance has also been reported to kidney[7], liver[8], bowel[9], and composite tissue (limb) grafts[10] in rats, kidney grafts in rabbits[11], dogs[12] and rhesus monkeys[13], and heart grafts in pigs[14]. In contrast to organ grafts, skin graft survival is dependent on the continued presence of CsA. Significant prolongations have been achieved in mice[15,16], rats[17,18], rabbits[19] and dogs[20,21]. However, skin graft rejection following withdrawal of CsA treatment is the rule.

The main variation in the requirement for CsA in the induction of tolerance to organ allografts in different species lies in the duration of the treatment schedule, which appears to be in proportion to the longevity of the species. Thus, a 14-day course of CsA has been shown to induce tolerance to accessory heart grafts in rats[22]; a 28-day couse was required for tolerance induction to kidney grafts in rabbits[23]; a 120-day course of CsA was found to be effective in inducing prolonged survival of orthotopic heart grafts in pigs[14], and a 336-alternate-day course induced tolerance to kidney grafts in dogs[12]. The successful induction of tolerance in a range of animal models has paralleled its immunosuppressive potency clinically. Since its introduction in the clinic in 1978[24], CsA has become the mainstay of immunosuppressive treatment in kidney[25-32], liver[33-38], pancreas[36], heart[37,38], and heart/lung transplantation[37].

A potential future role for CsA lies in the induction of allograft tolerance in man.

In this chapter a detailed account of the induction of tolerance by CsA, using a rodent heart allograft model, is provided. In particular the kinetics of induction, underlying mechanisms, requirements for maintenance, and the influence of concomitant treatments such as steroids and splenectomy is discussed in the context of current information on tolerance induction by CsA.

The criteria adopted here for the definition of tolerance includes specific, systemic, non-responsiveness to donor strain antigens as demonstrated by the ability of the animal in question to retain a skin graft of donor origin for more than 50 days. Tolerant rats bearing heart grafts always showed the ability to protect from rejection, donor-specific skin grafts but not third-party test skins. In practice, prolongation of donor-specific skins for more than 50 days was achieved in a majority, but never 100%, of tolerant animals. The cause of this is unclear, but probably reflects the biological variation to be expected in any such experiment, despite the genetic homogeneity involved.

CsA SCHEDULES IN TOLERANCE INDUCTION

It is known that a short course of CsA administered for either 1 week[39] or 2 weeks[17], at 15 mg kg^{-1} day^{-1} induces tolerance to heart allografts in rats. In order to identify a baseline requirement for CsA in the tolerizing process, these short-duration treatments were studied, along with serial measurements of CsA blood levels. DA hearts were grafted into PVG recipient rats. CsA, dissolved in olive oil at 25 mg/ml, was administered intramuscularly at a dose of 15 mg kg^{-1} day^{-1}, from day 0, for 1 week (group 1), and 2 weeks (group 2). Animals with heart grafts surviving beyond 100 days were classified as long-term survivors (LTS). LTS were tested for systemic tolerance, by grafting at day 100+, donor-specific, and third-party (WAG) skins. Blood samples were collected at weekly intervals for 7 weeks in group 1, and 10 weeks in group 2. CsA levels were measured by radioimmunoassay, using the ^{125}I immunonuclear kit.

We confirmed that short-term CsA treatment induced tolerance to heart grafts in the rat strains studied. A 2-week regime at 15 mg kg^{-1} day^{-1} produced indefinite heart graft survival in 69% of animals, and was twice as effective as a 1-week regime, which produced LTS in 35% of animals ($p < 0.02$) (see Table 5.1).

Table 5.1 Heart allograft survival with 1 week (group 1) and 2 weeks (group 2) of CsA treatment (Rx)

Group	Heart graft survival (days)	Median survival (days)
No Rx controls	7, 7, 7, 7, 7, 7, 8, 8, 8, 10	7.0
1	29, 32, 32, 33, 37, 40 42, 47, 56, 56, 84, 100 (× 6)	56.0
2	39, 46, 57, 58, 83, > 100 (× 11)	> 100.0

Specific tolerance was confirmed by the acceptance of donor-specific skin grafts for more than 50 days in 14 out of a total of 17 cases (six LTS in group 1, 11 LTS in group 2 (see Table 5.2). Two animals from group 1, and one animal from group 2, rejected their donor-specific skins on days 27 and 31, ..nd day 23 respectively; however, heart grafts continued to function indefinitely. Third-party skins were always rejected in these long-term survivors (MST 8.8 days).

With both treatment schedules, heart grafts rejected during a short, relatively well-defined 'risk period' of between 30 and 60 days for the 1-week group, and 40–60 days in the 2-week group (Figure 5.1). We found that the 'risk period' was entered when CsA levels fell below a threshold value of 200–300 ng/ml, in both treatment groups (Table 5.3). The increased incidence of graft rejection in group 1 could be attributed to the extra 10 days of 'risk' (as defined by loss of immunosuppressive levels of CsA) to which these animals were exposed (Table 5.3). Beyond 60 days, despite low to negligible levels of CsA in the blood, rejection episodes were rare, and the vast majority of grafts that survived beyond 60 days were accepted

Table 5.2 Survival of donor-specific (DS) and third-party (TP) skin grafts in CsA long-term survivors

Group	DS skin survival (days)	TP skin survival (days)
1 $n = 6$	26, 30, >50 (× 4)	8, 8, 9, 9, 9, 10
2 $n = 11$	22, >50 (× 10)	8, 8, 8, 8, 9, 9, 9, 9, 9, 9, 10

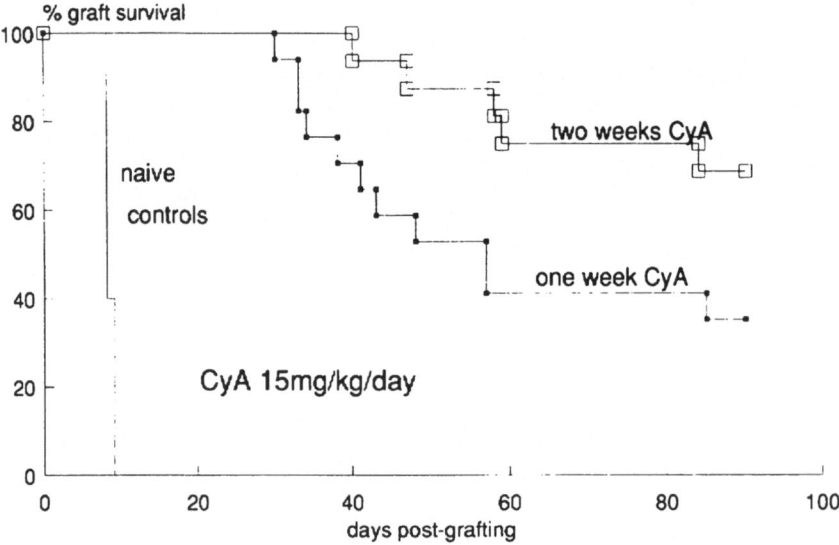

Figure 5.1 Survival of DA heart allografts in PVG recipients treated with 15 mg/kg of CsA for 1 week $n = 17$) and 2 weeks $n = 16$), compared with untreated allografts

84

Table 5.3 Mean CsA whole-blood levels (ng/ml) at weekly intervals in groups 1 (7 days CsA) and 2 (14 days CsA)

Group	CsA whole-blood levels (ng/ml), weeks 1–10									
	1	2	3	4	5	6	7	8	9	10
1	4574	1674	398	241	94	69	39	—	—	—
2	3655	5429	2410	772	329	271	196	218	185	164

indefinitely, indicating that the presence of CsA was no longer required after this time. Animals losing grafts did not have CsA levels that were significantly lower than those who retained their grafts, and the levels persisted for just as long as in tolerant rats.

The high CsA blood levels achieved in these rats (Table 5.3) may have been due to the cumulative effects of daily dosage. CsA was detected in the blood for much longer than anticipated; with 2 weeks of treatment CsA levels remained detectable for up to 10 weeks. The intramuscular administration of CsA may have been contributory, since this route results in a greater bioavailability of the drug compared with oral administration[40]. The observation of the persistence of CsA levels despite a cessation of therapy suggests that a lower total drug dose as obtained with alternate-day(s) regimes might have been used. Friedman *et al.*[41] reported that a 10 mg/kg alternate-day, intraperitoneal dose of CsA in rabbit produced a mean survival of 12.3 days for skin allografts, which was comparable to the results obtained in the same model, using a daily dose of 10 mg/kg (MST 14.8 days). An alternate-day regime of CsA and azathioprine has recently been shown to induce tolerance to renal allografts in mongrel dogs[12]. It would appear that a lower daily dose (< 15 mg/kg), or a spacing-out of treatment days, might avoid the high CsA levels seen in this study, whilst still maintaining immunosuppressive levels (> 200–300 ng/ml) throughout the tolerizing process.

The conclusion drawn from these data is that the induction of tolerance to heart grafts in the strains studied occurs during the 60 days following grafting, and is dependent on the presence of at least 200–300 ng/ml of CsA in the blood during this time. The question of whether this risk period can be overcome entirely by prolonging CsA cover (> 200–300 ng/ml of whole blood) to day 60, or whether this just further postpones it, was investigated. Based on the data obtained from CsA blood levels, a new intermittent 17-day CsA schedule was formulated. This schedule included 1 week of CsA treatment, followed by 2 weeks rest, then another week of treatment followed again by 2 weeks rest, and finally a 3-day mini-boost. CsA was administered on days 0–6, 21–27, and 42–4. During days 7–20, 28–41, and after day 44, no immunosuppression was given. In this way the total number of treatment days was kept to a minimum, whilst immunosuppressive levels of CsA were maintained (see Figure 5.2). The issue of whether the treatment schedule could be reduced further by a delay in the start of CsA administration has not been addressed. However, Homan and colleagues[7], using a rat kidney allograft model, have shown that the immunosuppressive effect of CsA is lost if treatment is delayed until day 4 post-grafting.

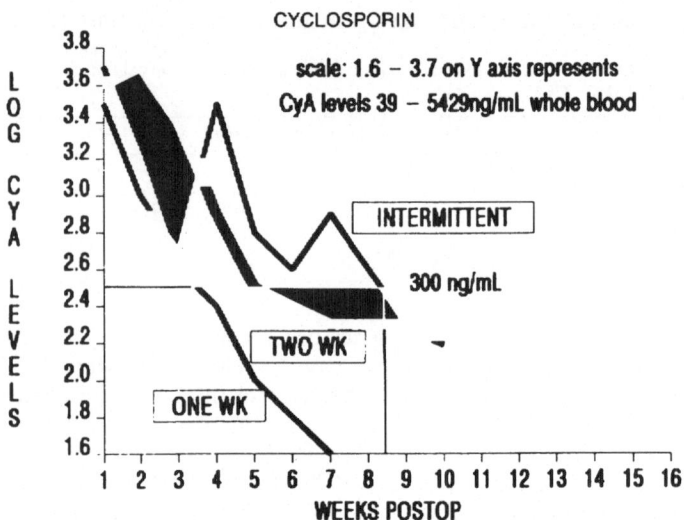

Figure 5.2 Log plot of mean, serial CsA whole-blood levels in groups of recipient PVG rats receiving 1 week, 2 weeks and 17 days (intermittent schedule) of CsA at 15 mg kg^{-1} day^{-1}. Horizontal line marks log 2.5 y axis) which is equivalent to 300 ng/ml; vertical line marks 60 days x axis) which represents the end of the 'risk period'

Using the 17-day intermittent CsA schedule, all heart grafts survived beyond 100 days. This represented a significant improvement in comparison with the 69% LTS achieved with 2 weeks of CsA ($p < 0.005$), and 35% LTS achieved using 1 week of CsA ($p < 0.001$) (see Figure 5.3). These long-term survivors were shown to be systemically tolerant, by the acceptance of donor-specific skin grafts in 17 out of 20 cases. Some (but not all) long-surviving heart graft were noted to atrophy with time (total observation period 24 months). Histological examination, however, revealed relatively good preservation of architecture with minimal evidence of ongoing rejection in several of these long-term (> 100 days) heart grafts (see Figure 5.4).

The experiments confirmed that in the DA to PVG strain combination the tolerizing process for heart grafts is not well established until day 60. After this time immunosuppressive levels of CsA are no longer necessary. Similar observations have also been made by others, though not based on CsA blood measurements. Nagao and colleagues[42], using the same rat strains, showed that the phase of specific unresponsiveness induced by CsA was not manifest until more than 50 days after cessation of 2 weeks of CsA treatment. Both Kupiec-Weglinski and colleagues[43], and Hall[6], using different strain combinations, also found that a specific and stable state of unresponsiveness induced by CsA developed only after 50 days following grafting.

THE INFLUENCE OF THE MAJOR HISTOCOMPATIBILITY COMPLEX (MHC) ON THE INDUCTION OF TOLERANCE BY CsA

To determine the influence of MHC components on tolerance induction by CsA, the PVG congenic series of rats was used[44]. Skins and hearts were grafted across the following mismatches with and without CsA therapy:

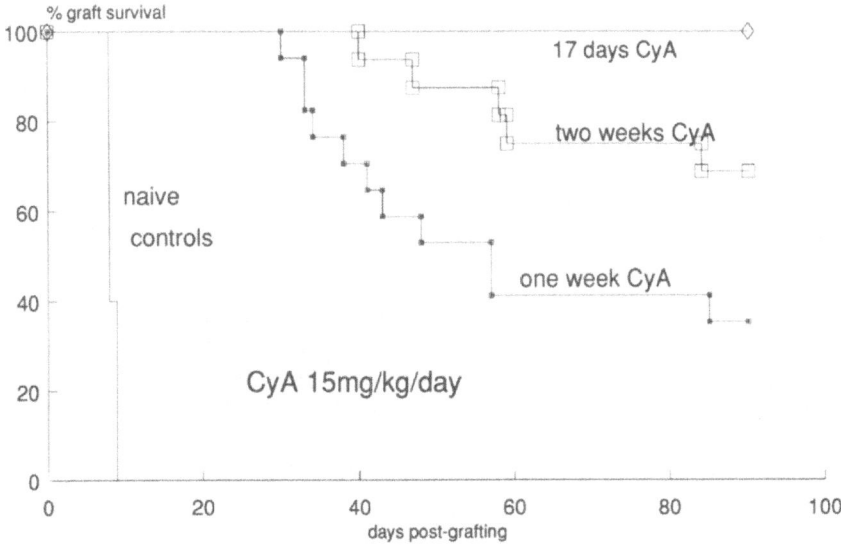

Figure 5.3 Survival of DA heart allografts in PG recipients treated with 15 mg kg^{-1} day^{-1} of CsA for 17 days $n = 20$), according to the intermittent schedule, compared with the groups receiving 1-week $n = 17$) and 2-week $n = 16$) treatment schedules

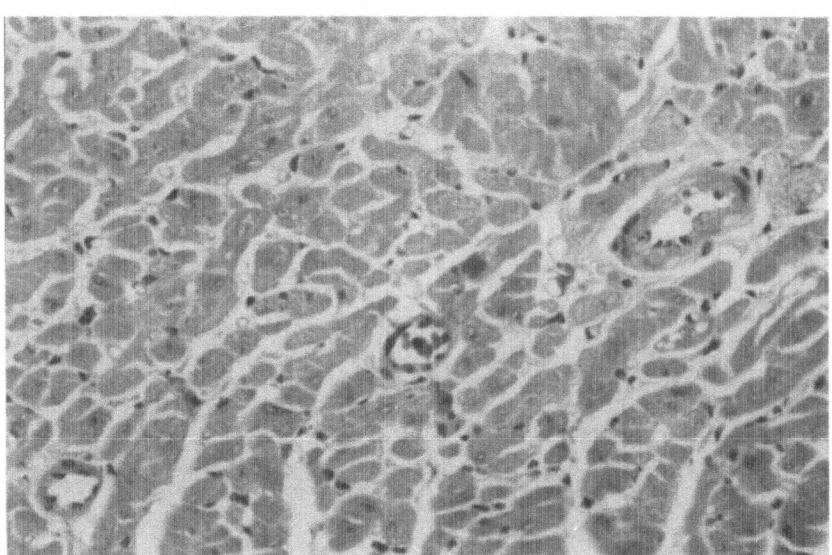

Figure 5.4 Histological section of a DA(RT1a) heart after 100 days in a CsA-treated PVG(RT1c) recipient. At the time of removal the heart was rhythmically contracting. Most areas were essentially unremarkable, with intact myocardial fibres (seen here in cross-section), normal vessels, no increase in interstitial fibrosis and no cellular infiltration (HE x 400)

87

major (classes I and II) only, class I only and class II only. The donor/recipient strain combinations used to achieve these mismatches are shown in Table 5.4.

In the absence of CsA treatment, skin grafts were rejected in the major mismatch (median survival 8.5 days), class I mismatch (median survival 12.0 days), and class II mismatch groups (median survival 9.0 days) (see Table 5.5). With 17 days of CsA, skin graft survival was significantly prolonged in the major (median survival 55.5 days), class I (median survival 100.0 days) and class II (median survival 62.5 days) mismatch groups. Whilst in the major mismatch and class II mismatch groups, LTS were achieved only sporadically (Table 5.5), in the class I mismatch group, tolerance to skins was achieved in 80% or 12/15 cases, as confirmed by the acceptance of donor-specific test skins (second skin grafts) for more than 50 days (Table 5.6). This is one of the very few examples known of tolerance being induced in adult animals by skin grafts.

Hearts grafted to include a class II incompatibility (major mismatch or class II mismatch alone), underwent acute rejection in the absence of CsA treatment (Table 5.7). In contrast, when hearts were grafted across a class II incompatibility, LTS were consistently achieved. This is consistent with

Table 5.4 Donor/recipient strain combinations used in this study

Group	Donor	Recipient	Area of mismatch
1	PVG-RT1a(a/a)	PVG(c/c)	Major (class I and II)
2	PVG.R1(a/c)	PVG(c/c)	Class I only
3	PVG-RT1a(a/a)	PVG.R1(a/c)	Class II only

Table 5.5 The influence of MHC and non-MHC components on the induction of tolerance to skin grafts

Mismatch	Skin graft survival CsA group (days)	Median survival of skins (days)	
		CsA group	Control group
Major (I and II) ($n = 10$)	33, 40, 40, 43, 55, 56, 64, 66, 69, 100	55.5	8.5
Class I ($n = 15$)	30, 45, 79, > 100 (x12)	100.0	12.0
Class II ($n = 10$)	44, 45, 49, 55, 59, 66, 68, 77, 79, 100	62.5	9.0

Table 5.6 Donor-specific (DS) and third-party (TP) test skin graft survival on CsA-treated rats tolerant of class I mismatched skin grafts

Group	DS skin survival (days)	TP skin survival (days)
Class I tolerant skins ($n = 12$)	> 50 (x12)	8, 8, 9, 9, 9, 9, 10, 10, 10, 10, 11, 11

Table 5.7 The influence of MHC and non-MHC components on the induction of tolerance to heart grafts

Mismatch	CsA group MST (days)	Control group MST (days)
Major	> 100 (n = 10)	6.3 (n = 10)
Class I	> 100 (n = 10)	100.0 (n = 10)
Class II only	> 100 (n = 10)	13.9 (n = 10)

reports of others that class I antigens represent weak transplantation barriers in rats[45–48]. With CsA treatment, heart graft survival was prolonged beyond 100 days (Table 5.7), and tolerance confirmed in all three groups (major, class I and class II mismatched groups) (Table 5.8). This represented a significant improvement in graft survival over controls, with the exception of the class I mismatched group where 100-day graft survivals were achieved both with and without CsA (Table 5.7).

We had earlier shown that with skin grafts it was difficult to induce tolerance across a class II incompatibility. A combination of both tissue-specific antigens, demonstrated by Lance and colleagues[49] in mice, and grafting methods (vascularized versus non-vascularized) described by Warren et al.[50], may account for the observed differences in survival of skin and heart grafts. The observation that different tissues and organs are not necessarily at equal risk when transplanted across the same histocompatibility barrier into normal hosts has previously been established[51–56].

AN ACTIVE REQUIREMENT FOR CsA IN TOLERANCE INDUCTION

Since the rejection of class I mismatched hearts does not occur in untreated recipients, this provided a model in which to study an active requirement for CsA in the induction of tolerance. We found that although these grafts 'reside' in non-immunosuppressed recipients for more than 100 days, such LTS were not tolerant, since they failed to retain donor-specific test skins for more than 50 days in any of the 10 cases studied (Table 5.8).

Was the failure to develop tolerance in this group due to a lack of appropriate antigenic stimulation or a lack of CsA? The answer to this question is provided by the observation that this same group (class I mismatch

Table 5.8 Donor-specific (DS) and third-party (TP) skin graft survival times on LTS bearing heart grafts > 100 days

Group of LTS	DS skin survival (days)	TP skin survival (days)
Major (I and II) (CsA)	20, 22, 38, 40, > 50 (x6)	8, 8, 9, 9, 9, 9, 10, 10, 10, 10
Class I (no CsA)	17, 17, 18, 19, 20, 22, 22, 22, 25, 25	9, 9, 10, 10, 10, 10, 11, 11, 11, 12
Class I (CsA)	58, 79, > 50 (x8)	9, 9, 9, 10, 10, 10, 10, 11, 11, 11
Class II (CsA)	18, 30, 32, 32, 33, > 50 (x5)	8, 10, 10, 10, 10, 11, 11, 11, 11, 11

alone) became systemically tolerant when treated with CsA (Table 5.8), despite this being unnecessary for the retention of the heart graft. Since the only difference between the two groups is the CsA treatment, it must be concluded that CsA plays an active part in the induction of allograft tolerance[57]. The results of this study are entirely novel, and serve to question the currently held belief[58] that CsA induces tolerance by preventing graft rejection and, in so doing, passively 'allows' the activation and proliferation of suppressor cells.

TOLERANCE IN THE FACE OF IMMUNITY

The ability of CsA to induce tolerance in immunized recipients was next investigated. Homan and colleagues[7] found that CsA was relatively ineffective in overcoming second set rejection of kidney allografts in rats. On the other hand, Deeg and colleagues[21] were able to obtain significant prolongation of skin grafts in sensitized dogs, and showed that the immunosuppression achieved was dependent on the continued presence of CsA, with cessation of therapy leading to graft rejection in all cases. It was of interest to note that CsA in high doses could significantly prolong skin graft survival in sensitized dogs[21], and there was a suggestion that the ability to do so might have been a consequence of the 'pulse' CsA schedule used by these authors. We therefore decided to investigate the ability of CsA to overcome the second set rejection of DA heart grafts in sensitized PVG recipients.

PVG rats were sensitized to DA donors by two sequential skin grafts, 3 weeks apart. One month following the rejection of the second skin graft, DA hearts were grafted into these sensitized recipients. They were then divided into three groups: a control group not receiving immunosuppression ($n = 10$), a CsA-treated group ($n = 10$) and a steroid treated group ($n = 10$). Rats in the CsA group were administered CsA intramuscularly at a dose of 15 mg $kg^{-1} day^{-1}$ commencing 48 h prior to heart grafting, and continued for a further 17 days according to the intermittent CsA schedule. A 48-h pretreatment schedule was included in order to achieve substantial blood levels of CsA at the time of heart grafting, since it is known that the kinetics of T cell reactivity and graft rejection are accelerated in presensitized animals[59]. A steroid-treated group was included, in order to compare the effectiveness of CsA to steroids, since the efficacy of short-term, high-dose steroids (20 mg/kg) in reversing allograft rejection in the clinic is well established[60-62]. Solumedrone (Upjohn) was administered intramuscularly to preimmunized rats, at a dose of 40 mg $kg^{-1} day^{-1}$ ($n = 10$) for 48 h preoperatively, and continued for 17 days, or up to the end-point of rejection, whichever came first.

In contrast to the first set rejection of hearts in naive controls (MST 7.4 days), heart grafts in the presensitized, no-treatment group underwent accelerated rejection (MST 3.7 days), confirming the effectiveness of the immunizing schedule (Table 5.9). With 40 mg $kg^{-1} day^{-1}$ of steroids, heart graft survival was prolonged to a MST of 5.0 days $p < 0.002$). In the CsA-treated group, although there was visible swelling of heart grafts on day 1

Table 5.9 Heart graft survival in presensitized rats – role of CsA compared with steroids

Group	Survival times (days)	MST (days)
Naive controls	7, 7, 7, 7, 7, 7, 8, 8, 8, 8	7.4 ± 0.52
Sensitized control	3, 3, 3, 4, 4, 4, 4, 4, 4, 4	3.7 ± 0.48
Sensitized CsA-treated	100 (x10)	100.0
Sensitized steroid Rx	3, 4, 4, 5, 5, 5, 5, 6, 6, 7	5.0 ± 1.2

post-transplant, this resolved by day 3, and all grafts then continued to beat beyond 100 days.

Of the 10 LTS, tolerance was confirmed in 50%, in contrast to the higher incidence of tolerance (85%) achieved by CsA in non-immunized animals (Table 5.10). Thus, using the CsA schedule described, it was possible not only to completely suppress the second set rejection of heart grafts, but also to achieve LTS in 100%, and systemic tolerance in 50% of sensitized recipients studied.

The presence of cytotoxic anti-donor antibody in these presensitized rats was also investigated. Blood samples were collected from preimmunized rats prior to CsA pretreatment, n day − 2 ($n = 8$), and on weeks 2 ($n = 5$) and 8 ($n = 5$) postoperatively. Sera obtained were assayed for the presence of anti-DA antibody using a chromium release cytotoxic assay. The specificity of the antibody for the different MHC products was determined by testing sera from PVG rats (RT1AcBc) against DA (RT1AaBa) targets, and PVG.R1 (RT1AaBc) targets. The lymphocytotoxic titre obtained using DA (RT1AaBa) targets measured the antibody present to both MHC class I and class II antigens. The lymphocytotoxic levels obtained using PVG.R1 (AaBc) targets measured the antibody present to class I antigens only.

It was found that day − 2 sera from all the preimmunized rats tested ($n = 8$), contained high titres of anti-DA lympocytotoxic antibody (see Figure 5.5). This provided further confirmation that a state of sensitization was present prior to heart grafting. In five of the rats tested, further serum samples were collected on weeks 2 and 8 post-grafting. The antibody titres in these animals were found to decline with time (see Figure 5.6). The results of assaying these sera on both DA (class I and II) and PVG.R1 (class I only) targets are illustrated in Figure 5.6, which shows the mean chromium release

Table 5.10 The survival of donor-specific (DS) and third-party (TP) test skin grafts on presensitized, CsA-treated LTS bearing heart grafts

Groups	DS skin survival (days)	TP skin survival (days)
Naive controls ($n = 10$)	8, 8, 8, 9, 9, 9, 9, 10, 10, 10	7, 7, 8, 8, 8, 8, 9, 9, 9
Tolerant (CsA) non-immunized ($n = 20$)	23, 37, 38, >50 (x17), 8 (x6), 9 (x9)	10 (x5)
Presensitized CsA–Rx, LTS ($n = 10$)	22, 24, 24, 29, 33, >50 (x5)	7, 7, 8, 8, 9, 9, 9, 9, 9, 9

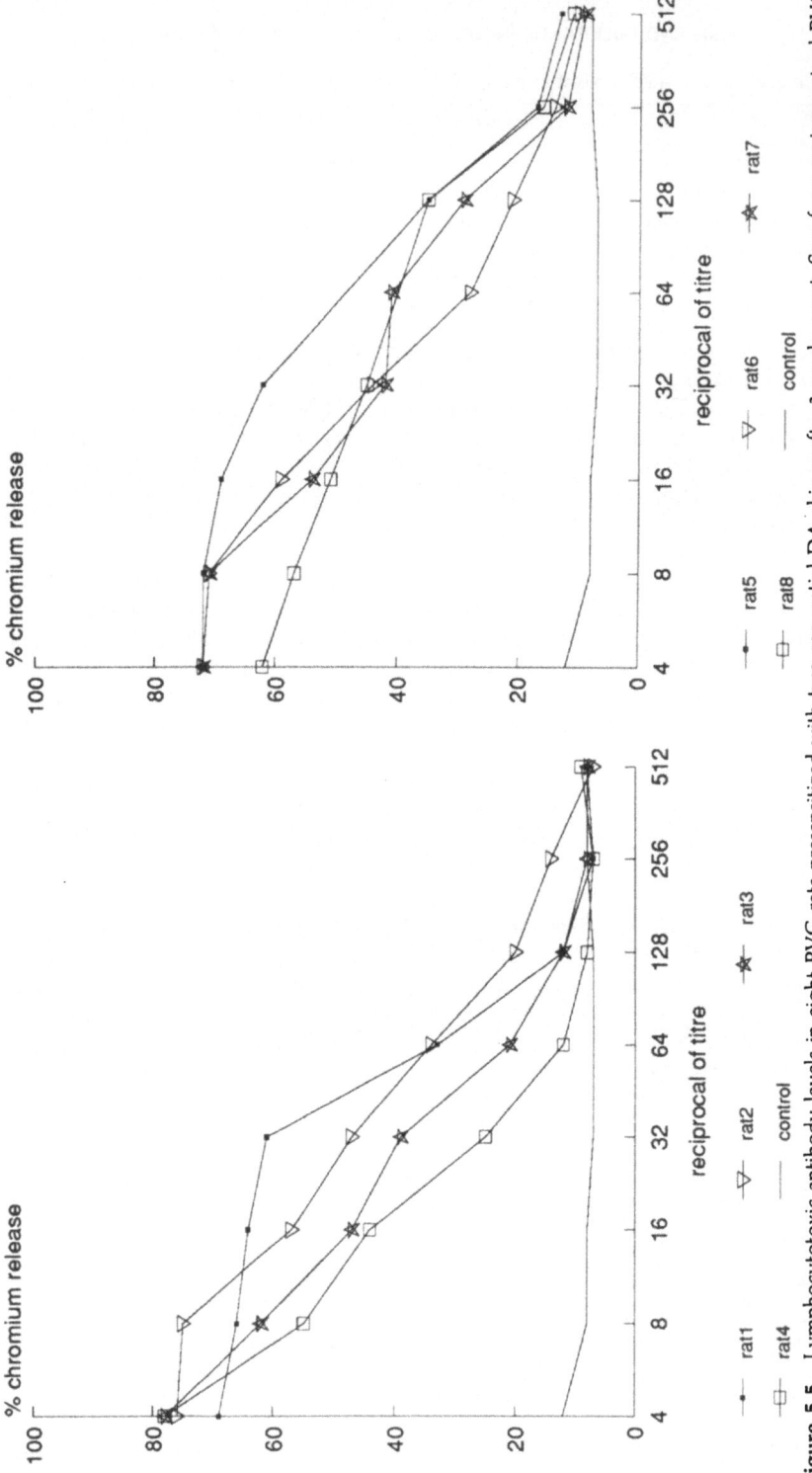

Figure 5.5 Lymphocytotoxic antibody levels in eight PVG rats presensitized with two sequential DA skin grafts, 3 weeks apart. Sera from preimmunized PVG rats were collected 1 month following rejection of second skin grafts, and prior to heart grafting for assay against DA lymphocyte targets in a chromium release assay

data for all five rats. It is seen that whilst, pre-transplant, the antibody contained a substantial anti-class I component, by week 8 this anti-class I antibody titre had declined to undetectable levels. However, antibody titres to DA (class I and II) targets were still present. From the genetics of the strain combinations used it may be concluded that the residual antibody titre obtained when DA targets were used must be anti-class II antibodies (see Figure 5.6).

The loss of anti-class I antibody may have been due to its absorption onto the graft, or to complexes formed with antigen liberated from the graft. In addition, antigen liberated from the graft, or the presence of the graft itself, may have been inhibitory for the further production of anti-class I antibody. A possible explanation for the persistence of the anti-class II antibody is that MHC class II antigen expression in the heart becomes substantially reduced by 8 weeks. Thus the existing antibody can no longer be absorbed by the graft, nor is there sufficient antigen remaining to down-regulate antibody production. It is tempting to speculate that this residual anti-class II antibody may have played a role in the induction of tolerance in these preimmunized rats. Indeed, Davies and Alkins[63] have demonstrated that passively transferred anti-class II antibody of the appropriate specificity enhances the survival, rather than causes the destruction, of rat heart allografts.

The absence of hyperacute rejection occurring in these preimmunized rats, despite the demonstrated presence of donor-specific (anti-DA) lymphocytotoxic antibody at the time of heart grafting is difficult to explain. Others[7], reporting similar findings, have attributed this either to defective complement pathways and/or defective complement fixation by rat alloantibody. In our model the complement pathway was found to be intact by the ability of the rat sera, without added guinea pig complement, to cause donor lymphocyte lysis at a titre of 1/4. In addition, it is known that hyperacute rejection of guinea pig hearts in PVG rats occurs within 10 min. Therefore a possible interpretation of the failure of the antibody to destroy heart allografts is probably strain-related, and can be explained by a difference in the distribution, expression or density of histocompatibility antigens on hearts, making complement activation difficult.

Using this sensitized model it was shown that steroids are of little value in preventing accelerated graft rejection. CsA, however, not only suppresses second set graft rejection by inhibiting pre-existing cellular immunity, but also induces tolerance in some of these sensitized rats. The mechanism of action is probably through an inhibition of pre-existing cellular rather than humoral immunity, since significant levels of anti-class II antibody have been detected, up to 8 weeks post-grafting. Whilst these experiments document the ability of CsA to induce tolerance in the face of presensitization, this achievement is probably possibly only in rat strains where antibody fails to destroy the graft.

MECHANISMS UNDERLYING CsA TOLERANCE

Possible mechanisms underlying CsA tolerance include clonal deletion, enhancing alloantibody, and suppressor cells. Clonal deletion has been

93

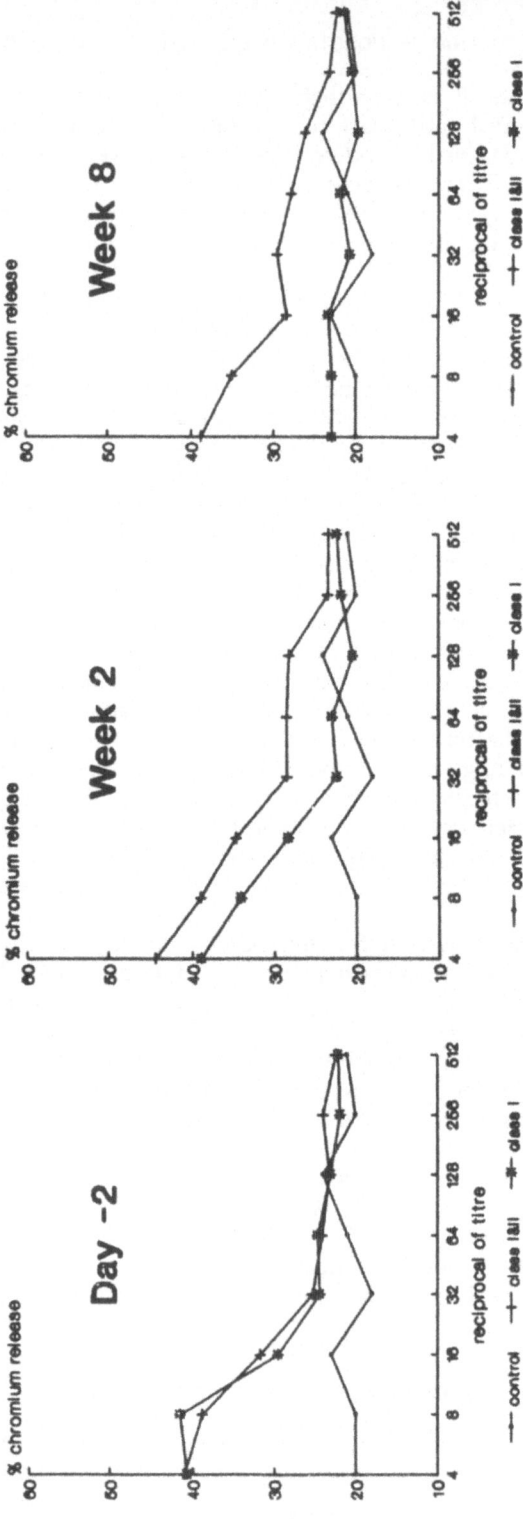

Figure 5.6 Serial assay of lymphocytotoxic antibody titres in immunized PVG (RT1AcBc) rats, at day -2, and weeks 2 and 8 post-heart grafting. Each point represents the mean percentage chromium release of five rats. The lymphocytotoxic antibody titre obtained using DA (Rî1AaBa) targets measured the antibody present to both MHC class I and II antigens, whilst that obtained using PVG.R1 targets measured the antibody present to class I antigens only

excluded since repopulation of tolerant animals with 1×10^8 naive, or immune, lymphocytes from a donor syngeneic with the recipient fails to break tolerance to heart grafts[64]. We investigated the presence of suppressor cells in CsA-tolerant rats by testing the ability of different doses (5×10^5, 1×10^6, 5×10^6, 1×10^7, and 5×10^7) of splenic lymphocytes to adoptively transfer suppression.

The lowest dose of splenic lymphocytes that achieved a significant prolongation of graft survival in comparison with irradiation controls was 1×10^6 ($p < 0.001$) (Table 5.11). Test heart graft survival times were noted to increase in proportion with increasing doses of splenic lymphocytes used. The lowest dose of splenic lymphocytes that achieved LTS in more than 50% of cases was 1×10^7. A role for serum factors is probably excluded since cells were washed twice, and resuspended in RPMI 1640 prior to adoptive transfer, thus removing any humoral component.

The specificity of the suppressor cells was tested, using donor strain or third-party heart grafts. This suppression was found to be specific; reconstitution with 5×10^7 tolerant lymphocytes, rather than prolonging survival, restored toward normal the rejection of third-party (WAG) heart grafts (median survival 13.5 days) (see Table 5.12).

The presence of suppressor cells in other lymphoid organs was also investigated. The tolerance-transferring ability of spleen, lymph node and thoracic duct lymphocytes was compared at two different doses, 5×10^7 and 1×10^7, to determine if a difference existed in the concentration or efficiency of suppressor cells in these lymphoid compartments. At a dose of 5×10^7 cells the adoptive transfer of suppression from the spleen, lymph nodes, and thoracic duct of tolerant donors was consistently demonstrated (median graft survival > 100 days for each) (see Table 5.13). This confirmed the presence of suppressor cells in all three compartments.

Table 5.11 A dose titration of splenic lymphocytes (Lys) in the adoptive transfer of tolerance, using a 550 rad model

Dose of Lys	Heart graft survival (days)	Median survival (days)
Nil–550 rad controls	11, 11, 16, 16, 17, 17, 18, 18, 20, 24	17.0
5×10^5	17, 17, 18, 18, 18, 19, 19, 22, 22, 22	18.5
1×10^6	19, 19, 20, 20, 22, 22, 25, 26, > 100 (x2)	22.0
5×10^6	19, 25, 35, 38, 39, 48, > 100 (x4)	43.5
1×10^7	35, 36, > 100 (x8)	> 100.0
5×10^7	> 100 (x10)	> 100.0
Nil-naive, no rad controls	7, 7, 7, 7, 7, 7, 8, 8, 8, 8	7.0

Table 5.12 Survival data for third-party (WAG) heart grafts in naive controls, irradiated (550 rad) only controls, and irradiated and reconstituted (5 x 10^7 splenic cells) PVG rats

Group	Third-party WAG heart graft survival (days)	Median survival (days)
Naive no rads	7, 7, 7, 8, 8, 8, 8, 8, 8, 8	8.0
550 rads no cells	12, 12, 13 15, 16, 18, 19, 19, 22, 22	17.0
550 rads + Lys*	10, 11, 11, 12, 13, 14, 14, 14, 14, 14	13.5

*These lymphocytes were obtained from standard, 100 + days CsA-treated PVG rats bearing DA (not WAG) heart grafts

Table 5.13 A comparison of the adoptive transfer of tolerance, using lymphocytes from spleen (SL), lymph nodes (LNL) and thoracic duct (TDL) of CsA-tolerant rats

Cell inocula	Heart graft survival (days)	Median survival (days)
Naive no rads	7, 7, 7, 7, 7, 7, 8, 8, 8, 8	7.0
550 rads no cells	11, 11, 16, 16, 17, 17, 18, 18, 20, 24	17.0
550 rads + SL (5 x 10^7)	> 100 (x10)	> 100.0
550 rads + SL (1 x 10^7)	35, 36, > 100 (x8)	> 100.0
550 rads + LNL (5 x 10^7)	> 100 (x10)	> 100.0
550 rads + LNL (1 x 10^7)	19, 20, 22, 22, 25, 26, 30, > 100 (x3)	25.5
550 rads + TDL (5 x 10^7)	> 100 (x10)	> 100.0
550 rads + TDL (1 x 10^7)	18, 18, 19, 19, 19, 19, 20, 20, 22, 22	19.0

With inocula of 1×10^7 cells the adoptive transfer of tolerance was achieved in 8/10 cases with lymphocytes from the spleen (median survival > 10 days) (Table 5.13). Lymph node lymphocytes prolonged heart graft survival to a median of 25.5 days, and adoptively transferred tolerance in 3/10 cases. The same dose of thoracic duct lymphocytes prolonged allograft survival to a median of 19.0 days, but failed to adoptively transfer tolerance. On a cell-for-cell basis, splenic lymphocytes were more efficient than thoracic duct lymphocytes ($p < 0.001$) or lymph node lymphocytes ($p < 0.005$) in the adoptive transfer of suppression (Figure 5.7).

These differences are the reverse of that observed with the adoptive transfer of rejection responses, where recirculating thoracic duct lymphocytes were found to be more efficient than lymph node and splenic lymphocytes in adoptively restoring allograft rejection (data not shown). This reverse hierarchy may be as a result of differing functional roles of lymphocytes in the different compartments. Thus thoracic duct and lymph node cells are actively involved in immune surveillance, whereas spleen cells may be more involved in antigen–cell contact resulting from efficient trapping of antigen by this organ[65]. By providing a conducive milieu for the interaction of alloantigen and suppressor cells, the spleen might be implicated as playing an important role in the maturation of these suppressor mechanisms.

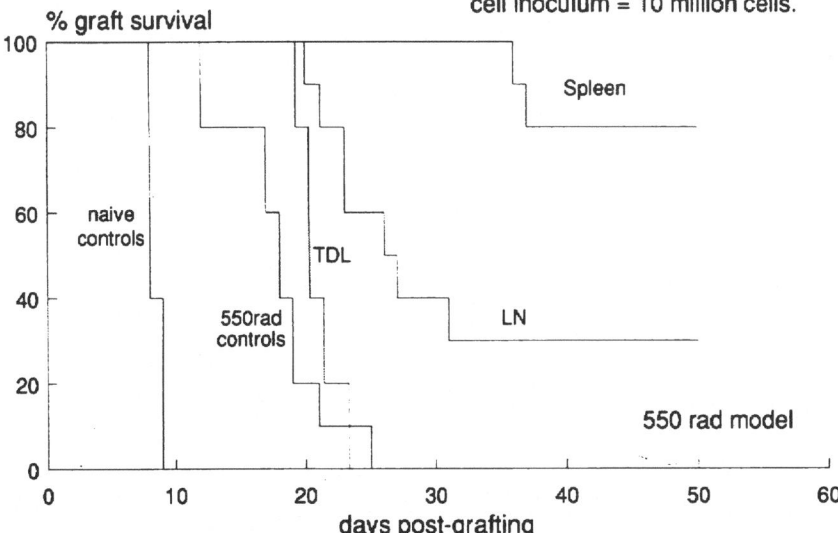

Figure 5.7 Adoptive transfer assay to compare the ability of 1×10^7 lymphocytes from the spleen, lymph nodes (LN) and thoracic duct (TDL) of CsA-tolerant rats to mediate suppression. Ten animals were included in each group. PVG rats were irradiated (550 rad) and reconstituted with a test inoculum of cells on day -1, and heart grafted (DA hearts) the next day. The median survival of heart grafts in naive controls (DA to PVG) is 7 days, and in 550 rad irradiated, but unreconstituted, controls is 17 days. At a dose of 1×10^7 cells, splenic inocula are more potent in adoptively transferring suppression than LN or TDL.

THE INFLUENCE OF STEROIDS ON THE INDUCTION OF TOLERANCE BY CsA

In clinical practice CsA is frequently used in combination with steroids in immunosuppressive schedules[66–68]. An important yet unresolved issue is whether the inclusion of steroids improves graft survival, and decreases the likelihood of rejection episodes. Recent controlled trials of steroids in CsA-treated renal transplant patients suggest that the inclusion of steroids may not be necessary[69–71]. Whilst the efficacy of steroids in the treatment of acute rejection episodes has been well documented both experimentally and clinically[62,72–74], its contribution to the induction of allograft tolerance by CsA has not been established. The influence of steroids both throughout the induction phase, and also at varying times during the risk period for tolerance induction, was investigated.

DA hearts were grafted into PVG rats on day 0. CsA was administered intramuscularly at 15 mg kg^{-1} day^{-1} for 14 days. This schedule produces 69% LTS, and was chosen because of its suitability for demonstrating either a beneficial ($>69\%$ LTS) or adverse ($<69\%$ LTS) effect of the steroid treatment on tolerance induction. Methyl prednisolone was administered intramuscularly at a dose of 5 mg kg^{-1} day^{-1}, in four different protocols (Table 5.14), to cover the risk period for CsA treatment (groups B and C), the induction phase of tolerance prior to the risk period (group D), and the

97

Table 5.14 CsA/steroid treatment schedules used in the study

Group	CsA dose (mg kg^{-1} day^{-1})	CsA Rx days	Steroid dose (mg kg^{-1} day^{-1})	Steroid Rx (days)
A	15	0–13	—	—
B	15	0–13	5	30–50
C	15	0–13	5	40–60
D	15	0–13	5	0–40
E	15	0–13	5	0–60
F	15	0–13	40	40–60
G	nil	—	5	0–60*

*This group received 5 mg/kg of steroids only from day − up until the time of established graft loss due to rejection

induction phase including the risk period (group E). The choice of this steroid dose is based on other studies using rodents, where steroids were combined with azathioprine in immunosuppressive protocols[75,76]. In addition, steroids were also used in large doses (40 mg kg^{-1} day^{-1}) in an attempt to prevent graft rejection during the risk period (group F). Control groups receiving 15 mg kg^{-1} day^{-1} of CsA only (group A), and 5 mg kg^{-1} day^{-1} of steroids only (group G), were included.

In the CsA-only control group (A), tolerance to heart grafts was achieved in 70% of cases. The addition of steroids to the CsA schedule (groups B–F) consistently reduced the number of grafts accepted long term (see Table 5.15). Steroid treatment during the risk period, both in low dose (5 mg kg^{-1} day^{-1} − groups B and C) and high dose (40 mg kg^{-1} day^{-1} − group F) merely postponed graft rejection to beyond the risk period. However, graft loss due to rejection ultimately occurred. Steroid treatment during the risk period did not increase the number of grafts going on to long-term survival; rather, these numbers decreased from 7/10 (CsA alone) to 6/10 (CsA and steroids − 5 mg/kg), and 5/10 (CsA and steroids − 40 mg/kg) (NS) (see Table 5.15).

The inclusion of steroids throughout the induction phase of CsA tolerance (groups D and E) reduced, though not significantly, the number of grafts accepted in the long term, compared with CsA treatment alone (Table 5.15). Whilst steroid treatment during days 0–40 (group D) led to a 50% graft acceptance rate, this was further reduced to 30% when steroid therapy was continued throughout the induction phase of CsA tolerance (days 0–60 − group E). Immunosuppression with steroids alone at a dose of 5 mg kg^{-1} day^{-1} failed to prolong graft survival beyond 11 days (Table 5.15).

The results of these studies suggest that steroids do not contribute to the induction of tolerance by CsA. Rather, they may actually inhibit the tolerizing process, possibly by preventing suppressor cells from being exposed to antigen through an inhibition of cell migration; by immunosuppressing the generation of suppressor cells, or through exerting a cytocidal effect on this cell subpopulation. Alternatively, the development of suppressor cells may not be impeded by steroids, but their subsequent function may be prevented by an immobilization of their cell membranes. The results of these studies

98

Table 5.15 The influence of steroid treatment on CsA-induced allograft tolerance in the rat

Groups	Survival times for heart grafts (days)	Percentage LTS
A (CsA only)	44, 45, 63, >100 (x7)	70
B (30–50d)	68, 71, 73, 78, >100 (x6)	60
C (40–60d)	46, 69, 73, 84, >100 (x6)	60
D (0–40d)	46, 50, 62, 62, 62, >100 (x5)	50
E (0–60d)	37, 37, 38, 63, 69, 83, 89, >100 (x3)	30
F (40–60d)*	60, 76, 78, 79, 88, >100 (x5)	50
G (steroids only)	7, 7, 7, 7, 8, 8, 10, 10, 11, 11	0

*Steroid dose 40 mg kg^{-1} day^{-1}

highlight the need to consider the influence of concomitant immunosuppressive drugs on the induction of tolerance by CsA.

THE ROLE OF GRAFT ADAPTATION IN CsA-INDUCED TOLERANCE

Whilst it may be assumed that CsA-induced suppressor cells are at least in part responsible for mediating allograft tolerance, they are probably not the only mechanisms involved. Graft adaption may also be an important factor contributing toward the prolonged survival of the graft. We investigated this possibility with the use of irradiation to eradicate the suppressor cell population in CsA-tolerant rats. The radiosensitivity of these cells was determined by subjecting splenic cell inocula from CsA-tolerant rats to 450 rad *in vitro*, prior to adoptive transfer. Whilst 1×10^8 unirradiated, splenic lymphocytes from CsA-tolerant rats consistently prolonged heart graft survival beyond 100 days, the same dose of irradiated cells, when adoptively transferred, achieved a median graft survival of only 15.0 days ($p < 0.01$) (Table 5.16). These data confirmed the susceptibility of alloantigen-specific suppressor cells to 450 rad of irradiation.

The tolerant status of CsA LTS bearing heart grafts was next challenged using the same dose of 450 rad whole-body irradiation. Previous studies have established that this dose is suitable for a significant elimination of the lymphoid population, without itself being a tolerizing dose. Tolerant rats

Table 5.16 The effect of *in vitro* irradiation (450 rad) on the tolerance-transferring ability of 1×10^8 splenic lymphocytes from CsA-tolerant rats

Cell inocula (1×10^8 spleen cells)	Heart graft survival (days)	Median survival (days)
Nil–550 rad controls	11, 11, 16, 16, 17, 17, 18, 18, 20, 24	17.0
550 rad + SL (unirradiated)	>100 (x10)	>100.0
550 rad + SL (irradiated)	10, 12, 12, 12, 15, 15, 18, 18, 20, 24	15.0
Nil–naive no rad controls	7, 7, 7, 7, 7, 7, 8, 8, 8, 8	7.0

bearing heart grafts for at least 100 days, and donor-specific test skin grafts for at least 50 days, were subjected to whole-body irradiation of 450 rad. Both grafts were monitored for 100 days following the procedure. Tolerant rats in the control (unirradiated) group continued to retain their heart grafts in all 10 cases, and test (donor-specific) skin grafts in 9/10 cases for at least 100 days. In the irradiated group all animals continued to retain both heart and skin grafts during this observation period (see Table 5.17).

Since suppressor cells have been shown to be radiosensitive, the results of these studies suggest that suppressor cells are not the only mechanism responsible for long-term graft acceptance. Indeed, graft adaptation may have also contributed to the indefinite survival of these hearts.

THE ROLE OF THE GRAFT IN THE MAINTENANCE OF SYSTEMIC TOLERANCE

As already described, the presence of a heart graft alone was not sufficient for the induction of systemic tolerance across a weak (class I only) histocompatibility barrier in rodents. Both short-term CsA treatment and the graft were required for the establishment of tolerance. Studies performed by Kasahara and colleagues[77] showed that continued antigen presence was important during the induction phase of CsA-induced unresponsiveness. These experiments were conducted between days 14 and 33 post-heart grafting. In the experiments described here a requirement for the presence of the heart graft in the maintenance phase (> 100 days) of systemic tolerance following cessation of CsA treatment was sought.

Heart grafts were removed from tolerant rats at day 100 +. Three weeks later these rats were challenged with donor-specific and third-party skin grafts. The survival of the skin grafts was documented. Donor-specific skins, grafted onto tolerant controls with heart grafts left in place, were accepted (> 50 days) in 80% of cases (Table 5.18). In contrast, when heart grafts were removed from CsA-tolerant rats, subsequent donor-specific skins were rejected in first set fashion (median survival 10.0 days $p < 0.001$). Third-party skin grafts were always rejected in both controls (with heart grafts) (median survival 8.5 days), and test groups (without heart grafts) (median survival 9.0 days) (Table 5.18). Thus a requirement for the presence of the graft in the maintenance of systemic tolerance induced by CsA was demonstrated. Removal of the graft consistently resulted in a loss of systemic tolerance to donor strain antigens.

Table 5.17 The effect of total-body irradiation (450 rad) on heart and test skin graft survivals in CsA-tolerant rats

Group	Survival (days) post-irradiation	
	Heart grafts	Skin grafts
Controls	> 100 (x10)	60, > 100 (x9)
450 rad	> 100 (x10)	> 100 (x10)

Table 5.18 Donor-specific (DS) and third-party (TP) skin survivals in CsA LTS with and without the presence of the heart graft

Group	Survival of DS skins		Survival of TP skins	
	Days	Median	Days	Median
LTS + heart	38, 45, > 50 (x8)	> 50	8 (x5), 9 (x4), 10	8.5
LTS − hear	8, 9, 10 (x5), 11, 12, 12	10	8 (x4), 9 (x6)	9.0

Similar observations have been made by Hall and colleagues[78], who showed that the removal of a long-standing graft (> 75 days) from a tolerant recipient resulted in a loss of suppressor activity after 1 week, using an adoptive transfer assay. In this study it was of interest to note that, even during a short space of 3 weeks, tolerance was lost. As such it is unlikely that chimerism could be advanced as an explanation for CsA-induced tolerance. If a state of chimerism existed in these animals, removal of the graft should not have led to the loss of tolerance. Assuming that suppressor cells are responsible for the maintenance phase of CsA tolerance, this observation supports the concept of the need for the continued presence of a graft to drive the suppressor circuit. Loss of antigen breaks the circuit, presumably by removing the stimulus for the maintenance of alloantigen-specific suppressor cells, and disrupts the tolerant state. Whether it is the graft itself, or the antigens released from the graft, that maintains the tolerant state could not be determined from these experiments.

A SEARCH FOR SUPPRESSOR CELLS AT DIFFERENT TIME PERIODS DURING THE INDUCTION OF CsA TOLERANCE

We have shown that suppressor cells are consistently demonstrated in the thoracic duct, lymph nodes and spleen of CsA-tolerant rats, 100 + days following heart grafting. Studies performed by Hutchinson[79] showed that suppressor cells could be demonstrated at different times during the induction phase of tolerance, and indeed, even in acutely rejecting allograft recipients on days 4–5 post-grafting. These suppressor cells formed a part of a suppressor circuit, and were called suppressor-inducers, suppressor-transducers, and suppressor-effectors. The existence of this circuit is an attractive hypothesis, and a search for suppressor cells was undertaken at two critical phases during the induction period: (a) during the first week, on day 7, and (b) during the risk period on day 40. In this manner it was hoped to establish a time period for the induction of specific suppressor cells in this model.

Inocula of 1×10^8 splenic lymphocytes were obtained from CsA treated (2-week schedule), heart-grafted rats during the first week, on day 7, during the risk period on day 40, and at > 100 days following heart grafting. The ability of these cells to adoptively transfer suppression in a 550 rad model was investigated ($n = 10$ for each). A control group reconstituted with 1×10^8 splenic cells from naive, ungrafted rats was included ($n = 10$). Whilst inocula of 1×10^8 splenic lymphocytes from tolerant rats (> 100 + days)

101

consistently prolonged graft survival beyond 100 days, inocula containing the same dose of cells obtained during the induction phase (on days 7 and 40) achieved median graft survivals of 16.0 and 17.0 days respectively (see Figure 5.8). This was not significantly different to graft survivals in irradiated but unrepopulated controls. While suppressor cells were consistently demonstrated in the spleens of CsA-tolerant rats (100 + days) on adoptive transfer, their presence during the induction phase (on days 7 and 40 post-grafting) could not be detected. On the other hand, these cell inocula (obtained on days 7 and 40 post-grafting) did not restore rejection responses toward normal in these adoptive recipients (Figure 5.8). Thus, a role for suppressor transducers as part of a suppressor circuit could not be ruled out; it is possible that alloreactive cells, present in the spleen, were in the process of losing their alloreactivity with respect to graft rejection, whilst at the same time acquiring suppressor activities, which have been shown to be fully established at day 100. The demonstration of a 'risk period' for graft rejection during the tolerizing period (60 days) lends support to the concept of a 'transit' phase between alloreactivity and allosuppression. This concept supports the existence of a polyfunctional cell type, that under appropriate circumstances may mediate either rejection or suppression. Alternatively, several subsets of monofunctional cells as part of a suppressor circuit may be involved.

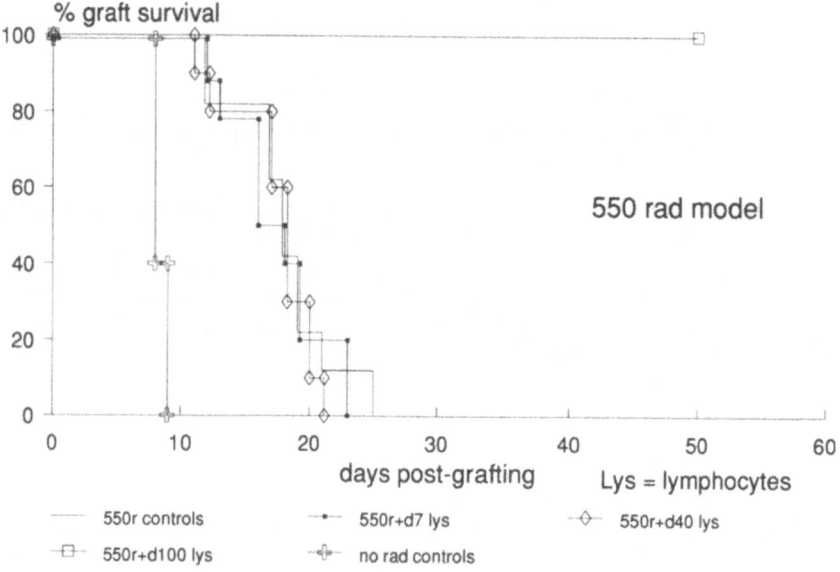

Figure 5.8 A search for suppressor cells in CsA-treated, heart-grafted rats at different times (days 7, 40 and > 100) post-grafting ($n = 10$ each). In the adoptive transfer assay PVG rats are irradiated (550 rad) and reconstituted with a test inoculum of cells on day − 1, and heart grafted (DA hearts) the next day. The median survival of heart grafts in naive controls (DA to PVG) is 7 days, and in 550 rad irradiated, but unreconstituted, controls is 17 days. Only test inocula obtained from 100-day CsA-treated, heart grafted rats adoptively transfer tolerance

SUPPRESSOR CELL PHENOTYPE IN CsA-TOLERANT RATS

The phenotype of the CsA-induced suppressor cell was investigated, using monoclonal antibodies and immunomagnetic beads. T(OX19 +), B(OX12 +), CD4 + (W3/25 +) and CD8 + (OX8 +) subsets obtained from inocula of 5×10^7 splenic lymphocytes from CsA-tolerant rats, were analysed by adoptive transfer. We found that negatively selected T cells or W3/25 + (CD4 +) cells from tolerant rats induced unresponsiveness to donor strain heart grafts in all instances (Figure 5.9). On the other hand, the adoptive transfer of B(OX12 +) lymphocytes (median survival 18.0 days) and OX8 + (CD8 +) cells (median survival 20.0 days) did not significantly prolong graft survival over 550 rad unrepopulated controls (median survival 17.0 days) (Figure 5.9). Therefore the phenotype of the suppressor cell in this model was identified as OX19 +, W3/25 +, OX8$^-$.

In CsA-treated rodents both OX8 + (CD8)[80] and W3/25 + (CD4)[81] suppressor cells have been identified. This apparent discrepancy in phenotypic characterization of CsA-induced suppressor cells is probably related to the timing of the assay with respect to the evolution of suppressor cell maturation. Whilst both the data reported here, and by Hall and colleagues[81], were obtained using tolerant rats > 75 days post-heart grafting, those described

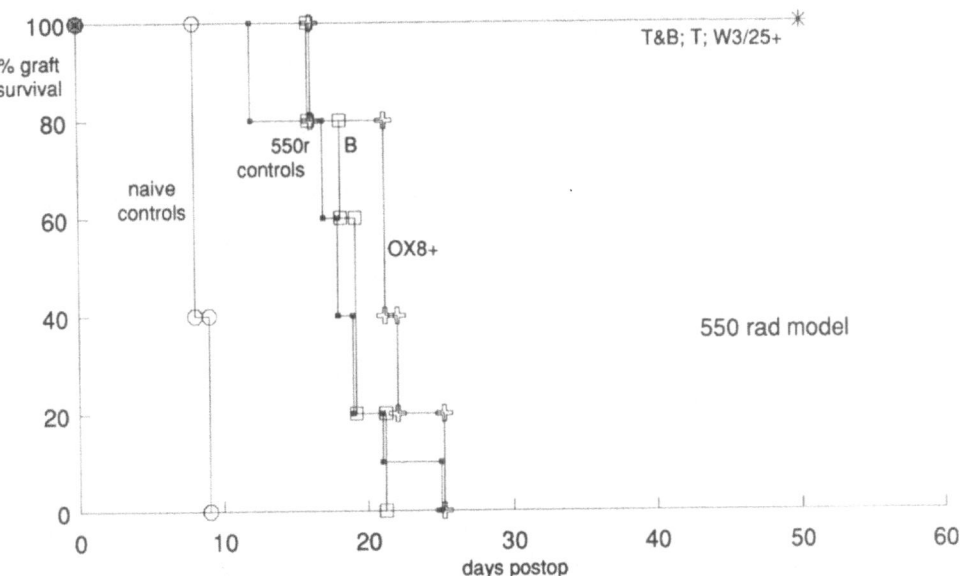

Figure 5.9 Identifying the phenotype of the suppressor cell in CsA-tolerant rats. Using a 550 rad assay, the adoptive transfer of tolerance is consistently achieved with inocula containing W3/25 + cells (inocula containing T and B cells, T cells only or W3/25 + cells only). OX8 + and OX12 + lymphocytes fail to confer tolerance in adoptive recipients. Cell separation was achieved using monoclonal antibodies and immunomagnetic beads. 5×10^7 lymphocytes from spleen, lymph node or thoracic duct were used. Five animals were included in each group. Only the negatively selected (free of beads) cell subpopulations were adoptively transferred

by Kupiec-Weglinski and colleagues[80] were derived from CsA-treated rats 20–30 days post-grafting. The presence of immunosuppressive levels of CsA at this time (20–30 days post-grafting), might have contributed to the detection of a different suppressor phenotype. Indeed, studies performed by Godden and colleagues[82] showed that a novel cell type carrying both W3/25 + (CD4 +) and OX8 + (CD8 +) markers appears in the blood of CsA-treated, heart-grafted rats during the first week of CsA treatment. This observation might explain the detection of different suppressor cell phenotypes at this time. Alternatively, variations in rat strains used may have contributed to the differences in results between different laboratories.

THE EFFECTS OF SPLENECTOMY ON CsA-INDUCED TOLERANCE

It is known that the spleen is a rich source of suppressor cells in several rodent models[83,84], and this has been confirmed in the studies described here, by the adoptive transfer of tolerance using splenic lymphocytes from CsA-tolerant rats. We therefore decided to investigate the effect of splenectomy on the induction and maintenance of CsA tolerance, and to determine the role of the spleen in the tolerizing process induced by CsA. DA hearts were grafted into PVG recipients, treated with 15 mg/kg of CsA intramuscularly for 14 days. As with the steroid experiment, this CsA schedule was selected since it produces 69% LTS and was therefore suitable for demonstrating either a beneficial or adverse effect of splenectomy on the induction of tolerance. Recipient PVG rats either underwent laparotomy alone ($n = 10$), or laparotomy and splenectomy ($n = 10$) on the day before heart grafting (day − 1). Graft survival was observed for 100 days.

Whilst in laparotomized-only CsA controls (spleen present), LTS were achieved in 70% of cases, in splenectomized PVGs LTS occurred in only 40% of cases treated with CsA (see Table 5.19). Thus there was a suggestion that the spleen may be required for the induction of suppressor mechanisms, since its absence prior to heart grafting reduced, though not significantly, the numbers of long-surviving heart grafts obtained. There are two possible reasons why the spleen may play an important role in the induction of tolerance by CsA:

1. It is the first effective site of contact between lymphocytes and antigen. Sprent and Miller[85] have shown that antigen-specific recruitment of immunocompetent cells to the spleen occurs 1–2 days after the intravenous injection of sheep erythrocytes in mice. In addition it is a prominent site for antigen localization and processing after transplantation of

Table 5.19   The influence of splenectomy on the induction of tolerance by CsA

Groups (n = 10)	Heart graft survival (days)	Percentage graft acceptance
Spleen present	40, 44, 49, > 100 (x7)	70.0
Spleen absent	40, 43, 60, 61, 65, 98, > 100 (x4)	40.0

vascularized organ allografts[65]. Thus it may be that the splenectomy results in the loss of this antigen-trapping capacity and thereby reduces the efficiency of the tolerizing mechanism.

2. The spleen is known to be a rich source of suppressor cells[83,84]. It may be that removal of the spleen reduces the number of potential suppressor cells below some critical threshold, and prevents the induction of tolerance.

Splenectomy performed during the maintenance phase of CsA-induced allograft tolerance led to the rejection of long-surviving heart grafts in 2/10 cases (see Table 5.20). The retention of heart grafts in the remaining eight animals did not necessarily imply that systemic tolerance was present, since other mechanisms such as graft adaptation might have accounted for the indefinite survival of these grafts. Indeed, this was confirmed by the results of donor-specific skin grafting (Table 5.21). The rejection of donor-specific skins in the eight splenectomized LTS contrasts with the prolonged (spleen present) controls $p < 0.005$) (Table 5.21). This confirms that a loss of tolerance has resulted from the splenectomy. This apparent phenomenon of 'split tolerance' to heart versus skin allografts in splenectomized LTS may be accounted for by the antigenicity of the fresh skin grafts resulting in rejection, compared with the retention of long-standing heart grafts (which are retained).

Further evidence for the loss of systemic tolerance following splenectomy was provided by the results of adoptive transfer using splenectomized LTS as cell donors. CsA-tolerant rats ($n = 10$) were subjected to splenectomy at day 100 +. Three months later these animals were subjected to thoracic duct cannulation. Inocula of 1×10^8 thoracic duct lymphocytes were adoptively transferred into 10 recipients (irradiated with 550 rad). Whilst the adoptive transfer of 1×10^8 thoracic duct lymphocytes from tolerant rats, whose spleens were present, consistently prolonged heart graft survival beyond 100 days, the same dose of TDL from splenectomized LTS resulted in the rejection of 8/10 heart grafts between 11 and 25 days (Figure 5.10). The difference in graft survivals obtained with TDL from CsA-tolerant rats with spleens present,

Table 5.20 The influence of splenectomy on the maintenance of CsA-induced allograft tolerance

Groups (n = 10)	Heart graft survival following splenectomy (days)	Percentage graft loss
Controls	> 100 (x10)	0
Spleen removed	64, 77, > 100 (x8)	20

Table 5.21 Donor-specific (DS) and third-party (TP) skin graft survivals in long-term survivors following either laparotomy only (controls), or laparotomy and splenectomy

Group	DS skin survival (days)	TP skin survival (days)
Controls	28, 33, 35, 44, > 50 (x6)	8, 8, 8, 8, 8, 8, 9, 9, 9, 9
Spleen removed	10, 10, 11, 18, 22, 38, 39, 44	8, 8, 8, 8, 9, 9, 9, 9

105

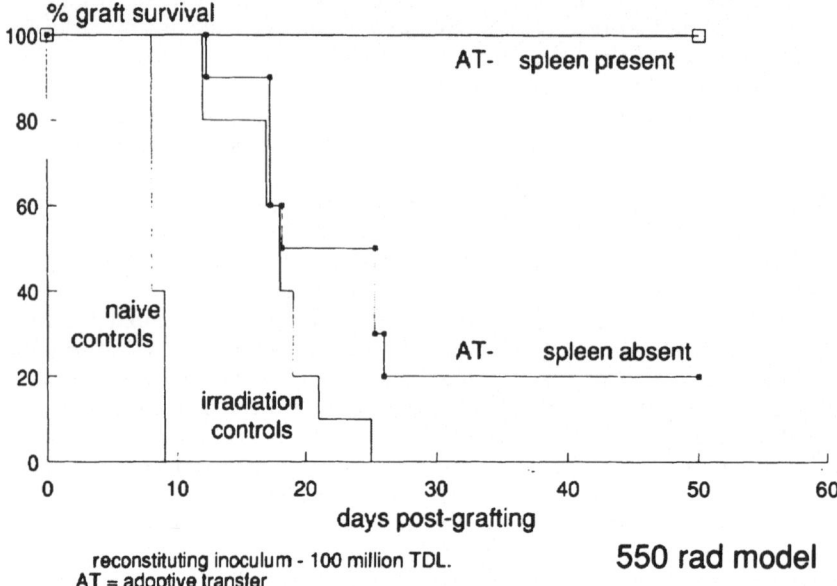

reconstituting inoculum - 100 million TDL.
AT = adoptive transfer

550 rad model

Figure 5.10 The effect of splenectomy (day 100+ post-grafting) on the adoptive transfer of suppression by thoracic duct lymphocytes (1×10^8) from CsA-tolerant rats. Ten animals were included in each group. PVG rats were irradiated (550 rad) and reconstituted with a test inoculum of TDL on day -1, and heart grafted (DA hearts) the next day. The median survival of heart grafts in naive controls (DA to PVG) is 7 days, and in 550 rad irradiated, but unreconstituted, controls is 17 days. TDL from CsA-tolerant rats (spleens present) regularly confers tolerance to adoptive recipients. In contrast, the same dose of cells from splenectomized CsA long-term survivors confers tolerance in 2/10 adoptive recipients

and CsA-'tolerant' rats with spleens absent was significant ($p < 0.001$), confirming that splenectomy abrogated the adoptive transfer of tolerance. This abrogation was incomplete, since in two cases LTS were achieved by adoptive transfer. This suggests that an incomplete depletion of suppressor cells was produced 3 months following splenectomy. Indeed, we have shown that suppressor cells are also present in the lymph nodes, in agreement with the findings of Cranston and colleagues[86], who have documented the presence of suppressor cells in lymph nodes of splenectomized rats.

The data presented here support the view that the spleen plays a central role in the maintenance of allograft tolerance. No other studies in the literature could be found of a detrimental effect of splenectomy on the maintenance phase of CsA tolerance. Its removal either results in a substantial decrease in the numbers of suppressor cells available directly, or by an alternation in suppressor cell trafficking, or abolishes the capacity of these cells to function as suppressors, by interfering in some way with the maturation process, perhaps by removing the milieu for interaction with alloantigen trapped in the spleen.

106

DISCUSSION

The ability of short-term CsA treatment to induce tolerance to heart grafts across all levels of MHC incompatibility, as well as in fully allogeneic rat strains, was confirmed by these studies. CsA was shown to be more effective than steroids in overcoming second set rejection and in inducing tolerance in preimmunized rats. A common denominator underlying the various permutations of CsA tolerizing schedules is the maintenance of adequate CsA levels ($> 200-300$ ng/ml) in the blood throughout the tolerizing process. In the rat strains studied this time period has been identified as 60 days, and encompasses a risk period, during which the incidence of graft rejection is high. there is a suggestion from the work of others[12,14] that the concept of a 'risk period', during which CsA cover is necessary, may also exist in other animal species.

We established an active requirement for CsA in the induction of tolerance, and showed that the presence of a graft alone was an insufficient stimulus for the induction of tolerance[57]. The kinetics of tolerance induction by CsA paralleled the maturation of a specific, suppressor cell population in these animals, detectable at the end of the tolerizing period (> 60 days), and in the absence of CsA therapy. Concomitant steroid therapy did not contribute toward the induction of tolerance by CsA. Rather there was a suggestion that steroids may have immunosuppressed the induction of suppressor cells, through their non-specific effects on lymphocytes.

Once these suppressor cells had been induced (> 60 days), CsA was no longer necessary for the maintenance of systemic tolerance. These suppressor cells were found to be of the W3/25 + phenotype, in agreement with the results of Hall[81], and were present in high concentration in the spleen, and to a lesser extent in lymph nodes and thoracic duct. Whilst their presence equated with systemic tolerance, we failed to demonstrate an absolute requirement for these radiosensitive cells in the maintenance of graft survival in the long term. That is, systemic tolerance was not an absolute prerequisite for continued graft survival in the long term. Rather, local factors, such as reduced graft immunogenicity, may have played a significant role. The presence of both the graft and a spleen was found to be essential for the maintenance of systemic tolerance. Removal of either organ consistently resulted in a loss of systemic tolerance. A need for continued graft presence suggests that CsA-induced alloantigen-specific suppressor cells require constant exposure to graft antigen to remain activated.

The adverse effects of splenectomy on systemic tolerance were attributed to the central role of this organ in the tolerizing process. We postulate that alloreactive cells interact with alloantigen present on the graft and trapped in the spleen. In the presence of CsA, alloreactivity is dampened, and allosuppression activated. A suppressor cell population thus matures in the spleen, and subsequently distributes to other lymphoid organs. In the absence of a spleen, other lymphoid organs such as the lymph nodes probably take on the role of providing a milieu for suppressor cell maturation, although this may be less efficient. During the maintenance phase the mechanism by which splenectomy abrogates systemic tolerance may include the bulk removal

107

of suppressor lymphocytes, and an alteration of trafficking of residual suppressor cells.

The success of CsA in the induction of tolerance in experimental models, in comparison to other immunosuppressive drugs, probably arises from its specific action on activated $CD4^+$ alloreactive lymphocytes. This is an apparent dichotomy since this subset also mediates suppression in this model. This issue may be explained by the existence of a polyfunctional subset of CD4 + cells, which under appropriate conditions mediates either 'help' or suppression. Alternatively, further subdivisions of monofunctional cells may exist within the $CD4^+$ subset. In either case a selective dampening of alloreactive cells is probably required initially. Meanwhile, the activation of alloantigen-specific suppressor cells occurs over time, and is detected once CsA therapy is withdrawn. An important question with relevance to the clinical situation is whether continued CsA treatment inhibits suppressor cell activity. This issue is currently being investigated.

REFERENCES

1. Borel, J. F. (1982) History of cyclosporin A and its significance in immunology. In White, D. J. G. (ed.), Cyclosporin A, pp. 5–17. (Amsterdam: Elsevier)
2. Kostakis, A. J., White, D. J. G. and Calne, R. Y. (1977) Prolongation of rat heart allograft survival by cyclosporin A. IRCS Med. Sci., 5, 280
3. Calne, R. Y. and White, D. J. G. (1977) Cyclosporin A – a powerful immunosuppressant in dogs with renal allografts. IRCS Med. Sci., 5, 595
4. Kawahara, K., Sutherland, D. E. R., Rynasiewicz, J. R. and Najarian, J. S. (1980) Prolongation of heterotopic cardiac allografts in rats by cyclosporin A. Surgery, 88, 594–600
5. Bordes-Aznar, J., Kupiec-Weglinski, J. W., Duarte, A. J. S., Milford, E. L., Strom, T. B. and Tilney, N. L. (1983) Function and migration of suppressor lymphocytes from cyclosporine-treated heart graft recipients. Transplantation, 35, 185
6. Hall, B. M., Jelbart, M. E. and Dorsch, S. E. (1984) Suppressor T cells in rats with prolonged cardiac allograft survival after treatment with cyclosporine. Transplantation, 37, 595
7. Homan, W. P., Fabre, J. W., Williams, K. A., Millard, P. R. and Morris, P. J. (1980) Studies on the immunosuppressive properties of cyclosporin A in rats receiving renal allografts. Transplantation, 29, 361
8. Engemann, R., Ulrichs, K., Thiede, A., Muller-Ruchholtz, W. and Hamelmann, H. (1983) Induction of liver graft tolerance in a primarily nontolerant rat strain combination with temporary treatment of cyclosporine. Transplant. Proc., 15, 2986
9. Kirkman, R. L., Lear, P. A., Madara, J. L. and Tilney, N. L. (1984) Small intestine transplantation in the rat – immunology and function. Surgery, 96, 280
10. Black, K. S., Hewitt, C. W., Fraser, L. A., Howard, E. B., Martin, D. C., Achauer, B. M. and Furnas, D. W. (1985) Composite tissue (limb) allografts in rats. II. Indefinite survival using low dose cyclosporine. Transplantation, 39, 365
11. Green, C. J. and Allison, A. C. (1978) Extensive prolongation of rabbit kidney allograft survival after short-term Cyclosporin A treatment. Lancet, 1, 1182
12. Collier, D. St J., Calne, R. Y., De Curtins, M., Thiru, S., White, D. J. G., Jamieson, N. V., Thick, M. and Barroso, E. (1987) Alternative-day cyclosporine A and azathioprine in experimental dog renal allografts. Transplant. Proc., 19, 1279
13. Borleffs, J. C. C., Neuhaus, P. and Balner, H. (1983) Cyclosporin A as optimal immunosuppressant after kidney allografting in rhesus monkeys. Heart Transplant, 2, 111–117
14. Calne, R. Y., Rolles, K., Smith, D. P. and Hebertson, B. M. (1978) Prolonged survival of pig orthotopic heart grafts treated with cyclosporin A. Lancet, 1, 1183
15. Borel, J. F., Feurer, C., Gubler, H. U. and Stahelin, H. (1976) Biological effects of cyclosporin A: a new antilymphocytic agent. Agents Actions, 6, 468–475

16. Lems, S. P. M. and Koene, R. A. P. (1979) Prolongation of mouse skin allograft survival by cyclosporin A: graft rejection after withdrawal of therapy. *IRCS Med. Sci.*, **7**, 184
17. White, D. J. G., Rolles, K. and Ottawa, T. (1980) CyA induced long-term survival of fully incompatible skin and heart grafts in rats. *Transplant Proc.*, **12**, 261
18. Towpik, E., Kupiec-Weglinski, J. W., Schneider, T. M., Tyler, D., Padberg, W., Araneda, D. and Tilne, N. L. (1985) Cyclosporine and experimental skin allografts. *Transplantation*, **40**, 714
19. Gratwohl, A., Forster, I. and Speck, B. (1981) Skin grafts in rabbits with cyclosporin A. Absence of induction of tolerance and untoward side effects. *Transplantation*, **31**, 136
20. Borel, J. F. and Meszaros, J. (1980) Skin transplantation in mice and dogs. Effects of cyclosporin A and dihydrocyclosporin C. *Transplantation*, **29**, 161
21. Deeg, H. J., Storb, R., Gerhard-Miller, L., Shulman, H. M., Weiden, P. L. and Thomas, E. D. (1980) Cyclosporin A, a powerful immunosuppressant *in vivo* and *in vitro* in the dog, fails to induce tolerance. *Transplantation*, **29**, 230
22. Lim, S. M. L., White, D. J. G. and Calne, R. Y. (1987) Identifying a susceptible period following cyclosporine A-induced tolerance of heart grafts in the rat. *Transplant. Proc.*, **19**(5), 4218
23. Green, C. J., Allison, A. C. and Precious, S. (1979) Induction of specific tolerance in rabbits by kidney allografting and short periods of cyclosporin A treatment. *Lancet*, **2**, 123
24. Calne, R. Y., White, D. J. G., Thiru, S., Evans, D. B., McMaster, P., Dunn, D. C., Craddock, G. N., Pentlow, B. D. and Rolles, K. (1978) Cyclosporin A in patients receiving renal allografts from cadaver donors. *Lancet*, **2**, 1323
25. Calne, R. Y., White, D. J. G., Evans, D. B. and Wright, C. (1982) Three years' experience with cyclosporin A in clinical cadaveric kidney transplantation. In White, D. G. (ed.), *A. Proceedings of an International Conference on Cyclosporin A.* (New York: Elsevier), pp. 347–353
26. Wood, R. F. M., Thompson, J. F., Allen, N. H., Ting, A. and Morris, P. J. (1983) The consequences of conversion from cyclosporine to azathioprine and prednisolone in renal allograft recipients. *Transplant. Proc.*, **15** (Suppl. 1), 2862
27. Starzl, T. E., Hakala, T. R., Rosenthal, J. T., Iwatsuki, S. and Shaw, B. W. Jr. (1983) The Colorado–Pittsburgh cadaveric renal transplantation study with cyclosporine. *Transplant. Proc.*, **15** (Suppl. 1), 2459
28. Najarian, J. S., Strand, M., Fryd, D. S., Ferguson, R. M., Simmons, R. L., Ascher, N. L. and Sutherland, D. E. R. (1983) Comparison of cyclosporine versus azathioprine antilymphocyte globulin in renal transplantation. *Transplant. Proc.*, **15**, 2463
29. Kahan, B. D., Buren, C. T. van, Flechner, S. M., Payne, W. D., Boileau, M. and Kerman, R. H. (1983) Cyclosporine immunosuppression mitigates immunologic risk factors in renal allotransplantation. *Transplant. Proc.*, **15**, 2469
30. Sells, R. A. (1983) A prospective, randomized substitutive trial of Cyclosporine as a prophylactic agent in human renal transplant rejection. *Transplant. Proc.*, **15**, 2495
31. Stiller, C. (1983) The requirements for maintenance steroids in cyclosporine-treated renal transplant recipients. *Transplant. Proc.*, **15** (Suppl. 1), 2490
32. Sheil, A. G. R., Hall, B. M., Tiller, D. J. *et al.* (1983) Australian trial of cyclosporine in cadaveric donor renal transplantation. *Transplant. Proc.*, **25**, 2485
33. Calne, R. Y., Williams, R., Lindop, M. J., Farman, J. V., Tolley, M. E., Rolles, K., MacDougall, B., Neuberger, J., Wyke, R. K., Rafferty, A. T., Duffy, T. J., Wight, D. G. D. and White, D. J. G. (1981) Improved survival after orthotopic liver grafting. *Br. Med. J.*, **283**, 115
34. Starzl, T. E., Iwatsuki, S., Klintmalm, G., Schroter, G. P. J., Weil, R., Koep, L. J. and Porter, K. A. (1981) Liver transplantation 1980, with particular reference to cyclosporin A. *Transplant. Proc.*, **13**, 281
35. Wonigeit, K., Brolsch, C., Neuhaus, P., Burdelski, M., Schmidt, E., Lang, W. and Pichlmayr, R. (1983) Special aspects of immunosuppression with cyclosporine in liver transplantation. *Transplant. Proc.*, **15**, 2586
36. Sutherland, D. E. R. (1983) Workshop on transplantation of the pancreas. *Transplant. Proc.*, **15**, 1509
37. Reitz, B. A., Bieber, C. P., Rainey, A. A., Pennock, J. L., Jamieson, S. W., Oyer, P. E. and Stinson, E. B. (1981) Orthotopic heart and combined heart and lung transplantation with Cyclosporin A immunosuppression. *Transplant. Proc.*, **13**, 373
38. Wallwork, J., Cory-Pearce, R. and English, T. A. H. (1983) Cyclosporine for cardiac

transplantation: UK trial. *Transplant. Proc.*, **15**, 2559

39. Hutchinson, I. V., Shadur, C. A., Duarte, A. J. S., Strom, T. B. and Tilney, N. L. (1981) Cyclosporin A spares selectively lymphocytes with donor-specific suppressor characteristics. *Transplantation*, **32**, 210

40. Wassef, R., Cohen, Z. and Langer, B. (1985) Pharmacokinetic profiles of cyclosporine in rats. *Transplantation*, **40**, 489

41. Friedman, A. L., Beyer, M. M., Josephson, A. S. and Schiffman, G. (1987) Alternate-day cyclosporine. *Transplantation*, **43**, 457

42. Nagao, T., White, D. J. G. and Calne, R. Y. (1982) Kinetics of unresponsiveness induced by a short course of cyclosporine A. *Transplantation*, **33**, 31

43. Kupiec-Weglinski, J. W., Filho, M. A., Strom, T. B. and Tilney, N. L. (1984) Sparing of suppressor cells: a critical action of cyclosporine. *Transplantation*, **38**, 97

44. Butcher, G. W. and Howard, J. C. (1977) A recombinant in the major histocompatibility complex of the rat. *Nature*, **266**, 362

45. Rozing, J., Bonthuis, F., Joling, P., Vaessen, L. M. B. and Lameijer, L. D. F. (1983) The influence of RT1 subregion differences on cardiac allograft survival. *Transplant. Proc.*, **15**, 1647

46. Katz, S. M., Liebert, M., Gill, T. J., Kunz, H. W., Cramer, D. V. and Guttmann, R. D. (1983) The relative roles of MHC and non-MHC genes in heart and skin allograft survival. *Transplantation*, **36**, 96

47. Stewart, R., Butcher, G., Herbert, J. and Roser, B. (1985) Graft rejection in a congenic panel of rats with defined immune response genes for MHC class I antigens. *Transplantation*, **40**, 427

48. Klempnauer, J., Steiniger, B., Marquarding, E., Vogt, P., Lipecz, A., Wonigeit, K. and Gunther, E. (1987) Effects of the RT1.C region in rat allotransplantation. *Transplant. Proc.*, **19**, 713

49. Lance, E. M., Boyse, E. A., Cooper, S. and Carswell, E. A. (1971) Rejection of skin allografts by irradiation chimaeras: evidence for a skin-specific transplantation barrier. *Transplant. Proc.*, **3**, 864

50. Warren, R. P., Lofgreen, J. S. and Steinmuller, D. (1973) Differential survival of heart and skin allografts in inbred rats. *Transplant. Proc.*, **5**, 717

51. Murray, J. E., Sheil, A. G. R., Moseley, R., Knight, P., McGavic, J. D. and Dammin, G. J. (1964) Analysis of mechanism of immunosuppressive drugs in renal homotransplantation. *Ann. Surg.*, **160**, 449

52. White, E., Hildemann, W. H. and Mullen, Y. (1969) Chronic kidney allograft reactions in rats. *Transplantation*, **8**, 602–617

53. Barker, C. F. and Billingham, R. E. (1970) Comparison of the fates of Ag-B locus compatible homografts of skin and hearts in inbred rats. *Nature*, **225**, 851

54. Bildsoe, P., Ford, W. L., Pettirossi. O. and Simonsen, M. (1971) GVH analysis of organ-grafted rats which defy the normal rules of rejection. *Transplantation*, **12**, 189

55. Salaman, J. R., Elves, M. W. and Festenstein, H. (1971) Factors contributing to survival of rats transplanted with kidneys mismatched at major locus. *Transplant. Proc.*, **3**, 577

56. Sorensen, S. F., Bildsoe, P. and Simonsen, M. (1972) Mixed lymphocyte culture and graft-versus-host analyses of organ-grafted rats that defy normal rules for rejection. *Transplant. Proc.*, **4**(2), 181

57. Lim, S. M. L. and White, D. J. G. (1988) Long-term residence of a graft is an insufficient stimulus for the induction of tolerance. *J. Exp. M ed.*, **168**, 807

58. Tilney, N. L. and Strom, T. B. (1986) Chemical suppression of the immune responses. In Morris, P. J. and Tilney, N. L. (eds), *Progress in Transplantation*, vol. 3 (Edinburgh: Churchill Livingstone), pp. 1–31

59. Guttmann, R. D. (1976) A genetic survey of rat cardiac allograft rejection in presensitized recipients. *Transplantation*, **22**, 583

60. Bell, P. R. F., Briggs, J. D., Calman, K. C., Paton, A. M., Wood, R. F. M., Macpherson, S. G. and Kyle, K. (1971) Reversal of acute clinical and experimental organ rejection using large doses of intravenous prednisolone. *Lancet*, **1**, 876

61. Turcotte, J. G., Feduska, N. J., Carpenter, E. W., Mcdonald, F. D. and Bacon, G. E. (1972) Rejection crises in human renal transplant recipients. *Arch. Surg.*, **105**, 230

62. Woods, J. E., Anderson, C. F., De Weerd, J. H. *et al.* (1973) High-dosage intravenously administered methylprednisolone in renal transplantation. *J. Am. Med. Assoc.*, **223**, 896

63. Davies, D. A. L. and Alkins, B. J. (1974) What abrogates heart transplant rejection in immunological enhancement? *Nature*, **247**, 294
64. White, D. J. G., Timmerman, W., Davies, H. ff. S., Nagao, T., Kasahara, K. and Plumb, A. (1981) Properties of cyclosporin-A-induced graft acceptance. *Transplant. Proc.*, **13**(1), 379
65. Ford, W. L. '1975) Lymphocyte migration and immune responses. *Progr. Allergy*, **19**, 1
66. Starzl, T. E., Weil, R. III, Iwatzuki, S. *et al.* (1980) The use of cyclosporin A and steroid therapy in 66 cadaver kidney transplants. *Surg. Gynaecol. Obstet.*, **151**, 17
67. Stiller, C. R., Keown, P. A., Sinclair, N. R. and Ulan, R. A. (1982) Immune responses and pharmacokinetics in the human renal allograft recipient treated with Cyclosporin A. In White, D. J. G. (ed.), *Cyclosporin A* (Amsterdam: Elsevier), pp. 379–86
68. Tilney, N. L., Milford, E. L., Aranajo, J-L., Strom, T. B., Carpenter, C. B. and Kirkland, R. L. (1984) Experience with cyclosporine and steroids in clinical renal transplantation. *Ann. Surg.*, **200**, 604
69. Johnson, R. W. G., Wise, M. H., Bakran, A., Short, C., Dyer, P., Mallick, N. P. and Gokal, R. (1985) A four-year prospective study of Cyclosporine in cadaver renal transplantation. *Transplant. Today*, **8**, 1197
70. Johnson, R. W. G., Mallick, N. P., Bakran, A., Pearson, R. C., Scott, P. D., Dyer, P., Donaghue, D. and Gokal, R. (1988) Cadaver renal transplantation without maintenance steroids. *Transplant. Proc.* (In press)
71. Griffin, P. J. A., Ross, W. B., Williams, J. D. and Salaman, J. R. (1987) Low-dose cyclosporine monotherapy in renal transplantation. *Transplant. Proc.*, **19**(5), 3685
72. Goodwin, W. E., Kaufman, J. J., Mims, M. M., Turner, R. D., Glassock, R., Goldman, R. and Maxwell, M. M. (1963) Human renal transplantation − I: Clinical experiences with six cases of renal homotransplantation. *J. Urol.*, **89**, 13
73. Clarke, A. G. and Salaman, J. R. (1974) Methylprednisolone in the treatment of renal transplant rejection. *Clin. Nephrol.*, **2**, 230
74. Gray, D., Shepherd, H., Daar, A., Oliver, D. O. and Morris, P. J. (1978) Oral versus intravenous high-dose steroid treatment of renal allograft rejection. The big shot or not? *Lancet*, **1**, 117
75. Bell, P. R. F., Briggs, J. D., Calman, K. C., Quin, R. O., Wood, R. F. M., Paton, A. and Macpherson, S. G. (1973) The immunosuppressive effect of large doses of intravenous prednisolone in experimental heterotopic rat heart and human renal transplantation. *Surgery*, **73**, 147
76. Salaman, J. R. (1983) Influence of steroid dosage on the survival of cardiac allografts in the rat. *Transplantation*, **35**, 510
77. Kasahara, K., White, D. J. G. and Calne, R. Y. (1982) Antigen dependence of cyclosporin A-induced allograft acceptance. *Transplantation*, **34**, 216
78. Hall, B. M., Gurley, K. and Dorsch, S. E. (1987) Specific unresponsiveness in rats with prolonged allograft survival is dependent upon the graft and suppressor T cells. *Transplant. Proc.*, **19**(1), 95
79. Hutchinson, I. V. (1986) Suppressor T cells in allogeneic models. *Transplantation*, **41**, 547
80. Kupiec-Weglinski, J. W. Bordes-Aznar, J., Lear, P. A., Strom, T. B. and Tilney, N. L. (1982) Cyclosporin A allows expression of specific T suppressor lymphocytes *in vivo. Surg. Forum.*, **33**, 336
81. Hall, B. M., Jelbart, M. E. and Dorsch, S. E. (1985) Function of W3/25 + Th cells in rats with prolonged cardiac allograft survival after treatment with cyclosporine. *Transplant. Proc.*, **17**(1), 1372
82. Godden, U., Herbert, J., Stewart, R. D. and Roser, B. (1985) A novel cell type carrying both Th and Tc/s markers in the blood of cyclosporine-treated, allografted rats. *Transplantation*, **39**, 624
83. Wood, M. L. and Monaco, A. P. (1980) Suppressor cells in specific unresponsiveness to skin allografts in ALS-treated, marrow-injected mice. *Transplantation*, **29**, 196
84. Hutchinson, I. V. (1986) Suppressor T cells in allogeneic models. *Transplantation*, **41**, 547
85. Sprent, J. and Miller, J. F. A. P. (1974) Effect of recent antigen priming on adoptive immune responses. *J. Exp. Med.*, **139**, 1
86. Cranston, D., Wood, K. J. and Morris, P. J. (1988) Splenectomy and renal allograft survival in the rat. *Br. J. Surg.*, **75**, 18

6
Prevention of graft rejection by cyclosporin A in man

Michael C. Jones and Graeme R. D. Catto

INTRODUCTION

Preventing graft rejection remains the single most important challenge facing the clinician in organ transplantation. Since the immunological basis of rejection was first recognized, attempts have been made to modify the host response to foreign antigens in order to prevent rejection and possibly engender graft tolerance – a state in which the graft is no longer recognized as foreign by the host. This ideal is not yet possible in clinical practice but a variety of techniques have evolved to suppress the patient's immune response and prevent or suppress rejection. In the 1950s immunosuppression in the form of total-body irradiation was used, but because of associated morbidity and mortality was superseded in the 1960s by drug therapy – most commonly using combined treatment with azathioprine and prednisolone. This combination enabled renal transplantation to become a successful mode of therapy for patients with end-stage renal disease such that by the late 1970s it could be said to be the most effective and economical form of treatment[1], allowing the patient to return to near-normal health and activities.

The results of transplantation of other organs, however, were not so encouraging. Although Starzl and colleagues had reported the first human liver transplantation in 1963[2] and Barnard the first human cardiac allograft in 1967[3], neither technique had been widely adopted during the subsequent decade, apart from a flourish in cardiac transplantation in the months following the first case report. This loss of interest and cessation of cardiac transplantation programmes occurred because initial graft and patient survival rates were, even in the best surgical hands, not good. Only Shumway in Stanford, California, continued to perform cardiac transplantation on a regular basis.

Improved surgical techniques, early accurate diagnosis of rejection, and the use of anti-thymocyte globulin achieved a 1-year cardiac graft survival rate of 67% by 1979, compared to 22% in 1968[4]. These graft survival figures rekindled an interest in cardiac transplants, and programmes were commenced at Papworth and Harefield in the UK in the late 1970s. Only the development and clinical use of cyclosporin A (CsA), however, has led to the widespread use of transplantation in the treatment of organ failure affecting heart, lungs, liver and pancreas.

REJECTION

Organ transplantation other than that performed between identical siblings will always present antigens, associated with the graft, which are foreign to the recipient. These are the tissue or histocompatibility antigens. Such antigens are recognized by the graft recipient's immune system and stimulate the activation and associated proliferation of the immune cells. A subsequent attack on the foreign cell will be mediated through these antigens, which act as targets for the effector mechanisms of the host's immune reaction.

Organ transplantation obeys the rules for blood transfusion; recipient and donor are usually compatible for the ABO antigens (see section on liver transplantation). Apart from these red cell antigens, it is recognized that the most important antigens in terms of transplantation immunology are those generated by the major histocompatibility complex (MHC) which occupies a 2 centimorgan segment on the short arm of chromosome 6. Individual genes within or closely linked to the MHC control many of the complement components (Bf, C2, C4, C6 and C8) as well as the antigens which are important in transplantation. These antigens originally detected on the surface of white cells are known as the HLA antigens (H, human; L, leucocyte; A, the first, as so far only, series of histocompatibility antigen to be described). The HLA system is extremely polymorphic and controlled by six genetic loci – HLA-A, B, C, D/DR, DP and DQ, of which B and DR seem to be most important in organ transplantation. The genes are codominant and each nucleated cell may then have two antigens for each allele, one inherited from each parent.

HLA-A, B and C are termed class I antigens, whereas HLA-D/DR, DP and DQ are class II antigens. Both antigens are glycoproteins which consist of two chains. Class I antigens have a heavy chain of molecular weight 44 Kd which is linked non-covalently to β_2-microglobulin (MW 12 Kd). The C-terminal of the heavy chain is positioned within the cell. Class II antigens have an α (MW 34 Kd) and β (MW 29 Kd) chain in a non-covalent association. The C-terminals of both chains are located within the cell (Figure 6.1). Class I antigens are expressed on all nucleated cells and platelets, class II antigens are expressed on B lymphocytes, macrophages, monocytes, Langerhans cells of skin, dendritic cells, histiocytes and activated T cells. The distribution of class II antigens is important, as may be seen when considering the activation of T lymphocytes.

THE IMMUNE RESPONSE

A foreign antigen is presented to the T cell by an antigen-presenting cell (APC), usually a macrophage. The APC expresses class II antigen and presents

113

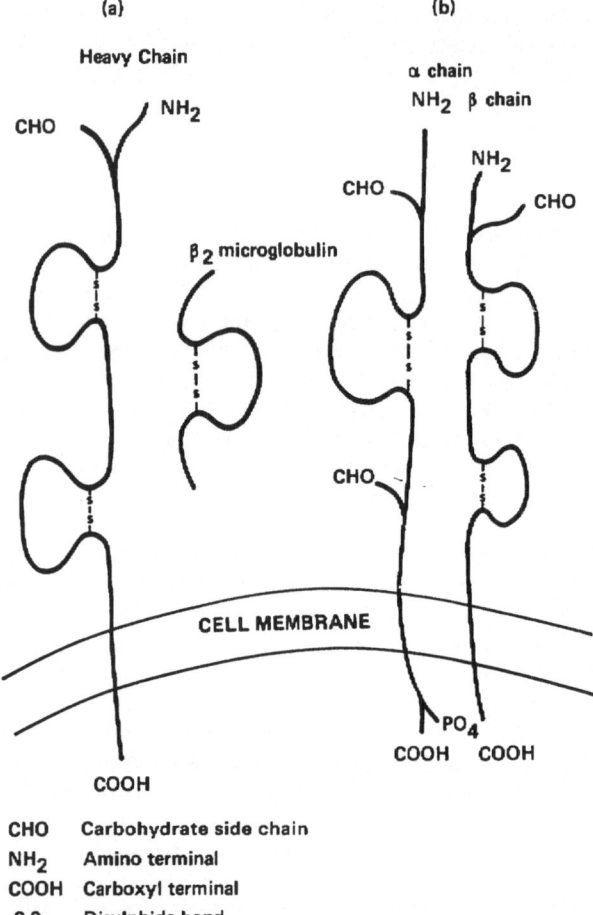

(a)   (b)

Heavy Chain

α chain

β chain

NH₂

β₂ microglobulin

CHO   Carbohydrate side chain
NH₂   Amino terminal
COOH   Carboxyl terminal
-S-S- Disulphide bond

Figure 6.1   Schematic representation of (a) class I and (b) class II antigens. S–S represents disulphide bonds

the foreign antigen in association with it. The recognition of foreign antigen and 'self' class II antigen triggers the cellular immune response leading to activation and proliferation of the T cells, thus emphasizing the importance of these cells in the immune mechanism. As well as being able to recognize the foreign antigen in association with its own MHC class II antigen, the T cell can recognize a foreign class II antigen alone with subsequent activation of an immune response. The T cells which recognize the foreign antigen in associated with self are of helper/inducer phenotype. When activated these cells undergo a biochemical change and secrete a number of substances (including interleukin-2 (IL-2)) termed lymphokines. Such activation of the T cell is aided by the production of interleukin-1 (IL-1) by the APC. The function of some of the important lymphokines in transplantation immunology are shown in Table 6.1. In general the lymphokines act by recruiting more cells into the immune response and activating an immune cascade to eliminate the foreign antigen. The specific reaction of T cells or the action of antibodies from B lymphocytes, primarily identify the antigen, and the associated inflammatory mediators, both cellular and chemical, destroy it.

Immune response in transplantation

Therefore in allograft rejection, as in any other form of immune response, antigens from the graft will be processed by the afferent limb of the immune response leading to activation of specific parts of the immune system, which in turn will lead to a reaction against the antigens presented these reactions are undertaken by the efferent limb of the immune response (Figure 6.2). The antigens from the graft may be presented in a variety of ways. 'Soluble' antigens, both from MHC antigens (class I and II) and other minor antigen systems, shed from the graft may be transported by the lymphatic or vascular systems to the spleen or other lymphoid aggregates where a specific immune response may develop. Similarly, antigens which remain associated with the graft may be recognized by circulating T and B lymphocytes and the primary immune response triggered *in situ*. Such antigens include the MHC class I and II antigens on nucleated graft cells, and MHC class I and II antigens on the vascular endothelium. When removed from the donor the graft is flushed with a solution to prevent vascular thromboses and to help preservation. Nevertheless, 'passenger cells' from the donor will still be present in the transplanted tissue. These cells – which are often highly immunogenic, expressing both class I and class II antigens – may be recognized by circulating lymphocytes and engender the host response. These mechanisms, if unchecked, can lead to acute rejection of the graft with its associated clinical manifestations, leading to the immunological destruction of 10–20% of all grafts in the first year[5].

Table 6.1 Lymphokines

Type	Effect
Macrophage-activating factor (MAF)	Enhances cytolytic activity of macrophages
Mononuclear phagocyte chemotactic factor (Migration inhibition factor)	Localization of macrophages
Interleukin-2	Promotes T cell clone proliferation
Interleukin-3	Colony-stimulating factor activity
Interferon (γ)	Inhibition of viral multiplication and as MAF
Mitogenic factor	T helper function
Lymphocyte-inhibitory factor	T suppressor function
B cell growth factor	Stimulates growth and differentiation of a B cell subset
Colony-stimulating factor	Supports growth and differentiation of monocytes

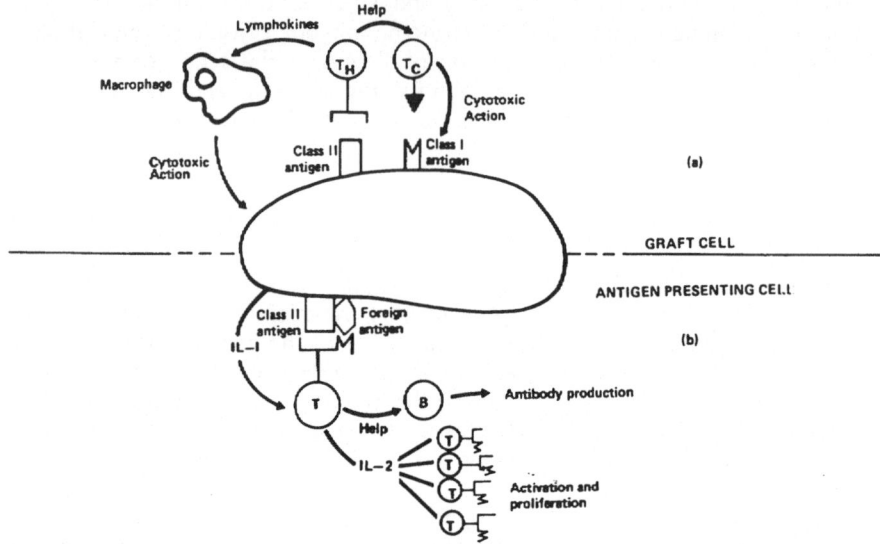

Figure 6.2 (a) Central cell represents graft cell. Class II antigen of donor is recognized by T helper (T_H) cell. Cytotoxic T cell (T_c) activated by help from T_H cell recognizes class I antigen and attacks graft cell. T_H also releases lymphokines to activate macrophages which contribute to the cytotoxic activity. (b) Central cell is antigen-presenting cell (APC) which has foriegn antigen associated with its own class II antigen. Interleukin-1 from the APC generates interleukin-2 production from the T cell leading to activation and proliferation of a T cell clone. In addition, T cell provides help for B cell antibody production. These developments are not mutually exclusive and during an immune response against an allograft all processes occur simultaneously

TYPES OF REJECTION

Rejection may be classified into three types – hyperacute, acute and chronic[6]. The immune mechanisms affecting human allografts have been best defined in association with the kidney, but similar mechanisms affect other vascularized grafts.

Hyperacute rejection

Hyperacute rejection is associated with the presence of preformed cytotoxic antibodies directed against donor antigens identified in the allografts. Such antibodies may have been stimulated by previous exposure to antigens in the form of pregnancy, previous transplantation or blood transfusion. In hyperacute rejection graft function usually ceases within the first 24 h, the organ becomes swollen and tender and the patient experiences fever with an associated leukocytosis and thrombocytopenia. The activation of the complement cascade by immune complexes leads to the generation of many mediators of inflammation, activates the coagulation system and leads to diffuse thrombus formation. Fibrin and fibrin degradation products appear in blood and urine, indicating active fibrin deposition with a subsequent marked

116

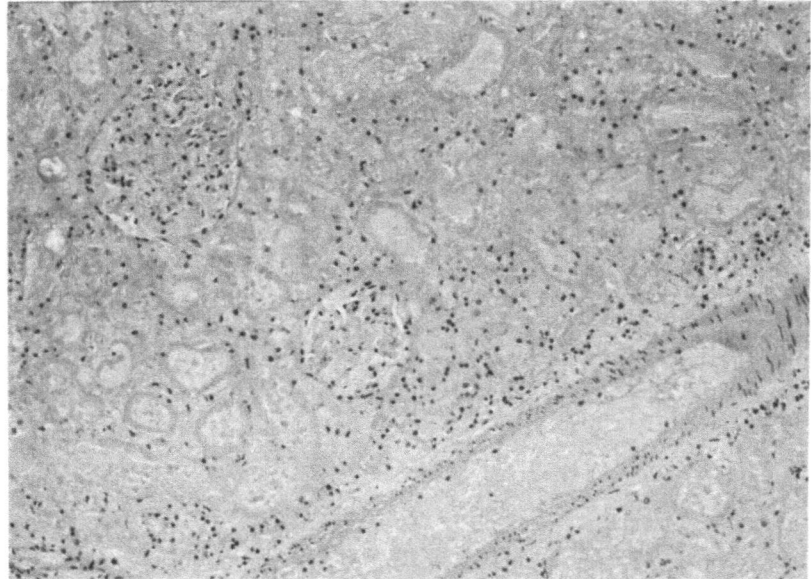

Figure 6.3 Hyperacute rejection. In this kidney removed several days after transplantation, there is infarction of the cortex. (H&E, x105)

deterioration in blood flow. Histological examination of such a kidney, as shown in Figure 6.3 reveals intense engorgement of the capillaries around the glomerulus and tubules, with aggregations of polymorphonuclear cells, red cells and platelets associated with thrombus formation. Immunopathological examination shows complement and antibody deposited in the same area.

There is no universally successful treatment for this type of rejection; anticoagulation with heparin has been tried but its benefit is questionable. Purified Malayan pit vipor venom has been used in a single human case with success[7], and intensive plasmapheresis has also been employed[8]. The best form of therapy is prevention. With the development of sensitive cross-matching techniques this form of rejection is now uncommon, although hyperacute rejection may still occur despite a negative cross-match[9].

Accelerated rejection

A subgroup of hyperacute rejection may be termed accelerated acute rejection, and usually occurs within the first 5 days of grafting. It is an antibody-mediated response and in terms of the immunological and inflammatory mechanisms observed relates more to hyperacute than to acute rejection.

Acute rejection

Acute rejection episodes, which may be experienced by up to 60% of patients, occur with greatest frequency during the first month following renal

117

transplantation[10]. They can and do occur, however, years after grafting. Prompt diagnosis and treatment is essential to minimize allograft damage. The clinical features experienced by the renal transplant patient on conventional immunosuppression, including fever and graft tenderness, are not so apparent when the patient receives CsA. Differentiation of rejection from CsA nephrotoxicity can be very difficult. This form of rejection has been intensively studied. Although many cell types are found the most important cellular element in acute allograft rejection is probably the T helper/inducer cell.

These cells, identified by the surface antigen T4, have a diversity of functions which include regulatory and effector mechanisms. T4 cells provide B cell help enhancing cytotoxic antibody production, but also induce suppressor cell production. The other major phenotypic group of T cells express the T8 antigen, the cytotoxic/suppressor cell. They are implicated in regulatory activity – suppressing both antibody synthesis and delayed-type hypersensitivity.

Histological examination of kidneys undergoing acute rejection demonstrates the various effects of activation of the immune system (Figure 6:4). Although the T cells are the important mediators of acute rejection, there is also marked interstitial oedema and intense focal infiltration with B lymphocytes, plasma cells and monocytes. An adverse prognostic feature is the presence of endothelial cell swelling of the glomerular capillaries. Sensitized T cells may be seen attached to the glomerular endothelium; thrombi and fibrinoid necrosis may subsequently develop.

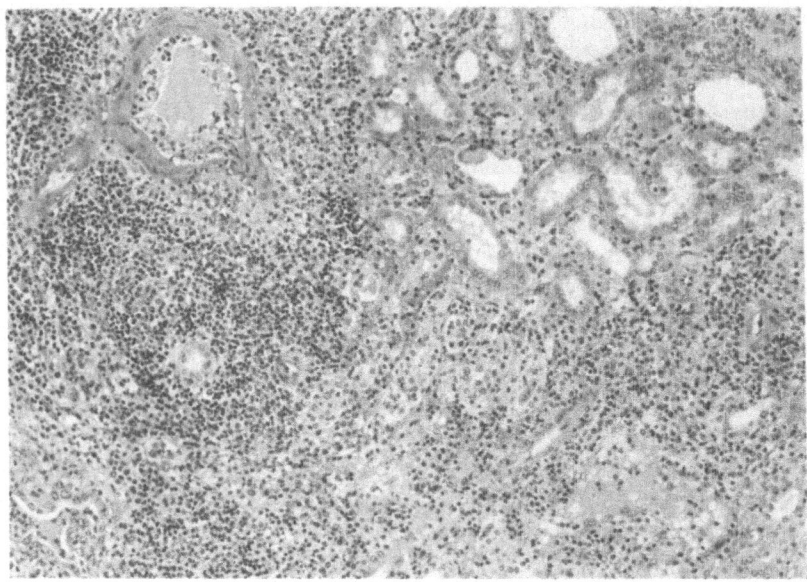

Figure 6.4 Acute (cellular) rejection. An extensive lymphoid infiltrate surrounds and infiltrates renal cortical tubules. Lymphoid cells are also present in the oedematous intima of an interlobular artery (top left). (H&E, x105)

Acute rejection may be treated in a variety of ways. Intravenous methylprednisolone 1 g daily for 3 days may successfully reverse approximately 75% of rejection episodes[11]. Alternatively, an increased dose of oral steroids commencing at 200 mg daily and reducing by 50 mg every 3 days to maintenance levels may also be effective[12]. Steroid-resistant acute rejection has previously been treated with anti-lymphocyte globulin, but more recently monoclonal antibodies have been used. OKT3 antibody directed against the pan-T cell antigen CD3 has been shown to be highly effective in reversing 94% of rejection episodes[13].

Chronic rejection

Chronic rejection occurs months to years after transplantation and probably represents a combination of factors which lead to progressive impairment of graft function and eventual failure. The immunological mechanisms involved have not been precisely identified; indeed it is likely that the renal injury of chronic rejection is due to both immunological damage and ischaemia. Clinically the patient may present with increasing hypertension, and is found to have deteriorating renal function; the most common cause of nephrotic syndrome after renal transplantation is chronic allograft rejection[14]. Histologically (Figure 6.5) there may be some evidence of cellular infiltration but the major features are interstitial fibrosis and thickening of the interlobular and arcuate vessels. The capillary turfs may show increased lobularity with

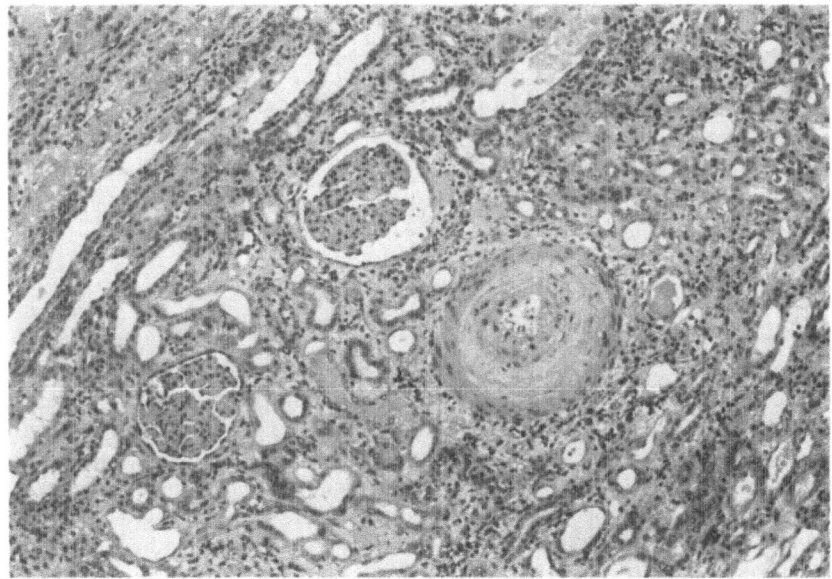

Figure 6.5 Chronic (vascular) rejection. Marked intimal fibrosis of an interlobular artery (centre right) has resulted in luminal narrowing with secondary atrophic changes in glomeruli and tubules. (H&E, x105)

expansion of the mesangial matrix, and the appearance may resemble mesangiocapillary glomerulonephritis. The glomerular size diminishes with time and the basement membrane becomes thickened. The underlying problem may represent a partially suppressed immune response with impaired T cell responses and with antibody/antigen complexes deposited in the graft. This low-grade immune response may generate a similarly low-grade inflammatory response which eventually leads to graft destruction. The impaired immune response may, of course, be related to the immunosuppressive regime prescribed to maintain graft function. In general, patients with chronic rejection do not respond to anti-rejection therapy. High-dose intravenous methylprednisolone may temporarily improve graft function but does not alter the eventual outcome.

REJECTION IN OTHER ORGANS

Rejection in other transplanted organs will present in a variety of ways related to the graft function.

Heart

In cardiac transplantation right heart catheterization and endomyocardial biopsies may be performed weekly during the first 4–6 weeks following transplantation, every second week for 6 weeks, monthly for 3 months and thereafter every 3 months. Using a combination of both clinical and histopathological data[15] the presence or absence of rejection is assessed. Mild interstitial mononuclear infiltrates are monitored carefully but without therapy unless more severe changes ensue. Moderate to severe monocyte infiltration, or the presence of myocyte necrosis, indicate a need for anti-rejection therapy which may take the form of pulsed intravenous methylprednisolone, anti-lymphocyte globulin or indeed OKT3. Chronic myocardial rejection resembles coronary arteriosclerosis and is diagnosed by right and left heart catheterization with coronary angiography.

Liver

Liver transplantation may be complicated by the three types of rejection mentioned above, although compared to renal transplantation the incidence is less. This may reflect the diminished expression of MHC class I and class II antigens on hepatocytes. Bile duct epithelium and sinusoids do express class II antigen, and in cases of rejection the cellular infiltrate is most marked in these areas. Acute rejection often initially presents as increasing biochemical abnormalities as the bilirubin, alkaline phosphatase and transaminase enzymes rise. These are non-specific findings, so the diagnosis is confirmed histologically[16]. Chronic rejection is manifest by progressive cholestasis and the so-called 'vanishing bile duct syndrome'. Acute liver rejection may be diagnosed when activated lymphocytes are found infiltrating the portal triads, and there is damage to bile duct epithelium and venous endothelium. As rejection becomes more severe the blood vessels become thrombosed and large areas of hepatocyte infarction may be seen.

Repeated biopsies may be used to monitor the response of acute rejection episodes to therapy. As with renal and cardiac allografts intravenous methyprednisolone may be effective in controlling the rejection but in cases of steroid resistance, OKT3 has been shown to be of considerable value[17].

Pancreas

Experience with pancreatic transplantation is more limited. There are many methods of performing pancreatic transplantation – from injection of islet cells into the portal vein to whole pancreatic grafts. A segmental pancreatic transplant, with a bladder anastomosis so that the urinary amylase can be monitored, is being increasingly undertaken. A drop in the urinary amylase concentration indicates pancreatic graft rejection and is a more accurate way of diagnosing rejection in a pancreatic allograft than is biopsy[18]. Many successful pancreatic allografts have also been performed, however, using other surgical techniques, including duct injection with neoprene or other polymers to promote atrophy of the exocrine part of the gland, and enteric drainage; the duct injection technique is, however, associated with a high incidence of late graft fibrosis and loss[19]. If biopsy is performed, a mononuclear cell infiltrate in the exocrine pancreas, or a vasculitis, may be noted; indeed it is believed that pancreatic rejection is initiated in the exocrine part of the gland[20]. The histological appearances of rejection in the pancreas are difficult to interpret as they may be similar to those found in pancreatitis, infection or associated with graft preservation techniques. Anti-rejection therapy is similar to that used in other types of organ transplantation.

IMMUNOSUPPRESSIVE AGENTS

In many areas of clinical practice prevention is better than cure. This is especially true when considering allograft rejection. Many experiments have demonstrated that it is difficult to inhibit an immune response which has been activated, whereas with appropriate therapy activation can be diminished. There are four major immunosuppressive agents in current clinical practice that are used to prevent activation of the immune response. These are CsA, azathioprine, prednisolone and, to a lesser extent, the various anti-lymphocytic antibodies. Cyclophosphamide has also been used but does not yield superior results to azathioprine in transplantation[21] and is both toxic and myelosuppressive. It is, however, the drug of choice in Wegener's granulomatosis[22] and therefore may have a role in renal transplantation if the patient suffers from this disease.

Cyclosporin A

CsA inhibits lymphocyte activation at numerous points in the cell cycle. Its precise modes of action are considered elsewhere. It may be administered

121

orally or intravenously although absorption is poor with a bio-availability of 20–50%. The maximum plasma level is reached 2–4 h after an oral dose. *In vitro* CsA is distributed among all the blood components including erythrocytes (55%), lymphocytes (5%), granulocytes (5%) and plasma (35%)[23]. As CsA is hydrophobic it must be dissolved in an organic solvent; the present preparation uses an olive-oil-based solution. This is not very palatable, and it is recommended that the patient takes the oral preparation in milk or juice. Large capsules of CsA have recently become available.

Over 70% of an oral dose is metabolized by the liver[24], utilizing the P-450 cytochrome oxidase system. Drugs which enhance this enzyme system may thus be associated with increased CsA clearance and possible allograft rejection[25]. The parent compound and metabolites are excreted into the bile, and usually eliminated in faeces but, enterohepatic circulation has been demonstrated[26] after transplantation.

Whole-blood trough levels are measured post-transplantation using either a radioimmunoassay or high-performance liquid chromatography. The initial polyclonal radioimmunoassay has recently been supplemented by a mono-clonal assay for the parent CsA molecule. Drug monitoring demonstrated that intramuscular administration is associated with poor and erratic drug absorption, and this route of administration is therefore no longer used[27]. Some centres have adopted a twice-daily dosage regime to achieve more uniform blood concentrations after oral administration.

Azathioprine

Azathioprine is the imidazole derivative of 6-mercaptopurine, which is the analogue of the purine base, hypoxanthine[28]. After absorption by the intravenous or oral route, azathioprine is converted to 6-mercaptopurine, which in turn is converted to thioinosinic acid. This compound competes with inosinic acid for conversion to xanthylic acid, an important step in DNA synthesis. The overall effect is to diminish DNA and RNA synthesis, *de novo* purine and protein synthesis and subsequently lymphocyte proliferation. This seems to effect mainly the T lymphocyte population and explains the efficacy of azathioprine in transplantation. Unfortunately, it can cause marrow suppression and has been associated with a variety of hepatic lesions including hepatitis and veno-occlusive disease[29].

Prednisolone

Prednisolone, and the other corticosteroids, penetrate the cell membrane[30] and bind to a cytoplasmic receptor in the lymphocyte. The steroid/receptor complex is transported to the nucleus of the cell and there inhibits DNA and RNA synthesis. In turn, macrophage-dependent liberation of interleukin 1 (IL-1) is attenuated and clonal expansion of antigen-activated cytotoxic T lymphocytes is prevented by inhibition of IL-2 production[31]. In addition, the anti-inflammatory action of corticosteroids diminishes macrophage chemotaxis and phagocytosis, reduces local prostaglandin production and superoxide radical release[32]. Steroids do have well-defined adverse effects (Table 6.2). In renal transplantation these have been greatly reduced by the pioneering work from Belfast indicating that low-dose prednisolone (20 mg/day) is as effective in reducing graft rejection as high dose (2 mg/kg daily)[11]. Prednisolone is usually given in a once-daily dose but has been administered on alternate days in an attempt to reduce the risks of infection[33] and growth retardation in children[34]. This latter approach, however, may be associated with decreasing glomerular filtration rates[35].

Anti-lymphocyte globulin

Anti-lymphocyte globulin prepared in rabbits, goats or horses by the injection of human splenocytes, lymphoblasts or thymocytes, is administered intravenously. It causes a lymphopenia and the dose is adjusted[36] to maintain a lymphocyte count of $0.5-2.5 \times 10^9/l$. There is, however, an increased risk of viral and fungal[37] infections, there may be significant batch-to-batch variations in potency, and the patient will receive a substantial amount of irrelevant globulin. Anti-lymphocyte globulins have been given prophylactically in transplantation – the largest experience of their use being in North America.

Monoclonal antibodies

OKT3, the previously mentioned monoclonal antibody, is not generally used prophylactically in renal transplantation as it is highly immunogenic and both the duration of therapy and the possibility of repeated courses are limited by the development of allotypic or idiotypic antibodies[38]. Whilst conventional anti-lymphocyte globulins are less immunogenic, repeated intravascular administration of any foreign protein may lead to sensitization and the risk of immunological reactions to any subsequent course of therapy.

TRANSPLANTATION RESULTS

Renal transplantation

Kidney transplantation was first successfully performed in 1954 between identical twins[39]. The subsequent development of immunosuppressive tech-

Table 6.2 Complications of steroid therapy

Growth retardation	Diabetes mellitus
Impaired wound healing	Peptic ulceration
Cushingoid appearance	Hypertension
Osteoporosis	Pancreatitis
Myopathy (especially proximal)	Colonic perforation
Hirsutism	Malignancy
Acne	Increased risk of infection
Cataracts	

niques enabled cadaveric renal transplantation to become established as the treatment of choice for patients with end-stage renal failure. One-year graft survival rates of around 60% were reported using a combination of azathioprine and prednisolone as maintenance immunosuppression.

During this period the so-called 'centre effect' became apparent. The chance of successful renal allografting was related to the centre in which the transplant was performed. In Belfast, graft survival rates of 78% at 1 year were reported using azathioprine and prednisolone alone; results from other units were, however, not so impressive, resulting in the overall average 1-year graft survival of 60%. At 5 and 10 years graft survival rates of 68% and 52.5% were reported by the Belfast group; these results compare well with those obtained by other units using CsA[40]. Figure 6.6 shows the actuarial graft survival of the Canadian multicentre trial over 5 years in patients treated with CsA. The data demonstrate that early graft function indicates that the chance of subsequent graft survival is improved[41]. This trial also showed that mismatching for B and DR HLA loci, increased donor age and presensitization were risk factors for graft loss.

Adjunctive anti-lymphocyte globulin with azathioprine and prednisolone improved the average graft survival rate to about 75–80% but was associated with increased infection rates[37]. Improving surgical techniques led to a slow

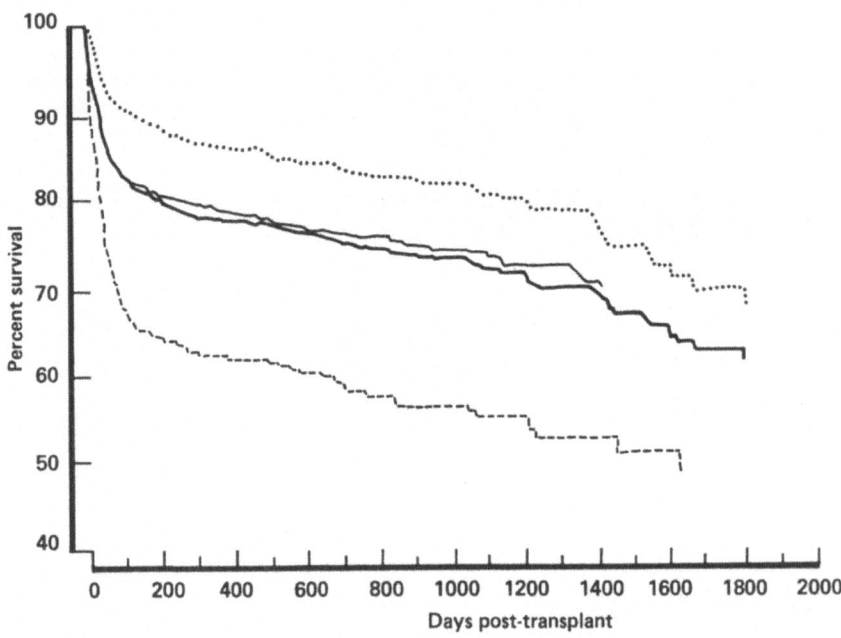

Figure 6.6 Actuarial graft survival rates in the total population of transplant patients with complete data (—), those divided into good (····) or poor (–––) early graft function, and in those with incomplete data —). (Reproduced from reference 41, with permission of the authors and publishers)

124

improvement in graft survival but rejection remained the major cause of graft loss. Attempts made to improve graft survival by minimizing antigenic differences between donor and recipient by good tissue typing, showed some benefit[42,43]. Furthermore it was reported somewhat paradoxically that exposure to foreign antigens, in the form of pre-transplant blood transfusions, could improve subsequent renal graft survival[44,45].

The CsA era

In 1978 Calne reported a renal graft survival rate of 86% at 1 year in poorly HLA matched patients[46]. This was a significant improvement in graft survival in the Cambridge unit and demonstrated that CsA, a then new immunosuppressive agent, was likely to prove of clinical value. Such good results led to the development of randomized clinical trials, comparing CsA with or without prednisolone against conventional immunosuppression therapy using azathioprine plus prednisolone combined in some centres with anti-lymphocyte globulins. Not all such trials confirmed a statistically significant improvement in renal allograft survival using CsA. The large European and Canadian multicentre trials, however, did show significantly higher 1-year graft survival figures in patients receiving CsA (72% vs 52%[47] and 80.4% vs 64%[48], respectively).

In the European trial the graft recipients were randomized to the trial only if, postoperatively, they achieved a diuresis of greater than 50 ml/h so that there could be a true trial of the immmunosuppressive effect of CsA whilst avoiding the common complication of nephrotoxicity that would more commonly occur in anuric patients. CsA was used without adjuvant immunosuppressive therapy in this trial but methylprednisolone was given for rejection episodes. In the Canadian multicentre trial CsA was given in combination with oral prednisolone. In both studies the improved graft survival rates in the CsA-treated groups were maintained at 3 years (European 66% vs 42%[49], Canadian 69% vs 58%[50]), and in the European study (55% vs 40%[51]) at 5 years. It is of note that, by 5 years, of the 117 patients originally commenced on CsA in the European study 43 (37%) had been converted to conventional immunosuppressive therapy and 54% of these still had functioning grafts. Only 34 patients were receiving CsA alone of the 64 patients with functioning grafts in the CsA groups. Furthermore, renal function was significantly poorer in the CsA group (mean serum creatinine 211 μmol/l vs 163 μmol/l).

The early trials that did not confirm superior renal graft survival using CsA require further examination. There were significant differences in the patients selected for these studies which were remarkable for the graft survival figures in the control groups of approximately 80%. These results were superior to those generally achieved using conventional therapy in cadaveric renal transplants. One of these studies performed in Minnesota used splenectomized multiply-transfused recipients, and compared CsA/prednisolone with azathioprine/prednisolone/anti-lymphocyte globulin regimes[52] In a recent follow-up review, graft survival figures after a mean of 47 months were 70% (CsA/prednisolone) vs 63% (azathioprine/prednisolone/ALG) – a difference in survival rates which is not statistically significant[53]. Moreover, 71% of those patients in the CsA group required a significant dose reduction of CsA with the addition of azathioprine or a switch to azathioprine therapy because of CsA nephrotoxicity. The mean serum creatinine concentration was significantly higher in the CsA group (1.73 ± 0.6 mg/dl vs 1.49 ± 0.59 mg/dl).

Overall the majority of trials have shown improved graft survival with the use of CsA. As in the European and Minnesota studies, however, the patients treated with CsA have higher mean serum creatinine concentrations, reflecting the nephrotoxic effects of this drug. Apart from the overall improvement in graft survival in renal transplantation, other factors which adversely affect graft outcome in conventionally treated patients have been reduced by CsA. Recipients over 55 years of age[54], strong immune responders[55], black patients and patients with a positive historical cross-match[56], have better graft survival when given CsA. Graft survival rates, however, are slightly poorer than those obtained in patients without these risk factors. HLA matching of recipient and donor in renal transplantation remains important to many units even when CsA is given. In the most recent analysis of the collaborative transplant study, Opelz demonstrated that matching for both HLA-B and -DR results in a significantly improved graft survival[57]. However, data from Minneapolis[58] and Scandinavia[59] show no benefit of matching for HLA-B or -DR.

The role of pre-transplant blood transfusions, however, remains controversial. Opelz initially suggested that the so-called blood transfusion effect was still apparent even if CsA was used[60]. Many centres therefore continued to transfuse dialysis patients in an attempt to improve subsequent graft survival. In a later report Opelz suggested that the blood transfusion effect was no longer demonstrable, but voiced caution that further randomized studies should be performed before the transfusion policies were abandoned[61]. The results of kidney re-transplantation using CsA have recently been reviewed, showing that on average second and third renal allografts demonstrate 10–30% lower graft survival rates than first grafts[62]. This reflects the importance of the immunological responsiveness of the recipient, although the 20-month graft survival rates of 58.5% on CsA compares favourably with the 40% obtained with conventional immunosuppression.

There are conflicting reports on the frequency and severity of acute rejection episodes. Many, but not all, trials have shown a lower frequency of these episodes in patients receiving CsA[52,55,63,47,48]. In living related transplantation, where the donor and recipient are likely to be haploidentical, CsA improves graft survival with graft survival rates of about 90% in the CsA group and 80% for those given conventional immunosuppression. Furthermore, in one centre using kidneys from living donors mismatched at two HLA haplotypes, the 1-year graft survival rate was 89%[64]. Another additional benefit from the use of cyclosporin is the ability to use the kidneys of cadaveric donors aged below 6 years with 85% 1-year graft survival rates[5]. This had not been possible using conventional immunosuppression.

Heart transplantation

No long-term, controlled, randomized trials comparing CsA with conventional immunosuppression have been reported in cardiac transplantation. However, a study from Richmond, Virginia, randomly assigned 25 patients to receive either conventional immunosuppression using azathioprine, anti-thymocyte globulin, prednisolone and pre-transplantation transfusions or CsA and prednisolone. The mortality was not different between the groups and there was no difference in rejection episodes per patient. Patients receiving conventional immunosuppression were found to have a greater number of serious infections, whereas those receiving CsA had a greater incidence of hypertension and impaired renal function[65]. A study of 56 heart transplants performed at the University of Arizona also compared conventional immuno-suppression with CsA. The first 32 patients in this trial received conventional immunosuppression while the subsequent 24 received CsA and prednisolone. Overall survival was similar in both groups but fewer rejection and infection episodes were recorded in survivors receiving the CsA therapy. Renal impairment and hypertension, however, were more commonly reported in this group[66].

Retrospective analysis of the results obtained by Shumway, who had continued to perform cardiac transplantation regularly during the 1970s, did demonstrate an improvement in graft survival at 1 and 2 years in the patients treated with CsA (80% vs 60% at 1 year, 75% vs 55% at 2 years)[67]. This group found that the graft survival rate had been achieved in association with a reduction in steroid doses and therefore fewer steroid side-effects were experienced. In particular, the postoperative mortality due to infectious complications was reduced. A further report using Stanford data recognizes the significance of heart transplantation as a modality for treatment of patients suffering from severe cardiac disease. This shows that patients accepted for transplantation, but for whom a donor did not become available, suffered 100% mortality rate at 1 year[68]. The 1-year patient survival figure using conventional immunosuppression was approximately 62%, a figure which is similar to the 5-year survival rate of patients immunosuppressed with CsA. A recent report from Papworth Hospital in England showed similar survival rates to those achieved in Stanford at 1 and 2 years when using CsA and their 5-year survival rate was 62.9%[69]. However, it was again noted that renal impairment was evident in all those who survived for at least 2 years.

The success of heart transplantation in the adult population has encouraged the development of cardiac transplantation in children and adolescents. Up to March 1986, 14 children aged between 2 and 16 had received cardiac transplants in the University of Pittsburgh, eight of whom had survived for between 4 months and 4 years after their transplantation and managed to return to age-appropriate activities[70]. Complications after paediatric cardiac transplantation include infection and rejection; as in adults both could prove fatal. Results from Philadelphia, however, showed that the majority of patients would survive their transplantation and return to normal function and, importantly, were found to have no developmental delays[71]. The impact of pre-transplant blood transfusion and HLA matching has not been extensively studied in cardiac allografts. A study from Texas, however, has demonstrated a beneficial effect from both pre-transplant blood transfusion and HLA matching on subsequent patient survival[72].

Some pathological processes which affect the heart may also involve other organs. The advent of CsA therapy, however, has enabled multiple-organ transplants to be performed with success. In homozygous familial hypercholesterolaemia there is rapidly progressive arteriosclerosis which would recur in a transplanted heart unless the liver were also replaced. Starzl reported the first case of heart/liver transplantation for this condition in 1984[73]. Many other multi-system diseases have proved amenable to multi-organ transplantation, and most of these would not have been thought appropriate prior to CsA. In heart transplantation the introduction of CsA has been associated with a reduction in serious morbidity; hence a shorter hospital stay and therefore reduced cost of transplant programmes quite apart from their increased success[74].

Liver transplantation

The use of CsA in hepatic transplantation has dramatically improved allograft survival. First used by Calne, and subsequently by Starzl, 1-year graft survival rates approximately doubled from 30 to 35% when the most common postoperative immunosuppressive regime consisted of azathioprine, prednisolone and anti-lymphocyte globulin, to 60–70% using a regime of CsA and low-dose prednisolone[75]. This improvement in survival rate with CsA is maintained over the years after grafting (Figure 6.7). The 5-year survival rate following hepatic transplantation in Starzl's unit is 62% in CsA-treated patients compared to 20% in those receiving conventional immunosuppression[76]. A diminution in the frequency and severity of rejection episodes was noted, as had also been reported with renal transplantation; only 25% of patients experienced such episodes[77]. These episodes, however, could lead to failure of the organ requiring re-transplantation. The most common indications for hepatic transplantation are biliary atresia, post-necrotic cirrhosis, primary biliary cirrhosis and sclerosing cholangitis[78]. Primary liver malignancy is also amenable to treatment by hepatic transplantation. Unfortunately, in these latter patients tumour recurrence is both common and rapid. Transplantation of the liver is also being increasingly used for patients suffering from inborn errors of metabolism, including patients with Wilson's disease, tyrosinaemia, α_1-anti-trypsin deficiency, glycogen storage disease, haemochromatosis and, as mentioned above, familial hypercholesterolaemia. Survival in these patients is excellent in one study at about 75% at 5 years. In this study 313 primary orthotopic liver transplants using CsA as the major immunosuppression agent, and 170 using azathioprine and steroids, were reported. Twenty per cent of patients required re-transplantation for rejection, technical failure or primary graft failure. Only four out of 21 patients receiving conventional immunosuppression following re-transplantation survived for 6 months. In comparison to this, 68 patients received re-transplants using CsA, 31 survived for at least 1 year, suggesting that an aggressive approach to re-transplantation is justified.

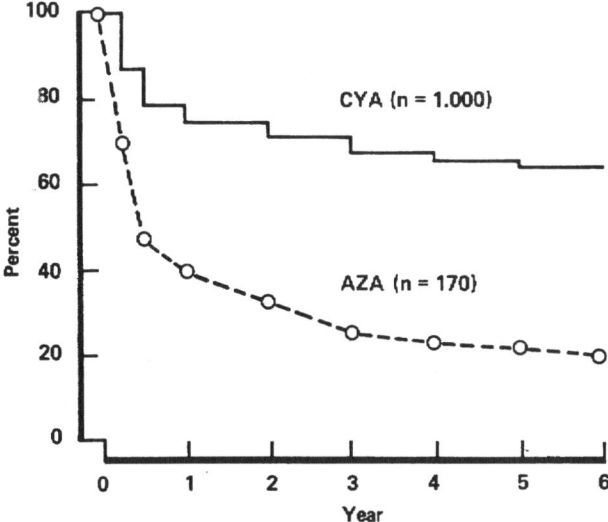

Figure 6.7 Overall actuarial survival rates of 1000 patients treated with CsA—steroid therapy in comparison with overall actual survival rates of 170 patients treated with azathioprine—steroid therapy following hepatic transplantation. (From ref. 76, with permission of the publisher)

Nephrotoxicity in patients receiving hepatic transplants does not seem to have been a significant problem and, as reported by Starzl, only 5% of adult patients in his series[79] have a serum creatinine greater than 117 mol/l. Results of hepatic transplantation in children have been shown to be at least as good as those achieved in adults, and many of these paediatric patients have tolerated very high doses of CsA without experiencing nephrotoxicity and were able to achieve a normal growth pattern[80]. A problem peculiar to hepatic transplantation is the altered absorption and metabolism of orally administered CsA, possibly because of poor hepatic metabolism of the drug. Monitoring whole-blood levels of CsA after hepatic transplantation is important as the reduced clearance in hepatic dysfunction increases the risk of nephrotoxicity, but similarly adequate absorption of the oral drug has to be demonstrated to avoid graft rejection[81]. Hepatic transplantation results are not affected by tissue-typing or matching, and indeed may be performed across ABO blood group barriers. This has enabled the development of emergency liver transplantation for fulminant hepatitis. A recent study reported the results in 17 patients transplanted between January 1986 and April 1987. Twelve of these patients were alive 2—15 months after transplantation[82]. Overall, the development of hepatic transplantation with improvements in surgical technique and postoperative care, combined with an effective immunosuppressive agent in the form of CsA, means that the 85% of adults who survive surgery are able to resume normal activity[83].

129

Heart/lung transplantation

Overall the results in renal, cardiac and hepatic transplantation have improved by between 20% and 40% with the use of CsA. In heart/lung and pancreatic transplantation, however, the CsA effect has been even more marked. Three human heart/lung transplants were performed between 1968 and 1979 with very poor patient survival. Only when CsA became available was such transplantation again performed in 1981. Survival rates at 1 year are now in the order of 65% using a combination of CsA, azathioprine, prednisolone and occasionally anti-thymocyte globulin[84]. At 5 years the success rate is 30–40%, the major cause of late failure being bronchiolitis obliterans, a manifestation of chronic rejection affecting the lungs. One study has shown that the introduction of azathioprine in addition to CsA steroid slows the rate of progression of bronchiolitis obliterans, and many units do use this form of triple therapy[85]. In a further attempt to avoid this complication HLA matching has been investigated, and it was found that patients with either one or no mismatch at the HLA-A antigen had a tendency towards less severe bronchiolitis obliterans than patients with two mismatches[86]. The increased success of heart/lung transplantation, therefore, during the CsA era, has offered patients suffering from otherwise universally fatal conditions such as Eisenmenger's syndrome, or primary pulmonary hypertension, a realistic chance of curative therapy[87].

Pancreatic transplantation

In pancreatic transplantation 1-year graft survival rates were approximately 3% between 1966 and 1977. Since CsA was introduced the 1-year graft survival rate has significantly improved, although the extent of improvement is affected by the surgical technique used. Although in many cases pancreatic transplantation is performed in insulin-dependent diabetics to replace the destroyed native islets of Langerhans, islet cell graft itself has not yet been very successful. If segmental or whole pancreatic grafting is undertaken the exocrine secretions have to be controlled either by drainage into the bladder or gut, or by injection of the pancreatic duct by polymers. Pancreatic grafts are also much more susceptible to vascular thrombosis or infection, threatening the viability of the graft. Techniques developed to combat these risks include the use of anti-coagulant protocols which may include single-dose heparin, aspirin and dipyridamole[88]. Prophylaxis against infection is achieved using a variety of antibiotic regimes. These developments, including CsA-based immunosuppression, have enabled the Minneapolis group to report a 72% 1-year graft survival rate when using living related donors. The overall 1-year graft survival rates between 1983 and 1986, which were reported to the International Pancreas Registry, showed minor variations according to the surgical technique used. One-year graft survival is 50% for urinary diversion, 41% for enteric diversion and 44% for duct-injected grafts[89]. The attrition rate for these grafts, especially those with duct injection, is high, and although results continue to improve pancreatic grafts which have survived longer than 5 years remain relatively few. As diabetes may be associated with failure of other organs, most noticeably the kidney, pancreatic transplantation is often performed in conjunction with renal transplantations. One-year kidney graft survival in these patients is similar to that achieved in the general diabetic population – about 64% on CsA therapy. Sutherland and Moudry[89] have commented on the effect pancreatic transplantation has had on other diabetic complications, and have found that neuropathy generally improved whereas retinopathy was not affected. The microscopic lesions of diabetic nephropathy in the patient's native kidneys were also seen to regress. This, however, did not correlate with an improvement in renal function whilst the patients were receiving CsA. Indeed, a further study showed that the administration of CsA after pancreatic transplantation in non-uraemic diabetic patients could produce a decline in glomerular infiltration rate which, after the initial fall, became stable, albeit at a lower level[90]. A more recent study looking at the effects of pancreatic transplantation and diabetic neuropathy attributed the improvement in neuronal function after pancreatic and renal transplantation to the relief of uraemia, concluding that normoglycaemia for 2 years after transplantation did not reverse the diabetic neuropathy to an important extent[91].

ADVERSE EFFECTS OF CsA

Although there is no doubt that the use of cyclosporin has generally improved survival of the various vascularized allografts, treatment is not without troublesome side-effects, the most notable of which is nephrotoxicity. This has been apparent from the earliest trials and is related to the dose and whole-blood trough levels. The problem may be especially troublesome after renal transplantation when the presentation of the patient with deteriorating graft function and decreasing urine volumes may be related either to acute rejection or CsA nephrotoxicity. The problem is compounded by the fact that the classical clinical rejection picture of a patient with pyrexia, hypertension and graft tenderness is seen much less frequently in CsA-treated renal allograft recipients. Nephrotoxicity has also been described in patients receiving bone marrow, liver and cardiac allografts; indeed one of the reports of CsA in cardiac transplantation revealed that two patients, from a population of 32, had developed end-stage renal disease after their cardiac allograft, and this deterioration in renal function was attributed solely to their CsA therapy[92].

In renal transplantation a number of ways have been developed to differentiate between acute rejection and CsA nephrotoxicity in the patient with deteriorating graft function. An attempt to correlate whole-blood trough CsA levels with rejection or nephrotoxicity showed that rejection episodes occurred at a median of 5 weeks after transplant surgery compared with the median of only 2 weeks for nephrotoxicity. Mean whole-blood CsA levels were 471 ng/ml in the group experiencing rejection and 891 ng/ml for the nephrotoxicity group (using a therapeutic range of 400–800 ng/ml measured by radioimmunoassay[93]). However, two of the 36 patients who were diagnosed as suffering rejection had an average level above 800 ng/ml. The diagnosis of rejection or nephrotoxicity was made retrospectively according to the response to therapy. As it is recognized that a proportion of patients may have both nephrotoxicity and rejection, it is apparent that whole-blood trough CsA levels provide only a rough guide of immunosuppression. It is, however, well recognized that an individual patient developing renal allograft dysfunction is more likely to be suffering from nephrotoxicity if there has been a recent sudden rise in trough CsA levels.

Unfortunately, conventional histopathological examination of a transplant biopsy may not be able to differentiate between rejection and nephrotoxicity. Fine-needle aspiration biopsies have demonstrated that class II MHC antigen expression in the cortical tubular cells increases more during rejection than CsA nephrotoxicity[94]. At the time of fine-needle aspiration biopsy interstitial pressure can also be measured by manometry, and it is suggested that an interstitial pressure exceeding 40 mmHg is indicative of acute rejection[95]. Both these techniques give some indication of the likely cause of allograft dysfunction, but cannot be regarded as providing the definitive diagnosis. The development of computer programs to take account of the patients' haemotocrit in relation to the whole-blood CsA concentration may make the differentiation of rejection from nephrotoxicity easier[96]. The release of urinary enzymes, especially N-acetyl-β-D-glucosaminidase, may also assist in the diagnosis of rejection[97].

Kahan developed an algorithm (Table 6.3) which takes into account the clinical history, physical signs of rejection, the overall clinical picture including biochemistry, perfusion of the kidneys as assessed by technetium 99 DTPA scans, urinary lymphocytes and trough serum CsA levels. This algorithm provides an assessment of the likelihood of nephrotoxicity and acute rejection for the individual patient[98]. In view of the concern that CsA nephrotoxicity may be progressive and irreversible, as demonstrated by the unfortunate cardiac transplantation patients who presented with normal renal function but eventually required dialysis[92], longer-term studies were undertaken to assess pathological changes in renal allografts treated with CsA. It was found that the degree of interstitial fibrosis correlated with high cumulative CsA dose during the first 6 months of treatment, as well as with the number of episodes of acute CsA nephrotoxicity[99]. These findings were confirmed in a more recent study comparing histological appearances in patients given either CsA or azathioprine; the increase in interstitial fibrosis in the CsA-treated group was found only 6 months after transplantation[100].

Dosage regimes

Nephrotoxicity and the long-term expense of CsA have led to many changes in dosage regimes, including conversion of patients from treatment with CsA to azathioprine and prednisolone. Studies in renal transplantation comparing graft survival rates in patients converted from CsA therapy to conventional immunosuppressive therapy are discussed subsequently.

Even from the earliest study there has been no agreement between units on the need for adjunctive therapy. In the first reported study Calne had used CsA as the sole initial immunosuppressive agent[46]. Initially it was administered

Table 6.3 Kahan's algorithm

Parameter	Percentage likelihood of	
	Nephrotoxicity	*Rejection*
CsA level	> 75	10–25
> 250 ng/ml ₹IA		
< 100 ng/ml RIA	10–25	50–75
Urinary output decrease		
< 25%	50–75	10–25
25–50%	25–50	25–50
> 50%	10–25	50–75
Signs of rejection physically	0–10	50–75
Adverse donor conditions	50–75	10–25
Rate of serum creatinine rise		
Fast	25–50	50–75
Slow	50–75	25–50
Extent of serum creatinine rise		
< 25%	> 75	25–50
25–50%	25–50	25–50
> 50%	25–50	50–75
Urea/creatinine ratio of 20/1	50–75	10–25
Decreased perfusion by radionuclide	10–25	50–75
Second transplants	10–25[a]	50–75
Time past transplant		
< 40 days	25–50	> 75
> 40 days	50–75	10–25
Urinary lymphocytes		
> 20%	10–25	50–75

[a] Except where patient high drug absorber and CsA used for first transplant
From ref. 98, with permission from the publishers

intramuscularly 25 mg kg^{-1} day^{-1} for the first 2 or 3 days, and orally thereafter, with subsequent slow tapering of dose. Many of these patients, however, developed anuria or oliguria, perhaps related to rejection, and additional treatment with a cyclophosphamide derivative and prednisolone was thus added to the CsA regime. This, however, led to a high incidence of infection, and lymphomas occurred in three patients[101]. A modified regime of 17.5 mg kg^{-1} day^{-1} CsA was adopted, and the intramuscular mode of administration discontinued. Only patients with an initial diuresis entered the randomized trial to receive CsA alone or azathioprine plus prednisolone.

Starzl used CsA with adjuvant steroid therapy in renal transplantation. He commenced with 17.5 mg kg^{-1} day^{-1}, gave the patient a 1 g bolus of methylprednisolone during surgery, and prednisolone was started at 200 or 160 mg a day and tapered within 1 week to a maintenance of 10–20 mg a day[102]. A similar regime was used by Starzl in his hepatic transplantation series. In cardiac transplantation the Stanford group commenced with a starting cyclosporin dose of 18 mg kg^{-1} day^{-1} given intramuscularly or intravenously at first, then orally; the patients were also given low-dose prednisolone and a short course of anti-thymocyte globulin[103]. In the Pittsburgh series of cardiac transplantation the initial daily dose of cyclosporin was again 17.5 mg kg^{-1} day^{-1} orally but in view of the observed renal impairment this was subsequently modified[14] to 10 mg $kg^{-1}\,day^{-1}$. From a relatively small number of variations in therapy, there is now a bewildering array of regimes, varying from CsA monotherapy with lower dosages, to therapy combined CsA with azathioprine, prednisolone and anti-lymphocyte globulin, although a consensus of opinion suggests that CsA should be used in lower dosage: a maximum of 14 mg $kg^{-1}\,day^{-1}$ as a starting dose reduced to 5–6 mg $kg^{-1}\,day^{-1}$ by day 180 after transplantation[98], and in many centres the initial CsA dose is often less than 10 mg $kg^{-1}\,day^{-1}$. Some transplant units now use an induction regime consisting of CsA in low doses, prednisolone, azathioprine and polyclonal or monoclonal antibodies; others avoid the use of CsA for the first few days after transplantation using prednisolone, azathioprine and polyclonal or monoclonal anti-thymocyte globulin. The induction therapy is then modified with withdrawal of the antibodies leading to therapy with CsA and prednisolone with or without azathioprine. Similarly in cardiac and renal transplantation some units avoid the use of CsA for the first 3 days after transplantation in an attempt to avoid renal and hepatic injury. Indeed, the aim of all the immunosuppressive regimes is to minimize the nephrotoxicity and hepatotoxicity of CsA whilst providing adequate immunosuppression during the immediate post-transplantation period[105].

DELAYED GRAFT FUNCTION

It has been reported that CsA may delay the onset of graft function in those patients whose kidneys fail to function immediately. This may be related to CsA-associated reduced renal blood flow[16], but is also associated with prolonged cold ischaemic times, prolonged anastomotic time and increasing age of the donor[107]. A recent study has shown that patients with delayed graft function have significantly higher serum creatinine concentrations at 1 month after transplantation, although actuarial graft survival rate and mean serum creatinine concentrations at 1 year were not adversely affected[108]. The results obtained in this study contrast with those obtained in the Canadian multicentre trial (Figure 6.6) where poor early graft function led to the loss of 5–10% of transplanted kidneys. In an attempt to decrease the time of delayed graft function anti-lymphocyte globulin has been advocated, but the use of azathioprine plus prednisolone in the immediate postoperative period has been shown to give equivalent graft survival. The azathioprine regime, however, was associated with a greater number of rejection episodes[109]. All patients were converted to CsA therapy when graft function was established. These regimes, however, have the theoretical disadvantage of losing the influence of CsA during the critical phase when the T-helper cell is first exposed to foreign antigen, although this does not seem to be a significant factor clinically. The present immunosuppressive regime in Aberdeen for renal transplantation consists of a combination of prednisolone, azathioprine and low-dose CsA with reduction in doses as shown in Figure 6.8.

At the time of writing (June 1988) such a regime for a 70 kg patient, assuming immediate graft function and freedom from episodes of acute

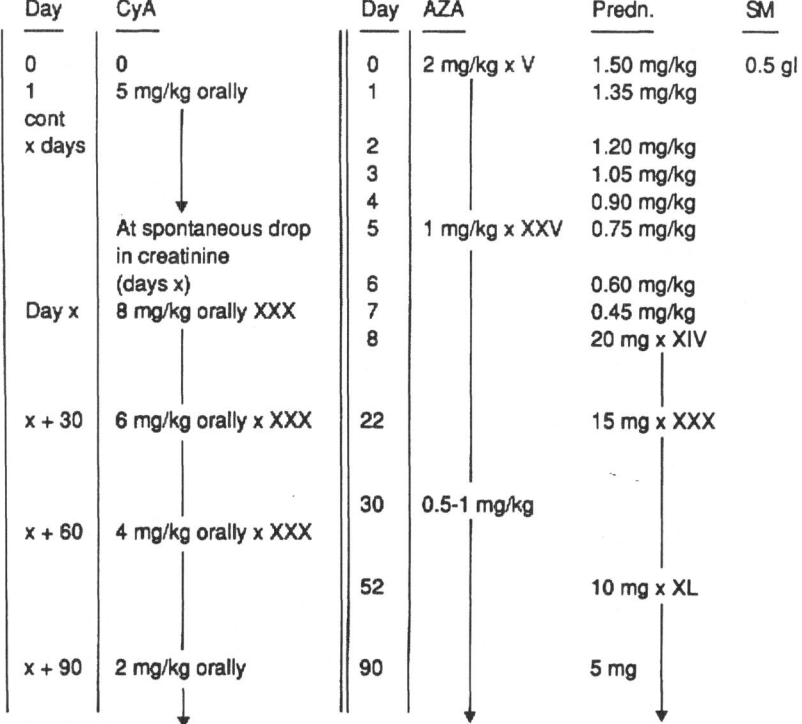

Day	CyA	Day	AZA	Predn.	SM
0	0	0	2 mg/kg x V	1.50 mg/kg	0.5 gl
1	5 mg/kg orally	1		1.35 mg/kg	
cont					
x days	↓	2		1.20 mg/kg	
		3		1.05 mg/kg	
		4		0.90 mg/kg	
	At spontaneous drop in creatinine	5	1 mg/kg x XXV	0.75 mg/kg	
	(days x)	6		0.60 mg/kg	
Day x	8 mg/kg orally XXX	7		0.45 mg/kg	
		8		20 mg x XIV	
x + 30	6 mg/kg orally x XXX	22		15 mg x XXX	
		30	0.5-1 mg/kg		
x + 60	4 mg/kg orally x XXX				
		52		10 mg x XL	
x + 90	2 mg/kg orally	90		5 mg	

- Trough whole blood levels

Month	ng/ml
< 1	100 - 200
1 - 3	75 - 180
4 - 6	50 - 150
> 6	40 - 100

Figure 6.8 Immunosuppressive regimen for recipients of renal grafts from cadaveric donors. *Key*: CYA, Cyclosporin A; AZA, azathioprine; Predn, prednisolone; SM, soluble methyl prednisolone. Roman numerals: V, 5; XIV, 14; XXV, 25; XXX, 30; XL, 40

rejection, would cost £2200 for 1 year. A regime using azathioprine and prednisolone for the same patient would cost £320. This considerable difference in cost provided the impetus to determine if patients could safely be converted from treatment with CsA to azathioprine.

CONVERSION REGIMES

Attempts to convert renal transplant recipients from treatment with CsA to azathioprine in order to avoid nephrotoxicity have met with varying success.

135

Indications for, and methods of, effecting the change have varied widely. The Oxford group converted 36 patients electively at 3 months after transplantation, 28 of whom were on CsA monotherapy. Three months after conversion a 48% fall in mean serum creatinine was noted among those on monotherapy and a 35% fall in mean serum creatinine in those on CsA and prednisolone[110]. In Munich, nine patients were electively converted, 14 were converted because of uncontrolled rejection and eight because of nephrotoxicity; of these groups three, nine and three patients respectively lost graft function after conversion[111]. Flechner converted 10 patients because of nephrotoxicity; two lost graft function[112].

The frequency of acute rejection episodes also varied. Wood and co-workers reported six episodes of rejection in 30 patients in the first 2 weeks after conversion[110] but Canafax *et al.*, using a protocol in which the CsA and azathioprine therapy overlapped for 5–7 days, noted only four acute rejection episodes in 28 patients followed for 2 years following conversion[113]. Twenty-five per cent of these patients also received anti-lymphocyte globulin during conversion, and five of these died from infective complications. A 32% rejection rate complicating conversion was demonstrated in a similar study, with the loss of one graft from a patient with previously stable renal function at the time of conversion[114].

Since these early studies, the conversion of patients with stable graft function has been assessed, again with varying success. Most centres attempting conversion, however, now wait longer than 3 months after grafting and ensure a significant overlap of CsA and azathioprine therapy.

Despite the almost universal finding of the lowered mean serum creatinine after conversion, some recent studies have cast doubts about the long-term viability of grafts after conversion. One study from Leicester observed that 36% of patients experiencing late rejection episodes of insidious onset after conversion and the 2-year graft survival rate in the conversion group was 73% compared to 86% for the long-term CsA group[115]. Similar results have been reported from Groningen[116].

In considering immunosuppressive regimes it is well recognized that the concomitant administration of other drugs can modify the metabolism of CsA and either provoke rejection by lowering CsA levels, or, conversely, induce CsA nephrotoxicity. Drugs which induce hepatic CsA metabolism (e.g. rifampicin[25], phenobarbitone and phenytoin) cause a decrease in CsA blood levels and may be associated with an increased frequency of rejection episodes, whilst others (e.g. erythromycin, ketoconazole, diltiazem and nicardipine) may increase blood levels. Some drugs may show synergistic nephrotoxicity, e.g. gentamicin, non-steroidal anti-inflammatory drugs, sulphonamides and trimethoprim. It has been suggested that some drugs, particularly the calcium channel antagonists verapamil and diltiazem[117], given when the donor kidney is being prepared after donor nephrectomy, may protect against subsequent delayed graft function. Furthermore, the concurrent administration of steroids with CsA to the graft recipient may also play a protective role. These results are largely derived from single studies, and should probably be confirmed before current clinical practice is modified.

Other unwanted CsA effects

Hypertension has been reported to be more frequent in patients receiving CsA following renal[118], hepatic[119] or cardiac[120] allografts. This may be a manifestation of nephrotoxicity; indeed, nephrotoxicity may be more pronounced in the presence of hypertension or in association with renal ischaemia; kidneys from an elderly donor, for example, are often more susceptible to CsA toxicity[41].

Hyperkalaemia has also been reported in renal allograft recipients treated with CsA[121] and may, if untreated, lead to serious cardiac dysrhythmias. It has been suggested that the hypertension and hyperkalaemia may be caused by alteration of the renin–angiotensin–aldosterone system by CsA.

There are reports of glomerular thrombi developing in renal allografts treated with CsA therapy[122]. This condition should be distinguished from haemolytic uraemic syndrome which may also develop after renal transplantation. The patient presents with renal failure associated with thrombocytopenia, bone marrow hyperplasia, a reticulocytosis, morphological abnormalities of the erythrocytes and evidence of a haemolytic process. The condition may respond to a reduction in CsA dose or conversion to azathioprine[123].

Hepatotoxicity, manifest as a transient rise in serum bilirubin usually in the first month after transplantation, was evident in up to 20% of patients in the European renal transplantation multi-centre trial[47]. Serum transaminases were less frequently elevated than the bilirubin but both abnormalities were related to high trough whole-blood CsA levels, or a cyclosporin dose in excess of $17 \text{ mg kg}^{-1} \text{ day}^{-1}$. The biochemical abnormalities responded to a reduction in dose. Hepatotoxicity is now seen less frequently using the present low-dose CsA regimens, and is of little significance clinically.

Non-T-cell lymphomas developed in six patients involved in the pilot studies of CsA[101,124]. Such lymphoproliferative disorders are associated with immunosuppressive therapy itself, and subsequent studies have demonstrated that the risk of developing a lymphoreticular malignancy is no greater in the patients receiving CsA than those treated with conventional immunosuppression. Furthermore, in virtually all the patients developing a lymphoproliferative disease previous infection with Epstein–Barr virus was apparent, and a nuclear antigen from the virus was expressed on the neoplastic cells, suggesting a possible aetiological role. The treatment for these lesions has included surgery, chemotherapy and radiotherapy. Starzl, however, provided evidence that regression of the neoplasm could occur with reduction or, if necessary, discontinuation of immunosuppression[125]. In the 5-year European multicentre trial four of the 117 CsA-treated patients developed neoplasia, two of which were renal malignancies.

Therapy with CsA is also associated with other side-effects which, whilst not life-threatening, may be distressing to an individual patient. In particular hirsutism, which occurs in approximately 30–40% of patients, may prove disturbing to a female patient[47,48]. It usually develops 2–8 weeks after transplantation, involves the face, arms and back and may respond to reduction in dose. If CsA is withdrawn hirsutism resolves within 1–2 months. Gingival hyperplasia[47,48], similar to that associated with phenytoin, occurs in up to

25% of renal transplant patients, but is again seen less frequently with low-dose CsA regimens. It rarely requires surgical therapy as it responds within 1–2 months to reduction of dose or discontinuation of CsA.

Neurological sequelae of CsA therapy are uncommon. Seizures have been reported in very few renal and cardiac transplant patients. Tremors and paraesthesiae are noted more frequently and may occur in about 10% of patients[48,119]. Indeed, the development of tremor in a patient after transplantation may be an easily detectable clinical sign of CsA toxicity which will respond to a reduction in dose. Other neurological manifestations include ataxia, hallucinations and encephalopathy.

Transient gastrointestinal symptoms occur quite commonly, including anorexia and nausea[48,119]; these respond to lowering the dose. The development of the capsule form of CsA should minimize the chance of the patient tasting the CsA and procipient, and may also lower the prevalence of nausea. Case reports have implicated CsA in the development of breast fibroadenomata[126] and haemolytic anaemia, but these problems have been observed in few patients to date.

SUMMARY

It is apparent that the initial enthusiasm associated with the advent of CsA into the world of transplantation was justified. The use of high doses in the initial trials led to the discovery of worrying adverse effects, mainly nephrotoxicity and the association with lymphoreticular malignancies. Fortunately, the lower-dose regimens now generally adopted have enabled improved graft survival rates with a reduced incidence of adverse effects. The higher mean serum creatinine concentrations found in many trials does not seem to be associated with progressive renal damage and the incidence of lymphomata or other malignancies is no greater with CsA than with conventional immunosuppression. New immunosuppressive agents are being developed but as yet remain experimental. Analogues of CsA such as CsG have not been associated with lower nephrotoxicity rates than the parent compound. Preliminary studies of techniques to diminish the antigenicity of the graft are encouraging[127]. A complement-binding monoclonal antibody which recognizes dendritic or passenger cells in renal allografts has been developed, and when used to prepare the donor kidney prior to transplantation has caused a decrease in subsequent episodes of acute rejection. Although specific tolerance remains the overall goal for any vascularized graft, the improved graft survival rates obtained with CsA have enabled an increasing number of patients with end-stage organ disease to obtain successful organ transplantation and the associated improved quality of life.

REFERENCES

1. Pincherle, G. (1979) Kidney transplantation and dialysis. In Rainsbury, R. (ed.), *Topics of our Time*, Vol. 2: *Kidney Transplants and Dialysis* (London: HMSO)
2. Starzl, T. R., Marchiero, T. L., Von Kaulla, K. N., Hermann, G., Brittain, R. S. and Waddell,

W. R. (1963) Homotransplantation of the liver in humans. *Surg. Gynecol. Obstet.*, **117**, 659–676

3. Barnard, C. N. (1987) A human cardiac transplant. *s. Afr. Med. J.*, **41**, 1271–1274
4. McGregor, C. G. A. (1987) Cardiac and cardiopulmonary transplantation. In Catto, G. R. D. (ed.), *Clinical Transplantation: Current Practice and Future Prospects* (Lancaster: MTP)
5. Sheil, A. C. R. (1988) The second international congress on cyclosporine. *Transplant. Proc.*, **20**(3), 1123–1131
6. Dunhill, M. S. (1979) Histopathology of rejection in renal transplantation. In Morris, P. J. (ed.), *Kidney Transplantation: Principles and Practice* (London: Academic Press)
7. Zhang, J., Munda, R. and Glas-Greenwalt, P. (1983) Prolongation of survival of a heart xenograft by defibrination with ancrod. *Transplantation*, **35**, 620
8. Flechner, S. M., Van Buren, C. and Kerman, R. H. (1984) The nephrotoxicity of cyclosporine in renal transplant recipients. In Kahan, B. D. (ed.), *Cyclosporine: Biological Activity and Clinical Applications* (New York: Grune and Stratton)
9. Morris, P. J., Mickey, M. R., Singal, D. P. and Terasaki, P. I. (1969) Serotyping for homotransplantation XXII specificity of cytotoxic antibodies developing after renal transplantation. *Br. Med. J.*, **1**, 758–759
10. Klintmalm, G., Ringden, O. and Groth, C. G. (1984) Clinical and laboratory signs in nephrotoxicity and rejection in cyclosporine treated renal allograft recipients. In Kahan, B. D. (ed.) *Cyclosporine: Biological Activity and Clinical Applications* (New York: Grune & Stratton). p. 599
11. Bell, P. R. F., Calman, K. C., Wood, R. F., Briggs, J. D., Paton, A. M., McPherson, S. G. and Kyle, K. (1971) Reversal of acute clinical and experimental organ rejection using large doses of intravenous prednisolone. *Lancet*, **1**, 876–877
12. McGeown, M. C., Douglas, J. F., Brown, W. A., Donaldson, R. A., Kennedy, J. A., Loughridge, W. G., Mehta, S., Nelson, S. D., Doherty, C. C., Johnstone, R., Todd, G. and Hill, C. M. (1980) Advantages of low dose prednisolone – from the day after renal transplantation. *Transplantation*, **29**, 287–289
13. Kreis, H. and Goldstein, G. (1985) Monoclonal antibodies for the treatment of acute rejection episodes in renal transplantation. *Transplant. Proc.*, **17**, 2751–2753
14. Cheigh, J.-S., Stenzel, K. H., Susin, M., Rubin, A. L., Riggioi, R. R. and Whitsell, J. S. (1974) Kidney transplant nephrotic syndrome. *Am. J. Med.*, **57**, 730–740
15. Billingham, M. E. (1981) Diagnosis of cardiac rejection by endomyocardial biopsy. *Heart Transplant.*, **1**, 25–30
16. Hubscher, S. G., Clements, D. G., Elias, E. and McMaster, P. (1985) Biopsy findings in cases of rejection of liver allograft. *J. Clin. Pathol.*, **38**, 1366-1373
17. Cosimi, A. B., Cho, S. I., Delmonico, F. L., Kaplan, M. M., Rohrer, P. J. and Jenkins, R. L. (1987) A randomised clinical trial comparing OKT3 and steroids for treatment of hepatic allograft rejection. *Transplant. Proc.*, **19**, 2431–2433
18. Prieto, M., Sutherland, D. E. R., Fernandez-Cruz, L., Heil, J. B. and Najarian, J. S. (1987) Rejection in pancreas transplantation. *Transplant. Proc.*, **19**, 2348–2349
19. Liu, T., Sutherland, D. E. R., Heil, J., Dunning, M. and Najarian, J. S. (1985) Beneficial effects of establishing pancreatic duct drainage into hollow organ (bladder, jejunum, stomach) compared to free intraperitoneal drainage or duct injection. *Transplant. Proc.*, **17**(1), 366–371
20. Sutherland, D. E. R., Casanova, D. and Sibley, R. K. (1987) Role of pancreas graft biopsies in the diagnosis and treatment of rejection after pancreas transplantation. *Transplant. Proc.*, **19**, 2329–2331
21. Jeffrey, J. R., Downs, A. R., Lye, C. and Ramsey, E. (1979) Immunosuppression with azathioprine, prednisolone and cyclophosphamide. *Transplantation*, **28**, 10
22. Wolf, S. M., Fauci, A. S., Horn, R. G. and Dale, D. C. (1974) Wegener's granulomatosis. *Ann. Intern. Med.*, **81**, 513
23. Beveridge, T. (1982) Pharmacokinetics and metabolism of cyclosporin A. In White, D. J. G. (ed.), *Cyclosporin A.* (Amsterdam: Elsevier). p. 35
24. Rogers, A. J. and Kahan, B. D. (1984) Mechanism of action and clinical application of cyclosporine in organ transplantation. *Clin. Immunol. Allergy*, **4**, 217–258
25. Van Buren, D., Wideman, C. A., Reid, M., Gibbon, S., Van Buren, G., Jarowenko, M., Flechner, S. M., Frazier, O. H., Cooley, D. A. and Kahan, B. D. (1984) The antagonistic effect of rifampicin upon cyclosporin bioavailability. *Transplant. Proc.*, **16**, 1642–1645

26. Kahan, B. D., Reid, M. and Newburger, J. (1983) Pharmacokinetics of cyclosporine in human renal transplantation. *Transplant. Proc.,* **5**, 446
27. Keown, P. A., Stiller, C. R., Ulan, R. A., Sinclair, N. R., Wall, W. J. and Carruthers, G. (1981) Immunological and pharmacological monitoring in the clinical use of cyclosporin A. *Lancet,* **1**, 686
28. Elion, G. B. (1967) Biochemistry and pharmacology of purine analogues. *Fed. Proc.,* **26**, 989
29. Jones, M. C., Best, P. V. and Catto, G. R. D. (1988) Is nodular regenerative hyperplasia of the liver associated with azathioprine therapy after renal transplantation. *Nephrol. Dialysis Transplant.,* **3**, 331–333
30. Neifield, J. P., Lippman, M. E. and Tormey, D. C. (1977) Steroid hormone receptors in normal human lymphocytes. *J. Biol. Chem.,* **252**, 2972
31. Larsson, E. L. (1980) Cyclosporine A and dexamethasone suppress T cell responses by selectively acting at distinct sites of the triggering process. *J. Immunol.,* **124**, 2828
32. Hong, S. L. and Levine, L. (1976) Inhibition of arachidonic acid release from cells as the biochemical action of anti-inflammatory corticosteroids. *Proc. Natl. Acad. Sci. USA,* **73**, 1730
33. Dumler, F., Levin, N. W., Szego, G., Vulpetti, A. T. and Prauss, W. E. (1982) Long term alternate-day steroid therapy in renal transplantation. *Transplantation,* **34**, 78–82
34. Soyka, L. F. and Saxena, K. M. (1965) Alternate-day steroid therapy for nephrotic children. *J. Am. Med. Assoc.,* **192**, 225–230
35. Breitenfield, F. V., Hebert, C. A., Lemann, J., Pirring, W. F., Kauffman, H. M., Sampson, D., Kalbfleisch, J. and Beres, J. A. (1980) Stability of renal transplant function with alternate day corticosteroid therapy. *J. Am. Med. Assoc.,* **244**, 151–159
36. Halloran, P. F., Lien, J., Aprile, M. and White, N. (1982) Preliminary results of a randomized comparison of cyclosporine and Minnesota anti-lymphoblast globulin. *Transplant. Proc.,* **14**, 627
37. Cosimi, A. B. (1983) The clinical usefulness of anti-lymphocyte antibodies. *Transplant. Proc.,* **15**, 583–589
38. Norman, D. J., Barry, J. M., Hennell, K., Funnel, M. B., Goldstein, G. and Bohannon, L. (1985) Reversal of acute allograft rejection with monoclonal antibody. *Transplant. Proc.,* **17**, 39–41
39. Merrill, J. P., Murray, J. R., Harrison, J. H. and Guild, W. R. (1956) Successful homotransplantation of human kidney between identical twins. *J. Am. Med. Assoc.,* **160**, 277
40. McGeown, M. G., Douglas, J. F., Donaldson, R. A., Hill, C. M., Kennedy, J. A., Loughridge, W. G. G. and Middleton, D. (1988) Ten year results of renal transplantation with azathioprine and prednisolone as only immunosuppression. *Lancet,* **1**, 983
41. Sinclair, N. R. St. C., Stiller, C. R., Jeffery, J. R. and Keown, P. A. (1988) Multivariate analysis of risk factor leading to kidney graft loss in cyclosporin treated patients. *Transplant. Proc.,* **20**, 350
42. Opelz, G. (1985) Correlation of HLA matching with kidney graft survival in patients with or without cyclosporine treatment. *Transplantation,* **40**, 240–243
43. Ting, A. and Morris, P. J. (1980) Powerful effects of HLA-Dr matching on survival of cadaveric renal allografts. *Lancet,* **2**, 282–285
44. Morris, P. J., Ting, A. and Stocker, J. (1968) Leucocyte antigens in renal transplantations. (1) The paradox of blood transfusion in renal transplantation. *Med. J. Aust.,* **2**, 1088–1090
45. Opelz, G., Sengar, P. D. S., Mickey, M. R. and Terasaki, P. I. (1973) Effect of blood transfusions on subsequent kidney transplants. *Transplant. Proc.,* **5**, 253–259
46. Calne, R. Y., White, D. J., Thiru, S., Evans, D.B., McMaster, P., Dunn, D. C., Craddock, G. N., Pentlow, B. N. and Rolles, K. (1978) Cyclosporin A in patients receiving renal allografts from cadaver donors. *Lancet,* **2**, 1323–1327
47. European Multicentre Trial Group (1983) Cyclosporine in cadaveric renal transplantations. One year follow up of a multicentre trial. *Lancet,* **2**, 986–989
48. Canadian Multicentre Transplant Study Group (1983) A randomised clinical trial of cyclosporin in cadaveric renal transplantation. *N. Engl. J. Med.,* **309**, 809–815
49. European Multicentre Trial Group (1986) Cyclosporine in cadaveric renal transplantation. Follow up at three years of a multicentre trial. *Transplant. Proc.,* **18**, 1229–1233

50. Canadian Multicentre Transplant Study Group (1986) A randomised clinical trial of cadaveric renal transplantation: analysis at three years. *N. Engl. J. Med.*, **314**, 1219–1225
51. Calne, R. Y. (1987) Cyclosporin in cadaveric renal transplantation: 5 year follow up of a multicentre trial. *Lancet*, **2**, 506–507
52. Najarian, J. S., Fryd, D. S., Strand, M., Canafax, D. M., Ascher, N. L., Payne, W. D., Simmons, R. L. and Sutherland, D. E. (1985) A single institution randomised prospective trial of cyclosporin versus azathioprine–antilymphocyte globulin for immunosuppression in renal allograft recipients. *Ann. Surg.*, **201**, 142–157
53. Johnson, C. P., Simmons, R. C., Sutherland, D. E. R., Canafax, D. M., Ascher, N. L. Payne, W. D., Flick, B., Najarian, J. S. and Fryd, D. S. (1988) A randomised trial comparing cyclosporine with antilymphocyte globulin–azathioprine for renal allograft recipients. *Transplantation*, **45**, 380–385
54. Ringden, O., Ost, C., Klintmalm, G., Tillegard, A., Fehrman, I., Wilczek, H. and Groth, C. G. (1983) Improved outcome in cyclosporine-treated renal transplant recipients above 55 years of age treated with cyclosporine and low doses of steroids. *Transplant. Proc.*, **15**, 2507–2512
55. Kahan, B. D., Van Buren, C. T., Flechner, S. M., Payne, W. D., Boileau, M. and Kerman, R. H. (1983) Cyclosporine immunosuppression mitigates immunologic risk factors in renal allotransplantation. *Transplant. Proc.*, **15**, 2469–2478
56. Kerman, R. H., Flechner, S. M., Van Buren, C. T., Lorber, M. I. and Kahan, B. D. (1985) Successful transplantation of cyclosporin treated allograft recipients with serologically positive historical but negative preoperative donor crossmatches. *Transplantation*, **40**, 615
57. Opelz, G. (1987) Effect of HLA matching in 10,000 cyclosporine treated cadaver kidney transplants. *Transplant. Proc.*, **19**, 641–646
58. Najarian, J. S., Migliori, R. J., Simmons, R. L., Ascher, N. L., Payne, W. D., Dunn, D., Sutherland, D. E. R. and Fryd, D. S. (1988) Effect of HLA matching in cadaver renal transplant. *Transplant. Proc.*, **20**(3), 249–256
59. Brynger, H., Persson, H., Flatmark, A., Albrechtsen, D., Frodin, L., Tufvesson, G., Gabel, H., Weibull, H., Moller, E., Lundgren, G. and roth, C. G. (1988) No effect of blood transfusion or HLA matching on renal graft success rate in recipients treated with cyclosporine–prednisolone or cyclosporine–azathioprine–prednisolone: the Scandinavian experience. *Transplant. Proc.*, **20**(3), 261–263
60. Opelz, G. (1985) Current relevance of the transfusion effect in renal transplantation. *Transplant. Proc.*, **17**, 1015
61. Opelz, G. (1987) Improved kidney graft survival in non-transfused recipients. *Transplant. Proc.*, **19**, 149
62. Stratta, R. J., Oh, C. S., Sollinger, H., Pirsch, J. D., Malayoglu, M. and Belzer, F. O. (1988) Kidney retransplantation in the cyclosporine era. *Transplantation*, **45**, 40–45
63. Bunzendahl, H., Wonigeit, K., Klempnawer, J., Brouch, C. and Pichlmayr, R. (1983) Cyclosporine and steroids: effects on clinical course after renal allotransplantation. *Transplant. Proc.*, **15**, 2531–2534
64. Sodal, G. A., Albrechtsen, D., Berg, K. J., Bondevik, H., Brekke, I. B., Fauchalf, P., Jakobsen, A., Talseth, T., Thorsby, E. and Flatmark, A. (1987) Renal transplantation from living donors mismatched for two HLA haplotypes. *Transplant. Proc.*, **19**, 1509–1510
65. Berenhart, G. R., Hastillo, A., Goldman, M. W. *et al.* (1985) A prospective randomised trial or pretransfusion and azathioprine and prednisolone vs cyclosporin and prednisolone immunosuppression in cardiac transplant recipients: preliminary results. *Circulation*, **72** (Suppl. II), 227–230
66. Emery, R. W., Costa, R., Christensen, R., Levinson, M. M., Icenogle, T. B., Riley, J., Ott, R. A. and Copeland, J. G. (1986) Cardiac transplant patients at one year: cyclosporin versus conventional immunosuppression. *Chest*, **90**, 29–33
67. Oyer, P. E., Stinson, E. B., Jamieson, S. W., Hunt, S. A., Perlroth, M., Billingham, M. and Shumway, N. E. (1983) Cyclosporine in cardiac transplantation. A two and a half year follow up. *Transplant. Proc.*, **15**, 2546–2552
68. Schroeder, J. S. and Hunt, S. (1987) Cardiac transplantation update 1987. *J. Am. Med. Assoc.*, **258**, 3142–3145
69. Hakim, M., Spiegelhalter, D., English, T., Caine, N. and Wallwork, J. (1988) Cardiac

141

transplantation with cyclosporine and steroids: medium and long term results. *Transplant. Proc.*, **20**(3), 327–332

70. Fricker, F. J., Griffith, B. P., Hardesty, R. L. *et al.* (1987) Experience with heart transplantation in children. *Pediatrics*, **79**, 138–146

71 Dunn, J. M., Gavarrocchi, N. C., Balsara, R. K. *et al.* (1987) Pediatric heart transplantation at St Christopher's Hospital for Children, Philadelphia. *J. Heart Transplant.*, **6**, 334–342

72. Kerman, R. H., Van Buren, C. T., Lewis, R. M., Frazier, O. H., Cooley, D. and Kahan, B. D. (1988) The impact of HLA'-A B and DR blood transfusions and immune responder status on cardiac allograft recipients treated with cyclosporine. *Transplantation*, **45**, 333–337

73. Starzl, T. E., Bilheimer, D. W., Balinson, H. T. *et al.* (1984) Heart/liver transplantation in a patient with familial hypocholesterolaemia: a case report. *Lancet*, **1**, 1382–2383

74. McGregor, C. G. A. (1987) Current state of heart transplantation. *Br. J. Hosp. Med.*, **37**, 310–318

75. Starzl, T. E., Iwatsuki, S., Van Thiel, D. H., Gartner, J. C., Zitelli, B. J., Macatack, J., Schade, R. R., Shaw, B. W. Jr., Hakala, T. R., Rosenthal, J. T. and Porter, K. A. (1982) Evolution of liver transplantation. *Hepatology*, **2**, 614–636

76. Iwatsuki, S. (1988) 1000 liver transplants using cyclosporin A. *Transplant. Proc.*, **20** (Suppl. 1), 499

77. Pichlamyr, R., Brolsch, C. and Neuhaus, P. (1983) Report on 68 human orthotopic liver transplantations with special reference to rejection phenomena. *Transplant. Proc.*, **15**, 1279–1283

78. Gordon, R. D., Shaw, B. W. Jr., Iwatsuki, S., Esquivel, C. O. and Starzl, T. E. (1986) Indications for liver transplantation in the cyclosporin era. *Surg. Clin. N. Am.*, **66**, 541–556

79. Iwatsuki, S, Starzl, T. E., Gordon, R. D., Esquivelco Todos, Tasakis A. G., Makowka, L., Marsh, J. W. and Miller, C. M. (1987) Late mortality and morbidity after liver transplantation. *Transplant. Proc.*, **19**, 2373–2377

80. Jamieson, N. V., Calne, R. Y., Rolles, K., Barnes, N. D. and Mowat, A. P. (1987) Results and problems in pediatric liver transplantation in the Cambridge/Kings College Hospital series 1968–July 1986. *Transplant. Proc.*, **19**, 2447–2448

81. Wonigeit, K., Brolsch, C., Neuhaus, P., Burdelski, M., Schmidt, E., Lang, W. and Pichlmayr, R. (1983) Special aspects of immunosuppression with cyclosporine in liver transplantation. *Transplant. Proc.*, **15**, 2586–2591

82. Bismuth, H., Samuel, D., Gugenheim, J., Castain, G. D., Barnuau, J., Rueff, B. and Benhamou, J.-P. (1987) Emergency liver transplantation for fulminant hepatitis. *Ann. Intern. Med.*, **107**, 337–341

83. Sabesin, S. M. and Williams, J. W. (1987) Current status of liver transplantation. *Hosp. Pract.*, **22**(7), 75–86

84. Burke, C. M., Theodore, J., Baldwin, J. C., Tazelaar, H. D., Morris, A. J., McGregor, C. G. A., Shumway, N. E., Robin, E. D. and Jamieson, S. W. (1986) An evaluation of the results of human heart lung transplantation. *Lancet*, **1**, 517–519

85. Glanville, A. R., Baldwin, J. C., Burke, C. M., Theodore, J. and Rabin, E. D. (1987) Obliterative bronchiolitis after heart–lung transplantation: apparent arrest by augmented immunosuppression. *Am. Intern. Med.*, **107**, 30–304

86. Harjula, A. L. J., Baldwin, J. C., Glanville, A. R. *et al.* (1987) Human leukocyte antigen (HLA) compatibility in heart–lung transplantation. *J. Heart Transplant.*, **6**, 162–166

87. Griffith, B. P., Hardesty, R. L., Trento, A. *et al.* (1987) Heart–lung transplantation: lessons learned and future hopes. *Ann. Thorac. Surg.*, **43**, 6–16

88. Sutherland, D. E. R., Goetz, C. and Najarian, J. S. (1987) Pancreas transplantation at the University of Minnesota: donor and recipient selection, operative and postoperative management and outcome. *Transplant. Proc.*, **19**(4), 63–74

89. Sutherland, D. E. R. and Moudry, K. C. (1987) Clinical pancreas and islet transplantation. *Transplant. Proc.*, **19**, 113–120

90. Casanova, D. (1987) The effect of cyclosporin on native kidney function in non-uraemic diabetic patients after pancreas transplantation. *Kidney Int.*, **32**, 619–620

91. Solders, G., Wilczek, H., Gunnarsson, R., Tyden, G., Persson, A. and Groth, C.-G. (1987) Effects of combined pancreatic and renal transplantation on diabetic neuropathy: a 2 year follow-up study. *Lancet*, **2**, 1232–1235

92. Myers, B. D., Ross, J., Newton, L., Luejcher, J. and Perlroth, M. (1984) Cyclosporine associated chronic nephropathy. *N. Engl. J. Med.*, **311**, 699–705
93. Holt, D. W., Marsden, J. T., Johnston, A., Bewick, M. and Taube, D. H. (1986) Blood cyclosporin concentrations and renal allograft dysfunction. *Br. Med. J.*, **293**, 1057–1059
94. Hayry, P. and Von Willebrand, E. (1986) The influence of the pattern of inflammatory and administration of steroids on class II MHC antigen expression in renal transplants. *Transplantation*, **42**, 358
95. Salaman, J. R. and Griffin, P. J. A. (1985) The use of fine-needle intrarenal manometry in the management of renal transplant patients receiving cyclosporine. *Transplantation*, **39**, 523
96. Hillis, A. N. (1985) The measurement of cyclosporin A in whole blood by HPLC in renal allograft recipients. In *Abstracts of the 22nd Congress of the European Dialysis and Transplantation Association*, p. 175
97. Jones, M. C., Whiting, P. W., Innes, A., Propper, D. J., Edward, N. and Catto, G. R. D. (1989) Biochemical abnormalities in serum and urine from renal transplant recipients receiving cyclosporin. *Transplant. Proc.* (In press)
98. Kahan, B. D. (1985) An algorithm for the management of patients with cyclosporin-induced renal dysfunction. *Transplant. Proc.*, **17** (Suppl. 1), 303–308
99. Klintmalm, G., Bohman, S.-O., Sundelin, B. and Wilczek, H. (1984) Interstitial fibrosis in renal allografts after 12 to 46 months of cyclosporin treatment: beneficial effect of low doses in early post-transplant period. *Lancet*, **2**, 950–954
100. Ruiz, P., Kolbeck, P. C., Scroggs, M. W. and Sanfilippo, F. (1988) Associations between cyclosporine therapy and interstitial fibrosis in renal allograft biopsies. *Transplantation*, **45**, 91–95
101. Calne, R. Y., Rolles, K., White, D. J. G., Thiru, S., Evans, D. B., McMaster, P., Dunn, D. C., Craddock, C. N., Henderson, R. G., Aziz, S. and Lewis, P. (1979) Cyclosporin A initially as the only immunosuppressant in 34 recipients of cadaveric organs: 32 kidneys, 2 pancreases, 2 livers. *Lancet*, **2**, 1033–1036
102. Starzl, T. E., Klintmalm, G. B., Weil, R. III, Porter, K. A., Iwatsuki, S., Schroter, G. P. J., Fernandez-Bueno, C. and MacHugh, N. (1981) Cyclosporin A and steroid therapy in sixty-six cadaver kidney recipients. *Surg. Gynecol. Obstet.*, **153**, 486–494
103. Oyer, P. R., Stinson, E. B. and Reitz, B. A. (1982) Preliminary results with cyclosporin A in clinical cardiac transplantation. In White, D. J. G. (ed.), *Cyclosporin A* (Amsterdam: Elsevier)
104. Griffith, B. P., Hardesty, R. C., Deeb, G. M., Starzl, T. E. and Bahnson, H. T. (1982) Cardiac transplantation with cyclosporin A and prednisolone. *Ann. Surg.*, **196** (No. 3 Suppl.), 324
105. Land, W. (1987) Immunosuppressive combination therapy. In Land, W. (ed.), *Optimal Use of Sandimmun in Organ Transplantation* (Berlin: Springer Verlag)
106. Fry, W. R., Davidson, I., Alway, C. C. and Rooth, P. (1988) Cyclosporine A induced decreased blood flow in cadaveric kidney transplants. *Transplant. Proc.*, **20**(3), 222–225
107. Neumayer, H.-H., Henkel, M. and Wagner, K. (1988) Cyclosporine immunosuppression and early kidney graft function. *Transplant. Proc.*, **20**(3), 226–232
108. Barry, J. M., Shiveley, N., Hubert, B., Hefty, Norman, D. J. and Bennett, W. M. (1988) Significance of delayed graft function in cyclosporine treated recipients of cadaver kidney transplants. *Transplantation*, **45**, 346–348
109. Matas, A. J., Tellis, V. A., Quinn, T. A., Glicklich, D., Soberman, R. and Veith, F. J. (1988) Individualisation of immediate post-transplant immunosuppression. *Transplantation*, **45**, 406–409
110. Wood, R. F. M., Thompson, J. F., Allen, H., Ting, A. and Morris, P. J. (1983) The consequence of conversion from cyclosporine to azathioprine and prednisolone in renal allograft recipients. *Transplant. Proc.*, **15**, 2862
111. Land, W., Castro, C., Hillebrand, G., Gunther, K. and Gokel, J. M. (1983) Conversion rejection consequence by changing the immunosuppressive therapy from cyclosporine to azathioprine after kidney transplantation. *Transplant. Proc.*, **15**, 2852
112. Flechner, S. M., Van Buren, C. T., Kerman, R. and Kahan, B. D. (1983) The effect of conversion from cyclosporine to azathioprine immunosuppression for intractable nephrotoxicity. *Transplant. Proc.*, **15**, 2869
113. Canafax, D. M., Sutherland, D. E. R., Ascher, N. C., Simmons, R. L. and Najarian, J. S.

(1983) Cyclosporin nephrotoxicity in renal allograft recipients: conversion to azathioprine to improve renal function. *Transplant. Proc.*, **15**, 2874

114. Rocher, L. L., Milford, E. L., Kirman, R. L., Carpenter, C. B., Strom, T. B. and Tilneu, N. L. (1984) Conversion from cyclosporine to azathioprine in renal allograft recipients. *Transplantation*, **38**, 669–674

115. Veitch, P. S., Taylor, J. D., Feehally, J., Walls, J. and Bell, P. R. F. (1987) Elective conversion from cyclosporine to azathioprine: long term follow up. *Transplant. Proc.*, **19**, 2017

116. Tegzess, A. M., Van Son W. J., Beelen, J. M., Sluiter, W. J., Meijer, S. and Sloof, M. J. H. (1987) Improvements of renal function after conversion from cyclosporine only to prednisolone-azathioprine followed by late onset graft failure in renal transplant patients. *Transplant. Proc.*, **19**, 2000–2004

117. Wagner, K. and Neumayer, H.-H. (1987) Influence of the calcium antagonist diltiazem on delayed graft function in cadaveric kidney transplantation: result of a 6-month follow up. *Transplant. proc.*, **19**, 1353–1357

118. Laupacis, A. (for the Canadian Transplant Study Group) (1983) Complications of cyclosporine therapy – a comparison to azathioprine. *Transplant. Proc.*, **15**, 2748–2753

119. O'Grady, J. G., Forbes, A., Rolles, K., Calne, R. Y. and Williams, R. (1988) An analysis of cyclosporine efficacy and toxicity after liver transplantation. *Transplantation*, **45**, 575–579

120. Hunt, S. A. (1983) Complications of heart transplantation. *Heart Transplant.*, **3**, 70–74

121. Adu, D., Turney, J., Michael, J. and McMaster, p. (1983) Hyperkalaemia in cyclosporine treated renal allograft recipients. *Lancet*, **2**, 370–372

122. Neild, G. H., Reuben, R., Hartley, R. B. and Cameron, J. S. (1985) Glomerular thrombi in renal allografts associated with cyclosporin treatment. *J. Clin. Pathol.*, **38**, 253–258

123. Van Buren, D., Van Buren, C. T., Flechner, S. M., Maddox, A. M., Verani, R. and Kahan, B. D. (1985) *De novo* hemolytic uremic syndrome in renal transplant recipients immunosuppressed with cyclosporine. *Surgery*, **98**, 54–62

124. Sweny, P., Farrington, K., Younis, F., Varghese, Z., Baillod, R. A., Fernando, O. N. and Moorhead, J. F. (1981) Sixteen months experience with cyclosporin-A in human kidney transplantation. *Transplant. Proc.*, **13**, 365–367

125. Starzl, T. E., Nalesnik, M. A., Porter, K. A., Ho, M., Iwatsuki, S., Griffith, B. P., Rosenthal, J. T., Hakala, T. R., Shaw, B. W., Hardesty, R. L., Atchison, R. W., Jaffe, R. and Bahnson, H. T. (1984) Reversibility of lymphomas and lymphoproliferative lesions developing under cyclosporin-steroid therapy. *Lancet*, **1**, 583–587

126. Rolles, K. and Calne, R. Y. (1980) Two cases of benign lumps after treatment with cyclosporine A. *Lancet*, **2**, 795

127. Taube, D., Welsh, K. I., Bewick, M., Dische, F. E., Palmer, A., Parsons, V. and Snowden, S. (1987) Pretreatment of human renal allografts with monoclonal antibodies to induce long term tolerance. *Transplant. Proc.*, **19**, 1961–1963

7
Cyclosporin A and bone marrow transplantation

Kerry Atkinson

SUMMARY

The use of cyclosporin A (CsA) in human marrow transplantation was first reported in 1978[1]. Shortly thereafter, its use in minimizing graft-versus-host disease (GVHD) by inducing graft–host tolerance was reported[2]. It has been shown to be effective in minimizing both the incidence of GVHD and marrow graft rejection. Both these complications of marrow transplantation are mediated by T cells, the former by those in the infused donor marrow and the latter by those of the recipient. CsA has been shown to be as effective as methotrexate, the previously used standard agent, in minimizing the incidence and severity of acute GVHD. The combination of CsA and methotrexate is superior in this regard compared to either drug used alone. CsA is also useful in treating both acute and chronic GVHD once they become established. The incidence of viral infections, including cytomegalovirus pneumonitis, is the same with each drug. CsA is associated with a faster rate of marrow engraftment and less oropharyngeal mucositis than methotrexate. However, it is associated with more nephrotoxicity and hypertension than methotrexate. Hepatotoxicity and neurotoxicity are also seen with its use in this patient population. In some prospective randomized trials, although not in others, the incidence of recurrent leukaemia in patients given CsA appears greater than in those given methotrexate. CsA has also been used as immunosuppression after mismatched family member and matched unrelated donor transplantation, and again it appears that the combination of CsA and methotrexate is useful. CsA interacts with a number of other medications commonly used in marrow transplant recipients, particularly aminoglycoside antibiotics and amphotericin B, sulphadimidine and trimethoprim, melphalan, ketoconazole, cimetidine, phenytoin, erythromycin, rifampicin and the contraceptive pill. If the use of these agents cannot be avoided, extra care in monitoring the patient's clinical course is required.

CsA IN EXPERIMENTAL BONE MARROW TRANSPLANTATION

Prevention of marrow graft rejection

Rejection of MHC-compatible bone marrow grafts is usually due to prior sensitization of the recipient to non-MHC antigens present on the donor cells. Commonly this sensitization is produced by preceding blood product transfusion. CsA dramatically reduced the incidence of marrow graft rejection in dogs given DLA-identical littermate marrow transplants after donor blood transfusion[3].

In contrast, rejection of MHC non-identical marrow is usually due to inherent allogeneic resistance, and is mediated by chemo-radiation-resistant recipient cells. In dogs given 9 Gy of total-body irradiation followed by a marrow transplant from DLA-non-identical unrelated dogs the combination of CsA and methotrexate (MTX) was successful in allowing donor marrow engraftment, while the use of either CsA alone or MTX alone in this model was associated with a high incidence of marrow graft rejection[4].

The induction of graft—host tolerance

In the above MHC-incompatible canine model, which represents a very severe test of immunosuppression, only the combination of CsA and methotrexate was able to minimize the severity of graft-versus-host disease and allow long-term survival[4]. CsA alone, however, was able to prevent GVHD after histocompatible canine littermate marrow grafts[4]. In both rodent[5,6] and canine[7] models of marrow transplantation using CsA as immune suppression, non-specific suppressor cells were detectable early post-transplant, with the later appearance of cells specifically suppressive of anti-host alloreactivity. It is possible that these observed specific suppressor cells are involved in the mediation of graft—host tolerance, as has also been observed in human recipients of HLA-identical sibling marrow transplants[8]. CsA has been previously described to favour the development of T cells with suppressor (as opposed to cytotoxic) function[9].

Induction of syngeneic GVHD

The initial descriptions of a clinical and histological syndrome identical to acute GVHD, but occurring after human syngeneic[10] or autologous[11] marrow transplantation were met with some scepticism. However, the development of animal models in which syngeneic GVHD can be readily reproduced has validated the clinical observations. The first such animal model was described in rats given syngeneic haemopoietic grafts and CsA[12]. The GVHD syndrome was manifested within 14—28 days of the cessation of CsA. Subsequently, similar findings were made in a murine model[13]. Syngeneic GVHD appears to represent an imbalance between autoreactive cytotoxic and suppressor cell mechanisms, resulting in failure to discriminate self from non-self. A severe autoaggression syndrome is the result. Autoreactive cytotoxic T cells with specificity for class II MHC antigens have been demonstrated[14], but the mechanism by which withdrawal of CsA facilitates the development of these cells is unclear. The syndrome can be transferred in irradiated recipients by the transfer of spleen plus lymph node cells[13] or thymocytes[15]. It may be that CsA treatment leads to altered self-recognition in the thymus, especially in view of the finding that CsA administration results in a rapid depletion of medullary thymocytes[13,16]. Additionally, in mice with CsA-induced syngeneic GVHD, there is a striking decrease in overall thymic Ia expression[13]. It is possible that the absence of self-class II MHC antigens in the thymus results in the failure of thymocytes to recognize self-class II MHC antigens as self.

The possibility of increasing the incidence of syngeneic or autologous GVHD for its possible graft-versus-leukaemia effect can now be exploited by administering, and subsequently withdrawing, CsA to appropriate human recipients.

CsA IN HLA-IDENTICAL SIBLING BONE MARROW TRANSPLANTATION

Prevention of marrow graft rejection

CsA appears capable of reducing the incidence of early graft failure to a level of approximately 10% in adults given HLA-identical sibling marrow transplants for severe aplastic anaemia[17], who are immunosuppressed immediately pre-transplant with cyclophosphamide 200 mg/kg. Graft rejection in this situation is due, at least in part, to previous sensitization to non-HLA antigens by preceding blood transfusion. Late graft rejection has also been described in these patients, usually occurring more than 6 months post-transplant, as the CsA dose is being tapered. This represents an argument for a very gradual reduction in dosage over a prolonged period of time for this patient population[18].

Prevention of acute GVHD

CsA has been shown to be as useful as methotrexate in minimizing the incidence and severity of acute GVHD after HLA-identical sibling marrow transplantation for haematological malignancy in a number of prospective randomized trials[19-23]. When the three trials from Seattle were combined[24], the overall incidence of moderate to severe acute GVHD in patients given CsA was 39%, while it was 55% in those given methotrexate (MTX) (not significant). Additionally, long-term survival was not significantly different between the two patient cohorts. More recently, several groups have reported the use of CsA in combination with MTX or prednisone. The combination of CsA and MTX has been shown to be superior to CsA alone in patients given HLA-identical sibling marrow transplants for acute non-lymphoblastic leukaemia (ANL) in first remission or chronic myeloid leukaemia (CML) in chronic phase[25]. This combination was also superior in patients given HLA-identical sibling transplants for severe aplastic anaemia when compared to MTX alone[26]. The combination of CsA and prednisone has been shown to

147

be superior to MTX and prednisone in minimizing the incidence and severity of acute GVHD in patients transplanted for leukaemia[27].

Treatment of established acute GVHD

Cyclosporin was found to be as effective as prednisone in treating established acute GVHD[28], and the combination of CsA and anti-thymocyte globulin (ATG) was considerably superior to the combination of CsA, ATG and prednisone. This superiority was apparently due to less infectious toxicity in the double, compared to the triple, regime[29].

Prevention of chronic GVHD

As with acute GVHD, there was no significant difference in the incidence of chronic GVHD in patients given marrow transplants for haematological malignancy and immunosuppressed either with CsA (incidence 42%) or MTX (incidence 48%)[24].

Treatment of established chronic GVHD

CsA and prednisone used on an alternating daily basis is able to salvage a proportion of patients with high-risk chronic GVHD refractory to therapy with prednisone alone, or prednisone and azothiaprine[30].

It is perhaps surprising that CsA is able to reverse established GVHD (acute and chronic) since, although it is able to inhibit T cell activation, it cannot prevent clonal proliferation once activation has occurred[31]. However, presumably its additional ability to suppress interleukin-2 secretion from activated T cells explains its capacity to reverse already-established T cell mediated disease (such as GVHD).

CsA and recurrent leukaemia after transplantation

The three prospective randomized trials[24] comparing CsA with MTX reported from Seattle showed no difference in the incidence of recurrent leukaemia in patients transplanted for either ANL in first remission, CML in chronic or accelerated phase or leukaemia in advanced stage. The overall incidence of leukaemic recurrence was 31% in CsA-treated patients and 36% in MTX-treated patients. When the three patient cohorts were analysed separately, the incidence of relapse in patients transplanted for ANL in first remission given CsA or MTX was 20% and 23% respectively; among patients with CML there was a moderately, but not significantly, lower incidence of relapse in CsA-treated patients (17%) compared to MTX-treated patients (55%) ($p = 0.16$). In patients with leukaemia in relapse at the time of transplant, the incidence of recurrence in CsA-treated patients was 75% compared with 30% in MTX-treated patients ($p = 0.06$). Although the latter difference also did not reach statistical significance, it is of interest that in two other prospective randomized trials, CsA-treated patients did have a significantly higher incidence of leukaemia recurrence post-transplant compared to those given MTX[22,23]. The first of these trials was restricted to patients with ANL or acute lymphoblastic leukaemia (ALL) in first remission[22], and the second included patients with acute leukaemia both in first remission and beyond first remission[23]. Additionally, multi-centre data from the International Bone Marrow Transplant registry suggest a higher incidence of leukaemic recurrence post-transplant in patients with ALL given CsA compared to those given MTX. Furthermore, CsA administration was thought to be one of the risk factors for the high incidence of leukaemic recurrence in patients with CML given T cell depleted HLA-identical sibling marrow grafts[32]. For the time being, therefore, this point remains controversial.

Although several cases have been reported[33,34], the occurrence of B cell lymphoma as a consequence of CsA immunosuppression appears much rarer after marrow transplantation than after solid organ transplantation.

CsA and the rate of marrow engraftment

CsA has been shown to be associated with more rapid marrow engraftment compared to MTX[19,23,35,36]. The time taken to achieve a given white cell count or neutrophil count post-transplant is consistently shorter. This reduced duration of neutropenia has resulted in less febrile days post-transplant. Also associated with the shorter duration of neutropenia has been a reduction in the severity of oropharyngeal mucositis[35].

CsA-associated nephrotoxicity after marrow transplantation

CsA-associated nephrotoxicity is commonly seen after allogeneic marrow transplantation[37–40]. Three different syndromes have been described. The commonest is an asymptomatic rise in the serum concentration of creatinine and urea. This complication is easily managed by lowering the dose of CsA, and is always reversible. Secondly, a syndrome characterized by clinical septicaemia, high blood concentrations of CsA, and acute renal failure often accompanied by hyperbilirubinaemia was seen not infrequently in the early years of CsA usage after marrow transplantation[37]. This syndrome is also reversible, although dialysis may be required temporarily. Caution should be exercised with the use of aminoglycoside antibiotics, and it may be preferable to use a double beta-lactam combination such as a semi-synthetic penicillin and a cephalosporin in patients immunosuppressed with CsA. Finally, a syndrome has been described predominantly in recipients of HLA-non-identical marrow transplants in which acute renal failure is characterized histologically by glomerular thromboses and multiple other organ complications, including fitting and pulmonary oedema. This syndrome resembles thrombotic thrombocytopenic purpura and is not usually reversible[37].

Examination of the urinary sediment can give a strong clue to the presence of CsA nephrotoxicity, with the presence of degenerative and necrotic abnormalities in proximal convoluted tubule cells[41].

CsA-associated hypertension after marrow transplantation

Diastolic hypertension is commonly seen with the use of CsA after marrow transplantation, and has been shown to be significantly commoner in CsA recipients compared to MTX recipients[37,42]. Interestingly, CsA-associated hypertension is relatively resistant to first-line anti-hypertensive therapy (diuretics and beta-blocking agents), but the use of the calcium antagonist nifedipine usually allows relatively easy control. CsA-associated hypertension is common, occurring in up to 70% of marrow transplant recipients. It may be linked to a renal magnesium-wasting syndrome which results in hypomagnesaemia[43]. Hypertensive encephalopathy can occur in young patients with a diastolic blood pressure of 100–110 mmHg, and the combination of this, together with thrombocytopenia makes cerebral haemorrhage a risk.

CsA-associated hepatotoxicity after marrow transplantation

CsA is also hepatotoxic, and this too is not infrequent in patients receiving 12.5 mg kg^{-1} day^{-1} CsA after marrow transplantation[44]. Again this is reversible, and it is not a particularly serious complication. The liver function test profile is characteristic in that the main abnormality is a conjugated hyperbilirubinaemia. Taken with the clinical picture, this enables CsA-associated hepatotoxicity to be distinguished from other causes of jaundice after marrow transplantation including GVHD, hepatitis, veno-occlusive disease of the liver and haemolysis (Table 7.1).

CsA-associated neurotoxicity

CsA-associated neurotoxicity is a rare but important complication of the drug in the marrow transplant recipient. While tremor is relatively common, the more serious neurological manifestations include paraparesis, a cerebellar-like syndrome characterized by severe ataxia, sometimes involving the larynx, and a Parkinsonian-like 'stunned' facies and poverty of movement[45]. All these serious manifestations are reversible on cessation of the drug, although this may take weeks to several months to occur; these syndromes therefore constitute a relative contraindication to its use. A switch to MTX immune suppression may be required and can be successful[46]. Other less common neurological complications that have been ascribed to CsA in this patient population include 'cotton-wool' retinal spots[47], paralysis of the deltoid muscle[48], mania[49], cerebral blindness and encephalopathy[50], and visual hallucinations[51]. Serious CsA neurotoxicity appears commoner after marrow than after solid organ transplantation, and this is likely due to the additional neurological insults to which marrow transplant recipients are exposed. These include the occurrence of meningeal leukaemia, the administration of intrathecal chemotherapy and total-body irradiation.

Table 7.1 Liver function test profiles in jaundice after marrow transplantation

Cause of jaundice	Serum values		
	Bilirubin	Alanine transaminase	Alkaline phosphatase
Cyclosporin hepatotoxicity	Raised	Moderately raised	Normal or minimally raised
Graft-versus-host disease	Raised	Moderately raised	High
Hepatic veno-occlusive disease	Raised	Moderately raised	High
Viral hepatitis	Raised	High	Moderately raised
Systemic infection	Raised	Moderately raised	Moderately raised
Haemolysis secondary to ABO incompatibility	Mildly raised (unconjugated)	Normal	Normal

CsA-associated changes in facial appearance

Facial dysmorphism has been described in renal transplant recipients immuno-suppressed with CsA[52], and similar coarsening and thickening of facial features has been noted in recipients of marrow allografts. CsA-associated hirsutism can further detract from the cosmetic appearance, as can oedema caused by fluid retention associated with the use of CsA.

CsA IN MARROW TRANSPLANTATION FROM DONORS OTHER THAN HLA-IDENTICAL SIBLINGS

Mismatched family member donor transplants

Although initial results were encouraging[53], subsequent follow-up of patients with haematological malignancy given non-T cell depleted mismatched family member marrow grafts and immunosuppression with CsA has been disappointing. When T cell depletion of the donor marrow was used to minimize the risk of GVHD (in addition to the post-transplant administration of CsA), results were again disappointing[54]. The incidence of marrow graft failure and GVHD was high in both studies. The degree of MHC disparity between donor and patient in these two reports was considerable (most haploidentical). In contrast, when donor and recipient differed phenotypically at only one MHC locus, the results were considerably better[55], especially when CsA and MTX were used in combination as prophylactic immunosuppression[56].

Matched unrelated donor transplants

Several centres are now reporting results of transplants in which the donor and recipient are unrelated but phenotypically matched for the MHC antigens. The donor is selected from a registry of volunteer marrow donors. In Seattle a miscellaneous group of patients with haematological malignancy were transplanted with matched unrelated bone marrow after preparation with cyclophosphamide 120 mg/kg and fractionated total-body irradiation 12 Gy. They were given non-T cell depleted marrow and CsA together with MTX as immunosuppression. Initial results are promising, with survival not significantly different from that using matched sibling marrow[57]. The apparent ability of matched unrelated marrow transplants to produce such results will make marrow transplantation available to a considerably greater number of patients with diseases of the bone marrow than previously, since only approximately one-third of individuals have a matched sibling to act as a donor.

CsA AND IMMUNE RECONSTITUTION POST-TRANSPLANT

Disappointingly, and in contrast to the more rapid haemopoietic reconstitution seen with the use of CsA, the rate of immune reconstitution does not differ significantly from that seen in patients given MTX[58,59]. This applies to both humoral and cell-mediated immunity. The main determinants for the rate of immune reconstitution remain the presence or absence of GVHD and the time elapsed post-transplant.

CYCLOSPORIN PHARMACOKINETICS AFTER HUMAN MARROW TRANSPLANTATION

Absorption

CsA is absorbed in the terminal ileum; approximately 40% of the ingested dose is absorbed. Approximately one-quarter of this is eliminated by the hepatic first-pass effect; thus 30% of the oral dose is bioavailable. Since diarrhoea is common in all recipients during the first 1 to 2 weeks post-transplant (due to chemoradiation enteritis, and subsequently also in those who develop acute GVHD of the gut), the intravenous route should be utilized in the initial post-transplant period. Markedly low serum concentrations of CsA have been noted in marrow transplant recipients with diarrhoea[60]. The intravenous preparation is stable in both normal saline and 5% dextrose, and retains its immunosuppressive capacity for 24 h in these vehicles[61]. If the oral route is used, it is important (since most of the 11 amino acids in the polypeptide are hydrophobic) that the drug be given in milk and not in juice, water or other soft drinks whose base is water.

Serum, whole blood and tissue levels

Peak plasma concentrations occur 2–4 h after an oral dose. The drug has two half-lives[62], one of between 2 and 4 h and the second between 10 and 27 h. In blood, 50% of the drug is bound to erythrocytes, 10% to leukocytes and 40% to lipoproteins in the serum[63]. The whole-blood concentration is approximately twice that of the serum concentration. The drug may be assayed either by radioimmunoassay, which measures CsA and its metabolites, or by HPLC which measures CsA alone. Either method is valid for monitoring marrow transplant recipients[64]. The drug has been found in all autopsy tissues analysed[65], and was detectable in these tissues in one case 14 days after the cessation of administration of the drug.

Correlation of serum or blood CsA concentration with toxicity

Most[66,67] but not all[68] studies suggest that there is a correlation between CsA serum or blood concentration and CsA-associated nephrotoxicity, although the strength of the correlation is not great. Likewise, one report[44] has demonstrated a weak correlation between CsA serum concentration and CsA-associated hepatotoxicity.

Correlation of serum of blood CsA concentration with efficacy

In contrast, most studies have been unable to find a correlation between CsA serum or blood concentration and the prevention of GVHD[66–68]. However, some studies have found a correlation between high levels of CsA and a decreased incidence of GVHD, and there is a general consensus that low concentrations (less than 200 ng/ml) are subtherapeutic. For practical purposes, careful monitoring of the serum creatinine concentration provides as good an indicator of toxicity as measuring blood or serum concentration of CsA. CsA concentration measurement is valuable for detecting subtherapeutic CsA concentrations, especially in patients with gut dysfunction not receiving the intravenous preparation of the drug.

INTERACTIONS BETWEEN CsA AND OTHER MEDICATIONS AFTER MARROW TRANSPLANTATION

Three types of interaction should be noted: firstly, interactions due to medications showing a similar spectrum of clinical toxicity to CsA. Secondly, interactions between CsA and medications that result in an increase in serum or blood CsA concentration (Table 7.2). Thirdly, interactions between CsA and medications that result in a decrease in the blood or serum CsA concentration (Table 7.2).

Medications used in marrow transplant recipients that produce toxicity additive to that of CsA include aminoglycoside antibiotics[38], amphotericin B[69] and melphalan[46], all of which can produce nephrotoxicity alone and can thereby exacerbate that produced by CsA.

Important medications that can potentiate CsA toxicity by increasing the CsA blood concentration include ketoconazole, cimetidine and erythromycin. Curiously, neither miconazole nor ranitidine have any such effect. A recent report has suggested that ketoconazole and CsA can be given concurrently if the CsA dose is markedly reduced[70]. Erythromycin is best avoided in this patient population, and there is normally an adequate alternative choice of antibiotic.

Finally, it should be noted that anaphylaxis to the intravenous preparation of CsA has been described, almost certainly related to the Cremophor in the vehicle[71]. Patients affected are usually able to continue to tolerate the oral preparation.

ACKNOWLEDGEMENTS

This work was supported by grants from the National Health and Medical Research Council of Australia and the New South Wales State Cancer Council.

Table 7.2 Drugs causing changes in CsA blood concentration

Increased CsA concentration	Decreased CsA concentration
Erythromycin	Phenytoin
Ketoconazole	Rifampicin
Contraceptive agents	Phenobarbitone
Cimetidine (?)	Sulphadimidine and trimethoprim
	Isoniazid (?)

REFERENCES

1. Powles, R. L., Barrett, A. J., Clink, H. M., Kay, H. E. M., Sloane, J. and McElwain, T. J. (1978) Cyclosporin A for the treatment of graft-versus-host disease in man. *Lancet*, **2**, 1327–1331

2. Tutschka, P. J. Beschorner, W. E., Allison, A. C., Burns, W. H. and Santos, G. W. (1979) Use of cyclosporin A in allogeneic bone marrow transplantation in the rat. *Nature*, **280**, 148–151

3. Storb, R., Deeg, H. J., Atkinson, K., Weiden, P. L., Sale, G. E., Colby, R. and Thomas, E. D. (1982) Cyclosporin A abrogates transfusion-induced sensitization and prevents marrow graft rejection in DLA-identical canine littermates. *Blood*, **60**, 524–526

4. Deeg, H. J., Storb, R., Weiden, P. L., Raff, R. F., Sale, G. E., Atkinson, K., Graham, T. C. and Thomas, E. D. (1982) Cyclosporin A and methotrexate in canine marrow transplantation. Engraftment, graft-versus-host disease, and induction of tolerance. *Transplantation*, **34**, 30–35

5. Tutschka, P. J., Hess, A. D., Beschorner, W. E. and Santos, G. W. (1981) Suppressor cells in transplantation tolerance. I. Suppressor cells and the mechanism of tolerance in radiation chimeras. *Transplantation*, **32**, 203–209

6. Tutschka, P. J., Ki, P. F., Beschorner, W. E., Hess, A. D. and Santos, G. W. (1981) Suppressor cells in transplantation tolerance. II. Maturation of suppressor cells in the bone marrow chimera. *Transplantation*, **32**, 321–325

7. Deeg, H. J., Severns, E., Raff, R. F., Sale, G. E. and Storb, R. (1987) Specific tolerance and immunocompetence in haploidentical, but not incompletely allogeneic, canine chimeras treated with methotrexate and cyclosporine. *Transplantation*, **44**, 621–632

8. Tsoi, M. S., Storb, R., Dobbs, S. and Thomas, E. D. (1981) Specific suppressor cells in graft–host tolerance of HLA-identical marrow transplantation. *Nature*, **292**, 355–357

9. Hess, A. D. and Tutschka, P. J. (1980) Effect of cyclosporin A on human lymphocyte responses *in vitro*. I. CsA allows for the expression of alloantigen-activated suppressor cells while preferentially inhibiting the induction of cytolytic effector lymphocytes in MLR. *J. Immunol.*, **124**, 2601–2608

10. Rappeport, J., Mihm, M., Reinherz, E., Lopansri, S. and Parkman, R. (1979) Acute graft-versus-host disease in recipients of bone marrow transplants from identical twin donors. *Lancet*, **2**, 717–720

11. Hood, A. F., Vogelsang, G. B., Black, L. P., Farmer, E. R. and Santos, G. W. (1987) Acute graft-versus-host disease. Development following autologous and syngeneic bone marrow transplantation. *Arch. Dermatol.*, **123**, 745–750

12. Glazier, A., Tutschka, P. J., Farmer, E. R. and Santos, G. W. (1983) Graft-versus-host disease in cyclosporin A treated rats after syngeneic and autologous bone marrow reconstitution. *J. Exp. Med.*, **158**, 1-8

13. Cheney, R. T. and Sprent, J. (1985) Capacity of cyclosporine to induce auto-graft-versus-host disease and impair intrathymic T cell differentiation. *Transplant. Proc.*, **17**, 528–520

14. Hess, A. D., Orwitz, L., Beschorner, W. E. and Santos, G. W. (1985) Development of graft-versus-host disease-like syndrome in cyclosporin-treated rats after syngeneic bone marrow transplantation. I. Development of cytotoxic T lymphocytes with apparent polyclonal anti-Ia specificity including autoreactivity. *J. Exp. Med.*, **161**, 718–730

15. Beschorner, W. E., De Gennaro, K. A., Hess, A. D. and Santos, G. W. (1987) Cyclosporine and the thymus; influence of irradiation and age on thymic immunopathology and recovery. *Cell. Immunol.*, **110**, 350–364

16. Boland, J., Atkinson, K., Britton, K., Darveniza, P., Johnson, S. and Biggs, J. (1984) Tissue distribution and toxicity of cyclosporin A in the mouse. *Pathology*, **16**, 117–123

17. Hows, J., Palmer, S. and Gordon-Smith, E. C. (1982) Use of cyclosporin A in allogeneic bone marrow transplantation for severe aplastic anaemia. *Transplantation*, **33**, 382–386

18. Hows, J., Palmer, S. and Gordon-Smith, E. C. (1985) Cyclosporine and graft failure following bone marrow transplantation for severe aplastic anaemia. *Br. J. Haematol.*, **60**, 611–617

19. Deeg, H. J., Storb, R., Thomas, E. D., Flournoy, N., Kennedy, M. S., Banaji, M., Applebaum, F. R., Bensinger, W. I., Buckner, C. D., Clift, R. A., Doney, K., Fefer, A., McGuffin, R., Sanders, J. E., Singer, J., Stewart, P., Sullivan, K. M. and Witherspoon, R. (1985)

155

Cyclosporine as prophylaxis for graft-versus-host disease; a randomised study in patients undergoing marrow transplantation for acute nonlymphoblastic leukaemia. *Blood*, **65**, 1325-1334

20. Storb, R., Deeg, H. J., Thomas, E. D., Applebaum, F. R., Buckner, C. D., Cheever, M. A., Clift, R. A., Doney, K. C., Flournoy, N., Kennedy, M. S., Loughran, T. P., McGuffin, R. W, Sale, G. E., Sanders, J. E., Singer, J. W., Stewart, P. S., Sullivan, K. M. and Witherspoon, R. P. (1985) Marrow transplantation for chronic myelocytic leukaemia. A controlled trial of cyclosporine versus methotrexate for prophylaxis of graft-versus-host disease. *Blood*, **66**, 698–702

21. Irle, C., Deeg, H. J., Buckner, C. D., Kennedy, M., Clift, R., Storb, R., Applebaum, F. R., Beatty, P., Bensinger, W., Doney, K., Cheever, M., Fefer, A., Greenberg, P., Hill, R., Martin, P., McGuffin, R., Sanders, J., Stewart, E., Sullivan, K., Witherspoon, R. and Thomas, E. D. (1985) Marrow transplantation for leukaemia following fractionated total body irradiation. A comparative trial of methotrexate and cyclosporine. *Leuk. Res.*, **9**, 1255–1261

22. Atkinson, K., Biggs, J. C., Concannon, A., Dodds, A., Downs, K. and Ashby, M. (1988) A prospective randomized trial of cyclosporin versus methotrexate after HLA-identical sibling marrow transplantation for patients with acute leukaemia in first remission: analysis 2.5 years after last patient entry. *Aust. NZ J. Med.*, **18**, 594–599

23. Ringden, O., Backman, L., Lohnqvist, D., Heimdahl, A., Lindholm, A., Bolme, P., Gahrton, G. (1986) A randomised trial comparing the use of cyclosporin and methotrexate for graft-versus-host disease prophylaxis in bone marrow transplant recipients with haematological malignancies. *Bone Marrow Transplant*, **1**, 41–51

24. Storb, R., Deeg, H. J., Fisher, L., Applebaum, F., Buckner, C. D., Bensinger, W., Clift, R., Doney, K., Irle, C., McGuffin, R., Martin, P., Sanders, J., Schoch, G., Singer, J., Stewart, P., Sullivan, K., Witherspoon, R. and Thomas, E. D. (1988) Cyclosporine versus methotrexate for graft-versus-host disease prevention in patients given marrow grafts for leukemia. Long term follow up of three controlled trials. *Blood*, **71**, 293–298

25. Storb, R., Deeg, H. J., Whitehead, J., Appelbaum, F., Beatty, P., Bensinger, W., Buckner, C. D., Clift, R. A., Doney, K., Farewell, V., Hansen, J., Hill, R., Lum, L., Martin, P., McGuffin, R., Sanders, J., Steweart, P., Sullivan, K., Witherspoon, R., Yee, G. and Thomas, E. D. (1986) Methotrexate and cyclosporine compared with cyclosporine alone for prophylaxis of acute graft-versus-host disease after marrow transplantation for leukemia. *N. Engl. J. Med.*, **314**, 729–735

26. Storb, R., Deeg, H. J., Farewell, V., Appelbaum, F., Beatty, P., Bensinger, W., Buckner, C. D., Clift, R., Hansen, J., Hill, R., Longton, G., Lum, L., Martin, P., McGuffin, R., Sanders, J., Singer, J., Stewart, P., Sullivan, K., Witherspoon, R. and Thomas, E. D. (1986) Marrow transplantation for severe aplastic anaemia. Methotrexate alone compared to a combination of methotrexate and cyclosporine for prevention of acute graft-versus-host disease. *Blood*, **68**, 119–125

27. Forman, F. J., Bloom, K. G., Trance, R. A., Miner, P. J., Metter, G. E., Hill, L. R., O'Donnell, M. R., Nademanee, A. P. and Snyder, D. S. (1987) A prospective randomised study of acute graft-versus-host disease in 107 patients with leukemia. Methotrexate/prednisone versus cyclosporin A/prednisone. *Transplant. Proc.*, **19**, 2605–2607

28. Kennedy, M. S., Deeg, H. J., Storb, R., Doney, K., Sullivan, K. M., Witherspoon, R., Applebaum, F., Stewart, P., Sanders, J., Buckner, C. D., Martin, P., Weiden, P. and Thomas, E. D. (1985) Treatment of acute graft-versus-host disease after allogeneic marrow transplantation. Randomised study comparing corticosteroids and cyclosporine. *Am. J. Med.*, **78**, 978–983

29. Deeg, H. J., Loughran, T. P., Storb, R., Kennedy, M. S., Sullivan, K. M., Doney, K., Appelbaum, F., Thomas, E. D. (1985) Treatment of human acute graft-versus-host disease with anti-thymocyte globulin and cyclosporine with or without methyl prednisolone. *Transplantation*, **40**, 162–166

30. Sullivan, K. M., Deeg, H. J., Storb, R., Nims, J., Witherspoon, R., Doney, K., Appelbaum, F. and Thomas, E. D. (1986) Alternating day cyclosporine and prednisone improves survival in patients with high-risk chronic graft-versus-host disease. *Exp. Hematol.*, **14**, 529 (abstract)

31. Andrus, L. and Lafferty, K. J. (1982) Inhibition of T cell activity by cyclosporin A. *Scand. J. Immunol.*, **15**, 449–458

32. Apperley, J. F., Mauro, F. and Goldman, J. M. (1987) Risk factors for relapse after bone marrow transplantation for chronic myeloid leukemia in first chronic phase. *Exp. Hematol.*, **15**, 535 (abstract)

33. Blume, K. G., Brenner, A. K., Sullivan, J. L., Chaganti, R. S., Dinsmore, R. and O'Reilly, R. (1985) Lymphoma of host origin in a marrow transplant recipient in remission of acute myeloid leuk.iemia and receiving cyclosporine. *Am. J. Hematol.*, **18**, 73–83

34. Forman, S. J., Sullivan, J. L., Ratech, H., Racklin, B. and Blume, K. G. (1987) Epstein–Barr related malignant B cell lymphoplasmacytic lymphoma following allogeneic bone marrow transplantation for aplastic anaemia. *Transplantation*, **44**, 244–249

35. Atkinson, K., Biggs, J. C., Ting, A., Concannon, A., Dodds, A. and Pun, A. (1983) Cyclosporin A is associated with faster engraftment and less mucositis than methotrexate after allogeneic bone marrow transplantation. *Br. J. Haematol.*, **53**, 265–270

36. Hows, J. M., Kaffaf, S., Palmer, S., Harris, R., Fairhead, S. and Gordon-Smith, E. C (1982) Regeneration of peripheral blood cells following allogeneic bone marrow transplantation for severe aplastic anaemia. *Br. J. Haematol.*, **52**, 551–'4558

37. Atkinson, J., Biggs, J. C., Hayes, J., Ralston, M., Concannon, A., Dodds, A. and Naidoo, D. (1983) Cyclosporin A nephrotoxicity in the first 100 days after marrow transplantation: 3 distinct syndromes. *Br. J. Haematol.*, **54**, 59–67

38. Hows, J. M., Chipping, P. M., Fairhead, S., Smith, J., Baughan, A. and Gordon-Smith, E. C. (1983) Nephrotoxicity in bone marrow transplant recipients treated with cyclosporin A. *Br. J. Haematol.*, **54**, 69–78

39. Gluckman, E., Devergie, A., Lokiec, F., Poirier, O. and Baumelou, A. (1981) Nephrotoxicity of cyclosporin A in bone marrow transplantation. *Lancet*, **2**, 144–145

40. Shulman, H., Striker, G., Deeg, H. J., Kennedy, M., Storb, R. and Thomas, E. D. (1981) Nephrotoxicity of cyclosporin A after allogeneic marrow transplantation; glomerular thrombosis and tubular injury. *N. Engl. J. Med.*, **305**, 1392–1395

41. Steller, F., Stoccoli, R., Steller, C., Biagoni, S., Giardiani, C., Baronconi, D. and Manenti, F (1987) Urinary cytologic abnormalities in bone marrow transplant recipients of cyclosporin. *Acta Cytol.*, **31**, 615-619

42. Loughran, T. P., Deeg, H. J., Dalberg, S., Kennedy, M. S., Storb, R. and Thomas, E. D. (1985) Incidence of hypertension after marrow transplantation among 112 patients randomised to either cyclosporin or methotrexate as graft-versus-host disease prophylaxis. *Br. J. Haematol.*, **59**, 547-553

43. June, C. H., Thompson, C. B., Kennedy, M. S., Loughran, T. P. and Deeg, H. J. (1986) Correlation of hypomagnesemia with the onset of cyclosporine-induced hypertension in marrow transplant patients. *Transplantation*, **41**, 47–51

44. Atkinson, K., Biggs, J., Dodds and Concannon, A. (1983) Cyclosporin A associated hepatotoxicity after allogeneic bone marrow transplantation; differentiation from other causes of post transplant liver disease. *Transplant. Proc.*, **25**, 2761–2767

45. Atkinson, K., Biggs, J., Darveniza, P., Boland, J., Concannon, A. and Dodds, A. (1984) Cyclosporine-associated central nervous system toxicity after allogeneic bone marrow transplantation. *Transplantation*, **38**, 34–37

46. Atkinson, K., Biggs, J., Concannon, A., Dodds, A., Dale, B. and Norman, J. (1986) Second marrow transplants for haematological malignancy. *Bone Marrow Transplant*, **1**, 159–166

47. Gloor, E., Gratwohl, A., Hahn, H., Kretzschmar, S., Robert, Y., Speck, B. and Daicker, B. (1985) Multiple cotton wool spots following bone marrow transplantation for treatment of acute lymphatic leukaemia. *Br. J. Ophthalmol.*, **69**, 320–325

48. Papa, G., Arcese, W., Bianchi, A., Mauro, F. R., Jandolo, B., Pompili, A., Gessini, L. and Mandelli, F. (1985) Cyclosporin-associated bilateral deltoid paralysis after allogeneic bone marrow transplantation for chronic myelogenous leukemia. *Haematologica*, **70**, 273–274

49. Wamboldt, F. W., Weiler, S. J. and Kellin, A. H. (1984) Cyclosporin-associated mania. *Biol. Psychol.*, **19**, 1161–1162

50. Rubin, A. M. and King, H. (1987) Cerebral blindness and encephalopathy with cyclosporin A toxicity. *Neurology*, **37**, 1072–1076

51. Katir, J. I. M. B. (1987) Visual hallucinations and cyclosporine. *Transplantation*, **43**, 768–769

52. Reznik, V. M., Jones, K. L., Durham, B. L. and Mendoza, S. A. (1987) Changes in facial appearance during cyclosporin treatment. *Lancet*, **1**, 1262–1263

53. Powles, R. L., Morganstern, G. R., Kay, H. E. M., McElwain, T. J., Clink, H. M., Dady, P.

J., Barrett, A., Jameson, B., Depledge, M. H., Watson, J. G., Sloane, J., Leigh, M., Lumley, H., Hedley, D., Lawler, S. D., Filshie, J. and Robinson, B. (1983) Mismatched family donors for bone marrow transplantation as treatment for acute leukaemia. *Lancet*, **1**, 612–615

54. Trigg, M. E., Billing, R., Sondel, P. M., Exten, R., Hong, R., Bosdech, M. J. Horowitz, S. D., Finlay, J., Moen, R., Longo, W., Erickson, C. and Peterson, A. (1985) Clinical trials depleting T lymphocytes from donor marrow for matched and mismatched allogeneic bone marrow transplants. *Cancer. Treat. Rep.*, **69**, 377–386

55. Beatty, P. G., Clift, R. A., Mickelson, E. M., Nispiros, B. B., Flournoy, N., Martin, P. J., Sanders, J. E., Stewart, P., Buckner, C. D., Storb, R., Thomas, E. D. and Hansen, J. A. (1985) Marrow transplantation from related donors other than HLA-identical siblings. *N. Engl. J. Med.*, **313**, 765–771

56. Beatty, P. G., Anasetti, C., Storb, R., Thomas, E. D., Hansen, J. A. (1988) Marrow transplantation from relatives other than HLA genotypically identical siblings. *J. Cell. Biochem.* (Suppl. 12c), **81** (abstract)

57. Beatty, P. G., Hansen, J. A., Storb, R. and Thomas, E. D. (1987) Cyclosporine plus methotrexate as prophylaxis for acute graft-versus-host disease in patients receiving marrow grafts from HLA-matched unrelated donors. *Blood*, **70**, 303a (abstract)

58. Witherspoon, R. P., Deeg, H. J., Lum, L. G., Ochs, H. D., Hansen, J. A., Thomas, E. D. and Storb, R. (1984) Immunologic recovery in human marrow graft recipients given cyclosporine or methotrexate for the prevention of graft-versus-host disease. *Transplantation*, **37**, 456–461

59. Atkinson, K., Luckhurst, E., Penny, R., Warren, H. and Biggs, J. (1983) Immunological reconstitution after allogeneic marrow transplantation in man. *Transplant. Proc.*, **15**, 474–479

60. Atkinson, K., Biggs, J. C., Britton, E., Farrell, C., Concannon, A. J. and Dodds, A. J. (1984) Oral administration of cyclosporin A for recipients of allogeneic bone marrow transplants. Implications of clinical gut dysfunction. *Br. J. Haematol.*, **56**, 223–231

61. Atkinson, K., Britton, K., Farrell, C. and Biggs, J. C. (1983) The chemical and immunosuppressive stability of cyclosporin A during continuous intravenous infusion. *Transplantation*, **36**, 590–592

62. Beveridge, T., Gratwohl, A. and Michot, F. (1981) Cyclosporin A pharmacokinetics after a single dose in man and serum levels after multiple dosing in recipients of allogeneic bone marrow grafts. *Curr. Ther. Res.*, **30**, 5–18

63. Atkinson, K., Britton, K. and Biggs, J. C. (1984) Distribution and concentration of cyclosporin in human blood. *J. Clin. Pathol.*, **3**, 1167–1171

64. Sonneveld, P., Kokenberg, E., Sizoo, W., Hagenbeek, A., van der Steuijt, K. and Lowenberg, B. (1987) Concentrations of ciclosporin in allogeneic bone marrow recipients. Comparison of assay methods. *Blut*, **55**, 467–472

65. Atkinson, K., Biggs, J. C. and Britton, K. (1982) Distribution and persistence of cyclosporin in human tissue. *Lancet*, **2**, 1196

66. Atkinson, K., Biggs, J. C., Britton, K. and Downs, K. (1985) Cyclosporine in human marrow transplantation: absence of a therapeutic window. *Transplant. Proc.*, **17**, 1239–1241

67. Gratwohl, A., Speck, B., Wenk, M., Forster, I. U., Muller, M., Osterwalder, B., Nissen, C. and Follath, F. (1983) Cyclosporin in human bone marrow transplantation. Serum concentration, graft-versus-host disease, and nephrotoxicity. *Transplantation*, **36**, 40–44

68. Lindholm, A., Ringden, O. and Lonnqvist, B. (1987) The role of cyclosporine dosage and plasma levels in efficacy and toxicity in bone marrow recipients. *Transplantation*, **43**, 680–684

69. Kennedy, M. S., Deeg, H. J., Segal, M., Crowley, J. J., Storb, R. and Thomas, E. D. (1983) Acute renal toxicity with combined use of ampotericin B and cyclosporine after marrow transplantation. *Transplantation*, **35**, 211–215

70. Schroeder, T. J., Nelvan, D. B., Clardy, C. W., Wadwa, N. K., Myra, S. A., Reising, J. M., Wolf, R. K., Collins, J. A., Pesc, E. and First, M. R. (1987) Use of cyclosporine and ketoconazole without nephrotoxicity in two heart transplant recipients. *J. Heart Transplant.*, **6**, 84–89

71. Habboush, H. W. and Hann, I. K. (1986) Anaphylactic reaction to cyclosporin in a bone marrow transplant recipient. *Br. J. Haematol.*, **62**, 195–196

8
Cyclosporin A and intraocular inflammatory disease

John V. Forrester, Janet Liversidge and Hamish M. Towler

INTRODUCTION

Although the benefits of cyclosporin A (CsA) therapy in various transplantation procedures had been clearly recognized for some time, the introduction of CsA to ophthalmology did not occur until 1980 when the drug was used on an experimental model of autoimmune ocular inflammation, namely experimental autoimmune uveoretinitis (EAU)[1]. That it was not first used for transplantation management in ophthalmology was in part due to the low rate of corneal graft rejection compared to renal or cardiac graft rejection and, if rejection did occur, it was often controlled satisfactorily with topical steroids provided it was diagnosed sufficiently early. However, the early use of CsA in EAU also reflected a continuing major clinical problem in ophthalmology, namely endogenous posterior uveitis. Posterior uveitis, a significant cause of blindness in the USA and other countries[2], is probably autoimmune in nature, at least in some of its clinical forms, and is often refractory to treatment even with systemic steroids. Some special forms of uveitis such as Behçet's disease are highly prevalent in certain geographical regions such as the Middle East, Turkey and Japan, and represent a considerable morbidity in these countries.

Since these early reports the use of CsA in other autoimmune diseases has become more widespread, including other ocular autoimmune diseases such as dysthyroid eye disease[3], and keratoconjunctivitis sicca, either alone or as part of Sjögren's syndrome[4]. Although much of the early data regarding CsA toxicity was derived from renal transplant studies, it has frequently been difficult to differentiate primary renal disease from drug toxicity; therefore studies in uveitis patients whose renal function was often considered normal, provided firm evidence of a dose-related CsA-induced renal impairment[5]. Within the limitations of its side-effects, however, the drug has proved valuable in reducing ocular inflammation and improving vision. In addition, it has been extremely valuable in cases of severe optic nerve compression due to thyroid orbital infiltration[3] and has benefited some patients with vernal keratoconjunctivitis[6].

The possible use of CsA in anterior segment eye disease such as severe vernal keratoconjunctivitis, and in corneal graft rejection, has further advanced the development of topical CsA preparations and the study of their pharmacokinetics. Newer topical preparations with better tissue penetrations have recently been reported[7]. In the present chapter, however, the discussion is restricted to a summary of the use of CsA in chronic posterior endogenous uveitis.

OCULAR PHARMACOLOGY OF CsA

Considerable experimental and clinical data are now available on the pharmacology of CsA after oral, subcutaneous or intramuscular administration (see Chapter 12). This highly hydrophobic drug is normally administered in an oil-based vehicle, and binds to and enters cells via the prolactin receptor. Two major intracellular CsA binding proteins have been described: calmodulin which controls Ca^{2+}-dependent cell activation pathways, and cyclophilin, the function of which is unknown, but which may act by concentrating CsA in lymphoid cells on which the drug exerts a selective inhibitory action (reviewed in reference 8). Tissues with a high lipid content also accumulate CsA and are susceptible to toxicity.

Studies of systemic administration of CsA have shown that it appears in ocular tissues in detectable levels within 24 h, but drug levels within the aqueous do not reach levels comparable with serum[9]. In contrast, experimental studies in rabbits indicate that topical administration of CsA leads to similar low levels in aqueous and serum, with high levels of the drug being retained within the corneal stroma[10]. It was therefore suggested that topical CsA may be useful for controlling corneal graft rejection while avoiding the side-effects of systemic CsA. Clearly, however, it would be of little value in the management of endogenous intraocular inflammation, either anterior or posterior uveitis, and this has been confirmed experimentally[11]. Failure of CsA to penetrate the corneal stroma is probably related to the hydrophilic nature of this layer, which would reject a hydrophobic compound like CsA[12]. However, considerably high levels of the drug persist in the cornea for 24 h after a single application[10].

Several studies have shown that topical[13], subconjunctival[14], retrobulbar[15] and intramuscular[16] injections of CsA are effective in experimental corneal allografts, but there have been few human studies and little is known regarding the effective tissue drug levels achieved by these routes. A recent study comparing topical and intramuscular administration of CsA in rabbits reported that similar levels were found in both plasma and aqueous by either route, but in both cases the levels achieved were below the therapeutic value[9], i.e. < 100 ng/ml. A separate study showed that epibulbar injection, as opposed to subconjunctival injection, achieved high levels of intraocular (aqueous) CsA[17] (360, 700 and 200 ng ml^{-1} at 2, 8 and 24 h after injection), but repeated administration via this route is unlikely to be acceptable to patients with chronic uveitis. Oral administration of CsA would therefore appear to be the preferred route, at least for such deep-seated conditions as endogenous uveitis. The possible use of intravitreal CsA has been considered after a rabbit toxicity study showed that high levels of intravitreal CsA alone (more than 5 times the required dose) produced minimal retinal damage[18]. No human trials have so far been attempted with this route.

Endogenous uveitis

Uveitis is a term applied to inflammatory disease of any part of the uveal tract. It is categorized by anatomical location into anterior uveitis (affecting the iris, 'iritis' or the iris and anterior ciliary body, 'iridocylitis') and posterior uveitis (affecting the choroid and retina). An intermediate form of uveitis affecting the posterior ciliary body (or pars plana) and vitreous base region of the eye also occurs and is known as intermediate uveitis or pars planitis (Figure 8.1). Uveitis may also be acute or chronic, and is exogenous when it is induced by some invasive organism, e.g. bacterial, viral or fungal agents. In contrast, endogenous uveitis occurs when there is no obvious aetiological agent. Traditionally, clinical uveitis has been categorized into granulomatous or non-granulomatous, depending on the nature of the cellular exudate which occurs in the anterior chamber of the eye and appears as deposits of white cells on the corneal endothelium (keratic precipitate) (Figure 8.2). However, this grading system has not been helpful in advancing our understanding of the pathogenesis, and is little used at the present time.

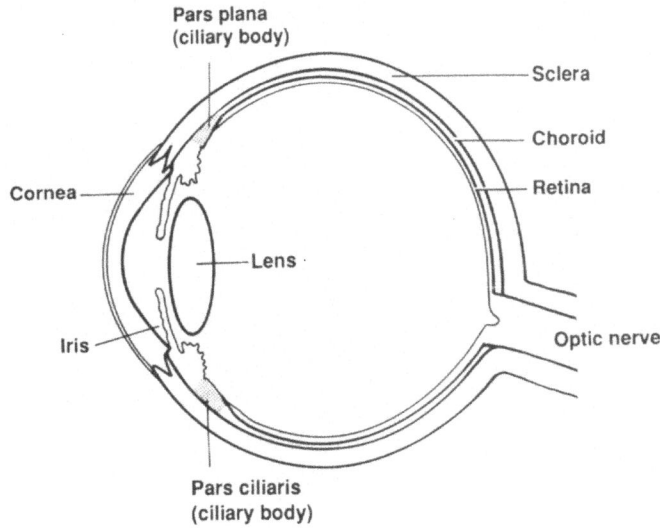

Figure 8.1 Diagram of the eye

161

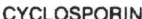

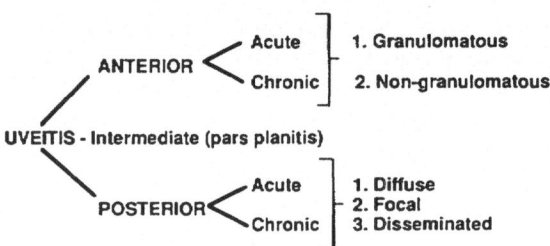

Figure 8.2 Flow diagram of classification of uveitis by anatomical location

CLINICAL FORMS OF UVEITIS

Anterior uveitis is pathogenetically a separate disorder from intermediate and posterior uveitis. Most forms of anterior uveitis occur as acute episodes and many are linked to ankylosing spondylitis in association with the HLA-B27 haplotype. In addition, there is considerable cross-association with other 'non-infectious' inflammatory disorders such as Reiter's syndrome and enterocolitis caused by *Yersinia* and *Klebsiella* (Figure 8.3). Immunological disturbances have been observed in some of these patients, but in general the uveitis is self-limiting or easily controlled with the use of topical steroids. Chronic anterior uveitis is much less common, but may occur in association with certain forms of pauci-articular arthritis and produces a particularly insidious form of ocular damage, with cataract, hypotension and band keratopathy.

The term endogenous uveitis is usually reserved for chronic intraocular

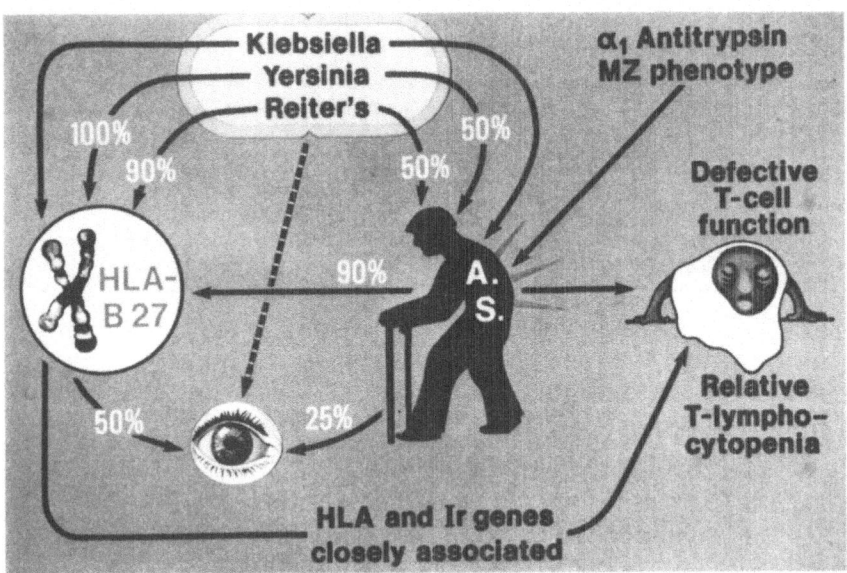

Figure 8.3 Interrelationships between anterior uveitis, ankylosing spondylitis, HLA-B27 and enterocolitis

Table 8.1   Endogenous posterior uveitis

Includes	Excludes
Diffuse uveitis	Anterior uveitis
Pan uveitis	Recurrent chorioretinitis (e.g. toxoplasmosis)
Focal chorioretinitis	Acute retinal necrosis
Retinal vasculitis	Endophthalmitis
Pars planitis	Lens-induced uveitis
Sympathetic opthalmia	
Birdshot choroidoretinopathy	
Behçet's disease	
Vogt–Koyanaga–Harada disease	
Some pigment epitheliopathies	

inflammation affecting the posterior segment, and includes a very wide variety of clinical syndromes (Table 8.1). The severity of the inflammation can vary from mild (as in pars planitis) to marked (as in Behçet's disease) with involvement of the retina, vitreous and choroid and frequently hyperacute episodes in which there is 'spill-over' of inflammation into the anterior chamber (secondary anterior uveitis). Endogenous uveitis may be found in association with certain systemic diseases such as sarcoidosis or multiple sclerosis, but no aetiological link has been demonstrated. Consideration of this heterogeneous set of disorders as a single entity remains controversial, and many believe that certain forms are discrete entities, such as retinal vasculitis, or Vogt–Koyanagi–Harada disease, or most recently, birdshot retino-choroidopathy in which the strongest HLA haplotype association for any human disease so far has been recorded (HLA.A29 in over 95% of cases)[19,20]. However, as will be discussed later, there is considerable logic in considering these disorders as a single group.

PATHOLOGY OF UVEITIS

Histopathological studies of uveitis have been rare, mainly because of the obvious difficulty in obtaining material during the active stage of the disease. Most of our information derives from studies of sympathetic ophthalmia, in which the uveitis develops in the fellow-eye after penetrating ocular injury[21]. This condition was probably the first autoimmune disease described in man[22], and led to the early searches for an ocular antigen[23]. The characteristic ocular lesion in sympathetic ophthalmia is the Dalen–Fuchs nodule, which is a microgranulomatous lesion occurring within a heavily lymphocyte-infiltrated choroid and involving the outer retinal layers (Figure 8.4). Immunohistochemical studies by several groups have shown that the lesions contain large numbers of MHC class II antigen-positive cells (presumably macrophages) and T cytotoxic cells[24,25] while the surrounding choroid is infiltrated with T helper cells. The Dalen–Fuchs nodule has considerable similarity to lesions induced experimentally in guinea pigs (Figure 8.5) and other animals by retinal S antigen, a 48 kd protein located in the photoreceptor rod outer segment[26-28], and known as experimental autoimmune uveoretinitis (EAU).

163

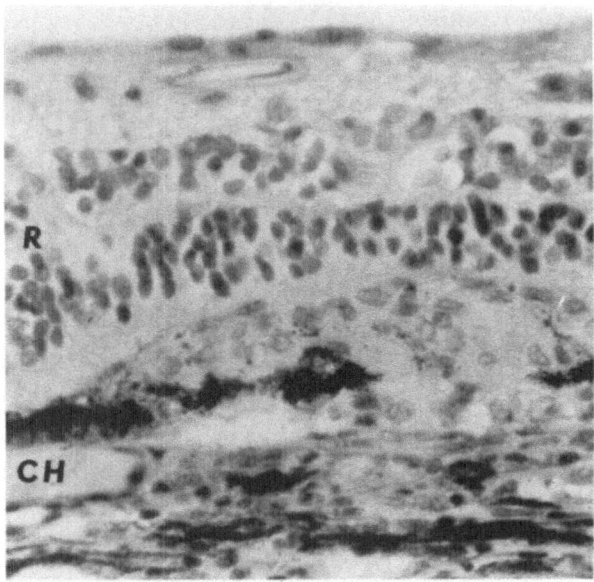

Figure 8.4 Dalen–Fuchs nodule in human sympathetic ophthalmia. R, retina; Ch, choroid. (Courtesy, Professor W. R. Lee)

After fruitless years of research for an autoantigen in uveal tissue[29], Wacker and Lipton[30] rediscovered the highly uveitogenic nature of retinal tissue and purified a soluble antigen, S antigen, from bovine retina in 1977[26]. The target organ in EAU is the rod outer segment[31], and the earliest lesions after immunization involve specific rod outer segment lysis. High doses of antigen produce acute and extensive photoreceptor loss[31] and eventually lead to replacement of the photoreceptor layer with fibroblast-like cells.

Since the discovery of retinal S antigen and the confirmation of endogenous uveitis as an autoimmune disorder, other retinal antigens such as rhodopsin[32] and interphotoreceptor retinal binding protein[33] have also been shown to induce ocular inflammatory disease[34]. Specific uveitogenic peptides both from retinal S antigen and from IRBP have been isolated and synthesized, and also induce EAU, particularly in the Lewis rat, although less so in other species[35–37].

EAU is a Th cell-mediated disease[38] and S antigen specific Th cell lines have been developed[39,40]. However, EAU induced by cell transfer is never as severe as that induced by the whole antigen, suggesting that other mechanisms regulate or contribute towards the expression of the disease. Certain monoclonal antibodies to S antigen inhibit the induction of EAU[41,42] (although they have less effect on pinealitis[42]) and studies in guinea pigs have shown that B cells and plasma cells predominate in end-stage or 'healed' EAU lesions[43].

The role of retinal antigens in human uveitis is less clear. Initial studies suggested that patients with endogenous uveitis, especially birdshot retino-choroidopathy, showed increased responsiveness to bovine and human retinal

164

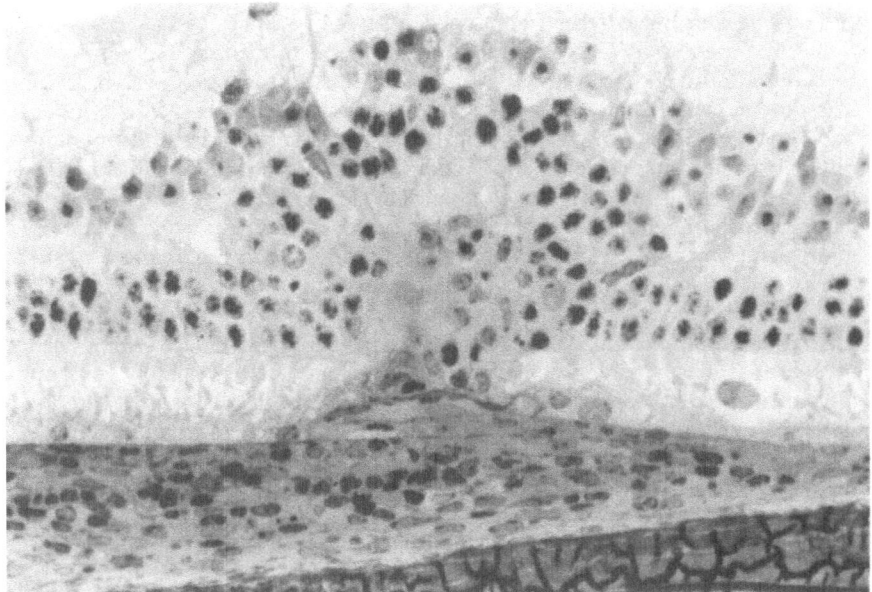

Figure 8.5 Experimental autoimmune uveoretinitis in the guinea pig induced by retinal S antigen. Note extensive photoreceptor damage and focal accumulation of cells in outer retinal layers

S antigen in a lymphocyte proliferation assay[44]. Since bovine and human retinal S antigen show a very high degree of sequence homology[45,46], these results were considered relevant. However, later studies have been less supportive[47,48], particularly when strict attention is paid to controls. Similarly, initial reports indicated that patients with uveitis (and other retinal disorders or injuries) showed elevated levels of antibodies to bovine retinal S antigen[49]. However, these results were not confirmed with human S antigen[50] and, indeed, high levels of antibodies to human and bovine S antigen have been found in the normal population[51]. It has been suggested that these 'natural' antibodies may have a protective function[51] and, indeed, there is some indirect evidence for this, since patients with retinal vasculitis have a disease severity index inversely proportional to their serum concentration of immune complexes[52]. To date, the most reliable data on immune responsiveness to S antigen in human uveitis have been shown by Doekes et al.[50], using a sensitive macrophage migration inhibition assay. Interestingly, some patients with retinitis pigmentosa, a slowly degenerative and frequently inherited group of retinal diseases, appear to have high levels of memory B cells for S antigen which can be stimulated to secrete antibodies if polyclonally activated by EB virus[53] or purified protein derivative[54], but the significance of this finding is unclear. In general, although the results of autoimmunity to retinal antigens in human uveitis remains equivocal, this is hardly surprising since the current tests are relatively insensitive or non-specific, since the percentage of specific autoreactive T or B cells in the circulating pool of lymphocytes will be low, and since exposure to retinal antigen is likely to be limited.

Despite the findings in clinical immunology, the model of EAU has served to promote our understanding of human uveitis considerably. For instance, it is now apparent that a single antigen such as retinal S antigen can induce a wide spectrum of clinicopathological changes closely resembling the range of uveitis syndromes seen in man[55] (Table 8.2). Thus, the precise inflammatory response depends on the dose of antigen, the species, strain, and even haplotype of the animal, the number and type of adjuvants and the state of immunosuppression. This has implications for the nature of human uveitic disease. It is likely that the retina and choroid have only a limited set of responses to immunological challenge and it is therefore on this basis that the various clinical forms of uveitis can be considered as a single entity. Most of these disorders have in common four clinical signs, namely vitreous inflammatory cells, focal choroido-retinal infiltration, micro- or macro-retinal vasculitis and macular oedema (Figure 8.6). Other signs may occur in addition to these, particularly in severe uveitis, but in general are merely extensions of the four basic signs.

CURRENT THERAPY FOR ENDOGENOUS UVEITIS

Endogenous uveitis is a difficult condition to treat. Patients with mild disease such as pars planitis frequently present as young adults with minimal symptoms of 'floaters' in one eye. The disease may persist at this level for many weeks or months and eventually recede spontaneously, or it may progress to produce significant cellular infiltrate in the vitreous with discrete opacities and macular oedema. Active intervention is usually considered when vision is affected, but a decision to treat is not taken lightly since the only effective form of therapy is some variant of immunosuppression. While topical steroids are uniformly ineffectual, systemic steroids usually in the form of prednisolone in a dosage of $1-2$ mg kg^{-1} day^{-1} as a single oral dose have proved to be effective in many cases of endogenous uveitis. However, it is not yet clear whether systemic steroid therapy leads to preservation of vision in the long term. In addition, steroids have considerable side-effects if used over prolonged periods; especially so in young patients during phases of growth[56]. It is not uncommon for a decision regarding adequate therapy to be postponed by default until the second eye becomes affected, by which time the macula of the first eye is irreversibly damaged by the development of a macular hole or other pathology.

At the other extreme, patients with severe endogenous uveitis such as retinal vasculitis, either idiopathic or as part of Behçet's disease, may require very high doses of systemic steroids to control their disease. Alternatively they may be steroid-resistant. In these cases other immunosuppressive regimes have been tried. Colchicine is commonly prescribed in a dose of 0.05 mg kg^{1} day^{-1} for patients with Behçet's disease in some parts of the world such as Japan[57]. Other drugs such as methotrexate and 6-mercaptopurine have been used but are usually second-line therapies. Considerable reliance has been placed on chlorambucil, cyclophosphamide and azathioprine. Most of these

Table 8.2 Correlation between clinical and experimental uveitis syndromes

	S-antigen-induced uveoretinitis			Human (?autoimmune) uveoretinitis		
Pathology	*Pathology*	*Species*	*Conditions*	*Pathology*	*Clinical*	*Severity*
Focal lesion	Focal lesion	Guinea pig	Low dose, bovine antigen	Focal chorioretiniti	Pars planitis	Mild
Focal lesion	Focal lesion	Guinea pig	High dose, complete depletion	Focal chorioretinitis	Sympathetic ophthalmia	Moderate
Focal lesion	Focial lesion	Rat	High dose, CsA	Focal chorioretinitis plus retinal vasculitis	Sarcoid, birdshot	Moderate
Focal lesion plus retinal vasculitis		Monkey	High dose			
Retinal vasculitis	Retinal vasculitis	Rat	High dose	Retinal vasculitis plus focal lesions	Idiopathic	Moderate to severe
Hypopyon uveitis	Hypopyon uveitis	Rat	High dose, double adjuvant	Hypopyon uveitis with retinal vasculitis	Behçet's disease	Severe
Panophthalmitis	Panophthalmitis	Guinea pg	High dose, guinea pig antigen	Retinal vasculitis, exudative detachment of retina	Vogt–Koyanagi–Harada	Severe

167

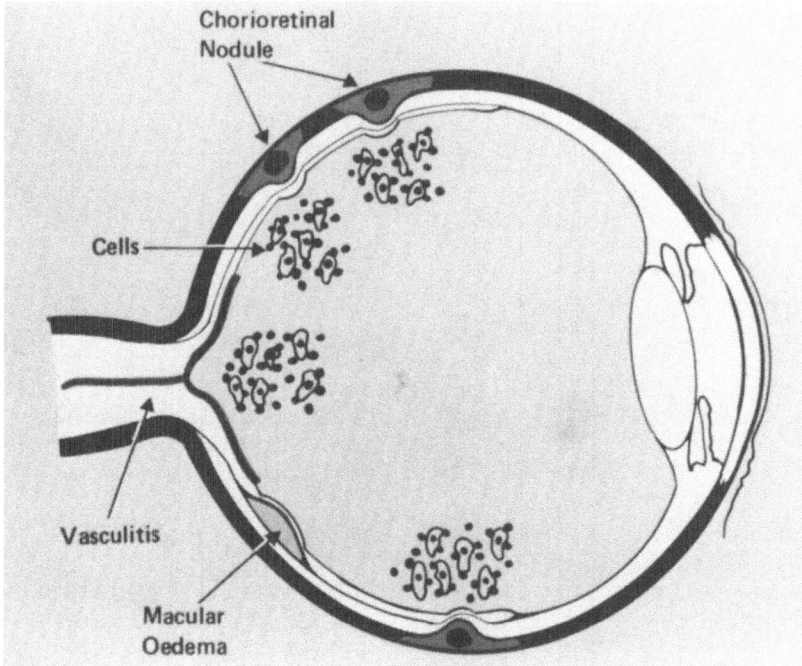

Figure 8.6 Diagrammatic representation of the four cardinal signs of endogenous posterior uveitis

are effective in reducing inflammation, but progressive visual loss still occurs and the side-effects of these drugs are frequently intolerable[58]. These include bone marrow depression, susceptibiity to infection, and tumour development as a result of chromosomal injury. In addition chlorambucil is associated with azoospermia. Several other therapies including levamisole, thymosin, BCG, transfer factor, γ-interferon and plasmapheresis have been tried (for review, see reference 58), but without benefit. The wide range of treatment modalities for this disorder, plus other severe forms of endogenous uveitis, attests to the difficulties of providing adequate therapy, particularly since none of these treatments has been tested in a clinically controlled manner. Clearly, alternative approaches are required.

CsA THERAPY IN EXPERIMENTAL UVEITIS

Since the original observation that CsA is effective in preventing retinal S-antigen-induced EAU[1,59] several further studies have addressed the questions of how CsA acts to reduce the inflammatory response and whether it is effective in inhibiting established disease. Nussenblatt *et al.*[59] showed that CsA could still inhibit EAU if the drug was administered a week after immunization but before the onset of clinical disease in rats. Further studies compared CsA with other anti-inflammatory drugs such as dexamethasone, cyclophosphamide, bredinin and colchicine[60]. Whereas CsA consistently inhibited EAU, at doses which produced little or no side-effects, the remaining drugs failed to prevent EAU in Lewis rats unless they were used at lethal doses. Colchicine had no effect whatsoever, while the other three drugs caused some delay in the onset of EAU. It was also of note that, in CsA-treated rats, although there was a decrease in DTH skin responses and lymphocyte blast transformation to S antigen, there was no inhibition of antibody production. In contrast, cyclophosphamide-treated animals showed a considerable decrease in antibody production as well as a reduced lymphocyte transformation reaction. These results indicate that although immunosuppression is effective in modulating EAU, not all aspects of the immune response are suppressed since all three components, namely the secretion of the antibody, the cell-mediated DTH and lymphocyte blast transformation, and the uveitogenic (or cytopathic) effect could be differentially affected. Indeed, recent studies of S antigen[61] and RIBP-induced[62] EAU have been shown that whereas several peptides from both molecules can evoke antibody responses, only a few can reproduce the uveitogenic response[63]. The use of CsA in such experiments may assist in improving our understanding of these immunological problems. Of greater clinical interest, however, is the question of whether CsA can inhibit established uveitis, since it is clearly not likely that CsA will be used prophylactically. Striph et al.[64] showed that CsA was more effective in reducing the severity of established EAU in guinea pigs than systemic steroids, and that a combination of both drugs was more effective than either alone, although there was no evidence of synergism. These results supported the use of CsA in human uveitis where treatment is only instituted in overt and severe inflammatory disease.

MODE OF ACTION OF CsA IN EXPERIMENTAL UVEITIS

Currently, CsA is considered to exert most of its activity by inhibiting the secretion of lymphokine from activated Th cells, thus inhibiting the activation of cytotoxic T lymphocytes whilst sparing the IL-2 independent activation and expansion of T suppressor cell clones[65]. CsA appears to have its effect at the level of mRNA transcription of lymphokine[66]; however, it has no effect on preformed lymphokine. Convincing evidence for the effect of CsA on nuclear transcription of lymphokine mRNA has been reported in DNA–RNA blotting experiments of cell extracts after phorbol myristate acetate stimulation[67]. The effect appeared to be specific for lymphokine gene expression. Other reports have suggested that CsA may have further activity at the cell membrane, for instance on phospholipase A_2 expression[68] and membrane potential[69]. Lymphokine secretion, particularly IL-1 and IL-2, is essential during the process of Th 'help' for T effector cells and B cells. However, although CsA inhibits Th-mediated cytotoxic responses, Th-independent antibody secretion may remain unaffected[60]. In contrast, calcium-dependent B cell functions are CsA-sensitive and distinct subsets of memory B cells, i.e. CsA-sensitive and resistant, have been demonstrated[70], suggesting that additional mechanisms of CsA action remain to be revealed.

Th cell activation requires antigen presentation in association with MHC class II antigen expression on antigen-presenting cells, a process which is also lyr·phokine-mediated. This activation may be inhibited by CsA by more than one mechanism. Macrophage antigen presentation is directly inhibited by CsA without any reduction in surface class II antigen[71]. CsA is also effective in indirectly inhibiting class II antigen expression on choroidal inflammatory cells in EAU, presumably via its effect on lymphokine production[72]. Although CsA inhibited clinical evidence of EAU and histopathologic evidence of retinal destruction, there was still a significant infiltrate of Tc/s cells in the choroid, but these and other choroid cells were class II negative. Recently, aberrant presentation of antigen by tissue cells, as opposed to circulating mononuclear cells, has been proposed as a mechanism of autoimmune disease induction in such conditions as thyroiditis[73] and diabetes mellitus[74]. Indirect evidence to support this notion has been provided by the expression of class II antigens on thyroid epithelial cells and pancreatic beta cells. Class II antigen expression on retinal pigment epithelial cells has also been observed in experimental[75,76] and clinical uveitis[77] and, more recently, on retinal microvascular endothelial cells[43,78]. Retinal pigment epithelial cells *in vitro* can be induced to express class II antigen in a dose-dependent response to interferon or lymphocyte-activated lymphokine[79], and human RPE cells may express the DP, DQ and DR antigen differentially in response to lymphokine[80]. Although CsA does not directly affect this *in vitro* class II antigen expression by RPE cells, CsA-treated lymphocytes fail to produce a class-II inducing lymphokine-rich supernatant[79]. It would thus appear that, if aberrant presentation of antigen by tissue cells is important in organ specific autoimmunity, then CsA would inhibit such a disease by its effects on lymphokine secretion.

CsA may have additional modes of action. Prolactin, the hypothalamic/pituitary hormone, is known to have a significant effect on lymphocyte responsiveness[81]. CsA competes with prolactin for receptors on T lymphocytes, and agents which stimulate prolactin secretion reduce the immunosuppressive effect of CsA. Bromocriptine, a specific inhibitor of prolactin secretion, has been shown to enhance the immunosuppressive effect of Csa in EAU[82], but its usefulness in the clinical situation is limited, and it may even have a deleterious effect, because prolactin levels in these patients are frequently low due to homeostatic negative feedback mechanisms.

CLINICAL USE OF CsA IN UVEITIS

Nussenblatt et al.[83] were the first to report on the clinical use of CsA in endogenous uveitis. In their study, 16 patients with active bilateral posterior uveitis of non-infectious origin who had failed to respond adequately to systemic steroids or cytotoxic agents were treated with CsA orally at a dose of 10 mg kg^{-1} day^{-1}. Fifteen of the patients showed an improvement in visual acuity even in some cases where there was persistent macular oedema as shown by fluorescein angiography. The types of patients treated in this initial study included the entire spectrum of uveitides (see above) from pars planitis to severe ocular Behçet's disease. Failure to respond adequately to conventional therapy was due either to continued visual loss in spite of therapy or an improved visual acuity, but only with unacceptably high doses of steroids and/or cytotoxic drugs. CsA therapy was continued for 2–18 months in this group of patients, and although some maintained good vision on a reduced dose of CsA, others required supplementation with systemic steroids or an increase in CsA dosage to 15 mg kg^{-1} day^{-1}.

Two important problems in the management of uveitis patients with CsA emerged from this study. First, some patients developed renal impairment as showed by elevated serum creatinine and reduced creatinine clearance, in spite of having renal function indices with the reference range prior to therapy. Of more general interest, however, regarding drug trials in posterior uveitis, it has become clear that there is no satisfactory grading system for measuring inflammation, and thereby response to therapy. Previous clinical grading systems have been restricted mainly to anterior uveitis[84], which may not reflect inflammatory activity in the posterior segment. In part the problem of grading posterior segment disease relates to the wide heterogeneity in types of posterior uveitis (see above). In spite of these limitations, most patients with posterior uveitis have some degree of vitreous opacification due to infiltration of the vitreous gel with inflammatory cells and exudate. A reduction in the degree of vitreous 'haze' can be seen in response to most therapies, and provides a usable measure of drug effectivity[85].

Several further 'open' studies have confirmed the effectiveness of CsA in endogenous uveitis[86–93]. In most of these studies, therapy was commenced at a dose of 10 mg kg^{-1} day^{-1} and gradually reduced to the minimum effective dose. Too rapid a withdrawal from the drug was associated with severe recurrences[89], and in some patients side-effects, particularly renal dysfunction (see below) necessitated cessation of the drug. In spite of these problems, the drug was effective in over 60% of cases in improving or maintaining vision, and its effects were manifested within 2–4 weeks of starting therapy.

In a study of Behçet's disease[90], short-term (3-month) therapy with oral CsA (10 mg kg^{-1} day^{-1}) was also found to be effective in controlling ocular inflammation, but severe recurrences developed after cessation of the drug and, in general, this form of therapy was not recommended.

Controlled trials of CsA versus conventional therapy have been attempted on a few occasions[94,95]. In the Dutch study[95] all patients were treated with a low dose of prednisone. Half of the patients also received CsA (10 mg kg^{-1} day^{-1}) in a randomized manner, with the remaining patients receiving placebo. CsA and steroid was found to be more effective in controlling inflammation and maintaining vision than prednisone alone, but the effect was lost on cessation of therapy. In this study, side-effects were few. A further study of patients with Behçet's disease in Turkey (Ussman, Y. and Yacizi, H., personal communication) compared cyclophosphamide versus CsA in (a) reducing the frequency of acute exacerbations and (b) maintaining visual acuity. In this study CsA also appeared to provide greater benefit. CsA was also more effective in the treatment of Behçet's disease than combination therapy of corticosteroids and azathioprine[94].

Although CsA has been found to be beneficial in ocular Behçet's disease, differences of opinion exist concerning its effectiveness in controlling the non-ocular manifestations such as arthralgia, gastrointestinal disease and mucocutaneous ulceration[90.94]. However, grading of severity of the non-ocular disease is even more difficult than the ocular disease, and further studies are required to assess this effect.

It would therefore appear that the major limitation of the use of CsA in uveitis is the risk of systemic and other side-effects[96]. Accordingly, several 'low-dose' studies of CsA in uveitis have been initiated. The regime of therapy is to commence with an oral dose of $5 \, \text{mg kg}^{-1} \, \text{day}^{-1}$ and to reduce this slowly over a period of several weeks to arrive at the minimum effective dose, usually $2-3 \, \text{mg kg}^{-1} \, \text{day}^{-1}$. The rationale behind this approach is the knowledge that nephrotoxicity, both experimentally[94] and clinically[97], is dose-dependent (see below). Currently there are at least five 'low-dose' open trials of CsA in endogenous uveitis. In the Scottish study, 13 patients with endogenous uveitis of various causes have been enrolled[98]. Treatment regimes to date have lasted from 3 to 40 months and average maintenance dose has been $3.5 \, \text{mg/kg}$ wt. In general, visual improvement has been achieved (Figure 8.7) and maintained for at least 12 months. Attempts to withdraw CsA have been successful in only a few cases, and in some patients acute recurrences of uveitis have been observed, requiring restitution of higher-dose therapies. In approximately half of the patients CsA therapy has been combined with low-dose systemic steroids (always less than $20 \, \text{mg}$ total dose prednisolone and usually less than $10 \, \text{mg}$) to achieve satisfactory control of the ocular

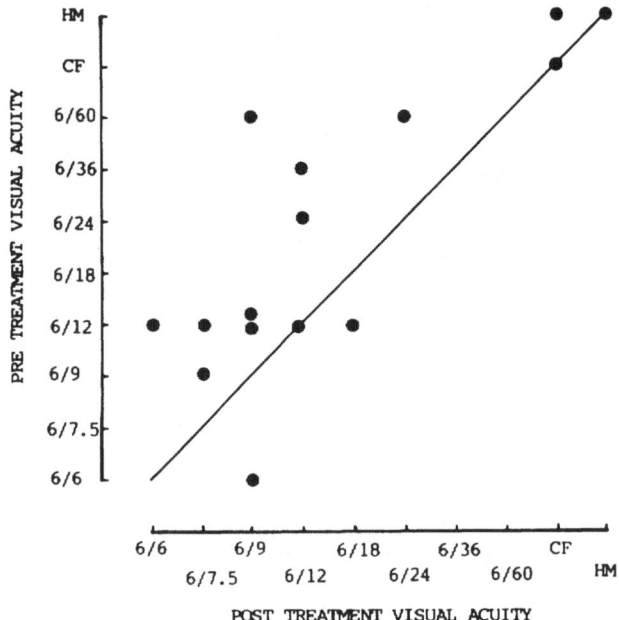

Figure 8.7 Effect of 12 months CsA therapy on visual acuity in patients with endogenous uveitis

inflammation. The hope that 'low-dose' CsA would prevent nephrotoxicity has not been fully realized, since in most of these patients there was a gradual rise in serum creatinine, plus changes in other renal function indices (see below). However, the problem is less serious with lower doses of CsA, is less evident in younger patients and may be reversible.

An obvious solution to the problem of CsA toxicity is either to monitor drug levels of CsA or to correlate effective immunosuppression as tested *in vitro* with the minimal effective dose of CsA. Methods of monitoring drug levels are dealt with elsewhere in this book. Briefly, they involve assaying CsA or its metabolites either chemically using high-pressure liquid chromatography (HPLC), or by immunological means using polyclonal or monoclonal antibody to CsA. Few studies of CsA therapy in uveitis have documented blood levels during treatment. Of those with data, no clear correlation with the dose of the drug or with clinical efficacy has been noted[89,98]. Probably it would be of greater relevance to measure local tissue concentrations such as in aqueous or vitreous samples, but it is still dubious whether the assay methods are sufficiently reproducible to provide results which could justify taking such samples routinely.

Monitoring CsA effectiveness by assaying lymphocyte responsiveness is also difficult in patients with uveitis. No specific or non-specific immunological abnormality has been detected in patients with posterior uveitis. Non-specific autoantibodies[99] and antibodies to retinal S antigen[50,51] occur with equal frequency in patients with uveitis as in normal, healthy volunteers. Some patients with posterior uveitis show enhanced lymphocyte responsiveness to S antigen (but not to IRBP[47]) and positive macrophage migration inhibition responses to S antigen[50], but the inherent variability of these biological assays is too great to be of use in monitoring CsA effects. Similarly, the levels of circulating T and B cells and their subsets are not sufficiently different between patients with uveitis and healthy controls to be of value in assaying CsA effects[48]. However, this approach to assaying CsA effects may still be possible. Recently, it has been shown that patients with uveitis have higher levels of circulating 'activated' T cells, as shown by their expression of IL-2 receptors and other markers[100]. Since CsA inhibits expression of IL-2 on T lymphocytes *in vitro*[101], it should be possible to demonstrate CsA effects by a reduction in the number of IL-2-positive cells. Such an approach has already been used in CsA-treated multiple sclerosis patients[102]. Interestingly, it was noted the CSF lymphocytes from CsA-treated patients showed no change in IL-2 expression, indicating that the drug failed to cross the blood–brain barrier in sufficient concentration to inhibit T cell activation locally. Since CsA is effective in endogenous uveitis (see above), it must be assumed that the drug can cross the blood–retina barrier, although presumably this barrier is already damaged or breached in uveoretinal inflammatory disease[103].

TOXICITY OF CsA IN UVEITIS

The side-effects of CsA in renal transplant patients and in patients with autoimmune disease have been extensively reviewed[104] (see Chapter 13) and include nephrotoxicity, gastrointestinal disorders, neurological complaints, hypertrichosis and gingival hyperplasia, hypertension, normochromic anaemia and hepatotoxicity. In the initial studies with CsA in uveitis, doses of 10 mg kg^{-1} day^{-1} and above were used, and side-effects were frequent, sometimes necessitating cessation of therapy[88,89]. Side-effects with low-dose CsA have been less severe[98], although nephrotoxicity and hypertension remain significant problems.

Nephrotoxicity during CsA therapy is considered to be an arteriolopathy[105] and may induce at least three types of kidney damage: interstitial nephritis, glomerular damage and tubular damage. Miescher et al.[106] found little evidence of renal damage in a series of 21 patients on combined steroid/low-dose CsA using renal biopsy to determine nephrotoxicity. In contrast, functional glomerular deficit has been observed in patients on low-dose CsA[98] as measured by a gradual rise in serum creatinine and a reduction in creatinine clearance. Furthermore, evidence of tubular renal damage has been shown by a deterioration in lithium clearance, correlated with a rise in urinary N-acetyl glucosaminidase[107], both of which are measures of tubular function[108,109]. The significance of these results is not clear since lithium clearance is a highly sensitive assay of renal function[110]. Furthermore, the deficit may reverse both for glomerular and tubular function upon cessation or lowering of the dose of CsA (Whiting et al., manuscript in preparation). Whether interstitial fibrosis is also reversible, however, has so far not been shown. It should also be noted that assumption of good renal function in uveitis patients cannot generally be made, since some have shown subclinical renal dysfunction on no therapy, which underscores the need for full medical assessment before initiating CsA, or indeed any systemic, treatment.

Low-dose CsA regimes have been associated with other side-effects such as hypertension, hypertrichosis and other minor complaints (cramps, hypomagnesaemia, skin rash[98]. An interesting experimental study has shown that in rats with renal transplants, CsA may be cataractogenic[111]. This may coincide with the observation that CsA treatment of uveitis patients is associated with an increase in cataract formation (R. B. Nussenblatt, personal communication), which is also a known complication of prolonged steroid use. A continuing concern has been to determine the risk of tumour, particularly lymphoma. However, in over 1000 uveitis patients now treated with CsA worldwide only two cases of tumour have been recorded, neither of which was lymphomatous (P. Timonen, personal communication). It must also be borne in mind that the potential side-effects of CsA therapy have to be weighed against the not inconsiderable, and sometimes life-threatening, side-effects, of more conventional therapeutic immunosuppressive agents.

CONCLUSION

Although there has been a considerable increase in our understanding of the immunology of autoimmune uveitis, clinical trials are hindered by the lack of a universally acceptable and reliable measure of occular inflammatory disease. Despite this, CsA is a useful addition to the therapeutic alternatives available for the treatment of severe sight-threatening endogenous uveitis. Although CsA therapy does not provide a cure, it can limit the destructive effects of the inflammatory process on vision. In addition, low-dose CsA therapy may have fewer side-effects while still achieving a therapeutic effect. CsA can also be combined with systemic steroids or other immunosuppressive agents to give an additive effect. A suggested protocol for CsA therapy in uveitis has been published[112]

REFERENCES

1. Wacker, W. B., Cavario, S. J., Salinas-Carmona, M. C. and Gery, I. (1981) Cyclosporin A. Inhibition of experimental autoimmune uveitis in Lewis rats. *J. Clin. Invest.*, **67**, 1228–1231
2. Ganley, J. P. (1980) Uveitis in current ocular therapy. In F. T. Freunfelder and F. H. Roy (eds.) *Ocular Pharmacology* (Philadelphia: W. B. Saunders), pp. 485–490
3. Kahaly, G., Schrezenmeir, J., Krause, V., Schwiekert, B., Meuer, S., Mulber, W., Dennebaum, R. and Beyer, J. (1986) Cyclosporin and prednisone v. prednisone in treatment of Graves ophthalmology: a controlled, randomized and prospective study. *Eur. J. Clin. Invest.*, **16**, 415–422
4. Droses, A. A., Skopouli, F. N., Costopoulos, J. S., Papdimitrou, C. S. and Montsopoulos, H. M. (1986) Cyclosporin A (Cya) in primary Sjögren's syndrome. A double blind study. *Ann. Rheum. Dis*, **45**, 732–735
5. Palestine, A. G, Austin, H. A., Barlow, J. E., Autonouych, T. T., Sabins, S. G., Preuss, H. G. and Nussenblatt, R. B. (1986) Renal histopathologic alterations in patients treated with cyclosporine for uveitis. *N. Eng. J. Med.*, **314**, 1293–1298
6. BenEzra, D. (1986) Cyclosporin eye drops for the treatment of severe vernal keratoconjunctivitis. *Am. J. Ophthalmol.*, **101**, 278–282
7. Newton, C., Gebhardt, B. M. and Kaufman, H. E. (1988) Topically applied cyclosporine in azone prolongs corneal allogaft survival. *Invest. Ophthalmol. Vis. Sci.*, **29**, 208
8. Thomson, A. W. and Webster, L. M. (1988) The influence of cyclosporin A on cell-mediated immunity. *Clin. Exp. Immunol.*, **71**, 369–376
9. Bell, T. A. G. and Hunnisett, A. G. (1986) Cyclosporin A: tissue levels following topical and systemic administration to rabbits. *Br. J. Ophthalmol.*, **70**, 852–855
10. Mosteller, M. W., Gebhardt, B. M., Hamilton, A. M. and Kaufman, H. E. (1985) Penetration of topical cyclosporine into the rabbit cornea, aqueous humour and serum. *Arch. Ophthalmol.*, **103**, 101–102
11. Nussenblatt, R. B., Dinning, W. J., Fujikawa, L. S., Chan, C.-C. and Palestine, A. G. (1985) Local cyclosporine therapy for experimental autoimmune uveitis in rats. *Arch. Ophthalmol.*, **103**, 1559–1562
12. Havener, W. H. (1974) *Ocular Pharmacology*, 3rd edn. (St Louis: C. V. Mosby)
13. Hunter, P. A., Garner, A., Wilhelmus, K. R. and Rice, N. S. C. (1982) Corneal graft rejections: a new rabbit model and cyclosporin A. *Br. J. Ophthalmol.*, **66**, 292–302
14. Kana, J. S., Hoffman, F., Buchen, R., Krolic, A. and Wiederhold, M. (1982) Rabbit corneal allograft survival following topical administration of cyclosporin A. *Invest. Ophthalmol. Vis. Sci.*, **22**, 686–690
15. Salisbury, J. D. and Gebhardt, B. M. (1981) Suppression of corneal allograft rejection cyclosporin A. *Arch. Ophthalmol.*, **99**, 1640–1643
16. Bell, T. A. G., Easty, D. L. and McGullagh, K. G. (1982) A placebo-controlled blind trial of cyclosporin A in prevention of corneal graft rejections in rabbits. *Br. J. Ophthalmol.*, **66**, 303–308
17. Behrens-Baumann, W., Theuring, S., Fry, F., Sostmann, H. and Bircher, J. (1986) Cyclosporin concentrations in the rabbit aqueous humour and cornea following subconjunctival administration: importance of the anatomical site of injection. *Graefe's Arch. Klin. Exp. Ophthalmol.*, **224**, 368–370
18. Grisolano, J. and Deyman, G. A. (1986) Retinal toxicity study of intravitreal cyclosporin. *Ophthalmic. Surg.*, **17**, 155–156

19. Nussenblatt, R. B., Mittal, K. K., Ryan, S., Green, W R. and Maumenee, A. E. (1982) Birdshot retinochroidopathy associated with HLA-A29 antigen and immuno-responsiveness to retinal S antigen. *Am. J. Ophthalmol.*, **94**, 147-158
20. Priem, H. A. and Oosterhuis, J. A. (1988) Birdshot choroiretinopathy; clinical characteristics and evaluation. *Br. J. Ophthalmol.*, **72**, 646-659
21. Peynard, M., Riffenburgh, R. S. and Maes, E. F. (1983) Effect of corticosteroid treatment and enucleation on the visual prognosis of sympathetic ophthalmia. *Am. J. Ophthalmol.*, **96**, 290–294
22. Elschnig, A. (1910) Studien zur sympathischen ophthalmis. Die antigene wirkung des augenpigmentes. *Albrect von Graefe's Arch. Ophthalmol.*, **76**, 509–546
23. Hess, C. and Romer, P.; cited by Faure, J. P. (1980) Autoimmunity and the retina. *Curr. Top. Eye Res.*, **37**, 613–625
24. Jakobiec, F. A., Marboe, C. C., Knowles, D. M., Iwamoto, T., Harrison, W., Chang, S. and Coleman, D. J. (1983) Human sympathetic ophthalmia. An analysis of the inflammatory infiltrate by hybridoma-monoclonal antibodies, immunochemistry, and correlative electron microscopy. *Ophthalmology*, **90**, 76–95
25. Chan, C.-C., BenEzra, D., Rodrigues, M.. M., Palestine, A. G., Hsu, S. M. and Nussenblatt, R. (1985) Immuno-histochemistry and electron microscopy of choroidal infiltrates and Dalen-Fuchs nodules in sympathetic ophthalmia. *Opthalmology*, **92**, 580–590
26. Wacker, W. B., Donoso, L. A., Kalsow, C. M., Yankeeloo, J. A. and Organisciack, D. T. (1977) Experimental allergic uveitis. Isolation, characterisation, and localisation of a soluble uveitopathogenic antigen from bovine retina. *J. Immunol.*, **119**, 1949–1958
27. Borthwick, G. M and Forrester, J. V. (1983) Purification of retinal S antigen by ion-exchange chromatography and chromatofocussing. *Exp. Eye Res.*, **37**, 613–625
28. McKechnie, N. M., Al-Madhawi, S., Dutton, G. and Forrester, J. V. (1986) Ultrastructural localisation of retinal S antigen in the human retina. *Exp. Eye Res.*, **42**, 479–487
29. Aronson, S. B., Schnellman, D. L. and Yamamoto, E. A. (1966) Uveal autoantibody in ocular disease. *J. Am. Med. Assoc.*, **196**, 225–228
30. Wacker, W. B. and Lipton, M. M. (1965) Experimental allergic uveitis: homologous retina as uveitogenic antigen. *Nature*, **206**, 253–254
31. Forrester, J. V., Borthwick, G. M. and McMenamin, P. G. (1985) Ultra-structural pathology of S-antigen uveoretinitis. *Invest. Ophthalmol. and Vis Sci.*, **26**, 1281–1287
32. Brockhuyse, R. M., Winkens, H. J., Kuhlman, E. D. and van Bugt, A H. M. (1984) Opsin-induced experimental autoimmune retinitis in rats. *Curr. Eye Res.*, **3**, 1405–1412
33. Gery, I., Wigert, B., Redmond, T. M., Kuwabasa, T., Crawford, M. A., Vistica, B. P. and Chader, G. J. (1986) Uveoretinitis and pinealitis induced by immunisation with interphoto receptor retinoid-binding protein. *Invest. Ophthal. Vis. Sci.*, **27**, 1296–1300
34. Gery, I., Mochizuki, M. and Nussenblatt, R. B. (1986) Retinal specific antigens and immunopathogenic processes they provoke. *Prog. Ret. Res.*, **5**, 75–109
35. Donoso, L. A., Merryman, C. F., Shinohara, T., Sery, T. H. and Smith, A. (1987) S antigen: experimental autoimmune uveitis following immunisation with a small synthetic peptide. *Arch Ophthal. Vis. Sci.*, **27**, 1296–1300
36. Sanui, H., Redmond, T. M., Hu, L. H., Kuwabara, T., Margalit, H., Cornette, J. L., Wiggert, B., Chader, G. J. and Gery, I. (1988) Synthetic peptides derived from IRBP induced EAU and EAP in Lewis rats. *Curr. Eye Res.*, **7**, 727–736
37. Singh, V., Yamaki, K, Donoso, L. and Shinohara, T. (1988) S antigen: experimental autoimmune uveitis induced in guinea pigs with two synthetic peptides. *Curr. Eye. Res.*, **7**, 87–92
38. Mochizuki, M., Kuwabara, T., McAllister, C., Nussenblatt, R. B. and Gery, I. (1985) Adoptive transfer of experimental autoimmune uveoretinitis in rats. *Invest. Ophthalmol. Vis. Sci.*, **26**, 1–9
39. Caspi, R. R., Roberge, F. G., McAllister, C. G., El-Saied, T. W., Gery, I., Hanna, E. and Nussenblatt, R. B. (1986) T cell lines mediating experimental autoimmune uveoretinitis (EAU) in the rat. *J. Immunol.*, **136**, 928–933
40. Gregerson, D. S., Obritsch, W. F., Fling, S. P. and Cameron, J. D. (1986) S antigen specific rat T cell lines recognise peptide fragments of S-antigen and mediate experimental autoimmune uveoretinitis and pinealitis. *J. Immunol.*, **136**, 2875–2882
41. deKozak, Y., Mirshahi, M., Boucheix, C. and Faure, J. P. (1987) Prevention of experimental

autoimmune uveoretinitis by active immunisation with auto-antigen-specific monoclonal antibodies. *Eur. J. Immunol.*, **17**, 541–545

42. Dua, H. S. and Forrester, J V. (1988) The effect of retinal S antigen specific monoclonal antibody therapy on experimental autoimmune uveoretinitis (EAU) and experimental autoimmune pinealitis (EAP). *Clin. Exp. Immunol.* (In press)

43. Liversidge, J. and Forrester, J. V. (1988) Experimental autoimmune uveitis (EAU): immunophenotypic analysis of inflammatory cells in chorioretinal lesions. *Curr. Eye. Res.* (In press)

44. Nussenblatt, R. B., Gery, I., Ballintine, E. J. and Wacker, W. B. (1980) Cellular immune responsiveness of uveitis patients to retinal S antigen. *Am. J. Opthalmol.*, **89**, 173–179

45. Shinohara, T., Dietzschold, B., Craft, C. M., Early, J. J., Donoso, L. A., Horwitz, J. and Tao, R. (1987) Primary and secondary structure of bovine retinal S antigen (48-KDa protein). *Proc. Natl. Acad. Sci. USA*, **84**, 6975–6979

46. Shinohara, T. cited by Donoso, L., Merryman, C., Sery, T. WE., Shinohara, T., Dietzschold, B., Smith, A. and Kalsow, C. M. (1987) S-antigen: characterisation of a pathogenic epitope which mediates experimental autoimmune uveitis and pinealitis in Lewis rats. *Curr. Eye Res.*, **6**, 1151–1159

47. Hirose, S., Tanaka, T., Nussenblatt, R. B., Palestine, A. G., Wiggert, B., Redmond, T. M., Chader, G. J. and Gery, I. (1988) Lymphocyte responses to retinal specific antigens in uveitis patients and healthy subjects. *Curr. Eye. Res.*, **7**, 393–402

48. Froebel, K. S., Armstrong, S., Cliffe, A. M., Urbaniak, S. J. and Forrester, J. V. (1988) An investigation of the general immune status and specific immune responsiveness to retinal S-antigen in patients with chronic posterior uveitis. *Eye* (In press)

49. Gregerson, D. S., Abrahams, I. J. and Thirkill, C. E. (1981) Serum antibody levels of uveitis patients to bovine retinal antigens. *Invest. Ophthalmol. Vis. Sci.*, **21**, 669–680

50. Doekes, G., van der Graag, R., Rothova, A., van Kooyk, Y., Broersman, L., Zaal, M. J. M., Dijkman, G., Fortuin, M. E., Baarsma, G. S. and Kiljstra, A. (1987) Humoral and cellular immune responsiveness to S-antigen in uveitis. *Curr. Eye Res.*, **6**, 909–919

51. Forrester, J. V., Stott, D. and Hercus, K. (1988) Naturally occurring antibodies to bovine and human retinal S antigen: a comparison between uveitis patients and healthy volunteers. *Br. J. Ophthalmol.* (In press)

52. Dumonde, D. C., Kasp-Grochowska, E., Graham, E., Thillaye, B., deKozak, Y. and Faure, J. P. (1982) Anti-retinal autoimmunity and circulating immune complexes in patients with retinal vasculities. *Lancet*, **2**, 787–792

53. Reid, D. M., Campbell, A. M. and Forrester, J. V. (1988) EB-virus transformed lymphocytes from uveitis and retinitis pigmentosa patients secrete antibodies to retinal antigens. *J. Clin. Lab. Immunol.*, **26**, 107–111

54. Froebel, K., Armstrong, S., Williamson, T., Urbaniak, S. and Forrester, J. V. (1988) (In preparation)

55. Forrester, J. V. (1985) Chronic intraocular inflammation. *Trans. Ophthalmol. Soc. UK*, **104**, 250–255

56. BenEzra, D. (1980) Inflammation of the retina and its vessels. In Michaelson, I. C. (ed.), *Michaelson's Textbook of the Fundus of the Eye*, 3rd edn. (Edinburgh: Churchill Livingstone), pp. 351–388

57. BenEzra, D., Nussenblatt, R. B. and Timonen, P. (1988) *Optimal Use of Sandimmum in Endogenous Uveitis* (Berlin: Springer-Verlag) p. 7

58. Tabbara, K. F. (1983) Chlorambucil in Behçet's disease: a reappraisal. *Ophthalmology*, **90**, 906–908

59. Nussenblatt, R. B., Rodrigues, M. R., Salinas-Carmona, M. C., Gery, I., Cevario, S. J. and Wacker, W. B. (1982) Modulation of experimental autoimmune uveitis with cyclosporin A. *Arch. Ophthalmol.*, **100**, 1146–1149

60. Mochizuki, M., Nussenblatt, R. B., Kuwabara, T. and Gery, I. (1984) Effects of cyclosporine and other immunosuppressive drugs on experimental allergic uveoretinitis in rats. *Invest. Ophthalmol. Vis. Sci.*, **26**, 226-232

61. Donoso, L. A., Merryman, C. F., Shinohara, T., Dietzschold, B., Wistow, G., Craft, C., Morley, w. and Henry, R. T. (1986) S-antigen: of the MA6A9-CT6 monoclonal antibody binding site and the uveitopathogenic sites. *Curr. Eye. Res.*, **12**, 995–1004

62. Fox, G. M., Kuwabara, T., Wiggert, B., Redmond, T. M., Hess, H. H., Chader, G. J. and Gery, I. (1987) Experimental autoimmune uveoretinitis (EAU) induced by retinal

interphotoreceptor retinoid-binding protein (IRBP): differences between EAU induced by IRBP and by S-antigen. *Clin. Immunol. Immunopathol.*, **43**, 256–264

63. Gregerson, D. S., Obritsch, W. F. and Fling, S. P. (1987) Identification of a uveitogenic cyanogen bromide peptide of bovine retinal S antigen and preparation of a uveitogenic peptide-specific T cell line. *Eur. J. Immunol.*, **17**, 405–411

64. Striph, G., Doft, B., Rabin, B. and Johnson, B. (1986) Retina S-antigen-induced uveitis: the efficacy of cyclosporine and corticosteroids in treatment. *Arch. Ophthalmol.*, **104**, 114–117

65. Converse, P. J. and Hess, A. D. (1985) Effect of cyclosporine and IL-2 on the restoration of *in vitro* immune responses to cytomegalovirus. *Scand. J. Immunol.*, **21**, 109-118

66. Borel, J. V. and Ryffel, B. (1986) The mechanism of action of cyclosporin: a continuing puzzle. In Schindler, R. (ed.) *Cyclosporin in Autoimmune Diseases* (Berlin: Springer-Verlag), pp. 24–31

67. Giranelli-Piperno, A, Andrews, L. and Steinwan, R. M. (1986) Lymphokine and non-lymphokine mRNA levels in stimulated human T cells: kinetics, mitogen requirements, and effects of cyclosporin A. *J. Exp. Med.*, **163**, 922–937

68. Miwa, Y., Kanp, T., Tanigueli, S., Miyadis, Y and Sakane, T. (1986) Effect of cyclosporin A on the membrane-associated events in human leukocytes with special reference to the similarity with dexamethasone. *Biochem. Pharmacol.*, **35**, 947–951

69. Damjanovich, S., Aszalos, A, Mulhern, S., Balazs, M. and Matyus, L. (1986) Cytoplasmic membrane potential of mouse lymphocytes is decreased by cyclosporins. *Mol. Immunol.*, **23**, 175-180

70. Dongworth, D. W. and Klaus, G. G. (1982) Effects of cyclosporin A on the immune system of the mouse. I. Evidence for a direct selective effect of cyclosporin A on B cells responding to anti-immunoglobulin antibodies. *Eur. J. Immunol.*, **12**, 1018

71. Palay, D. A., Cliff, C. W., Wentworth, P. A. and Ziegler, H. K. (1985) Cyclosporine inhibits macrophage-mediated antigen presentation. *J. Immunol.*, **136**, 4348–4353

72. Liversidge, J., Thomson, A. W., Sewell, H. F. and Forrester, J. V. (1987) EUA in the guinea pig: inhibition of cell-mediated immunity and Ia antigen expression by cyclosporin A. *Clin. Exp. Immunol.*, **69**, 591-600

73. Bottazzo, G. F., Pujol-Borell, R., Hanafusa, T. and Feldmann, M. (1983) Role of aberrant HLA-DR expression and antigen presentation in induction of endocrine autoimmunigy. *Lancet*, **2**, 1115-1117

74. Bottazzo, G. F., Dean, B. M., McMalhy, J. M., Mackay, J. M., Swift, P. G. F. and Gamble, D. R. (1985) *In situ* characterisation of autoimmune phenomena and expression of HLA-DR molecules in the pancreas in diabetic insulitis. *N. Engl. J. Med.*, **313**, 353–360

76. Chan, C.-C., Caspi, R. R., Roberge, R. F. and Nussenblatt, R. B. (1988) Dynamics of experimental autoimmune uveoretinitis induced by adoptive transfer of S antigen-specific T cell line. *Invest. Ophthalmol. Vis. Sci.*, **29**, 411–418

77. Chan, C.-C., Detrick, B., Nussenblatt, R. B., Palestine, A. G., Fujikawa, L. S. and Hooks, J. J. (1986) HLA-DR antigens on retinal pigment epithelial cells from patients with uveitis. *Arch. Ophthalmol.*, **104**, 725–729

78. Fujikawa, L. S., Chan, C.-C., McAllister, C., Gery, I., Hooks, J. J., Detrick, B. and Nussenblatt, R B. (1987) Retinal vascular endothelium expresses fibronectin and MHC Class II antigens in EAU. *Cell Immunol.*, **106**, 139–150

79. Liversidge, J., Sewell, H. F., Thomson, A. W. and Forrester, J. V. (1988) Lymphokine-induced MHC class II antigen expressions on cultured retinal pigment epithelial cells and the influence of cyclosporin A. *Immunology*, **63**, 313–318

80. Liversidge, J., Sewell, H. V. and Forrester, J. V. (1988) Human retinal pigment epithelial cells differentially express MHC Class II (HLA DP, DR and DQ) antigens in response to *in vitro* stimulation with lymphokine or purified IFN-gamma. *Clin. Exp. Immunol.*, **73**, 489-494

81. Hiestand, P. C., Mekler, P., Nordmann, R., Grieder, A. and Dermongkol, C. (1986) Prolactin as a modulator of lymphocyte responsiveness provides a possible mechanism of action for cyclosporine. *Proc Natl. Acad. Sci. USA*, **83**, 2599–2603

82. Palestine, A. G., Muellenberg-Coulombre, C. G., Kim, M. K., Gelato, M. C. and Nussenblatt, R. B. (1987) Bromocriptine and low-dose cyclosporine in the treatment of experimental autoimmune uveitis in the rat. *J. Clin. Invest.*, **79**, 78–81

83. Nussenblatt, R. B., Palestine, A. G. and Chan, C. C. (1983) Cyclosporin-A therapy in the

treatment of intra-ocular inflammatory disease resistant to systemic corticosteroids and cytotoxic agents. *Am. J. Ophthalmol.*, **93**, 275–281

84. Hogan, M. J., Kimura, S. J. and Thygeson, P. (1959) Signs and symptoms of uveitis I. Anterior uveitis. *Am. J. Ophthalmol.*, **47**, 155–170 (Suppl.)

85. Nussenblatt, R. B., Palestine, A. G., Chan, C.-C. and Roberege, F. (1985) Standardisation of vitreal inflammatory activity in intermediate and posterior uveitis. *Ophthalmology*, **92**, 467–471

86. Nussenblatt, R. B., Rook, A. H., Wacker, W. B., Palestine, A. G., Scher, I. and Gery, I. (1983) Treatment of intraocular inflammatory disease with cyclosporin A. *Lancet*, **2**, 235–238

87. Nussenblatt, R. B., Palestine, A. G., Chan, C. C., Mochizuki, M. and Yancey, K. (1985) Effectiveness of cyclosporin therapy for Behçet's disease. *Arthritis Rheum.*, **28**, 671–679

88. Graham, E., Sanders, M. D., James, D. G., Hamblin, A., Grochowska, E. D. and Dumonde, D. (1985) Cyclosporin A in the treatment of posterior uveitis. *Trans. Opthalmol. Soc. UK*, **104**, 146–151

89. Binder, A. I., Graham, E. M., Sanders, M. D., Dinning, W., James, W. G. and Denman, A. M. (1987) Cyclosporin A in the treatment of severe Behçet's disease. *Br. J. Rheumatol.*, **26**, 285–291

90. Muftuoglu, A. V., Pazarli, H., Yurdakul, S., Yazic, H., Ulku, B. Y., Tuzun, Y., Serdaroglu, S., Altug, E., Bahcecioglu, H. and Gungen, G. (1987) Short term cyclosporin A treatment of Behçet's disease. *Br. J. Ophthalmol.*, **71**, 387–390

91. Nussenblatt, R. B. (1988) The use of cyclosporin in ocular inflammatory disorder. *Transplant. Proc.*, **20**(3) (Suppl. 4), 114–121

92. BenEzra, D., Cohen, E., Rakotomalala, M., de Courten, C., Harris, W., Chajek, T., Friedman, G. and Matamuros, N. (1988) Treatment of endogenous uveitis with cyclosporin A. *Transplant. Proc.*, **20**(3) (Suppl. 4), 128-130

93. Le Hoang, P., Girard, B., Deray, G., Le Minh, H., De Kozak, Y., Thillaye, B., Faure, J. P. and Rousselic, F. (1988) Cyclosporine in the treatment of birdshot retinochoroidopathy. *Transplant. Proc.*, **20**(3) (Suppl. 4), 128–130

94. BenEzra, D., Brodsky, M., Pe'er, J., Chajek, T., Pizanti, S., Vertman, E. and Sachs, U. (1985) Cyclosporin A versus conventional therapy in Behçet's disease. Preliminary observations of a masked study. In Schindler, R. (ed.) *Cyclosporin in Autoimune Disease* (Berlin: Springer-Verlag), pp. 158–161

95. De Vries, J., Baarsma, G. S., Zaal, M. J. W., Boen-Tan, Rothova, A., Buitenhuis, H. J., Schweitzer, C. M. C., de Keizer, R. J. W. and Kijlstra, A (1987) Cyclosporine in the treatment of idiopathic posterior uveitis. *Second International Congress on Cyclosporine*, *Washington*, p. 55 (Abstract)

96. Whiting, P. H., Thomson, A. W., Blair, J. T. and Simpson, J. G. (1982) Experimental cyclosporin A nephrotoxicity. *Br. J. Exp. Pathol.*, **63**, 88-94

97. Palestine, A. G., Austin, H. A. and Nussenblatt, R. B. (1985) Cyclosporine-induced nephrotoxicity in patients with autoimmune uveitis. *Trans. Proc.*, **17** (Suppl. 1), 209–214

98 Towler, H. M. A., Cliffe, A. M., Whiting, P. H. and Forrester, J. V. (1988) Low dose cyclosporin A therapy in chronic posterior uveitis. Submitted to *Eye*

99. Murray, P. (1986) Serum autoantibodies and uveitis. *Br. J. Opthalmol.*, **70**, 266–268

100. Deschennes, J., Char, D. H. and Kaleta, S. (1988) Activated T lymphocytes in uveitis. *Br. J. Ophthalmol.*, **72**, 83–88

101 Lillehoj, H. S., Malek, T. R. and Shevach, E. M. (1984) Differential effect of cyclosporin A on the expression of T and B lymphocyte activation antigens. *J. Immunol.*, **133**, 244–250

102. Calder, V. L., Bellamy, A. S., Owen, S., Lewis, C., Rudge, P., Davison, A. N. and Feldmann, M. (1987) Effects of cyclosporin A on the expression of IL-2 and IL-2 receptors in normal and multiple sclerosis patients *Clin. Exp. Immunol.*, **70**, 570–577

103. Lightman, S. L., Palestine, A., Rapoport, S. and Rechthand, E. (1987) Quantitative assessment of the permeability of the rat retina to small water soluble non-electrolytes. *J. Physiol.*, **389**, 483–490

104. Van Graffenried, B. and Krupp, P. (1986) Side effects of cyclosporine in renal transplant recipients and in patients with autoimmune disease. *Transplant. Proc.*, **18**, 876–883

105. Mihatsch, M. J., Thiel, G. and Ryffel, B. (1986) Morphology of cyclosporin nephropathy. In Borel, J. (ed.) *Cyclosporin: Progress in Allergy*, vol. 38 (Basel: Karger), pp. 447–465

179

106. Miescher, P. A., Faure, H., Chatelauat, F. and Mihatsch, M. J. (1987) Combined steroid–cyclosporin treatment of chronic autoimmune diseases. *Klin. Wochenstr.*, **65**, 727–736
107. Whiting, P., Towler, H., Cliffe, A. M. and Forrester, J. V. (1988) Renal tubular dysfunction following cyclosporin A treatment in patients with chronic posterior uveitis (Submitted)
108. Thomsen, K. and Oleson, O. V. (1984) Renal lithium clearance as a measure of the delivery of water and sodium from the proximal tubule in humans. *Am. J. Med. Sci.*, **288**, 158–161
109. Whiting, P. H., Ross, I. S. and Borthwick, L. J. (1979) N-acetyl-beta-D-glucosaminidase levels and diabetic microangiopathy. *Clin. Chim. Acta*, **97**, 191–195
110. Thomsen, K. (1984) Lithium clearance: a new method for determining proximal and distal tubular reabsorption of sodium and water. *Nephron*, **37**, 217–223
111. Dieperink, H., Steinbruchel, D., Kemp, E., Svendson, P. and Sarklint, H. (1987) Cataractogenic effect of cyclosporin A: a new adverse effect observed in the rat. *Nephrol. Dial. Transplant.*, **1**, 251–253
112. BenEzra, D., Nussenblatt, R. B. and Timonen, P. (1988) *Optimal Use of Sandimmun in endogenous Uveitis* (London: Springer-Verlag), p. 18

9
Cyclosporin A in insulin-dependent diabetes

Jean-François Bach

More than 500 recent-onset diabetics have been treated with cyclosporine A (CsA) in an attempt to induce remission of the disease. All published reports have shown a favourable effect but problems persist which still preclude large-scale use of this new clinical application of CsA. In this article we shall review the main features of the use of CsA in experimental and clinical diabetes mellitus.

CsA COMPLETELY PREVENTS THE ONSET OF DIABETES IN RODENTS

NOD mice and BB rats develop diabetes at the age of 3–6 months. When CsA is given before the onset of diabetes, the disease is totally prevented[1,2]. The effect is obtained at non-toxic doses and is maintained for several months, as long as treatment is continued. However, in some but not all cases (approximately 50%), the disease relapses when CsA is stopped after short-term treatment (10 days)[3]. The effect is not observed when treatment is started late after the onset of clinically overt diabetes[4]. Intermediate results are obtained when CsA treatment is started at the very beginning of the period of hyperglycaemia. It is interesting to recall here that similar results have been reported in these two animal strains with other immunosuppressive methods selectively acting on T cells, as does CsA (neonatal thymectomy, anti-CD4 monoclonal antibodies, polyclonal anti-lymphocyte antibodies)[4].

CsA INDUCES LONG-TERM CLINICAL REMISSION OF DIABETES

Not long after the pilot studies performed in Canada[5] and in Paris[6], two major placebo-controlled randomized trials were set up on a large scale (350 patients), one in France[7], the other in Canada and Europe[7a]. The objective was to assess the incidence of complete remission after 9 or 12 months of treatment. Remissions were defined on the basis of decrease in insulin requirement (total drop-off in the case of complete remission) in patients with satisfactory metabolic control.

Results obtained in both trials clearly showed that CsA does induce (or prolong) the remission seen in a small percentage of placebo-treated patients. The precise incidence of remission closely depends on the patients selected for treatment. In the French trial (CDF, for Cyclosprine Diabetes France), 26% of all patients were in complete remission at 9 months but the proportion reached 37% when considering only patients having received efficient CsA dosage (total trough blood level > 300 ng/ml). Conversely, no more than 5% of placebo-treated patients were in remission at 9 months and none at 12 months.

Similar results were obtained in the Canadian–European trial with the important difference, however, that a higher rate of spontaneous remissions was observed in placebo-treated patients. These discrepancies pose the problem of the precise definition of remission. Table 9.1 presents the definition of remission in the two randomized trials.

Interesting results have also been reported in children in a series of 40 patients (recently extended to 100), with an incidence of remissions reaching 50% for complete remission and 75% for complete plus partial remission at 12 months[8]. This study was not randomized but a placebo-controlled trial is in progress.

CsA-INDUCED REMISSION RESTORES EXCELLENT (THOUGH NOT NORMAL) GLUCOSE METABOLISM

CsA-induced remissions have been studied in detail both in the three major trials described above and in open pilot studies. Remissions are associated with excellent metabolic control as assessed by glycaemia and HbA_{1c} levels. In fact these parameters even appear to be on the average better than in conventionally insulin-treated patients. One should not assume, however, that metabolic control is totally normalized. HbA_{1c} levels are still usually significantly higher than normal values, of the order of 6–6.5% versus 5–5.5% in controls, and C peptide production after glucagon stimulation

Table 9.1 Definition of remissions

	Insulin dosage (U kg^{-1} day^{-1})	Metabolic control (glycaemia, HbA_{1c})
French trials		
Complete remissions	0	Excellent (HbA_{1c} < 7.5%)
Partial remissions	< 0.25	Excellent (HbA_{1c} < 7.5%)
Failures	> 0.25	Indifferent
Unclassified	< 0.25	Insufficient (HbA_{1c} > 7.5%)

Canadian–European trial

Either Stimulated C peptide level in plasma ≥ 6 nmol/l, a value attained in > 90% of normal subjects (mean normal value ± SEM: 1.1 ± 0.01)

Or Non-insulin receiving state with adequate metabolic control remains depressed although much higher than in non-CsA-treated diabetics. This is not a really surprising observation since it is known that a large proportion of β cells is already destroyed when CsA treatment is initiated, and there is no experimental argument suggesting that β cells can regenerate in adults. This comment already suggests earlier treatment.

THE INCIDENCE OF REMISSION IS HIGHLY LINKED TO THE PRECOCITY OF TREATMENT: IMPLICATIONS FOR THE PATHOGENESIS OF REMISSION

All three studies reported above have convincingly shown that the rate of remission was directly linked to the duration of disease before the beginning of CsA treatment. This was consistently found whatever the parameter chosen to evaluate this duration:

1. date of first clinical symptoms (polydipsia, polyuria, polyphagia);
2. weight loss;
3. first detection of hyperglycaemia;
4. HbA_{1c} value;
5. existence of ketoacidosis (biological or clinical);
6. C peptide production (basal and glucagon-stimulated);
7. duration of insulin administration.

A multivariate analysis performed in the paediatric trial has revealed, not surprisingly, that all these factors were linked, with the exception of C peptide production whose low level is predictive of remission essentially independent of other factors[8].

This tight relationship between duration of disease and induction of remission is not surprising at first glance. One may argue, however, that it does not fit well with the putative time course of β cell aggression usually considered to represent a progressive attack of β cells over several years with at least 70% destruction at the time of clinical diagnosis (contemporary with glycosuria). How can one explain the apparent importance of the few days following clinical diagnosis in giving CsA its best chance of action? It appears that as few as 2–4 weeks after the first clinical manifestations of hyperglycaemia represent a significant predictive response factor. In other words, the β cell lesion which occurs during this time may create a state of definitive unresponsiveness to CsA, after which the β cell mass to be saved is too limited for clinical remission to take place. Several explanations can be brought to this paradox:

1. There are already very few β cells left when hyperglycaemia is manifested; any additional loss in incompatible with remission of insulin dependency.
2. The time of clinical diagnosis is associated with a burst of autoimmunity leading to accelerated destruction of β cells. In this acute disease phase the daily rate of β cell destruction may reach that of the previous weekly or monthly rate.
3. Hyperglycaemia (or insulinopenia), which characterizes the disease once clinical signs are present, suddently accentuates β cell destruction. This interpretation, which is supported by the delaying of diabetes onset

183

observed in BB rats after insulin therapy in prediabetic rats[9], is the basis of the attempts made by several authors to induce remission by early intensive insulin therapy[10].

In any case the main explanation for resistance to CsA in diabetes is thus probably excessive β cell destruction at the time of beginning CsA. One cannot exclude, however, that in some patients resistance is due to autoimmune hyperreactivity (as suggested by Lafferty's observations[11] showing, in an islet graft model in NOD mice, that anti-islet autoimmunity becomes more resistant to CsA late in life). Alternatively, a minority of patients might present a non-autoimmune form of diabetes, particularly those who are neither HLA DR3 nor DR4[+] and have not anti-islet cell antibodies.

A last point of interest is a comparison of the mechanisms of spontaneous and CsA-induced remission. If β cell function was exclusively dependent on β cell number one would expect that, when one reaches a given threshold, patients would become unable to maintain glycaemia levels within normal values. However, loss of glycaemia control could be due to a reversible increase in insulin needs. Such sudden and transient increase in insulin needs may occur at the time of infection, stress (for example, post-traumatic), or pregnancy. Additionally, part of the β cell acute aggression that led to insulin dependency is probably reversible, whatever the basis of this reversibility: participation of an inflammatory process reversibly inhibiting insulin release? deleterious role of hyperglycaemia? This reversibility is illustrated by the recovery of C peptide production noted in spontaneous remissons. CsA is assumed to stop the autoimmune β cell attack but it could also show an anti-inflammatory effect whether or not linked to T cell action. The existence of such an anti-inflammatory effect, linked or not to T cell action, has already been discussed in other settings[1] notably in murine[12] and human[13] lupus. Finally, CsA could act: (1) by preserving the residual β cell mass (whether or not the individual β cell function improves due to the relief from non-immunological factors e.g. correction of hyperglycaemia), and/or (2) by slowing the β cell inflammation.

It is important to realize that out of the four mechanisms discussed above preservation of remaining β cell mass; decrease of β cell inflammation; improvement of β cell function (secondary to normalization of glycaemia; decrease in insulin needs) the two latter mechanisms may occur spontaneously without CsA treatment, whereas CsA-treated patients can benefit from all four mechanisms. In any case, in the long term, in the absence of CsA treatment, β cell aggression will resume and β cell number and function will progressively decrease even in the absence of hyperglycaemia and/or abnormal insulin need. Consequently, only CsA-treated patients will maintain a good level of β cell function as assessed by C peptide production.

CsA TREATMENT MUST USUALLY BE CONTINUED TO MAINTAIN REMISSION: MECHANISMS AND HANDLING OF RELAPSES

Even if this is not a totally remote possibility, as will be discussed further, very long-term immunosuppression is worrisome in diabetics; hence the attempts to decrease CsA dosage or even stop the treatment.

By and large, decreasing of CsA dosage below 5 mg $kg^{-1}day^{-1}$, or more precisely below dosages providing trough blood levels lower than 200 ng/ml, is associated with a high risk of relapses (as assessed by reappearance of insulin requirement). The relapse does not occur rapidly, usually 1–4 months after stopping CsA treatment, but it is observed in the majority of cases. Only a few cases of absence of relapses in spite of CsA cessation have been reported (three cases in our experience with remissions now lasting more than 24 months after CsA stop). Not all these relapses are irreversible. In a significant number of cases rescue treatment using high-dose steroids and reinstitution of CsA can lead back to remission[14].

Relapses may also occur during CsA treatment, at effective doses (without tapering). This has been notably observed in a significant fraction of the children mentioned above after 18 months of treatment (P. Bougnères, personal communication) as well as in some of our adults. Importantly, in both cases, the insulin requirement was limited, less than that of non-CsA treated patients. Additionally, the relapse was not associated with a drop in C peptide production, at variance with relapses observed after stopping CsA treatment when C peptide production is lost (P. Bougnères, personal communication).

Taken together these observations indicate that relapses may be due to several different mechanisms:

1. Insufficient control of anti-islet cell autoimmunity due to inappropriate decrease of CsA dosage.
2. Progressive erosion of β cell mass due to insufficient immunosuppression from the beginning. In this case immunosuppression was sufficient to slow down the anti-islet attack but unable to stop it completely.
3. Functional degradation of metabolic control in spite of the control of the autoimmune β cell attack. Several factors, already discussed above in other settings, could contribute to this functional degradation: insulin resistance, increase of insulin needs (notably in growing children), decreased β cell function and possibly β cell destruction due to chronic hyperglycaemia or self-evolving post-autoimmune fibrosis.

THE VAST MAJORITY OF TYPE I DIABETICS ARE POTENTIAL CsA RESPONDERS

It is important to determine whether certain subgroups of type I diabetics respond better than others to CsA, independent of the duration of disease at the time of beginning CsA or of CsA blood levels, two factors that are not intrinsic to the patients but are related to the modalities of medical treatment. In fact, no factor has appeared to be really predictive of sensitivity to CsA.

The distribution of HLA antigens among CsA responders and non-responders has been thoroughly investigated in the three studies described above. Some correlation has been reported between the presence of HLA DR3 and CsA response[15], but we did not confirm this correlation[16]. In fact the only significant correlation we observed was a low rate of remission in

185

the small minority of patients who were neither DR3 nor DR4 ($p < 0.05$)[16]. Nor was any difference found when comparing the incidence of remission with sex or age (for the same duration of disease).

Interestingly, immunological markers did not provide any predictive factor (is et cell antibodies, anti-insulin antibodies, islet cell inhibitory T cells, activated T cells), again with the exception of non-DR3, non-DR4 patients who showed low frequency of anti-islet cell antibodies.

Our inability to recognize any predictive factor using major genetic and immunological markers of type I diabetes suggests that all DR3$^+$ and/or DR4$^+$ patients are potential responders to CsA provided they are treated early enough.

CsA IMMUNOSUPPRESSIVE EFFECT IS ESSENTIALLY DIRECTED TO CELL-MEDIATED IMMUNITY

CsA depresses both cell-mediated immunity and antibody formation, but the immunosuppressive effect is more readily observed on cell-mediated immunity. Abnormal antibody production is inhibited only when treatment is started before antigen administration. It is interesting to note that we have not observed a significant decrease in anti-islet cell antibody titres during CsA treatment[17], whereas T cell-mediated immunity as assessed by the insulin release inhibition assay was clearly and rapidly depressed[18]. These data fit with the concept that type I diabetes is probably linked to β cell aggression by activated islet cell specific T cells rather than to anti-islet antibodies[19].

There is an acute need for an *in vitro* assay to monitor the level of anti-islet cell pathogenic autoimmunity. Such an assay would permit guiding the administration of CsA in patients in remission. Unfortunately the only assay so far available (the insulin release inhibition assay mentioned above) is tedious and difficult to use on a large scale. Levels of activated T cells are not informative, nor are those of IL-2 production or circulating IL-2 receptor[20]. For T cell assays this failure is probably partly related to the rapid reversibility of the effects of CsA: lymphocytes from CsA treated patients recover their competence within a few hours when cultured *in vitro* in the absence of CsA. We are actively seeking an *in vitro* assay rapid enough to circumvent this difficulty. Two lines of research have proven promising in this regard: the level of IL-2 receptor RNA messenger[21] and Ca^{2+} influx[22], but we have not yet applied these two assays to CsA-treated diabetics.

CsA TOXICITY MAY BE MINIMIZED BUT TOTAL ABSENCE OF CHRONIC TOXICITY IS DESIRABLE IN THE LONG TERM

CsA is known to induce a number of side-effects. Only one of them, nephrotoxicity, has been of sufficient clinical significance to prompt stopping treatment or decreasing the dosage. Other complications, such as hypertension, hypertrichosis, hyperkalaemia, anaemia, etc., have not been observed or have remained modest.

It is remarkable that no opportunistic infection was observed in spite of the use of dosages providing clear-cut immunosuppression as assessed by the induction of disease remission, depression of T cell-mediated insulin release and inhibition of anti-insulin antibody production following exogenous insulin injections[17]. Several hypotheses can be put forward to explain this surprising and fortunate observation. It may be due to the fact that CsA has no effect on phagocyte function or on secondary immune responses which could play the predominant role in anti-infectious defence. It may also be that, at the doses used, CsA alters T cell function only very partially, sufficiently to decrease the above-mentioned immune parameters but not T cell-mediated anti-infectious defence. The observation of viral infection, notably due to cytomegalovirus or Epstein–Barr virus, in patients receiving higher CsA doses, is compatible with this interpretation.

Nephrotoxicity is commonly observed in CsA-treated patients, and was indeed observed in a significant number of adult patients of the two placebo-controlled randomized trials. No nephrotoxicity was, however, seen in children[8], probably because of the lower dosage used and because of a lower sensitivity to CsA nephrotoxicity in children.

Nephrotoxicity in adult CsA-treated diabetics is most generally mild and is at most moderate (Table 9.2). The incidence of an early increase in creatininaemia depended, not surprisingly, on the dosage administered and on CsA blood levels[23]. However, renal biopsy studies have revealed that these two factors were not totally reliable for avoiding the onset of nephrotoxicity, which was notably observed in some patients having received moderate doses $(5-7 \text{ mg kg}^{-1} \text{ day}^{-1})$ with adequate blood trough levels (300–500 mg/ml). On a practical basis two factors appear the best predictors of chronic nephrotoxicity:

1. Duration of treatment. Nephrotoxicity is very rarely seen when treatment is not continued with blood levels > 500 ng/ml for more than 4–6 months.
2. Early increase in creatininaemia. Such renal failure, which corresponds to acute nephrotoxicity, is usually reversible (is not associated with irreversible histological lesions). However, it has been our observation that patients who show significant early and sustained increase of creatininaemia most often are those who show chronic toxicity (as assessed by renal biopsy).

When these two factors are well controlled (which does not exclude a good remission rate), chronic nephrotoxicity appears to be very rare and to remain minimal.

Table 9.2 Nephrotoxicity of CsA in IDDM patients

Study	Dose $(\text{mg kg}^{-1} \text{ day}^{-1})$	Remissions at 12 months (%)	Fibrosis
CDF*	7.5 (first 6 months)	17.5	1/7
CDF†	7.5 (maintained)		7/23
Paediatric (St Vincent de Paul)	7.5	50	0/19
Open—adult‡	4–7.5	31	0/30

*Entered 1984–June 1985
†Entered July 1985–September 1986
‡Entered October 1986–May 1987

One should also mention at this stage the risk of EBV-associated lymphoma in patients treated with CsA for a long period of time. No case of lymphoma was observed in our patients; nor was there any increase in anti-EBV antibody titre or restriction of immunoglobulin heterogeneity. This is certainly reassuring, all the more so since a large fraction of CsA-associated lymphomas observed in transplanted patients regresses spontaneously when CsA treatment is stopped[24], but does not absolutely exclude the risk of lymphoma in the long term. One should remain cautious in using long-term CsA treatment in diabetics, and should maintain careful clinical and biological monitoring.

CsA HAS OPENED THE WAY, BUT MANY IMMUNOTHERAPEUTIC ALTERNATIVES EXIST

Present results obtained with CsA therapy in diabetes are interesting and promising, but not sufficiently convincing to justify its generalization to all recent-onset diabetics. Three major problems remain unsettled:

1. The persistence of a high proportion of failures;
2. The relapses of the disease, even in many cases without reduction of CsA treatment;
3. The risk of toxicity (nephrotoxicity, lymphomas) in case of continuous long-term treatment as could be required by the frequency of relapses observed after CsA tapering. This risk is very much limited but not suppressed by the careful monitoring discussed above.

Four alternative approaches can be considered

1. *Drug combinations* permitting use of CsA at lower (non-toxic) dosage or reducing CsA nephrotoxicity. Lines of research in this direction include conventional drug associations (azathioprine, steroids) and bromocriptin[25] Our own attempts to use steroids in combination with CsA have proven to be only partially successful[26], although showing a favourable trend. They must be confirmed on a larger scale.
2. *Improvement of the 'non-immunological' context*, notably administering insulin, perhaps at intervals, in order to prevent the deleterious effects of insulinopenia and/or hypoglycaemia
3. *Consecutive use of different agents.* CsA treatment could be preceded or followed by administration of other immunotherapeutic agents such as monoclonal anti-T cell antibodies, immunomodulators or thymic hormones. Recent experimental data obtained with anti-T cell monoclonals in the NOD mouse[27] are very encouraging and could be extended to human diabetes. Our trial with OKT3 has been hampered by the severe initial side-effect of the antibody, but other trials can be considered using other antibodies (notably anti-CD4 antibodies) or with OKT3 if the initial systemic reaction due to a massive release of cytokines[28] can be prevented.
4. *Earlier treatment.* All the evidence discussed above indicates that the earlier the treatment the higher the incidence of remission. One may assume that earlier treatment, before the onset of insulin dependency, could also allow

use of lower immunosuppression and limit the risk of relapse. In this vein it is interesting to mention that two prediabetic children have been treated before insulin treatment with long-term success (2 years).

CONCLUSIONS: PREVENTION OF DIABETES BY IMMUNOTHERAPY WILL BE ACHIEVED WHEN THE RISK/BENEFIT RATIO IS ACCEPTABLE

Experimental and clinical results obtained with CsA in type I diabetes indicate that immunosuppression can indeed at least transiently stop the autoimmune process responsible for insulin-dependent diabetes. The duration of treatment was too short to objectively reveal prevention of degenerative complications. The common occurrence of relapses observed in the present conditions of treatment (late start of CsA therapy, use of relatively low doses to avoid toxicity) might even cast some doubt on the feasibility of inducing long-term remissions. In fact data obtained in the experimental models of the NOD mouse and the BB rat with CsA and monoclonal antibodies, as well as the very long term follow-up of renal allograft recipients successfully treated with low-dose drug combinations, are reassuring. There is still much work to be done, but there is good reason to believe that the final goal of immunotherapy for disease prevention is accessible.

REFERENCES

1. Laupacis, A., Gardell, C., Dupré, J., Stiller, C. R., Keown, P., Wallace, A. C. and Thibert, P. (1983) Cyclosporin prevents diabetes in BB Wistar rats. *Lancet*, **1**, 10–12
2. Mori, Y., Suko, M., Odudaira, M., Matsuba, I., Tsuruoka, A., Sasaki, A., Yokoyama, M., Tanase, T., Shida, T., Nishimura, M., Terada, E. and Ykeda, Y. (1986) Preventive effects of cyclosporin on diabetes in NOD mice. *Diabetologia*, **29**, 244–247
3. Like, A. A., Dirodi, V., Thomas, S., Guberski, D. L. and Rossini, A. A. (1984) Prevention of diabetes mellitus in the BB/W rat with cyclosporin A. *Am. J. Pathol.*, **117**, 92–97
4. Boitard, C. and Bach, J. F. (1986) Experimental models of type I diabetes. *Pathol. Immunopathol. Res.*, **5**, 384–415
5. Stiller, C. R., Dupré, J., Gent, M., Jenner, M. R., Keown, P. A., Laupacis, A., Martell, R., Rodger, N. W., Granffenried, B. V. and Wolfe, B. M. J. (1984) Effects of cyclosporine immunosuppression in insulin-dependent diabetes mellitus of recent onset. *Science*, **223**, 1362–1367
6. Assan, R., Feutren, G., Debray-Sachs, M., Quiniou-debrie, M. C., Laborie, C., Thomas, G., Chatenoud, L. and Bach, J. F. (1985) Metabolic and immunological effects of cyclosporin in recently diagnosed type I diabetes mellitus. *Lancet*, **1**, 67–71
7. Feutren, G., Papoz, L., Assan, R., Vialettes, B., Karsenty, G., Vexiau, P., Du Rostu, H., Rodier, M., Sirmai, J., Lallemand, A. and Bach, J. F. (1986) Cyclosporin increases the rate and length of remissions in insulin-dependent diabetes of recent onset. *Lancet*, **1**, 119–123
7a. Canadian–European Diabetes Study Group (1988) Cyclosporin-induced remission of IDDM after early intervention: association of 1 year of cyclosporin treatment with enhanced insulin secretion. *Diabetes*, **37**, 1574–1582
8. Bougnères, P. H., Carel, J. C., Castano, L., Boitard, C., Gardin, J. P., Landais, P., Hors, J., Mihatsch, M. J. and Paillard, M. (1988) Factors determining early remission of type 1 diabetes in children treated with cyclosporin A. *N. Engl. J. Med.*, **318**, 663–670
9. Gotfredsen, G. F., Buschard, K. and Frandsen, E. K. (1985) Reduction of diabetes incidence of BB Wistar rats by early prophylactic insulin treatment of diabetes-prone animals. *Diabetologia*, **28**, 933-935

10. Shah, S. C., Malone, J. I. and Simpson, N. E. (1989) A randomized trial of intensive insulin therapy in newly diagnosed insulin-dependent diabetes mellitus. *N. Engl. J. Med.*, **320**, 550–554

11. Wang, Y., McDuffie, M., Nomikos, I. N., Hao, L. and Lafferty, K. J. (1988) Effect of cyclosporine in immunologically mediated diabetes in nonobese diabetic mice. *Transplantation*, **46**, 101S–106S (Suppl. 5).

12. Mountz, J. D., Smith, H. R., Wilder, R. L., Reeves, J. P. and Steinberg, A. D. (1987) CsA therapy in MRL-lp/lpr mice: amelioration of immunopathology despite autoantibody production. *J. Immunol.*, **138**, 157–163

13. Feutren, G., Querin, S., Noel, L. H., Chatenoud, L., Beaurain, G., Tron, F., Lesavre, P. and Bach, J. F. (1987) Effects of cyclosporine in severe systemic lupus. *J. Pediatr.*, **111**, 1063–168

14. Dupré, J., Stiller, C. R., Gent, M., Donner, A., Von Graffenreid, B., Murphy, G., Heinrichs, D., Jenner, M. R., Keown, P. A., Laupacis, A., Mahon, J., Martell, R., Rodger, N. W. and Wolfe, B. W. (1988) Effects of immunosuppression with cyclosporine in insulin-dependent diabetes mellitus of recent onset: the Canadian open study at 44 months. *Transplant. Proc.*, **20**, 184–192

15. Molvig, J., Mandrup-Poulson, T., Andersen, H. U., Spinas, G. A., Helqvist, S. and Munck, M. (1988) Ciclosporin immunotherapy in Type 1 (insulin-dependent) diabetes: importance of HLA-DR phenotype for the clinical and immunological response (abstract). In: *Abstracts Meeting Immunomodulation in Autoimmune Disease*, Paris, June 1988

16. Hors, J., Papoz, L., Eschwege, E., Vexiau, P., Geutren, G., Boitard, C. and Bach, J. F. (1988) HLA and responsiveness to cyclosporin A in treated IDD patients (abstract). In: *Abstracts Meeting Immunomodulation in Autoimmune Disease*, Paris, June 1988

17. Boitard, C., Feutren, G., Castano, L., Debray-Sachs, M., Assan, R., Hors, J. and Bach, J. F. (1987) The effect of cyclosporin A treatment on the production of antibody in insulin-dependent (type I) diabetic patients. *J. Clin. Invest.*, **80**, 1607–1612

18. Debray-Sachs, M., Sai, P., Feutren, G., Lang, F., Maugendre, D., Boitard, C., Hors, J. and Bach, J. F. (1988) Inhibition of insulin release *in vitro* mediated by mononuclear cells from cyclosporin A or placebo treated diabetic patients. *Diabetes*, **37**, 873–877

19. Bach, J. F. (1988) Mechanisms of autoimmunity in insulin-dependent diabetes mellitus. *Clin. Exp. Immunol.*, **72**, 1–8

20. Chatenoud, L., Feutren, G., Nelson, D. L., Boitard, C., Charron, D. J. and Bach, J. F. (1988) T cell mediated immunity in insulin dependent diabetic patients: effect of cyclosporin. *Diabetes* (In press)

21. Caillat-Zucman, S., Chatenoud, L. and Bach, J. F. (1988) Differential *in vitro* and *in vivo* action of cyclosporin A on the induction of IL-2 receptor α and β chains. *Clin. Exp. Immunol.* (in press)

22. Chatenoud, L., Dugas, B., Damais, C. and Bach, J. F. (1988) *In vivo* cyclosporine A treatment inhibits spleen cell mitogen-triggered free (Ca2+) increase. *Transplant. Proc.*, **20**, 170–172

23. Feutren, G. (1988) Functional consequences and risk factors of chronic cyclosporine nephrotoxicity in Type I diabetes trials. *Transplant. Proc.*, **20**, 356–366

24. Starzl, T. E., Porter, K. A., Iwatsuki, S., Rosenthal, J. T., Shaw, B. W. Jr., Atchinson, R. W., Nalesnik, M. A., Ho, M., Griffith, B. P., Hakala, T. R., Hardesty, R. L. and Jaffe, R. (1984) Reversibility of lymphomas and lympho-proliferative lesions developing under cyclosporin-steroid therapy. *Lancet*, **1**, 583–587

25. Mahon, J. L., Gunn, H. C., Stobie, K., Gibson, C., Garcia, B., Dupré, J. and Stiller, C. R. (1988) The effect of bromocriptine and cyclosporine on spontaneous diabetes in BB rats. *Transplant. Proc.*, **20**, 197–200

26. Assan, R., Feutren, G. and Sirmai, J. (1988) Cyclosporine trials in diabetes: updated results of the French experience. *Transplant. Proc.*, **20**, 178–183

27. Shizuru, J. A., Taylor-Edwards, C., Banks, B. A., Gregory, A. K. and Fathman, C. G. (1988) Immunotherapy of the nonobese diabetic mouse: treatment with an antibody to T-helper lymphocytes. *Science*, **240**, 659–661

28. Chatenoud, L., Ferran, C., Reuter, A., Franchimont, P., Legendre, C., Kreis, H. and Bach, J. F. (1988) Clinical use of OKT3: the role of cytokine release and xenosensitization. *J. Autoimmunity*, **1**, 631–640

10
Cyclosporin A and skin disease

Anne V. Powles, Barbara S. Baker and Lionel Fry

The treatment of skin diseases traditionally involves an empirical approach since neither the pathogenesis of the disease nor the mode of action of the treatments employed is well understood in most cases. In contrast the potential benefits of treating psoriasis with cyclosporin (CsA), a potent immunosuppressive drug widely used in organ transplantation because of its selective effect on T lymphocytes, were predicted because of the increasing evidence in support of psoriasis as a T cell-mediated disease.

PSORIASIS AS A T CELL-MEDIATED DISEASE

In the 1970s there were several reports describing defects of cell-mediated immunity in psoriasis. *In vivo* these include a depressed responsiveness to sensitization with chemicals that induce an allergic contact dermatitis, which corrects with therapy[1], and decreased delayed reactivity to intradermal challenge with antigen[2]. *In vitro*, the proliferative response by psoriatic lymphocytes to mitogens has been reported to be depressed. Whilst one group showed that the greater the extent of skin lesions, the lower the response to phytohaemaglutinin[3] (PHA), another found lymphocyte transformation with PHA to be relatively normal in psoriatic patients but noted a marked decrease in lymphocyte response to concanavalin A (Con A[4]. Furthermore, Goan and colleagues[5] recently showed that peripheral blood mononuclear cells from psoriatic patients showed impaired γ-interferon (γ-IFN) production with Con A, but not PHA or pokeweed mitogen, stimulation, suggesting that psoriatic lymphocytes are unable to respond to weak mitogen stimuli. It was proposed that the disproportionate depression of Con A versus normal PHA reactivity might indicate a deficiency of T suppressor cells; this could explain the occurrence of autoantibodies, immune complexes and elevated levels of immunoglobulins in psoriasis[4]. However, conflicting results for T suppressor, and indeed total and helper T cell numbers in peripheral blood of patients with psoriasis have been reported. Any reduction is probably secondary to the extent of lesions[6].

191

Thus patients with psoriasis appear to have an altered cell-mediated immune status which is not secondary to abnormal numbers of T lymphocytes or subclasses of T lymphocytes. This could result in defective elimination of antigens which have been postulated to accumulate in the skin of psoriatic individuals[7].

Both early and fully developed psoriatic lesions are characterized by an infiltrate of T lymphocytes and macrophages, with very few B lymphocytes or neutrophils[8]. With the advent of monoclonal antibodies this infiltrate has been characterized further[6,9,10]. Staining with Leu 2a (specific for CD8[+] suppressor/cytotoxic T cells) and Leu 3a (specific for CD4[+] helper/inducer T cells) monoclonal antibodies showed that the dermal infiltrate consists of approximately twice as many CD4 as CD8 T cells and that, judged by class II major histocompatibility antigen (HLA-DR) expression, most of the activated T cells are of the CD4 T cell subset[10]. Small numbers of T lymphocytes are also present in the epidermis of psoriatic lesions[10]. Unlike normal epidermis, in which T lymphocytes are almost exclusively of the CD8 phenotype, the epidermis of pinpoint lesions biopsied within 2 days of their eruption contains moderate numbers of CD4 T cells, some of which are activated (HLA-DR positive)[10]. These T cells are situated in the basal layer of the epidermis and are mostly in contact with the dendritic processes of antigen-presenting Langerhans cells. The latter are increased in total numbers and in the proportion expressing HLA-DR compared to normal skin, and tend to occur in small suprabasal aggregates. Epidermal CD8 T cells are not increased in these early lesions and remain inactive as judged by the absence of HLA-DR molecules.

However, in the epidermis, in late guttate lesions which are resolving spontaneously CD8 T cells again become more prominent than CD4 T cells and, in contrast to the erupting lesions, nearly all activated T cells are of the CD8 phenotype[10]. This trend was confirmed in sequential biopsies from a single patient with guttate psoriasis in whom fading of the lesions coincided with increasing numbers of HLA-DR positive CD8 T cells[10].

Chronic psoriatic plaques which had remained static in size for at least 1 year show a similar epidermal CD4/CD8 T cell ratio to resolving guttate lesions, and also markedly increased numbers of Langerhans cells. However, in contrast to the spontaneously resolving lesions, persistent plaques contain approximately equal numbers of activated CD4 and CD8 T cells[11].

These findings argue strongly for an on-going specific immune response in the psoriatic lesion. The presentation of antigen (in association with HLA-DR antigen) by an antigen-presenting cell to antigen-specific CD4 T cells results in activation of the latter and the subsequent release of lymphokines that can stimulate many different cell types including macrophages[12], osteoclasts[13] and keratinocytes[14]. This has formed the basis for a hypothesis by Valdimarsson and colleagues[7] which proposes that psoriasis is a disorder of keratinocyte proliferation mediated by T lymphocytes. Although the nature of the putative antigen in psoriasis is unknown, one possibility is streptococcal antigen, since a streptococcal infection is a well-documented trigger for guttate psoriasis[15]. Furthermore, the cross-reactivity of monoclonal antibodies against streptococcal antigens to the epidermal compartment of skin suggests that a streptococcal infection could lead to an autoimmune reaction against self antigens[16]. In support of this notion are the findings of a recent study[17] which showed that lesional psoriatic epidermal cells are more active in stimulating autologous T cell proliferation than cells from uninvolved psoriatic or normal epidermis.

An abnormal proliferative response by psoriatic keratinocytes to cytokines produced by activated T lymphocytes may also contribute to the disease process. Recent evidence in our laboratory suggests that γ-IFN has a less inhibitory effect on psoriatic than normal keratinocyte proliferation (Baker, B. S., Powles, A. V., Valdimarsson, H. and Fry, L., submitted manuscript).

Further support for the involvement of T lymphocytes in the pathogenesis of psoriasis is their rapid disappearance from the epidermis, prior to clinical and histological improvement, during treatment with psoralens plus UVA irradiation, or topical steroids[11,18]. Although these treatments probably have more than one site of action, it is more likely (based on these observations) that they exert their beneficial effects on immunocompetent cells in the lesion rather than directly inhibiting processes concerned with cell division of the keratinocyte.

The findings described above provide convincing support for the concept of psoriasis as a T cell-mediated disease and prompted its treatment with CsA, a drug known to selectively inhibit T lymphocyte function. In turn, the beneficial effects of CsA, even at low doses[19,20], further support a central role for T cells in the pathogenesis of psoriasis.

MECHANISM OF ACTION OF CsA

Effects of CsA on T cell activation

Cellular level

The stimulation of a resting CD4 T cell into an activated state involves two signals. The first is the recognition of a foreign antigen, in association with HLA-DR molecules, on the surface of an antigen-presenting cell. This activates the T cells from the G_0 resting phase and stimulates their expression of receptors for the T cell growth factor, interleukin-2 (IL-2). At the same time the antigen-presenting cell releases interleukin-1 (IL-1), the second signal required for T cell activation. The activated CD4 T cell is thus induced to release IL-2 which binds to the IL-2 receptors resulting in proliferation. Activated CD4 T cells also release several other lymphokines which affect a variety of different cell types. CsA interferes with an early step in T lymphocyte activation following initial antigen presentation. As a result, the T cells remain in the resting phase of the cell cycle, are unable to transform and release lymphokines, and are therefore unable to induce and mount an immune response.

Recent evidence suggests that the antigen-presenting function of macrophages[21] and epidermal Langerhans cells[22] may also be affected by CsA. However, the demonstration of this effect may depend upon the source of antigen-presenting and T cells used in the study[23].

193

CsA acts selectively on CD4 T cell function inhibiting the synthesis and release of IL-2[24], but with minimal effects on the expression and function of the receptor for IL-2[25]. The production of other lymphokines such as γ-IFN[26], interleukin-3 (IL-3)[27], migration-inhibition factor (MIF) and lymphocyte-derived chemotactic factor (LDCF)[28] are also inhibited. However, CsA does not interfere with the effects of these lymphokines on target lymphocytes such as IL-2-dependent T cell proliferation[27], or on the phagocytic, migratory and monokine-releasing activity of granulocytes or macrophages[28]. The maturation and generation of precursor cytotoxic T cells are also sensitive to the effects of CsA[24], whilst the cytolytic effector function of cytotoxic T cells already generated is completely resistant. In contrast, the activation and amplification of the T suppressor cell subpopulation appears to be spared by CsA[29]; this may contribute to the induction of specific tolerance to allograft tissue in experimental animal systems.

Although CsA was first thought to act only on T lymphocytes, it is now known that the drug will inhibit the *in vitro* activation of human and murine B cells by anti-Ig antibodies[30] which are believed to mimic the early effects of antigen on B cells. As in the case of T lymphocytes, CsA appears to inhibit an early event resulting from ligation of the surface Ig receptors; the mode of action of CsA may be similar, if not identical, in the two cell types.

Subcellular level

The binding of foreign antigen in association with HLA-DR antigen to the T cell receptor results in an increase in intracellular calcium and activation of the enzyme protein kinase C (PKC)[31]. A single receptor-mediated event, the hydrolysis of a membrane phospholipid, phosphatidylinositol bisphosphate (PIP$_2$) can stimulate both intracellular pathways. The turnover of PIP$_2$ generates two products with second messenger capabilities: inositol 1,4,5-triphosphate which mobilizes intracellular Ca^{2+}, and diacylglycerol which activates PKC[31]. One immediate consequence of the T cell receptor-mediated increase in Ca^{2+} is enhanced activity of the plasma membrane Na^+/H^+ exchanger, leading to an increase in intracellular pH[32]. This effect has been implicated as an important signalling mechanism in the stimulation of resting cells by growth factors, and in B lymphocyte differentiation. It is not clear how the subsequent activation of a certain set of genes, such as those coding for the oncogenes c-myc and c-fos, the IL-2 receptor, and a variety of lymphokines including IL-2 and γ-IFN, takes place. Activation may be in response to the second messengers described above, or perhaps more likely via further factors which can bind to targeted sequences and regulate gene expression.

It has been suggested that CsA inhibits T cell activation by interfering with the early activation of plasma membrane phospholipid metabolism[33]. However, since the intracellular rise[34] in Ca^{2+} and activation of PKC[35] are unaffected by CsA whilst the increase in intracellular pH[36] and synthesis of mRNA coding for various lymphokines including IL-2 and γ-IFN (but not mRNA synthesis in general[25]) are inhibited, the drug's site of action must lie between these two sets of events in the activation sequence. Furthermore, as mRNA for IL-2 is induced within a few hours of T cell stimulation, the drug-sensitive phase appears to be quite short. Since the intracellular CsA concentration was found to be markedly higher than its concentration in the medium[37], it has been suggested that CsA diffuses passively through the cell membrane into the cytoplasm without the requirement for a receptor. However, CsA will bind to lymphocyte prolactin receptors in competition with prolactin, a hormone which appears to regulate cell-mediated immune responses[38]. Recent reports suggest that, once inside the cell, CsA binds to and inhibits calmodulin, a cytoplasmic calcium-binding protein involved in the activation of second messengers and enzymes required for cell proliferation and function[39]. However, since three different isomers of CsA exhibited equivalent binding to calmodulin regardless of their different immunosuppressive activities, the biological significance of CsA inhibition of calmodulin-dependent processes has been questioned[40]. Furthermore, the selective action of CsA on T lymphocytes cannot be explained by its binding to this ubiquitous protein which is found in cells throughout the body. Another CsA-binding cytoplasmic protein, cyclophilin, has also been identified[41]. In contrast to calmodulin, a good correlation was observed between the binding of nine CsA derivatives to cyclophilin and their immunosuppressive activity[40]. Although it has been proposed that cyclophilin may play a role in concentrating CsA in the cytosol of lymphoid cells, the involvement of cyclophilin in the mechanism of action of CsA remains unclear. Thus CsA aborts lymphocyte activation at an early stage *in vitro*, before the onset of DNA synthesis. In contrast, studies of the effects of CsA *in vivo* have shown that, in animals, T cells (and perhaps B cells) can become primed and even proliferate in the presence of fully immunosuppressive levels of CsA[42]. However, priming under cover of CsA has not been described as yet in man. Other *in vivo* effects of the drug, such as immune enhancement[43] and exacerbation of experimental autoimmunity[44], have also not been adequately explained. Clearly there is much to learn about the mode of action of CsA *in vivo* which may prove to be considerably more complex than its effects *in vitro*.

THERAPEUTIC STUDIES OF CsA

A large proportion of current disorders seen in a dermatology clinic have an immunological basis. Therefore, drugs which affect immunological function may well prove helpful both in therapy and helping to unravel the pathogenic mechanisms of disease. CsA has proved to be just such a drug, particularly in psoriasis, and the majority of the work to date has been on this disease.

PSORIASIS

The immunosuppressive effects of CsA were described in 1976[45]. The first report of a beneficial effect of CsA in skin disease was a chance observation. Meuller and Hermann in 1979[46] were studying the effects of CsA on rheumatoid arthritis and decided to investigate the response of patients with psoriatic arthritis. They studied four patients who had both joint and skin involvement. They used high doses (450–900 mg daily), and found that the skin lesions cleared within a week and relapsed to their previous state within

2 weeks when CsA was discontinued. These observations were similar to those of Gubner and his colleagues[47] some 30 years previously, who were investigating the effects of folic acid antagonists on arthritis, and observed that in a patient with psoriatic arthritis the skin lesions cleared but there was only minimal improvement of the arthropathy. Because it has been assumed over the past 30 years that anti-psoriatic drugs exert their beneficial effect by a direct anti-mitotic effect on the hyperproliferation of the epidermal cells in psoriasis, the observations made by Mueller and Hermann were not pursued or appreciated. However, during the early 1980s it was shown that immunological processes involving activated T helper cells were probably playing a central role in the development of psoriatic skin lesions. These studies led to the hypothesis that psoriasis was a disorder of keratinocyte hyperproliferation mediated by T helper cells[7], and thus made it logical to use CsA in psoriasis. Apart from two case reports of the effect of CsA in psoriasis[48,49] there have now been several studies showing the beneficial effects of CsA on psoriasis[19,20,50-55]. Unfortunately, like other systemic therapeutic agents which are beneficial in psoriasis (e.g. methotrexate, etretinate, hydroxyurea, razoxane), CsA is not without side-effects. The principal ones are hypertension and nephrotoxicity, and these have been reported to be dose-dependent. Thus if CsA is to have a role to play in the treatment of psoriasis it must be effective in a dosage regime which has a low incidence of serious side-effects. In addition, if side-effects do occur then ideally they should be reversible when the dose is lowered or the drug discontinued.

Clinical response and dosage

There have been two double-blind cross-over studies demonstrating the effectiveness of CsA in psoriasis[20,52]. In the first study[52] there were 21 patients and CsA was given in a very high dose, i.e. 14 mg kg^{-1} day^{-1} for a 4-week period. Of the 11 patients who received CsA the psoriasis cleared in two, there was considerable improvement in six, moderate in two and minimal in one. In the 10 controls there was either no or only minimal improvement. When the controls were crossed over to CsA there was considerable improvement in their psoriasis. Of the 21 patients who received CsA, 17 (81%) had significant improvement at 1 week and 20 (95%) at 4 weeks. In the second study[20] 20 patients were in the trial and the mean dose of CsA was 5.5 mg kg^{-1} day^{-1}. Assessment of the psoriasis was made using the PASI (psoriasis area severity index) score[56]. (The advantage of the PASI score is that it takes into account not only the area of skin affected with psoriasis, but also the features of erythema, scaling and palpability. The range of PASI score is 0-72, but the improvement of psoriasis during treatment is usually given as a percentage reduction of the PASI score.) There was a significant difference at the end of the 4-week study between the two groups, the mean percentage reduction of the PASI score being 74% in the CsA-treated group, but no significant improvement in the placebo group. When the latter was treated with CsA for 4 weeks there was a 90% reduction in the PASI score.

Thus these double-blind studies show that CsA is effective in improving psoriasis over a 4-week period. It is important to note that virtually similar improvement was obtained at the 4-week point in time in both studies and yet the dose in one was 14 mg kg^{-1} day^{-1} and in the other 5.5 mg kg^{-1} day^{-1}[120]. However, there was a quicker response in the study using the higher dose. This was also observed in the original four patients of Mueller and Hermann[46] when they used approximately the equivalent of 14 mg kg^{-1} day^{-1} and reported clearing in a week.

Because of the nephrotoxicity, which is thought to be dose-related, two open studies have looked at the response of psoriasis to very low-dose CsA[19,51]. In the first study[19] 10 patients were treated for a period of 12 weeks. The initial dose was 2 mg kg^{-1} day^{-1} in eight and 3 mg kg^{-1} day^{-1} in two. The dose was increased by 1 mg kg^{-1} day^{-1} after a 2-week period if there was no significant improvement. At 4 weeks there was a 50% reduction in the PASI score, 68% at 6 weeks, 78% at 8 weeks and 84% at 12 weeks. The mean dose of CsA was 2.2 mg at the start of the study, 3.1 mg at 6 weeks and 3.5 mg at 12 weeks. In the second study[51] there were eight patients who were treated for periods ranging from 6 to 24 weeks. The initial dose was 1 mg kg^{-1} day^{-1} and was increased every 2 weeks by 1 mg kg^{-1} day^{-1} if there was no improvement. The mean time clearance was 7.4 weeks and the average dose 3.3 mg kg^{-1} day^{-1}. Thus these two studies have demonstrated that low doses of CsA are able to clear psoriasis and the higher doses used in other studies, 14 mg kg^{-1} day^{-1}[52], 5–15 mg kg^{-1} day^{-1}[53], and 7.5–8.5 mg kg^{-1} day^{-1}[54], are not necessary. However, the speed of clearance does appear to be dose-related in that clearance is slower with the 3–4 mg kg^{-1} day^{-1} than with the higher ones. However, in the two low-dose studies the initial starting doses were either 1 or 2 mg kg^{-1} day^{-1} in the majority of patients, and if the starting dose had been 3-4 mg/kg clearance may have been quicker. Thus it would seem at the present that the initial starting dose for treating psoriasis should be 3 mg kg^{-1} day^{-1} and this should be adjusted according to the clinical response. With this regime, significant clearance should occur within a month.

As yet there have been no long-term published studies of CsA in psoriasis, but these will almost certainly appear in the future as several groups are conducting such studies to determine (1) if the improvement obtained with CsA can be maintained long term, and (2) the incidence and severity of side-effects. We have at St Mary's been treating patients with psoriasis with long-term CsA and these results will shortly be published[55]. To date, 13 patients have been followed up for periods ranging from 60 to 120 weeks (mean 104). The mean reduction in PASI score was 72% at 4 weeks, 80% at 16 weeks and 80% at 24 weeks. The mean reduction at 104 weeks of follow-up was 84%. The results were achieved with a mean starting dose of 2.7 mg kg^{-1} day^{-1} at 8 weeks, 3.3 at 16 weeks, and 3.2 at 104 weeks. Thus these results have shown that it is possible to achieve significant improvement in psoriasis and maintain it over a long period of time. In addition, there was no evidence of tachyphylaxis, which may happen with topical steroid treatment of psoriasis.

CsA was stopped at the end of the two studies[19,52]. In all patients there was a relapse of psoriasis. In the group who received high doses the relapse of the psoriasis was gradual and began after periods of 2 weeks to 3 months[52]. In the 10 patients treated with low-dose CsA the recurrence began at intervals varying from 3 days to 2 months. No rebound was noted in any patients in either study.

Thus in summary of the clinical effects of CsA in psoriasis it appears that (1) low dosage, i.e. 3 mg kg^{-1} day^{-1} is effective in clearing and maintaining improvement over a long period; (2) gradual relapse occurs in all patients to date when the drug is stopped, but there is no rebound.

CsA blood levels and clinical response

It is difficult to compare the published reports of CsA blood levels because the various centres have not used the same methods for estimating CsA. Some centres have used HPLC and others have used a radioimmunoassay. In addition, some studies have measured plasma and others have used whole-blood trough levels. Finally, a polyclonal antibody to CsA was used in the past for the radioimmunoassay, in which metabolites of CsA have reacted in addition to the parent compound. Unfortunately, the various methods have given different therapeutic ranges and levels at which toxicity may be expected. It is surprising therefore that in many of the published reports on CsA in psoriasis the figures for the therapeutic range and toxicity levels have not been given and thus the blood levels reported are meaningless. In the future it is to be hoped that most centres will adopt the same technique for measuring CsA blood levels using the new monoclonal antibodies in a radioimmunoassay which measures the parent compound and metabolites separately.

In the studies[19,52,55] in which the methods were given for estimating CsA blood levels and therapeutic range, there was no correlation between clinical response and blood levels. In the study[52] using a HPLC method measuring whole-blood trough levels, those above 350 ng/ml were considered to be toxic. Of the five patients in whom the psoriasis cleared completely, three had blood levels which were amongst the lowest for all patients, never exceeding 205 ng/ml. The other two had blood levels near the average for the entire group (267 ng/ml). Among the four patients with less than 50% improvement, three had blood levels that remained low (< 200 ng/ml). In the other studies[19,55] CsA was measured by radioimmunoassay as whole-blood trough levels, and the normal therapeutic range was 400–800 ng/ml. In the initial study[19] of 12 weeks there was no correlation between the clinical response and blood levels. Four of the 10 patients had levels above 700 ng/ml at some stage of the study, and in three of these the patients had previously received methotrexate. One patient with early hepatic fibrosis, considered to be due to methotrexate, had levels above 800 ng/ml, but the reduction in his PASI score was only 69% at the end of the study compared to the mean 85% for the group as a whole. In the long-term study of 13 patients there was also no correlation between mean blood levels and clinical response. Five of the 13 patients had blood levels above 800 ng/ml on at least one occasion, all five had received methotrexate previously, and four of the five had abnormal liver function tests when CsA was commenced. The mean dosage of CsA for the patients with high trough blood levels was the same as with lower (i.e. 3 mg kg^{-1} day^{-1}), and in all patients the dose never exceeded 5 mg kg^{-1} day^{-1}.

CsA is metabolized by the cytochrome P-450 enzyme system which is found predominantly in the liver. If there has been impairment of liver function from previous methotrexate or alcohol, this may well interfere with liver enzymes and result in high CsA blood levels. It may well not be advisable to initiate therapy with methotrexate and subsequently switch to CsA. It may be better to use CsA as a first-line drug if systemic therapy is justified for psoriasis.

Side-effects

Hypertension

This is a well-recognized side-effect of CsA therapy. In transplantation subjects (particularly renal) it has been difficult to determine whether the rise in blood pressure has been caused by drugs other than CsA or a rejection phenomenon. In the short-term studies in the treatment of psoriasis mild hypertension has been reported in some patients. Three of the 10 patients developed mild hypertension at some stage with a mean dose of approximately 3 mg kg^{-1} day^{-1} over a 12-week period[19]. However, in one of the three patients the blood pressure returned to normal despite continuing CsA. In an 'open study' by Van Joost and his colleagues[50] on five patients with a dose of 5 mg kg^{-1} day^{-1}, two developed hypertension during the 4-week course. In a double-blind study by the same group of workers with a similar dose and duration, five of 18 (28%) patients developed hypertension[20]. In the study with the high dose of 14 mg k^{-1} day^{-1}, there was a rise in blood pressure from 121/72 to 133/88 over a 4-week period[52]. In the long-term study with a mean follow-up period of nearly 2 years[55], despite the mean average dose being 3 mg kg^{-1} day^{-1}, and no patient receiving more than 5 mg kg^{-1} day^{-1}, seven of the 13 patients (54%) developed hypertension at some stage. In two the blood pressure returned to normal without discontinuing CsA. In another two patients CsA was discontinued, the blood pressure returned to normal and CsA was reintroduced because of relapse of the psoriasis. Three patients were eventually treated with hypotensive drugs. The high incidence of hypertension with low-dose CsA when taken for a long period is disconcerting. However, six of the seven had high blood trough levels at some stage, which appeared to be related to previous methotrexate therapy.

The mechanism by which CsA causes a raised blood pressure is not fully understood. CsA has been shown to have a direct vasoconstrictor effect as well as a direct nephrotoxic one. It is difficult to know which is the more important mechanism, but at present in patients with psoriasis the raised blood pressure does appear to be reversible when the drug is discontinued. It appears likely that in part the effect of CsA may be idiosyncratic, for only a small proportion of patients develop a raised blood pressure in short-term studies with the same dose. It would be valuable, and interesting from a pathogenic standpoint, to be able to know which patients are at risk of developing hypertension when taking CsA.

Hype trichosis

This is a well-recognized side-effect of CsA although the biological mechanisms are not known. In the short-term studies ranging from 4 to 12 weeks, the incidence was 4/21[52], 2/18[20] and 3/10[19]. However, in the long-term study[14], approaching 2 years of CsA, the incidence was seven of 13 patients. Two of these were males and the hypertrichosis took the form of extension of the hair line to the forehead and neck, and increase in terminal hair on the trunk and limbs. In the five female subjects there was lanugo-type hair on the face and increase in terminal hair on the limbs. In none of the patients was hypertrichosis severe, and all patients considered the benefit from CsA far outweighed the hypertrichosis.

Other side-effects

The other common side-effects reported have been nausea, gingival hypertrophy, paraesthesia, malaise and headache. In none of the reported studies[19,20,5-55] were these effects severe, and they certainly did not warrant the discontinuation of CsA. In our experience the subjective symptoms of headache, malaise and nausea have usually been of a temporary nature and have ceased despite the patient continuing with CsA. In the long-term study of 13 patients[55], three had headache, one paraesthesia, two nausea and one malaise.

Malignancy

None of the short-term studies reported any development of malignancy, but they were of very short duration as most were designed simply to show the effectiveness of the drug in psoriasis. However, one patient in our short-term study[19] has subsequently developed multiple lesions of Bowen's disease on the penis. Whether this is directly related to CsA treatment is debatable, as the patient had previously been treated with PUVA and methotrexate, which may also be possibly implicated in the aetiology. In our long-term study[55] one of the 13 patients has developed two carcinomata, one a squamous-cell carcinoma at the margin of the anal canal which appeared 24 weeks after starting CsA. The lesion was surgically excised and there has been no recurrence despite continuing with CsA for a further 82 weeks. He has also developed a basal-cell carcinoma on his back, which appeared after 60 weeks of treatment and this was also treated surgically. This particular patient had a 60-year history of psoriasis, so although there is no certain way of knowing, it is possible he may have had arsenic in the past. In addition, he has had PUVA therapy and methotrexate, the latter for 11 years. CsA has been the most successful therapy he has had, and as he has very severe psoriasis, it has been considered justified to continue with the drug. In this patient it is also difficult to be dogmatic as to what part CsA may have played in the development of these malignant lesions.

Renal function

It has been generally accepted that renal toxicity from CsA is dose-dependent in organ transplantation[57]. It is thought that there are two possible mechanisms by which renal damage is produced. First, vasoconstriction of the renal arterioles occurs at an early stage, and second, tubular damage with subsequent interstitial fibrosis occurs at a later stage. The latter is thought to be due to the prolonged effect on the vasculature of the kidneys. The vasoconstriction leads to functional impairment early on, but at what stage irreversible damage occurs is difficult to ascertain without detailed functional and histological studies.

In retrospect it is unfortunate that none of the studies of CsA in psoriasis has included accurate tests of renal function. All the studies[19,20,50-55] have relied on the serum creatinine level as a measure of renal function and toxicity, and all have shown a rise in serum creatinine levels with varying incidence and levels. In the high-dose study (14 mg kg^{-1} day^{-1})[52] four of 21 patients had serum creatinine levels above the normal upper limit after a month, and there was a mean rise of 25% for the group. In the study giving 5.5 mg kg^{-1} day^{-1} for a month[20], seven of 18 (39%) patients had raised serum creatinine levels, but less than 40% of their original value, and in all the patients the levels returned to normal when CsA was discontinued. In the long-term study[55], 10 of 13 patients had raised creatinine levels of > 10% at their final assessment compared to their initial value, but in none did the level rise above the upper limit of normal.

It is now accepted[58] that the glomerular filtration rate (GFR) may fall by 20% without any rise in serum creatinine level. In a study of non-transplant patients it has been shown that with a dose of CsA of 10 mg kg^{-1} day^{-1} the GFR falls by 20% in the first week and by 40% at 4 weeks. In addition, the effective renal plasma flow (ERPF) is significantly reduced in a similar period. However, these effects are reversible and had returned to near-normal levels after stopping CsA for 2 weeks, having been taken for 12 weeks. It would seem imperative in future that, if patients with psoriasis are to be treated with CsA, both the GFR and ERPF should be measured before starting treatment and monitored throughout the study period. If they are significantly reduced the drug should be stopped and the tests repeated 1 month later. If the tests do not improve, renal biopsy will be necessary before the CsA can be recommenced.

Liver function tests

In two short-term studies[20,50] there was no biochemical evidence of liver toxicity. In the study in which a high dose of CsA was used (14 mg kg^{-1} day^{-1})[52], two of the 21 patients had raised bilirubin levels at the start of the study, but nine had raised levels at the end. However, these raised levels had returned to normal 2 weeks after stopping CsA. There was no significant change in the serum liver enzyme levels. In the long-term study[55], seven of the 13 patients had one or more abnormal liver function tests at the beginning of the study, and it may be significant that six of the seven had previously been treated with methotrexate. The main abnormalities were raised alkaline phosphatase and/or aspartate transaminase levels. These levels did not rise

201

further with CsA treatment; in fact of five patients who had raised alkaline phosphatase levels at the beginning of treatment, only two had raised levels at the end. Of five patients with raised aspartate transaminase levels at the beginning of the study, only three had raised levels at the end. Thus liver fun..tion tests actually improved in a number of patients during long-term treatment with CsA. It would appear therefore that CsA is not hepatotoxic in the dosage and duration in which the drug was used.

Haematological parameters
None of the studies so far published in the treatment of psoriasis has reported any haematological abnormalities.

Comparison with other current treatments

Unfortunately at present there are no treatments for psoriasis which appear to influence the natural history and activity of the disease. If the disease is active, it will soon recur when treatment is stopped. Currently, the therapeutic modalities for severe psoriasis are photochemotherapy, etretinate (a retinoid), methotrexate and CsA. Of the oral preparations CsA has the least subjective side-effects and nine of the 10 patients in our short-term study[19] thought CsA was the most effective drug they had been given, and we would endorse these views expressed by the patients. If long-term studies with low-dose CsA show that there is no permanent renal damage and no significant increase of malignant lesions, then in our opinion it should be the first-line systemic treatment in the management of severe psoriasis.

Topical and intralesional CsA in psoriasis

As systemic CsA may cause renal damage and induce hypertension, the chance of these side-effects would be greatly diminished if CsA were effective topically. However, as yet topical CsA has not been shown to be effective[59-61]. In the latter study CsA was used under polythene occlusion, but there was still no clinical improvement, although biopsies revealed a decrease in the polymorphonuclear leukocytes in the epidermis. These cells are usually found high in the epidermis, and this possibly implies topical CsA is only reaching this area and not the lower epidermis. The CsA may be bound to the upper epidermis in psoriasis. Topical CsA has been reported to be effective both in humans[62-64] and animals[65], so it is possible there is a difference between psoriatic and normal epidermis which does not allow penetration of CsA in psoriasis.

The other possible explanation for the lack of effect of topical CsA in psoriasis is that it is a metabolite and not the parent drug which is therapeutically active in psoriasis. To answer this question, Powles *et al.*[66] carried out a double-blind trial of intralesional CsA versus placebo in symmetrical plaque psoriasis and showed that intralesional CsA was indeed effective in clearing psoriasis. Thus it appears to be lack of penetration of CsA in psoriasis which accounts for the failure when topically applied. If there is binding of CsA in the upper epidermis, alteration of the vehicle for the topical preparation may not alter the clinical response.

ECZEMA

Atopic eczema

It is highly likely that atopic eczema is a T cell-mediated disease and therefore likely to improve with CsA. There have been two reports of the beneficial effect of CsA in atopic eczema[67,68]. Van Joost et al.[67] reported virtual clearance in two patients with severe atopic eczema after 4 weeks of treatment with a dose of 5 mg kg^{-1} day^{-1}. The other report[68] found significant improvement with 5 mg kg^{-1} day^{-1} in two patients. These reports are promising enough to be pursued.

Contact eczema

Borel, in his original experiments demonstrating the immunosuppressive effects of CsA, showed that intraperitoneal CsA inhibited delayed hypersensitivity in animals. Topical CsA has been shown to inhibit contact eczema in animals[64] and in humans[62]. In the latter study, however, the effect was demonstrated in only four of 18 patients with nickel sensitivity. The clinical response to CsA in these patients was accompanied by a diminution of the T cell infiltrate.

MYCOSIS FUNGOIDES AND SEZARY SYNDROME

Both mycosis fungoides and the Sezary syndrome are considered to be cutaneous T cell lymphomas. There have been a number of reports of CsA in both conditions[69-74]. It appears that initially there is a rapid improvement of associated pruritus and erythroderma, but this is not always sustained. Histologically there is often improvement in the initial stages of treatment and there are fewer features of the cutaneous lymphoma. However, it is disconcerting in that of the seven patients reported in the above studies, four had a flare-up of their disease and died within a short time of discontinuing CsA. In addition, another patient had a flare-up whilst taking CsA and required electron-beam therapy. There is a suggestion that tachyphylaxis occurs in CsA therapy in patients with cutaneous T cell lymphomas. Thus at present it would appear that CsA may not be appropriate for cutaneous T cell lymphomas and there seems to be accumulating evidence that the disease may be converted into a more malignant phase.

PEMPHIGUS AND PEMPHIGOID

These two disorders are autoimmune skin diseases with circulating antibodies directed against the cell membrane of the keratinocytes in pemphigus and the basement membrane zone in pemphigoid. Pemphigus is the more serious disease and requires very high doses of steroids for suppression of the skin lesions. Thus side-effects from this treatment are common. Pemphigoid is also treated with systemic steroids, but is easier to control. There have now been a number of reports claiming that CsA has a beneficial effect in both diseases. In the largest study[75] seven patients with pemphigoid and eight with pemphigus were treated with CsA. The dosage of CsA was 6–8 mg kg^{-1} day^{-1}. Of the seven patients with pemphigoid, four were treated initially with CsA alone, and two cleared. Prednisone 0.5 mg kg^{-1} day^{-1} was added in the other two patients and one cleared. Three other patients not responding to steroid therapy had CsA added to their regime and they all cleared. However, when the CsA was discontinued in the six patients who were clear, only two remained so. Of the eight patients with pemphigus, four were treated with CsA alone, but only one cleared. Prednisone 0.5 mg kg^{-1} day^{-1} was added to the treatment regime for the other three, and in two the disease cleared. In the other four patients the disease was steroid-resistant and in these the addition of CsA to their treatment resulted in clearance of the lesions. Of the seven who cleared, four remained so when treatment was discontinued. Other successful treatments of pemphigus with CsA have been reported[76,77].

ALOPECIA AREATA

Topical CsA has been used in alopecia areata, and although some regrowth of both vellus and terminal hairs has been reported, the results are not impressive[78,79]. There is a report of oral CsA for severe alopecia areata with a dose of 6 mg kg^{-1} day^{-1} for 3 months[80]. Some regrowth of terminal hair did occur, but this was already being lost 2 months after CsA had been discontinued. Unless a good reponse to a topical preparation is achieved it is unlikely that systemic CsA will be used for alopecia areata because of side-effects that are likely to be encountered with long-term therapy.

OTHER DISORDERS

CsA has been claimed to be beneficial in a number of systemic disorders with dermatological features. These include systemic sclerosis, dermatomyositis, systemic lupus erythematosus and Behçet's disease. The reports on systemic sclerosis and dermatomyositis are for the most part single case reports. There is good evidence that CsA is of help in Behçet's disease, particularly for the eye problems.

MECHANISM OF ACTION OF CsA IN PSORIASIS

The mechanism of action of CsA in psoriasis remains to be elucidated; however, the limited evidence obtained to date indicates a preferential effect on T lymphocyte function within the psoriatic lesion.

Although CsA appears to inhibit the proliferation of squamous cells *in vitro*[81], it does not inhibit epidermal cell growth at therapeutic levels[82,83]. In contrast, inhibition of keratinocytes grown on plastic in serum-free medium (but not cultured on collagen in the presence of serum) has been demonstrated[84]; the relevance of such findings to the *in vivo* situation where serum is present is, however, questionable. Similarly, the proliferation of fibroblasts, which have been suggested to play a pathophysiological role in psoriasis[85], are also inhibited *in vitro* in the absence but not presence of foetal calf serum[86].

CsA applied topically to psoriatic lesions resulted in the significant reduction of neutrophil aggregates present within the stratum corneum (Munro abscesses) but neither affected the T lymphocyte infiltrate nor inhibited the psoriatic process[61]. The lack of beneficial effects of topically applied CsA probably results from insufficient penetration of the drug preventing access to target cells. Thus it is unlikely that any modulation of neutrophil function by CsA is responsible for the clearing of psoriasis; indeed these observations argue against a primary role for neutrophils in the pathogenesis of this disease.

In contrast, effective treatment of psoriasis patients with oral CsA resulted in a marked decrease in CD4 and CD8 T cells both in the epidermis and dermis of psoriatic lesions (Figures 10.1, 10.2)[52,87]. However, activated (HLA-DR +) CD4 T lymphocytes persisted in the epidermis even after 12 weeks treatment[87]. As discussed earlier, CsA inhibits IL-2 production by activated CD4 T cells; furthermore, it suppresses the release of IL-1[24]. Both IL-1 and keratinocyte-derived ETAF (epidermal thymocyte-activating factor)[88], present in the epidermis, have been shown to be chemotactic for T cells. Thus the reduction in epidermal CD4 and CD8 T cell numbers may result from inhibition of IL-2 production or the effects of CsA on recruitment of further effector cells or both. Indeed, CsA has been shown to inhibit the accumulation of lymphocytes into the lymph nodes of rats following innoculation with sheep red cells[89]. The mechanism(s) for the selective persistence of activated CD4 T cells in the epidermis is, however, unclear. It has been postulated that the function of these cells is 'paralysed' and that, when the drug is withdrawn, they resume synthesis of factors responsible for stimulation of keratinocyte growth in

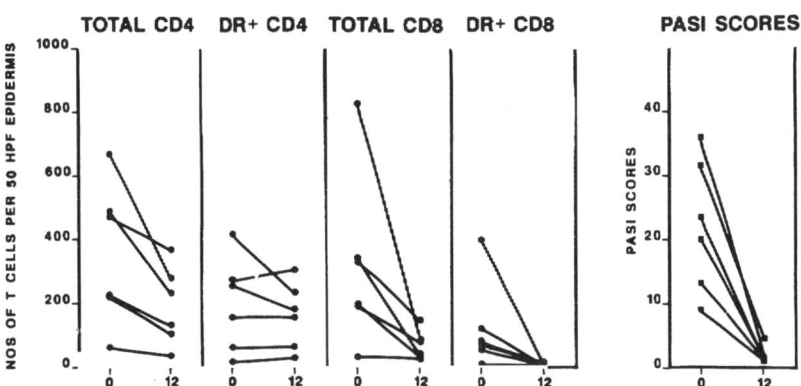

Figure 10.1 Numbers and HLA-DR expression of T lymphocytes in the lesional *epidermis* of six psoriasis patients before and 12 weeks after cyclosporin treatment. (Reproduced by kind permission of the *British Journal of Dermatology*)

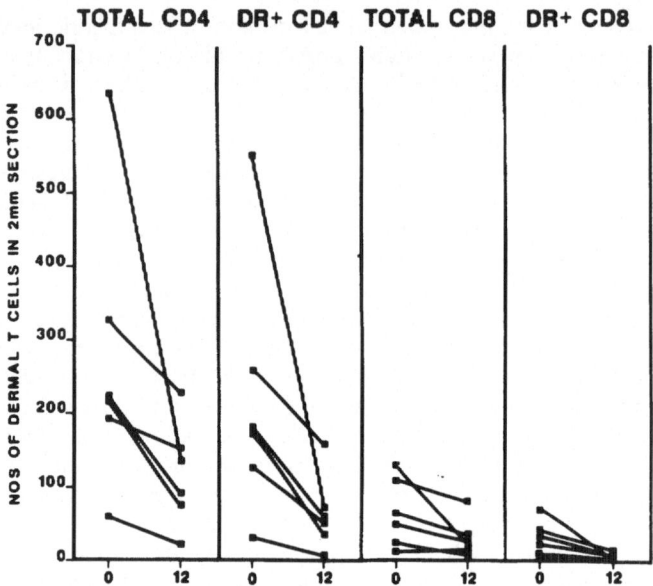

Figure 10.2 Numbers and HLA-DR expression of T lymphocytes in the lesional *dermis* of six psoriasis patients before and 12 weeks after cyclosporin treatment. (Reproduced by kind permission of the *British Journal of Dermatology*)

psoriasis[90]. This could explain the rapid relapse of the disease when CsA therapy is discontinued[19,52].

Epidermal HLA-DR + dendritic cells which lack the CD1 antigen characteristically expressed by Langerhans cells were also selectively depleted by systemic CsA treatment before clinical improvement was apparent and at a rate which correlated with clearance of psoriasis (Figure 10.3)[87]. (This dendritic cell subpopulation is observed in lesional, but not uninvolved, psoriatic or normal epidermis.) Although CsA has been shown to affect HLA-DR expression by monocytes[91], this is an unlikely explanation for these observations because numbers of the DR + CD1 + subpopulation were unchanged at the end of the treatment period[87]. It was postulated therefore that the disappearance of the DR + CD1 − dendritic cell subpopulation may be secondary to the effects of CsA on CD4 T cell function[87].

When CsA was injected into psoriatic lesions[92], similar changes in the T and dendritic cell subpopulations were observed, with two exceptions; epidermal DR + CD4 T cells did not persist and there was a significant increase in DR − CD1 + dendritic cells once the lesions had cleared. These observations probably result from a larger concentration of CsA present in the skin after injection than when the drug is taken orally. This may result in more profound effects on the CsA-sensitive CD4 T cell population. Thus the inhibition of γ-IFN production (and that of other lymphokines) by activated CD4 T cells, which has been shown to be concentrated dependent *in vitro*[93], could prevent the induction of HLA-DR on Langerhans cells[94] leading to increased DR − CD1 + dendritic cell numbers. Furthermore, antigen

206

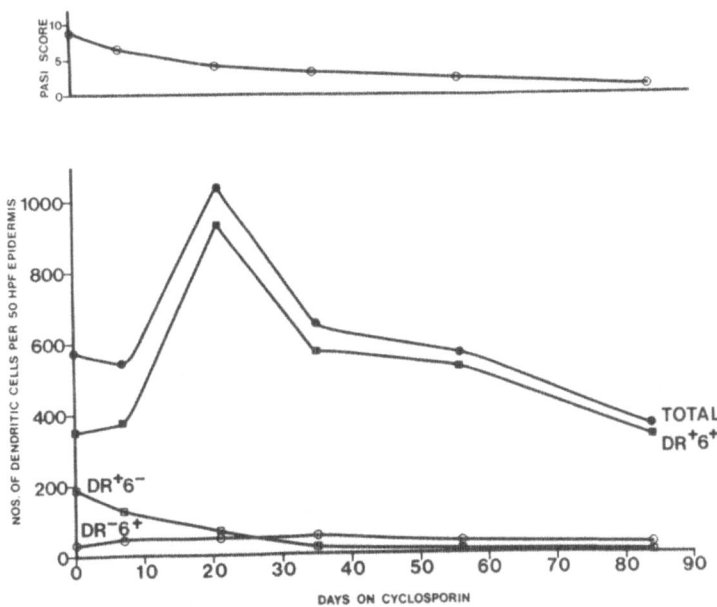

Figure 10.3 Typical changes in epidermal dendritic cell subpopulations and PASI (psoriasis area and severity index) scores in a single patient during cyclosporin treatment. (Reproduced by kind permission of the *British Journal of Dermatology*)

presentation by Langerhans cells may also be affected[22].

Alternative sites of action of CsA in psoriasis include phospholipase a_2 and the calcium-binding calmodulin. Phospholipase A_2 activity and leukotriene B_4 levels are elevated in psoriasis, and it has been proposed that the latter may be responsible, in part, for the increased epidermal proliferation and inflammation in the psoriatic lesion. A decrease in leukotriene B_4 levels in the psoriatic lesions of patients treated with CsA[52] may result from inhibition of phospholipase A_2 activity which has previously been shown to be susceptible to the drug's action[95]. Since calmodulin levels are also elevated in psoriatic epidermis[96] and CsA is a calmodulin antagonist *in vitro*, at least part of the effectiveness of CsA in inducing remission of psoriasis may be due to its action as a calmodulin antagonist *in vivo*. However, other calmodulin antagonists, including phenothiazines and mepacrine[97], have not been demonstrated to be effective in psoriasis. Indeed, propranolol, another calmodulin antagonist, can induce or exacerbate psoriasis. On the other hand, a recent study indicated that dithranol, widely used topically for the treatment of psoriasis, may also be a calmodulin antagonist[98]. The biological relevance of CsA inhibition of calmodulin-dependent processes has, however, been question, as discussed earlier.

Thus the mode of action of CsA in psoriasis has still to be determined. However, the evidence obtained to date supports an inhibitory effect on T lymphocyte and possibly Langerhans cell function, rather than a direct antiproliferative effect on psoriatic keratinocytes. This may involve inhibition of antigen presentation, lymphokine production, phospholipase A_2 or calmodulin activity, or a combination of these effects. The beneficial effects of CsA in psoriasis provides strong support for the concept that psoriasis is a T cell-mediated disease.

CONCLUSIONS

CsA has been shown to be a highly effective drug in psoriasis, and is the first therapeutic agent for this disease to be used for logical and scientific reasons, rather than empiricism which has characterized dermatological therapy up until now. Whether it will gain wide acceptance will depend on the risk of hypertension and nephrotoxicity when used over long periods, even in low dosage. Long-term studies and careful monitoring will be required, and the drug should be used with caution and by those with experience of its use. Its value in other dermatological conditions has yet to be determined, and far more clinical data are needed before its use can be recommended, but it looks promising in the bullous disorders, i.e. pemphigus and pemphigoid, and also in severe atopic eczema. Unfortunately at present the drug has not proved to be effective topically, particularly in psoriasis, and whether this is due to lack of penetration or other factors, remains to be determined. However, if a topical preparation can be made effective, particularly in psoriasis, it will have a significant impact on the treatment of this disease.

REFERENCES

1. Obalek, S., Haftek, M. and Glinski, W. (1977) Immunological studies in psoriasis. Dermatologica, **155**, 13–23
2. Krueger, G. G., Hill, H. R. and Jederberg, W. W. (1978) Inflammatory and immune cell function in psoriasis — a subtle disorder. 1. In vivo and in vitro survey. J. Invest. Dermatol., **71**, 189–194
3. Levantine, A. and Brostoff, J. (1975) Immunological responses of patients with psoriasis and the effect of treatment with methotrexate. Br. J. Dermatol., **93**, 659–668
4. Guilhou, J.-J., Clot, J. and Meynadier, J. (1977) T cell defect in psoriasis: further studies on membrane markers and T cell functions from 60 patients. Arch. Dermatol. Res., **260**, 163–166
5. Goan, S.-R., Volk, H. D., Eichhorn, I. and Diezel, W. (1986) Differences in interferon-gamma response of psoriatic lymphocytes to stimulation with various mitogens. Biomed. Biochim. Acta, **45**, 903–906
6. Baker, B. S., Swain, A. F., Valdimarssón, H. and Fry, L. (1984a) T-cell subpopulations in the blood and skin of patients with psoriasis. Br. J. Dermatol., **110**, 37–44
7. Valdimarsson, H., Baker, B. S., Jonsdottir, I. and Fry, L. (1986) Psoriasis: a disease of abnormal keratinocyte proliferation induced by T lymphocytes. Immunol. Today, **7**, 256–259
8. Bjerke, J. E., Krogh, H. K. and Matre, R. (1978) Characterisation of mononuclear cell infiltrate in psoriatic lesions. J. Invest. Dermatol., **71**, 340–343
9. Bos, J. D., Bulsebosch, H. J., Krieg, S. R., Bakker, P. M. and Cormane, R. H. (1983) Immunocompetent cells in psoriasis: in situ immunophenotyping by monoclonal antibodies. Arch. Dermatol. Res., **275**, 181–189
10. Baker, B. S., Swain, A. F., Fry, L. and Valdimarsson, H. (1984) Epidermal T lymphocytes and HLA-DR expression in psoriasis. Br. J. Dermatol., **110**, 555–564

11. Baker, B. S., Swain, A. F., Griffiths, C. E. M., Leonard, J. N., Fry, L. and Valdimarsson, H. (1985) Epidermal T lymphocytes and dendritic cells in chronic plaque psoriasis: the effects of PUVA treatment. *Clin. Exp. Immunol.*, **61**, 526–534

12. Mackaness, G. B. (1969) The influence of immunologically committed lymphoid cells on macrophage activity *in vivo*. *J. Exp. Med.*, **129**, 973-992

13. Horton, J. E., Raisz, L. G., Simmons, H. A., Oppenheim, J. J. and Mergenhagen, S. E. (1972) Bone resorbing activity in supernatant fluid from cultured human peripheral blood leukocytes. *Science*, **177**, 793–795

14. Korszum A.-K., Wilton, J. M. and Johnson, N. W. (1981) The *in vivo* effects of lymphokines on mitotic activity and keratinisation in guinea pig epidermis. *J. Invest. Dermatol.*, **76**, 433–437

15. Whyte, H. J. and Baughman, R. D. (1964) Acute guttate psoriasis and streptococcal infection. *Arch. Dermatol.*, **89**, 350–356

16. Swerlick, R. A., Cunningham, M. W. and Hall, N. K. (1986) Monoclonal antibodies cross-reactive with Group A streptococci and normal and psoriatic human skin. *J. Invest. Dermatol.*, **87**, 367-371

17. Schopf, R. E., Hoffman, A., Jung, M. Morsches, B. and Bork, K. (1986) Stimulation of T cells by autologous mononuclear leukocytes and epidermal cells in psoriasis. *Arch. Dermatol. Res.*, **279**, 89–94

18. Baker, B. S., Swain, A. F., Griffiths, C. E. M., Leonard, J. N., Fry, L. and Valdimarsson, H. (1985) The effects of topical treatment with steroids or dithranol on epidermal T lymphocytes and dendritic cells in psoriasis. *Scand. J. Immunol.*, **22**, 471–477

19. Griffiths, C. E. M., Powles, A. V., Leonard, J. N., Baker, B. S., Valdimarsson, H. and Fry, L. (1986) Clearance of psoriasis with low dose cyclosporin. *Br. Med. J.*, **293**, 731–732

20. Heule, F., Meinardi, M. M. H. M., van Joost, T. and Bos, J. D. (1988) Low-dose cyclosporine effective in severe psoriasis a double-blind study. *Transplant. Proc.*, **20**, 32–41

21. Palay, D. A., Cluff, C. W., Wentworth, P. A. and Ziegler, H. K. (1986) Cyclosporine inhibits macrophage-mediated antigen presentation. *J. Immunol.*, **136**, 4348–4353

22. Furue, M. and Katz, S. (1988) The effect of cyclosporine on epidermal cells. 1. Cyclosporine inhibits accessory cell functions of epidermal Langerhans cells *in vitro*. *J. Immunol.*, **140**, 4139–4143

23. Lu, C. Y., Lemay, P. A. and Lombardi, M. J. (1988) Inhibition of antigen-specific activation of an L3T4+ T cell line by cyclosporine with maintenance of macrophage-mediated antigen-presentation. *Transplantation*, **45**, 187–193

24. Bunjes, D., Hardt, C., Rollinghoff, M. and Wagner, H. (1981) Cyclosporine A mediates immunosuppression of primary cytotoxic T cell responses by impairing the release of interleukin 1 and interleukin 2. *Eur. J. Immunol.*, **11**, 657–661

25. Granelli-Piperno, A., Inaba, A. K. and Steinman, R. M. (1984) Stimulation of lymphokine release from T lymphoblasts. Requirement for mRNA synthesis and inhibition by cyclosporin A. *J. Exp. Med.*, **160**, 1792–1802

26. Reem, G. H., Cook, L. A. and Vilcek, J. (1983) Gamma interferon synthesis by human thymocytes and T lymphocytes inhibited by cyclosporin A. *Science*, **221**, 63–65

27. Lafferty, K. J., Borel, J. F. and Hodskin, P. (1983) Cyclosporine-A (CS): models for the mechanism of action. *Transplant. Proc.*, **15**, 2242–2247

28. Thomson, A. W., Moon, D. K., Geczy, C. L. and Nelson, D. S. (1983) Cyclosporin A inhibits lymphokine production but not the response of macrophages to lymphokines. *Immunology*, **48**, 291–299

29. Kupiec-Weglinski, J. W., Filho, M. A., Strom, T. B. and Tilney, N. L. (1984) Sparing of suppressor cells: a critical action of cyclosporine. *Transplantation*, **38**, 97–101

30. Klaus, G. G. B. and Hawrylowicz, C. M. (1984) Activation and proliferation signals in mouse B cells. II. Evidence for activation (G_0 to G_1) signals differing in sensitivity to cyclosporine. *Eur. J. Immunol.*, **14**, 250–254

31. Berridge, M. J. and Irvine, R. F. (1984) Inositol triphosphate, a novel second messenger in cellular signal transduction. *Nature*, **312**, 315–321

32. Rosoff, P. M. and Cantley, L. C. (1985) Stimulation of the T3-T cell receptor-associated Ca^{++} influx enhances the activity of the Na^+/H^+ exchanger in a leukaemic human T cell line. *J. Biol. Chem.*, **260**, 14053–14059

33. Kroggel, R., Goppelt-Strube, M., Martin, M. and Resch, K. (1987) The immunosuppressive activities of different cyclosporins are correlated to inhibition of the early membrane

phospholipid metabolism in activated lymphocytes. *Immunobiology,* **175**, 159–171

34. Metcalfe, S. (1984) Cyclosporine does not prevent cytoplasmic calcium changes associated with lymphocyte activation. *Transplantation,* **38**, 161–164

35. Wiskocil, R., Weiss, A., Imboden, J., Kamin-Lewis, R. and Stobo, J. (1985) Activation of a human T cell line: a 2 stimulus requirement in the pretranslational events involved in the coordinate expression of IL-2 and gamma-interferon genes. *J. Immunol.,* **134**, 1599–1c03

36. Rosoff, P. and Teres, G. (1986) Cyclosporin inhibits Ca^{++} dependent stimulation of Na^+/H^+ antiport in human T cells. *J. Cell Biol.,* **103**, 457–463

37. Merker, M. M. and Hanschumacher, R. E. (1984) Uptake and nature of the intracellular binding of cyclosporine A in a murine thymoma cell line, BW 5147. *J. Immunol.,* **132**, 3064–3070

38. Larson, D. F. (1986) Larson, D. F. (1986) Mechanism of action: antagonism of the prolactin receptor. *Progr. Allergy,* **38**, 222–238

39. Colombani, P. M., Robb, A. and Hess, A. D. (1985) Cyclosporin A binding to calmodulin: a possible site of action on T lymphocytes *Science,* **228**, 337–339

40. Legrue, S. J., Turner, R., Weisbrodt, N. and Dedman, J. R. (1986) Does the binding of cyclosporine to calmodulin result in immunosuppression? *Science,* **234**, 68–71

41. Hanschumacher, R. E., Harding, M. W., Rice, J. and Drugge, R. J. (1984) Cyclophilin: a specific cytosolic binding protein for cyclosporin A. *Science,* **226**, 544–547

42. Klaus, G. G. B. and Kunkle, A. (1983) Effects of cyclosporin on the immune system of the mouse. *Transplantation,* **36**, 80-84

43. Kunkle, A. and Klaus, G. G. B. (1980) Selective effects of cyclosporin A on functional B cell subsets in the mouse. *J. Immunol.,* **125**, 2526–2531

44. Shevach, E. M. (1985) The effects of cyclosporin A on the immune system. *Ann. Rev. Immunol.,* **3**, 397–423

45. Borel, J. F., Feurer, C., Gibner, H. U. and Stahelein, N (1976) Biological effects of cyclosporin A: a new antilymphocytic agent. *Agents Actions,* **6**, 468–475

46. Meuller, W. and Hermann, B. (1979) Cyclosporin A for psoriasis. *N. Engl. J. Med.,* **301**, 555

47. Gubner, R., August, S. and Gincberg, V. (1951) Therapeutic suppression of tissue reactivity. II. Effect of aminopterine in rheumatoid arthritis and psoriasis. *Ann. J. Med. Sci.,* **221**, 688–699

48. Harper, J. I., Keat, A. C. S. and Staughton, R. C. D. (1984) Cyclosporin for psoriasis. *Lancet,* **2**, 981–982

49. Van Hooff, J. P., Leunissen, K. M. L. and Staak, W. V. D. (1985) Cyclosporin for psoriasis. *Lancet,* **1**, 335

50. Van Joost, T. H., Heule, F., Stolz, E. and Beukers, R. (1986) Short-term use of cyclosporin A in severe psoriasis. *Br. J. Dermatol.,* **114**, 615–620

51. Marks, J. M. (1986) Cyclosporin A treatment of severe psoriasis. *Br. J. Dermatol.,* **115**, 745–746

52. Ellis, C. N., Gorsulowsky, D. C., Hamilton, T. A., Billings, J. K., Brown, M. D., Headington, J. T., Cooper, K. D., Baadsgard, O., Duell, E. A., Annesley, T. M., Turcotte, J. G. and Vorhees, J. J. (1986) Cyclosporine improves psoriasis in a double-blind study. *J. Am. Med. Assoc.,* **256**, 3110–3116

53. Wentzell, J. M., Baughman, R. W., O'Connor, G. T. and Bernier, G. M. (1987) Cyclosporine in the treatment of psoriasis. *Arch. Dermatol.,* **123**, 163–165

54. Picascia, D. D., Garden, J. M., Freinkel, R. K. and Roenigk, H. H. (1987) Treatment of resistant severe psoriasis with systemic cyclosporine. *J. Am. Acad. Dermatol.,* **17**, 408–414

55. Griffiths, C. E. M., Powles, A. V., McFadden, J. P., Baker, B. S., Valdimarsson, H. and Fry, L. (1989) Long-term cyclosporin for psoriasis. *Br. J. Dermatol,* **120**, 253–260

56. Fredriksson, T. and Petterson, V. (1978) Severe psoriasis oral therapy with a new retinoid. *Dermatologica,* **157**, 238–244

57. Calne, R. Y., White, D. J. G. and Thiru, S. (1978) Cyclosporin A in patients receiving renal allografts from cadaver donors. *Lancet,* **2**, 1323–1327

58. Tegzess, A. M. (1988) Ciclosporin and renal function. In van Joost, T. H. and Heule, F., Bos, J. D. (eds), *Ciclosporin (Sandimmune) in Psoriasis,* (Uden: Sandoz), pp. 128–136

59. Schauder, C. S. and Gorulowsky, D. C. (1986) Topical cyclosporine A in the treatment

of psoriasis. *Clin. Res.*, **34**, 1007A

60. Griffiths, C. E. M., Powles, A. V., Baker, B. S., Fry, L. and Valdimarsson, H. (1987) Topical cyclosporin and psoriasis. *Lancet*, **1**, 806

61. Schulze, H. J., Mahrle, G. and Steigleder, G. K. (1988) Topical application of ciclosporin in psoriasis. In van Joost, Th., Heule, F. and Bos, J. D. (eds), *Ciclosporin (Sandimmune) in Psoriasis* (Leiden: Sandoz), pp. 102–104

62. Aldridge, R. W., Sewell, H. F., King, G. and Thomson, A. W. (1986) Topical cyclosporin A in nickel contact hypersensitivity: results of a preliminary clinical immunohistochemical investigation. *Clin. Exp. Immunol.*, **66**, 582–589

63. Parodi, A. and Rebora, A. (1987) Topical cyclosporine in alopecia areata. *Arch. Dermatol.*, **123**, 165

64. Thomson, A. W., Aldridge, R. D. and Sewell, H. F. (1986) Topical cyclosporin in alopecia areata and nickel contact dermatitis. *Lancet*, **2**1, 971–972

65. Aldridge, R. A., Thomson, A. W., Rankin, R., Whiting, P. H., Cunningham, C. and Simpson, J. G. (1985) Inhibition of contact sensitivity reactions to DNFB by topical cyclosporin application in the guinea pig. *Clin. Exp. Immunol.*, **59**, 23–28

66. Powles, A. V., Baker, B. S., McFadden, J. P., Rutman, A., Griffiths, C. E. M. and Fry, L. (1988) Intralesional injection of cyclosporin in psoriasis. *Lancet*, **1**, 537

67. Van Joost, T. H., Stolz, E. and Heule, F. (1987) Efficacy of low dose cyclosporine in severe atopic skin disease. *Arch. Dermatol.*, **123**, 166–167

68. Camp, R. D. R. and Logan, R. A. (1987) Cyclosporine in atopic dermatitis. In *The Second International Congress of Cyclosporine*. (Texas: The University of Texas Health Science Centre). Abstracts, p. 51

69. Jensen, J. R., Thestrup-Pedersen, K., Zachariae, H. and Sogaard, H. (1987) Cyclosporin A for therapy for mycosis fungoides. *Arch. Dermatol.*, **123**, 160–163

70. Thomson, K. and Wantzin, G. L. (1987) Extracutaneous spreading with fatal outcome of mycosos fungoides in a patient treated with ciclosporin A. *Dermatologica*, **174**, 236–238

71. Catterall, M. D., Addis, B. J. and Smith, J. L. (1983) Sezary syndrome: transformation to a high lymphoma after treatment with cyclosporine A. *Clin. Exp. Dermatol.*, **8**, 159

72. Puttick, L., Pollack, A. and Fairburn, E. (1983) Treatment of Sezary syndrome with cyclosporine A. *J. R. Soc. Med.*, **76**, 1063–1065

73. Moreland, A. A., Robertson, W. B. and Heffner, L. T. (1985) Treatment of cutaneous T cell lymphoma with cyclosporin. *J. Am. Acad. Dermatol.*, **12**, 886–887

74. Totterman, T. H., Scheynius, A., Killander, A., Danersuna, A. and Alm, G. V. (1985) Treatment of therapy-resistant Sezary syndrome with cyclosporine A. *Scand. J. Haematol.*, **34**, 196–203

75. Barthelemy, H., Biron, F., Claudy, A., Souterland, P. and Thivolet, J. (1986) Cyclosporine: a new immunosuppressive agent in bullous pemphigoid and pemphigus. *Transplant. Proc.*, **18**, 913–914

76. Cunliffe, W. J. (1987) Pemphigus foliaceus and response to cyclosporin. *Br. J. Dermatol.*, **117** (Suppl. 32), 114–116

77. Balda, B. R. and Rosenzweig, D. (1985) Treatment of bullous dermatoses with cyclosporin. In Schindler, R. (ed.), *Ciclosporin in Autoimmune Diseases*. (Berlin: Springer), pp. 209–214

78. de Prost, Y., Teillac, D., Paquez, F., Carrugi, C., Bachelez, H. and Touraine, R. (1988) Treatment of severe alopecia areata by topical applications of cyclosporine. *Transplant. Proc.*, **20** (Suppl. 4), 112–113

79. Mauduit, G., Lenvers, P., Barthelemy, H. and Thivolet, J. (1987) Treatment of alopecia areata with topically applied cyclosporin A. *Ann. Dermatol. Venereol.*, **114**, 507–510

80. Gupta, A. K., Ellis, C. N., Tellner, D. C. and Voorhees, J. J. (1988) Cyclosporine A in the treatment of severe alopecia areata. *Transplant. Proc.*, **20** (Suppl. 4), 105–108

81. Lucia, M. G., Woan, M. C., Scheizer, R. T., Kosciol, C. M., Johnson, R. L. and Sharpe, R. J. (1986) Cyclosporine inhibits the proliferation of squamous cells. *Fed. Proc.*, **45**, 272

82. Katp, N., Halprin, K. M. and Taylor, J. R. (1987) Cyclosporin A does not inhibit epidermal cell growth at therapeutic levels. *J. Invest. Dermatol.*, **88**, 52–54

83. Kelly, G. E., Sheil, A. G. R., Wass, J. and Zbroja, R. A. (1986) Effects of ultraviolet radiation and immunosuppressive therapy on mouse epidermal cell kinetics. *Br. J. Dermatol.*, **114**, 197–208

84. Fisher, G. J., Duell, E. A., Nickoloff, B. J., Annesley, T. M., Kowalke, J. K., Ellis, C. N. and Vorjees, J. J. (1988) Levels of cyclosporin in epidermis of treated psoriasis patients

differentially inibit growth of keratinocytes cultured in serum free versus serum containing media. *J. Invest. Dermatol.,* **91,** 142–146

85. Saiag, P., Coulomb, B., Lebreton, C., Bell, E. and Dubertret, L. (1985) Psoriatic fibroblasts induce hyperproliferation of normal keratinocytes in a skin equivalent model *in vitro.* *Science,* **230,** 669–672

86. N.:koloff, B. J., Fisher, G. J., Mitra, R. S. and Vorhees, J. J. (1988) Direct cytopathic effects of cyclosporin A on rapidly proliferating cultured keratinocytes and dermal fibroblasts. *Transplant. Proc.,* **20,** 85–90

87. Baker, B. S., Griffiths, C. E. M., Lambert, S., Powles, A. V., Leonard, J. N., Valdimarsson, H. and Fry, L. (1987) The effects of cyclosporin A on T lymphocyte and dendritic cell subpopulations in psoriasis. *Br. J. Dermatol.,* **116,** 503–510

88. Sauder, D. N., Monick, M. M. and Hunninghake, G. W. (1985) Epidermal cell-derived thymocyte activating factor (ETAF) is a potent T-cell chemoattractant. *J. Invest. Dermatol.,* **85,** 431–433

89. Ali, A. T. M. M., Morley, J. and Rumjanek, V. M. (1982) Inhibition of lymphocyte accumulation by cyclosporin A. *Br. J. Pharmacol.,* **75,** 126P

90. Griffiths, C E. M., Powles, A. V., Baker, B. S., Fry, L. and Valdimarsson, H. (1987) Combination of cyclosporine A and topical corticosteroid in the treatment of psoriasis. *Transplant. Proc.,* **20,** 50–52

91. Whisler, R. L., Lindsey, J. A., Proctor, K. V. W., Newhouse, Y G. and Cornwell, D. G. (1985) The impaired ability of human monocytes to stimulate autologous and allogeneic mixed lymphocyte reactions after exposure to cyclosporin. *Transplantation,* **40,** 57–61

92. Baker, B. S., Powles, A. V., Savage, C. R., McFadden, J. P., Valdimarsson, H. and Fry, L. (1988) Intralesional cyclosporin A in psoriasis: effects on T lymphocyte and dendritic cell subpopulations. *Br. J. Dermatol.* (In press)

93. Buurman, W. A., Daeman, A. J. J. M., van der Linden, C. J. and Kootstra, G. (1987) Clinically used concentrations of cyclosporin A only partially inhibit interferon-gamma production by activated T lymphocytes. *Transplantation,* **19,** 1193

94. Berman, B., Duncan, M. R., Smith, B., Ziboh, V. A. and Palladino, M. (1985) Interferon enhancement of HLA-DR antigen expression on epidermal Langerhans cells. *J. Invest. Dermatol.,* **84,** 54–58

95. Fan, T.-P. D. and Lewis, G. P. (1985) Mechanism of cyclosporin A-induced inhibition of prostacyclin synthesis by macrophages. *Prostaglandins,* **30,** 735–747

96. Tucker, W. F. G., MacNeil, S., Bleehan, S. S. and Tomlinson, S. (1984) Biologically active calmodulin levels are elevated in both involved and uninvolved epidermis in psoriasis. *J. Invest. Dermatol.,* **82,** 298–299

97. Iizuka, H., Hashimoto, Y., Hirokawa, M., Matsuo, S., Mizumoto, T. and Ohkawara, A. (1985) Pig-skin epidermal calmodulin: effects of antagonists of calmodulin on DNA-synthesis of pig-skin epidermis. *Arch. Dermatol. Res.,* **278,** 133–157

98. Tucker, W. F. G., MacNeil, S., Dawson, R. A., Tomlinson, S. and Bleehan, S. S. (1986) An investigation of the ability of anti-psoriatic drugs to inhibit calmodulin activity: a possible mode of action of dithranol (anthralin). *J. Invest. Dermatol.,* **87,** 232–235

11
Cyclosporin A (Sandimmun®) in autoimmune disorders

Beat von Graffenried, David Friend, Nicholas Shand, Wilfried Scheiss and Pentti Timonen

RATIONALE FOR THE USE OF SANDIMMUN® IN AUTOIMMUNE DISEASES

Since the effect of Sandimmun® (cyclosporin A) was established in organ transplantation some years ago, increasing interest has been shown in studying its potential in autoimmune diseases. As of June 1988, about 5000 patients suffering from many different clinical syndromes have been treated in more than 100 clinical studies.

The main reasons for this interest, and for the high expectations in Sandimmun® are: (1) the mechanism of action of the drug, (2) the promising results in many animal models of autoimmunity, (3) the advantages over conventional immunosuppression as demonstrated in clinical transplantation and (4) the unsatisfactory situation with presently available therapy of many autoimmune diseases.

It is likely that most, if not all, of the effects of Sandimmun® which are the basis for its clinical efficacy in transplantation and autoimmunity are due to the abrogation of the production of lymphokines secreted by activated T cells[1,2]. These effects are rapid in onset, dose-dependent and quickly reversible. The activation of T lymphocytes requires two signals: the recognition of antigen presented in association with class II major histocompatability complex (MHC) products on the surface of an antigen-presenting cell and interleukin-1 (IL-1). Thus stimulated, the T helper cell synthesizes receptors to interleukin-2 (IL-2). IL-1 further stimulates the T helper cell to produce IL-2 as well as other lymphokines. IL-2 stimulates the replication of those T cells carrying the IL-2 receptor, regardless of the sub-population of T cells to which the cell belongs[3]. This IL-2-induced clonal expansion and maturation of cytotoxic T cells leads not only to direct destruction of target cells by interaction with antigen (again requiring expression of MHC products) but also to secretion of lymphokines other than IL-2: interferons (INF), macrophage-activating factors and colony-stimulating factors that encourage macrophage growth and activity. Other lymphokines in this same cascade stimulate B cell differentiation and antibody production.

Thus specific activation of the immune system can produce an autoimmune inflammatory response through cytotoxic T cells, antigen–antibody interactions, the release of lymphokines and other chemical mediators, notably leukotrienes and prostaglandins, all of which act on non-specific inflammatory cells or on target cells at the inflammatory site.

As shown in Figure 11.1 the principal effect of Sandimmun® is to shut off the production of IL-2 and other lymphokines in T cells[1,2]. The further recruitment of cytotoxic T cells is arrested by blocking IL-2 synthesis, and inflammatory effector mechanisms dry out in the absence of other lymphokines. Through inhibition of gamma-INF (γ-INF) production, the expression of MHC products will also be diminished, thereby inhibiting both inducer and effector mechanisms[4].

In therapeutic doses Sandimmun® is not cytotoxic, it probably does not influence the expression of the IL-2 receptor and also does not directly affect suppressor T cells. This lack of effect on suppressor function might be an important contribution to obtaining immunological quiescence. Although the T-dependent priming step of B cell activation is susceptible to inhibition by Sandimmun®, the drug has only limited effects on already activated, antibody-producing cells[2,5].

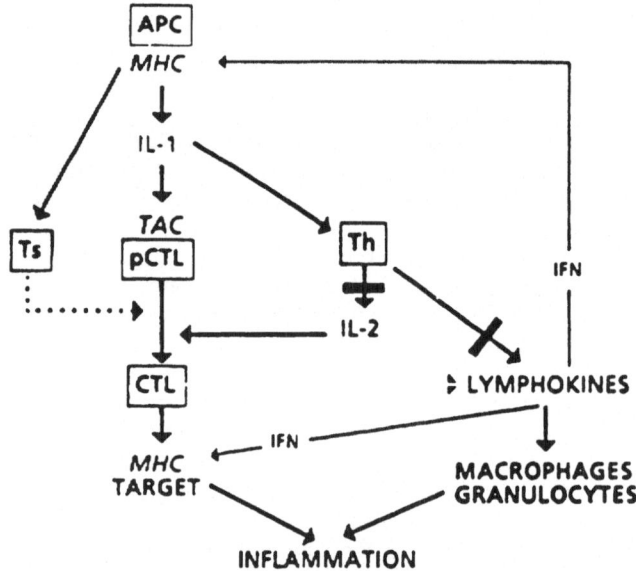

Figure 11.1 Mechanism of action of Sandimmun® in autoimmune disease. APC = antigen-presenting cell; MHC = major histocompatibility complex; IL = interleukin; TAC = IL-2 receptor; pCTL = precursor cytotoxic T-lymphocyte; Th = T helper lymphocyte; Ts = T suppressor lymphocyte; IFN = gamma interferon; ▬▬ indicates site of action of Sandimmun®

The inhibition of lymphokine synthesis by Sandimmun® is the result of its action at the nuclear level where it prevents the transcription of mRNA for IL-2[6,7].

Sandimmun® is the first of a new generation of immunosuppressive drugs. Its selective action on T lymphocytes confers it with several relevant clinical advantages over the older, conventional immunosuppressants because it lacks the mutagenic and bone marrow depressant effects of cytostatic drugs, and it does not paralyse most components of the immune system as do glucocorticoids, which inhibit macrophage and neutrophil function in addition to lymphocyte effects.

Apart from theoretical considerations based on the mechanism of action of Sandimmun® indicating that the drug could be useful both for induction and for maintenance of remission in autoimmune diseases, further encouragement to start clinical trials has come from a large series of experimental studies in animal models of autoimmunity in which Sandimmun® was active not only when given prophylactically but, at least in some, also therapeutically[8].

PROBLEMS OF CLINICAL TESTING IN AUTOIMMUNE DISEASES

The clinical pharmacologist is faced with difficult problems when preparing a clinical trial programme in autoimmune disease:

1. There are no sensitive and reliable immune parameters which could be used for dose-finding on short-term therapy in normal volunteers and which would be predictive of therapeutic efficacy in the patient.
2. Because of the variability of the spontaneous course of the many remitting—relapsing autoimmune diseases, the lack of homogeneity of patients within the same disease, and the difficulty in assessing the extent of reversible, potentially responsive pathology in an individual patient, uncontrolled pilot studies are of limited value.
3. Furthermore, in many autoimmune diseases clinical trial methadology is not well established, and reliable and sensitive parameters to assess efficacy are not available or not uniformally accepted.
4. Finally, in diseases where the aim is to prevent further progression, since already present symptomatology is largely irreversible (e.g. multiple sclerosis, primary biliary cirrhosis), only long-term studies in large patient numbers and with adequate control groups are meaningful.

Initial pilot studies with Sandimmun® (cyclosporin A) have mainly been conducted in therapy-resistant patients. Only after initial promising results has the use of Sandimmun® now started to be shifted cautiously to patients in less advanced disease stages which are more suitable to the study of drug effects. Pilot studies have been followed up with randomized controlled trials in larger numbers of patients, often involving multiple centres to provide for adequate statistical power (see Table 11.1). It is important to differentiate between clinical trials intended to study 'efficacy' of Sandimmun® and those which aim at evaluating 'benefit'. The demonstration that Sandimmun® reduces the number of T cells in broncho-alveolar lavage of patients with

Table 11.1 Randomized controlled trials with Sandimmun® in autoimmune diseases (status June 1988)

Versus placebo	Versus standard therapy
Rheumatoid arthritis 1, 2	Rheumatoid arthritis 1, 2
Uveitis posterior 1	Uveitis posterior 1
Insulin-dependent diabetes 1, 2	Behçet's disease 2
Multiple sclerosis 1, 2	Multiple sclerosis 1
Myasthenia gravis 1	Myasthenia gravis 2
Nephrotic syndrome 2	Nephrotic syndrome 2
Glomerulonephritis (chronic) 2	Psoriasis 2
Psoriasis 1, 2	Severe aplastic anaemia 2
Crohn's disease 1, 2	Endocrine ophthalmopathy 2
Primary biliary cirrhosis 2	
Sjögren's disease 1	

1 = studies completed; 2 = studies ongoing

pulmonary sarcoidosis is an indicator of efficacy and an important first step, but it does not necessarily mean that it is beneficial to prescribe the drug. A study demonstrating improvement in lung function and other disease symptoms is needed for that. The fact that Sandimmun® decreases serum alkaline phosphatase levels in patients with primary biliary cirrhosis may indicate efficacy. This should then be followed up by a formal study to assess the beneficial aspect of this observation by altering the natural course of the disease (progression of histological alteration, reduction of mortality). In insulin-dependent diabetes mellitus, proof of efficacy (induction of complete remission) still leaves open the question of the extent to which this is beneficial in terms of preventing vascular complications. These examples demonstrate that in the evaluation of therapies for many autoimmune diseases, a time-consuming stepwise procedure is needed.

In the following, the results of Sandimmun® are summarized separately for several autoimmune diseases (status June 1988).

RHEUMATOID ARTHRITIS

There is good evidence to suggest that, apart from antibody-mediated mechanisms, T lymphocytes and lymphokines are involved in the pathogenesis of rheumatoid arthritis (RA). Lymphokine-producing T cells are found in the cavity of affected joints during flare-ups[9], T helper cells that recognize self proteins such as collagen have been isolated and cloned from the joints of RA patients, and the synovial membrane contains predominantly clusters of T helper cells in close contact with large, HLA-DR positive, macrophage-like, interdigitating cells[10]. The synovial membrane effectively assumes the aspect of a peripheral lymphoid organ, manifesting a delayed hypersensitivity type of reaction with a preponderance of T helper cells. IL-1 and other lymphokines are known to stimulate the activity of osteoclasts and chondrocytes that synthesize collagenases to resorb bone and cartilage. Synovial cells, polymorphonuclear cells and macrophages in the synovial membrane and fluid, activated by lymphokines and complement, participate in the inflammatory activity releasing further proteolytic enzymes, oxygen free radicals, prostaglandins, etc. An overall picture can be constructed arguing a self-perpetuating process of immunological activation, inflammation and joint destruction which in turn feeds the system with antigen derived from self tissue[11,12].

Consequent y, the use of immunosuppressant drugs in this disease is rational and indeed the efficacy of cyclophosphamide, azathioprine and methotrexate, as well as steroids, supports this idea. Through inhibition of lymphokine secretion, Sandimmun® should exert clinical anti-inflammatory effects in RA, and by interrupting the immunological activation processes perhaps exert 'disease-modifying' effects.

Sandimmun® has been shown to be effective in a variety of animal models of RA such as adjuvant arthritis[13], arthritis induced through immunization of rats with type II collagen[14] and streptococcal cell wall antigen[15]. In these models Sandimmun® can prevent the appearance of the disease when given before the insult or it can improve the already established disease symptomatically. In addition to reducing joint swelling, Sandimmun® prevents radiologically assessed joint destruction in rats with adjuvant arthritis[16].

The first attempt to treat arthritic patients was in 1978, when Herrmann and Müller were able to obtain appreciable improvement in five out of six patients treated with Sandimmun® for up to 10 months[17].

To date, a total of 272 RA patients have participated in 14 published clinical studies, 215 of them receiving Sandimmun®. In ongoing studies, most of which are controlled, randomized studies comparing Sandimmun® to placebo, azathioprine and d-penicillamine, a further 200 patients are receiving Sandimmun® therapy. All these patients had failed previously on conventional disease-modifying drugs, had 'active' disease and were generally at functional and anatomic stages Steinbrocker II or III. The initial dosage of Sandimmun® employed varied from 5 to 10 mg kg^{-1} day^{-1}, which was then adjusted according to efficacy, tolerability and, in some, drug concentrations in blood. In one study[18] a control group was employed with a dosage of 1 mg kg^{-1} day^{-1}. In ongoing studies the initial dose is between 2.5 and 5 mg kg^{-1} day^{-1}.

Of the 14 published studies, 10 were open and uncontrolled, one controlled study compared two doses, one open study compared Sandimmun® treatment to that with azathioprine, and two double-blind studies were placebo-controlled. These are summarized in Table 11.2. In the 10 open, uncontrolled studies[17,19–27], plus the dose comparison study[18] improvements were reported in pain and morning stiffness by 43–87%, joint tenderness (Ritchie or ARA joint index) 38–67%, and grip strength 15–98%.

Taking the percentage of patients remaining in the study (i.e. not withdrawn because of side-effects and showing appreciable symptomatic improvement) as a rough guide to response, an overall 'responder rate' of between 17% and 95% is found (average 70%). The reduction of concomitant steroid dosage reported in some studies suggests the possible use of the drug in a 'steroid-sparing' capacity[28]. Cessation of treatment in responsive patients was followed by recurrence of symptoms within 2 to 10 weeks in the majority of patients[21,22].

It became obvious from these studies that the dosage is limited by side-effects (essentially nephrotoxicity). The early series of studies started with

Table 11.2 Sandimmun® in rheumatoid arthritis

Main author (date)	Reference	Trial design	n total	n Sandimmun®	Average dose (mg kg^{-1} day^{-1}) Initial	Final	Duration (months)
Herrmann (1979)	17	Open, uncontrolled	6	6	10	6	5–10
Dougados (1985)	20	Open, uncontrolled	6	6	8.5	7.8	3
Dougados (1987)	22	Open, uncontrolled	9	9	5	5.2	12
Weinblatt (1987)	21	Open, uncontrolled	10	10	6	6.1	6
Weinblatt (1987)	24	Open, uncontrolled	7	7	3		3
Tugwell (1987)	23	Open, uncontrolled	20	20	4.6	4.3	6
Bowles (1987)	19	Open, uncontrolled	10	10	6	3.9	6
Madhok (1988)	25	Open, uncontrolled	20	20	5	6	6–30
Miescher (1988)	26	Open, uncontrolled	25	25	5	3–5	6–18
Yoshinoya (1988)	27	Open, uncontrolled	23	23	3	2–5	4–18
Yocum (1987)	18	Double-blind, dose comparison	31	15	10	4.6	6
				16	1	0.85	
Van Rijthoven (1986)	29	Double-blind, placebo-controlled	36	17	10	5	6
Forre (1987)	28	Open, control vs azathioprine	24	12	10	6.4	6
Dougados (1988)	30	Double-blind, placebo controlled	52	26	4.6	4.6	4

218

$10 \, \text{mg} \, \text{kg}^{-1} \text{day}^{-1}$, and this dose must now be regarded as too toxic in most patients. With reduction of dose in studies started more recently (2.5–5 $\text{mg} \, \text{kg}^{-1} \text{day}^{-1}$), the side-effect profile is much improved while efficacy is still retained. The time till onset of effect, however, is clearly delayed with the lower doses. In successive studies from the same author the onset of action increased from 15 days[20] at $8.5 \, \text{mg} \, \text{kg}^{-1} \text{day}^{-1}$ to 1–2 months[22] at $5 \, \text{mg} \, \text{kg}^{-1} \text{day}^{-1}$. Tugwell et al. found the onset to occur at between 3 and 4 months at the latter dose[23]. In their low-dose ($1 \, \text{mg} \, \text{kg}^{-1} \text{day}^{-1}$) group, Yocum et al. were unable to demonstrate clinical benefit over 6 months[18]. Weinblatt et al.[24] retreated patients at $3 \, \text{mg} \, \text{kg}^{-1} \text{day}^{-1}$ over 3 months but found the therapeutic effect much less convincing than at the higher dose of $6 \, \text{mg} \, \text{kg}^{-1} \text{day}^{-1}$.

Two double-blind studies have compared the effects of Sandimmun® to that of placebo. Van Rijthoven et al.[29] showed significant improvements in some but not all clinical parameters over a 6-month period, at the initial dose of 10, decreasing to $5 \, \text{mg} \, \text{kg}^{-1} \text{day}^{-1}$. There was a high withdrawal rate in both groups, mainly because of side-effects in the Sandimmun® group and inefficacy in the placebo group. With a lower starting dose of $5 \, \text{mg} \, \text{kg}^{-1} \text{day}^{-1}$ and a treatment period of 4 months, Dougados et al.[30] had far fewer withdrawals. In the statistical analysis Sandimmun® was superior to placebo for five of seven clinical parameters (assessing pain, function and joint symptoms) and for overall responder rate (54% on Sandimmun®, 7% on placebo).

C-reactive protein values have been seen to decrease[25,28,30]; however, a fall in the erythrocyte sedimentation rate (ESR) seen in two early pilot studies[22,25] has not been reproduced in other studies. Also no reductions in rheumatoid factor or immunoglobulin concentrations have been found. Where measured, the T lymphocyte helper to suppressor ratio has remained unchanged[28]. The adverse event profile of Sandimmun® in RA is similar to the general one in autoimmune diseases which is presented in the section on 'side-effects'.

Of the patients treated with Sandimmun® in RA 24% had to be withdrawn because of SEs, i.e. mainly for GI intolerance and impaired renal function. Sandimmun®-treated RA patients appear to have a higher incidence of GI symptoms than non-RA patients. There is also a trend to more pronounced acute nephrotoxicity in RA. Both of these increases in SEs may be related to the concomitant use of NSAIDs. The highest serum creatinine increases were seen in the early studies that employed the highest dose. In all cases, dose reduction resulted in improved function so that only 12 withdrawals were seen (7% of those treated). In the six publications that give relatively detailed information on reversibility of renal dysfunction[20,21,23,28–33], complete reversibility was established, although sometimes only after several months. The few exceptions[31,32] were all from the higher-dose studies and demonstrated high serum creatinine increases. It appears that with the low-dose regimen ($2.5–5 \, \text{mg} \, \text{kg}^{-1} \text{day}^{-1}$, good monitoring of kidney function and reduction of Sandimmun® dose, if serum creatinine has increased by more than 30–50% over baseline, nephrotoxicity can be managed. In 14 patients with RA, kidney biopsies performed after 18 months of Sandimmun® therapy showed an absence of histological signs of chronic Sandimmun®-associated nephrotoxicity[26]. No lymphoma or serious infectious complications have been reported in Sandimmun®-treated RA patients (status June 1988).

In summary, the presently available data suggest that Sandimmun® is efficacious in the treatment of active RA used either alone or with cortico-steroids as a 'steroid sparer'. As a selective immunosuppressant, Sandimmun® has anti-inflammatory and may have 'disease-modifying' properties. Acting at a dosage of 2.5–5 mg kg^{-1}day^{-1} the onset of action is between 1 and 4 months. Results of the large, multi-centre, controlled studies, currently ongoing in Europe and Canada (vs. placebo and conventional therapy), will be available during 1989, and are needed to make more firm conclusions on the risk/benefit ratio of Sandimmun® in RA. The place of Sandimmun® in the hierarchy of drug treatment in RA still remains to be determined, and will no doubt require many years of further experimentation.

ENDOGENOUS UVEITIS

Endogenous uveitis is usually an acute phenomenon triggered by infectious or non-specific (endotoxins and other mediators of inflammation) agents. The chronicity of the process is mediated by immune mechanisms[34]. Experimental autoimmune uveitis (EAU) has been induced in rats following immunization against retinal S antigen[35]. Cellular immune mechanisms observed in human sympathetic ophthalmia[36] and EAU in rats[37] are similar. EAU has been transferred to naive Lewis rats by T cell lines derived from immunized Lewis rats of the same strain, while active induction of the disease was not possible in the T cell-deficient nude rats[38]. A high concentration of interleukin-1 (IL-1) and interleukin-2 (IL-2) has been detected in aqueous humour and vitreous taps from patients with ocular Behçet's disease[39]. These findings strongly support the idea of a pivotal role for T cell-mediated immune responses in these diseases.

Experimentally, Sandimmun® prevents the induction of EAU[40]. EAU can also be cured following treatment with Sandimmun®[41]. Immunocompetent cells invading the uvea in endogenous uveitis produce high levels of interleukins into the ocular fluids[42]. Therefore, it has been assumed that Sandimmun® might be a potentially effective drug to use for the treatment of this condition.

Several clinical studies have been carried out in order to evaluate the efficacy of Sandimmun® in the treatment of severe sight-threatening intermediate and posterior endrogenous uveitis. In 11 uncontrolled studies, over 200 patients suffering from endogenous uveitis refractory to treatment with systemic steroids and cytotoxic drugs have been treated with Sandimmun®[43–49]. In four controlled double-blind studies from Israel[50], Japan[51], the USA and the Netherlands[52], a further 210 patients were randomly assigned to receive Sandimmun®, conventional therapy (prednisone[50], chlorambucil[50], colchicine[51]), or placebo[52]. The most frequently studied subgroups of endogenous uveitis were Behçet's disease involving the posterior segment of the eye, 'idiopathic' uveitis, pars planitis, retinal vasculitis, Vogt–Koyanagi–Harada uveitis, birdshot chorioretinopathy and sarcoid uveitis.

Most patients receiving Sandimmun® had an initial loading dose of $5-10 \, mg \, kg^{-1} day^{-1}$ followed by a dose reduction according to ocular inflammatory activity and tolerability. Treatment duration was up to 36 months.

An evaluation of the data from the above studies has recently been summarized[53]. Improvement of intraocular inflammation and visual acuity was observed in over 60% of patients within the first 2–4 weeks. In many non-responders, failure may partly be due to irreversible changes that developed before the initiation of Sandimmun® therapy. Sandimmun® lowered the incidence and intensity of exacerbations; however, in many cases relapses of the inflammatory processes have been observed when discontinuation of Sandimmun® has been attempted.

Steroid-sparing is one of the most relevant effects of Sandimmun®. In Behçet's disease with ocular involvement, Sandimmun® has a remarkable therapeutic effect on the intraocular inflammatory process, prolonging the periods of remission and thereby arresting the inevitable gradual loss of vision. The beneficial effects on the systemic manifestations of the disease, however, are less obvious. Therefore, a combined Sandimmun® and steroid regimen has to be considered in patients demonstrating active extraocular manifestations of the disease.

The overall side-effects of Sandimmun® therapy, especially at high doses, are numerous and include hyper- and paraesthesia and numbness (50%), hypertrichosis (39%), gastrointestinal discomfort (37%), renal dysfunction (31%), fatigue and general malaise (31%), gingival overgrowth (27%), hypertension (16%), headache (16%), hepatic dysfunction (9%), anaemia (5%) and muscle cramps (4%). Practically every patient under Sandimmun® therapy will show one or more of the above complications during the treatment period. In most cases these side-effects are mild to moderate, tolerated by the patient and reversible on dose reduction.

Sandimmun®-associated structural kidney changes with arteriolopathy, interstitial fibrosis and tubular atrophy have been reported in uveitis patients treated with high doses for prolonged periods[54]. The extent of the histological alterations was correlated with the time during which serum creatinine was elevated more than 50% above baseline. Therefore, careful dosage adjustments with the aim of limiting creatinine increase to less than 50% over baseline is essential. For more details of renal side-effects, see section 'side-effects'.

Sandimmun® can be recommended for patients suffering from severe sight-threatening uveitis refractory to conventional therapy (steroids, cyto-static agents) and for those developing severe side-effects of such treatment, and especially patients with Behçet's disease involving the posterior segment of the eye. Only patients with active intraocular inflammation and at least partially reversible pathology will profit from Sandimmun®, and only those with a normal renal function should be considered for Sandimmun® therapy. Detailed treatment guidelines have been published[53].

INSULIN-DEPENDENT DIABETES MELLITUS

The hypothesis that autoimmune mechanisms are involved in the destruction of pancreatic beta cells in insulin-dependent diabetes mellitus (IDDM)[55], and

221

the findings that immune intervention with Sandimmun® is capable of modifying the natural course of the disease in animal models[56,57], has led to an exciting new era in clinical research of IDDM. The possibility of a new therapeutic principle is emerging, i.e. the preservation of residual insulin-secreting pancreatic tissue by immunosuppression. This may prevent not only insulin dependency but, more important, the devastating vascular complications of IDDM which, despite optimized insulin therapy, are still a considerable threat to patients[58].

The problem of immune intervention in IDDM is that at the time of clinical diagnosis the disease is in its end-stage with extensive beta-cell destruction[55]. The aim is to prevent the autoimmune destruction of the few remaining beta cells. It is very likely that continuous immunosuppression is necessary to do so.

The presently available experience with Sandimmun® is encouraging in that there can be no doubt that the natural course of the disease can be influenced in the expected direction. Table 11.3 gives an overview of the eight published clinical studies. Two double-blind, randomized studies[59-61] have confirmed the initial pilot study data in adults[62-65]: with Sandimmun® doses of 7.5–10 mg kg^{-1} day^{-1} significantly more patients were in complete remission (defined as good metabolic control without exogenous insulin) at 6–12 months than patients treated with placebo (see Table 11.4). In children, complete remission rates of up to 50% at 12 months have been reported in open studies[66,67]. A placebo-controlled study in very early-onset IDDM children is ongoing.

Clinical remission in Sandimmun® was associated with an increase in endogenous secretion of insulin as assessed by C-peptide measurements. Whereas in placebo-treated patients there was only a small and transient initial recovery of C-peptide, followed by a gradual decline, glucagon-stimulated C-peptide levels in Sandimmun®-treated patients rose to the near-normal range and could be maintained at least 12 months as long as Sandimmun® therapy was continued[60-62]. This documents that insulin secretion can be maintained, implying that immunosuppression has in actual fact arrested autoimmune isletitis.

The effect of Sandimmun® appears to be dose-dependent. In the French placebo-controlled study[59], the remission rate was higher when Sandimmun® whole-blood levels (RIA, polyclonal ABs) were maintained above 300 ng/ml; relapses occurred in all patients if Sandimmun® blood levels were below 200 ng/ml for 3 months or longer[60]. A further important predictive factor is the time of intervention. In the Canadian/European controlled study[61], the remission rate was greater in patients entering the study after less than 6 weeks with symptoms, and less than 2 weeks of insulin therapy. The same has been reported to be the most important predictive factor in children[67]. Initial C-peptide secretion and immunological parameters were not predictive.

The major problem in all patient series was that clinical remissions were rapidly lost after withdrawal of Sandimmun®, followed by progressive decline of stimulated C-peptide secretion. Relapse of insulin-dependency has also occurred when Sandimmun® was continued on either reduced dosage (because of toxicity), or even unchanged dosage. This is partly due to the

Table 11.3 Sandimmun® in insulin-dependent diabetes mellitus, published studies

Investigator(s)	References	Design	Number of patients	Duration of treatment (months)
Dupré, Stiller et al.	62, 63, 65	Open, no control	94	6–44
Assan, Bach et al.	64	Open, no control	12	3–12
Multi-centre, France (CDF)	59, 60	Double-blind, vs. placebo	122 (63)	6–12
Multi-centre, France (CDF)	60	Open, no control	79	3–12
Canadian–European Multicenter (CEDSG)	61	Double-blind, vs. placebo	187 (93)	12
Czernichow et al.	66	Open, no control	40	3–12
Bougnères et al.	67	Open no control	40	3–12
Assan, Bach et al.	60	Open, Sandimmun® vs. Sandimmun® + prednisone	25	3–12

Figures in parentheses show no. of patients on Sandimmun®

223

Table 11.4 Main results of two placebo-controlled studies with Sandimmun ® in IDDM

Investigator	Reference	Complete remission (percentage of patients)	
		Sandimmun ®	Placebo
CDF[a]	59, 60	n = 63	n = 59
	Month 6	25%	19%
	Month 9	22%	6%
	Month 12	17%	0%
CEDSG[b]	61	n = 93	n = 94
	Month 6	39%	19%
	Month 12	24%	10%

[a]CDF = French Multi-centre Study Group
[b]CEDSG = Canadian–European Diabetes Study Group

development of insulin-resistance. It has been possible to reinduce remission by increasing Sandimmun ® dosage[65], but the side-effect profile of Sandimmun ® often will not allow this, and it is likely that each relapse substantially reduces the chance of long-term maintenance of endogenous insulin secretion.

The side-effect profile of Sandimmun ® in IDDM is similar to that in other diseases, and will be described in more detail in the section on 'side-effects'. No serious infectious complications and no malignancies have occurred (status June 1988). However, dose-dependent and reversible renal dysfunction was common, and moderate degrees of structural changes were seen in 17/90 (19%) renal biopseis performed in Sandimmun ®-treated IDDM patients[68]. The most important factor influencing the histopathological alterations was the extent of renal dysfunction: in patients in whom serum creatinine did not increase more than 50% over baseline, the renal biopsy changes were much less pronounced[68]. It is especially encouraging that no relevant changes were found in biopsies of the French study in children[67] who achieved good remission rates with Sandimmun ® trough whole-blood levels below 300 ng/ml.

In summary, although well-controlled studies have clearly indicated that immunosuppression with Sandimmun ® can influence the natural course of the disease, and has thus opened a new dimension for treatment of IDDM, major problems still remain unsolved. The most important one is to establish a safe therapy which is able to maintain β cell function. The potential hazards of chronic immunosuppresssion must be balanced against the potential breakthrough of 'causal' therapy, perhaps preventing vascular complications. It is obviously very difficult to assess the risk–benefit situation; therefore therapy with Sandimmun ® in IDDM must still be regarded as an experimental procedure only justified within a limited number of controlled clinical trials[69].

NEPHROTIC SYNDROME

Most patients with nephrotic syndrome (hypoalbuminaemia due to massive proteinuria with oedema) who have been treated with Sandimmun ® had 'idiopathic' nephrotic syndrome (NS). This includes minimal-change nephropathy (MCN) and focal-segmental glomerulosclerosis (FSGS). Less frequently, Sandimmun® was also used to treat patients with NS due to IgM nephropathy, mesangiocapillary glomerulonephritis (GN), membranous GN, IgA nephropathy, and SLE. The empirical treatment of this heterogeneous patient group consists primarily of corticosteroids which are very effective, especially in MCN[70,71]. Usually renal function remains normal in MCN. In FSGS most patients are steroid-resistant[72]. FSGS is ofen associated with hypertension, and the natural outcome is renal failure within 1–15 years of diagnosis. Steroid-resistant patients, and steroid sensitive patients with frequent relapses, and/or who relapse while tapering off of steroids (steroid-dependent) are subgroups in need of alternative therapy. Immunosuppression with alkylating agents is used in such problem patients with relatively good results in children with steroid-dependent NS (MCN)[73]. However, much poorer results are obtained in FSGS[74].

NS occurs both in children and adults. MCN accounts for more than 80% of NS under the age of 10 and for about 20% in adults[75]. In adults, FSGS, membranous GN and mesangio-capillary GN each contribute approximately 20% of cases[76].

In contrast to the well-established role of immune complexes in some forms of GN (e.g. SLE), the mechanisms leading to idiopathic NS are not clear, and the rationale for the use of immunosuppressants, including Sandimmun®, is far from evident. In 1974 Shalhoub postulated that T cell dysfunction was invoked in the pathogenesis of idiopathic NS[77]. Lymphokines have been identified which might lead to alterations in the glomerular anionic sites, resulting in increased permeability for albumin[78]. Eyres et al.[79], using a leukocyte migration test, demonstrated that nephrotic syndrome patients have evidence of T cell sensitization. Lagrue et al.[80] have identified the presence of a lymphokine in the supernatant of lymphocytes taken from patients with the nephrotic syndrome. Plasma from relapsing NS patients was shown to inhibit autologous lymphocyte reaction to mitogens[81], and it has been postulated that a further lymphokine, called soluble immune response suppressor, is responsible for the immunosuppressed state of relapsing NS[82]. Finally, IL-2 was found to be increased in NS patients during relapse[83]. The lymphokine concept would obviously explain the efficacy of Sandimmun®, since Sandimmun® is known to inhibit the synthesis of a series of lymphokines by T cells.

In animal models of GN, Sandimmun® was shown to be effective in NZB/W mice[84], anti-GBM nephritis in rats[85] and mice[86], and immune-mediated interstitial nephritis[87].

Clinical studies with Sandimmun® in idiopathic NS have been performed almost exclusively in either steroid-resistant patients (mostly FSGS) or steroid-dependent patients (mostly MCN). Many of these patients were also resistant to main alkylating agents. In steroid-resistant NS the main aim was to induce remissions, and to study relapse rate after stopping Sandimmun®. In most steroid-dependent patients, remission was induced by the standard steroid regimen, after which Sandimmun® was given with the aim of maintaining remission despite dosage reduction and eventually withdrawal of steroids.

The published data stem mostly from uncontrolled studies[88–110]. A series of randomized controlled studies is still ongoing in idiopathic NS: in steroid-resistant NS vs. placebo or 'no treatment'; and in steroid-dependent NS vs. chlorambucil and cyclophosphamide. No results are yet available from these controlled studies. Interim results have, however, been reported of a randomized study in children (steroid status not reported), comparing high-dose prednisone with Sandimmun® in combination with low-dose prednisone[111]. Finally, a placebo-controlled study in IgA nephropathy has been conducted[112]. The overall results of the published data in 311 patients are summarized in Tables 11.5–11.7 (status June 88).

In steroid-dependent idiopathic NS (Table 11.5) positive outcome was reported in over 80% of patients. In the majority of these patients, steroid-induced remissions could be maintained despite withdrawal of steroids. In one study[88], relapse rates were compared during 6-month periods before, during and after Sandimmun® therapy. In seven patients mean relapse rate per month was reduced from 0.66 before Sandimmun® to 0.12 on Sandimmun® (in four patients no relapses) with relevant reduction of cumulative steroid dosage. After stopping Sandimmun®, relapse rate increased again to 0.45/month. In one group of children, Sandimmun® was used to induce remissions, which was possible in 11/13 (85%) patients within 2–8 weeks[93]. The starting dose of Sandimmun® ranged from 100 to 150 mg/m^2 or 5–17 mg/kg in children, and 3–8 mg/kg in adults. In most studies an attempt was made to adjust doses to maintain trough whole-blood levels between 200 and 500 ng/ml (RIA, polyclonal ABs)[75]. Treatment duration ranged from 3 to 24 months.

Relapses usually occurred within a few weeks of stopping or lowering the dose of Sandimmun®. Steroid-dependency was therefore replaced by Sandimmun®-dependency. In one study[93], however, sustained remissions were seen in 40% of responders. The lowest still effective dose seems to be variable.

In steroid-resistant idiopathic NS, complete remissions were achieved in 27%, and partial remissions in an additional 27% (Table 11.6). In patients with only slight reduction in proteinuria the effect may be related to Sandimmun®-

Table 11.5 Sandimmun®-idiopathic nephrotic syndrome (MCN, IgM-N, MCGN, FSGS), steroid-dependent

	n	'Success'[a]	Failure
Children[b]	66	59 (89%)	7 (11%)
Adults[c]	31	24 (77%)	7 (23%)
All	97	83 (86%)	14 (14%)

[a]Success = Complete remission or maintenance of steroid-induced remission after dose reduction or withdrawal of steroids.
[b]Refs 88, 89, 90, 91, 92, 93
[c]Refs 94, 95, 96, 98, 99, 100, 101
MCN = minimal change nephropathy;
IgM-N = IgM nephropathy;
MCGN = mesangio-capillary glomerulonephritis;
FSGS = focal–segmental glomerulosclerosis

Table 11.6 Sandimmun®-idiopathic nephrotic syndrome (MCN, IgM-N, MCGN, FSGS), steroid-resistant

	n	Complete remission	Partial remission	Failure
Children[a]	44	11 (25%)	6 (14%)	27 (61%)
Adults[b]	109	30 (27%)	36 (33%)	43 (39%)
All	153	41 (27%)	42 (27%)	70 (46%)

[a]Refs 88, 89, 90, 92, 93, 102
[b]Refs 96, 97, 99, 100, 101, 103, 104, 105, 106, 109
MCN   = minimal change nephropathy;
IgMN   = IgM nephropathy;
MCGN = mesangio-capillary glomerulonephritis;
FSGS   = focal–segmental glomerulosclerosis

induced reduction in glomerular filtration rate[106], however, clearly not in patients achieving remissions. Sandimmun® was usually used as a mono-therapy in doses ranging from 5 to 10 mg kg^{-1}day^{-1}. Treatment duration was 2–29 months. If Sandimmun® induced remissions this was usually achieved within the first 3–6 months, i.e. clearly less rapidly than in steroid-dependent NS. After stopping Sandimmun® most patients relapsed within a few weeks, and the best strategy to maintain remissions (Sandimmun® alone? Sandimmun® combined with low-dose steroids?) is unknown. It is also too early to assess if Sandimmun®-induced remissions in FSGS alter the natural history of disease, i.e. if Sandimmun® can prevent progression to renal failure.

Interim results have recently been reported of a randomized study in idiopathic nephrotic syndrome, in which Sandimmun® combined with low-dose prednisone is compared to high-dose prednisone[111]. Treatment duration was limited to 8 weeks. Children were entered with NS of less than 1 year of duration. Steroid status was not reported. Whereas remission rate was slightly higher in the Sandimmun® group (12 of 13 patients vs. seven of 10 patients in the control group), duration of remission appears to be shorter on Sandimmun® (3.8 months vs. 5.2 months on high-dose prednisone).

Table 11.7 summarizes the results in other forms of glomerulonephritis (mostly steroid-resistant). In IgA nephropathy, Sandimmun® was significantly more effective in reducing proteinuria than placebo[112]. In 10 out of the 12 Sandimmun®-treated patients, proteinuria was reduced by more than 50%

Table 11.7 Sandimmun®-nephrotic syndrome, various forms of glomerulonephritis (GN)[a], excluding MCN, IgM-N, MCGN and MCN, mostly steroid-resistant

	n	Complete remission	Partial remission	Failure
Adults[b]	61	10 (16%)	21 (34%)	30 (49%)

[a]Membranous GN, membranoproliferative GN, IgA, SLE, others
[b]Ref. 103, 106, 107, 108, 109, 110, 112
MCN   = minimal change nephropathy;
IgMN   = IgM nephropathy;
MCGN = mesangio-capillary glomerulonephritis;
FSGS   = focal–segmental glomerulosclerosis

within 4 weeks of Sandimmun® treatment. Serum IgA levels fell in nine of 12 patients.

The side-effect profile of Sandimmun® in NS is similar to that in other autoimmune diseases (see section on 'side-effects'). In patients with normal baseline renal function, especially in MCN, renal dysfunction was not more pronounced than in other autoimmune patients, and was fully reversible. However, several patients with FSGS, especially if renal function was abnormal at the start of Sandimmun® therapy, showed marked deterioration of renal function[88,89,92] and in some cases without improvement after stopping Sandimmun®. It is difficult to assess if this was due to Sandimmun® or rather to the natural course of disease[88].

In one patient a Hodgkin lymphoma developed after 22 months of continuous Sandimmun®-therapy (data on file, Sandoz; status June 1988).

Renal biopsies have been performed in 42 patients after 2–18 months of continuous Sandimmun® therapy[88,89,92,96,104,113]. Niaudet[92] reported slight–moderate changes suggestive of Sandimmun® nephrotoxicity in five of 22 biopsies, whereas no relevant changes were reported in the other series. However, in some biopsies progression of FSGS was recorded despite Sandimmun®-therapy[89,92,104].

In summary, experience in over 300 patients indicates that Sandimmun® is very effective in steroid-sensitive patients, and to a clearly lesser extent in steroid-resistant NS. Many questions relating to the optimal use, however, remain open[75]. Despite this, it appears that Sandimmun® can provide benefit for steroid-sensitive patients with steroid toxicity and resistance to conventional therapy, and that a therapeutic trial can be considered in steroid-resistant NS.

PSORIASIS

The cause of psoriasis is unclear. Trauma, infections, drugs, stress, and possibly hormonal factors may trigger the development of psoriasis[114]. Biochemical alterations and immunological phenomena have been described, and genetic factors are also thought to be involved.

It is unclear whether the hyperproliferative epidermis represents a primary defect in keratinocyte growth regulation or whether the increased population of proliferating keratinocytes is due to dermal influences. Similar controversy exists as to whether dermal abnormalities, such as the leukocytic inflammatory cell infiltrates and dilated capillaries, which might promote epidermal hyperplasia, do in fact represent a secondary response to inflammatory factors released from epidermis. More recently, autoimmune reactions have been suggested[115]. The appearance of psoriatic lesions is associated with the influx to the epidermis of antigen-presenting Langerhans cells and T helper cells. It is suggested that the activated T helper cells secrete lymphokines which stimulate proliferation of keratinocytes. These then generate factors which help to attract further T cells from the dermis into the epidermis, and this results in a vicious circle that might be responsible for the persistence and enlargement of the lesions. Spontaneous remission coincides with activation of T suppressor cells which redress the balance[115]. Further possible mechanisms involve γ-IFN and activation of macrophages with secretion of IL-1[116]. IL-1 results in direct proliferation of keratinocytes or indirectly through induction of eicosanoids[117].

Many of these abnormalities are corrected after therapy with Sandimmun® [118]. For a more comprehensive review of mechanisms of psoriasis and Sandimmun® in this disease, see Bos[119]. The clinical effect of Sandimmun® in psoriasis was detected by pure chance. Müller and Herrmann[120] studied Sandimmun® in arthritis and included four patients with psoriatic arthropathy into their trial. The quite dramatic effect of Sandimmun® on the skin lesions has since been confirmed by 10 further investigator groups in 129 published patients[116,121–136] (status June 1988). For design, dosage, treatment duration and main results see Table 11.8.

Eleven uncontrolled and two double-blind, placebo-controlled studies have been conducted in patients with severe, generalized psoriasis. Most patients had longstanding disease and had been treated previously with either PUVA, methotrexate or/and retinoids. With doses of about $5\,\mathrm{mg\,kg^{-1}day^{-1}}$ the majority of reported cases have reached complete or near-complete clearance of lesions within 4 weeks of therapy. A dose of $5\,\mathrm{mg\,kg^{-1}day^{-1}}$ of Sandimmun® was found to be significantly more effective than placebo[131]. According to the PASI (psoriasis area and severity index) scale of grading psoriasis, a mean PASI reduction of 75% by week 4 of treatment with Sandimmun® was observed versus only 3% on placebo[131]. The PASI quantifies the extent of skin surface involved, and the degree of erythema, infiltration and desquamation of psoriatic plaques[137]. Presently in large European multi-centre studies, dosing of $2.5\,\mathrm{mg\,kg^{-1}day^{-1}}$ is being studied. Initial results show PASI reductions of $\geqslant 75\%$ in approximately 50–60% of patients by week 12 of study. These results seem to confirm the data of some of the earlier studies which suggested that doses below $5\,\mathrm{mg\,kg^{-1}day^{-1}}$ are effective[121,125,126]. This is especially attractive, since clearly less renal side-effects have been seen in such low doses. Unfortunately, most patients brought into remission have relapsed within 2–10 weeks after therapy is withdrawn. This indicates the need for continued investigation of maintenance treatments of psoriasis on low doses of Sandimmun®, and possibly combining Sandimmun® with other forms of psoriasis treatment. It has been suggested that the high relapse rate seen in clinical studies with Sandimmun® is due to the fact that most patients studied so far had very severe disease which would relapse quickly on any therapy[138]. After stopping Sandimmun®, psoriatic lesions have returned to baseline severity. With a single exception[139], no exacerbations or transformations to pustular psoriasis have been reported.

The side-effect profile of Sandimmun® in psoriasis is similar to that seen in other non-transplant patients, and is described in more detail in the section on 'side-effects'. A squamous cell carcinoma at the anal margin, which was successfully removed, developed after 6 months of Sandimmun® in a 74-year-old patient with long-standing disease and 10 years of methotrexate therapy[132]. A benign modular cutaneous T lymphocyte infiltrate[140] was reported to develop within 2 weeks of high-dose Sandimmun® therapy; the lesion resolved spontaneously upon withdrawal of Sandimmun®. Finally, a

Table 11.8 Sandimmun® in psoriasis

Main author	Reference	n No. of patients	Dose (mg kg^{-1} day^{-1}) (mean or range)	Duration	Efficacy and comments
(a) In uncontrolled studies					
Mueller	120	4	300–400 (weight not given)	Up to 2 months	Dramatic reduction in psoriatic plaques
Harper	121, 135	5	2–5 (range)	1–3 years	All patients with exception of no. 4 with excellent clinical response. Patient no. 4 suspected non-compliance; two patients with marked improvement of psoriatic arthritis
Van Hoof	122	1	transplant doses	Unknown	Complete clearing within first week
Van Joost	123	5	5 (mean)	4 weeks	Mean PASI ↓84% (PASI = psoriasis area and severity index); grading of psoriasis on scale of 0–72; dependent on skin surface involved, erythema, infiltration and desquamation of psoriatic plaques[137]
Wakeel	124	1	5		Total clearance within 1 week.
Marks	125, 136	12	1–5 (range) Mean dose of responders: 3.3	24 weeks	Seven patients completely cleared (mean time to clearance 7.4 weeks), two patients improved, one patient with widespread pustular psoriasis without response, two patients off study during first 2 weeks with unrelated illness
Griffith	126	10	2.1 (mean)	12 weeks	Five patients completely cleared, five patients appreciable clearing, all by 8 weeks; no relation found between Sandimmun® trough levels and clinical response
Brookes	127	7	1–3 (range)	4 weeks	Six patients with rapid response; one patient found Sandimmun® unacceptable
Wentzell	129	14	5–15 (range)	2.5–8 weeks	Three patients completely clear, nine patients markedly clear; two patients' treatment discontinued due to rapid rise in serum creatinine; T_4 (helper) to T_8 (suppressor) ratios declined

230

Table 11.8 continued

Main author	Reference	n SIM/n total	Dose (mg kg^{-1} day^{-1}) (mean or range)	Duration	Efficacy and comments
(a) continued					
Picascia	130	6	7.5–8.5 initial dose then ↓	1.5–8 weeks	Four patients complete clearing, two patients good clearing
	134				
Fry	132	8	1–4 (range)	30–66 weeks	Mean ↓78% in PASI
Brown	116	11	14	4 weeks	8/11 (73%) marked improvement or cleared at 4 weeks (50–100% improvement)
(b) In double-blind, placebo-controlled, randomized studies					
Ellis	128	11/21	14 (mean)	4 weeks	SIM statistically significantly more effective than placebo Placebo group showed no change or minimal improvement. Placebo group at 4 weeks begun on SIM 6 mm skin biopsy before and after Sandimmun® treatment showed ↓86% mitoses, ↓32% epidermal thickness, mononuclear cells (including activated T-cells) and PMNS markedly reduced. No relation found between Sandimmun® trough levels and clinical response. 17/21 (81%) showed marked improvement or complete clearing on Sandimmun® (50–100% improvement from baseline at week 4)
Van Joost	131	10/20	5.6 (mean)	4 weeks	SIM statistically significantly superior to placebo Placebo group 3% reduction in mean PASI at week 4. 15/18 Sandimmun® treated patients 75% reduction mean PASI at week 4 Placebo group (with exception of two patients) began Sandimmun® week 4

231

mycosis-fungoides-like lesion was detected after 6 weeks of Sandimmun®
treatment, and also resolved completely within 2 months of stopping
Sandimmun® without specific therapy (data on file, Sandoz; status June 1988).
In addition to oral Sandimmun®, topical Sandimmun® is presently being
investigated for the treatment of psoriasis. Published reports have demonstrated disappointing efficacy[141-143], however, intralesional injection of Sandim-
mun® has been shown to be efficacious[144].

In summary, all presently available data indicate that Sandimmun® is
remarkably efficacious in doses of 2.5–5 mg kg^{-1}day^{-1} in patients with severe
generalized psoriasis. Although the drug is full of potential and promise, it
must be used with caution until ongoing studies have assessed the best and
safest way to use this powerful agent.

VARIOUS OTHER AUTOIMMUNE DISEASES

Gastroenterology, hepatology

Results of several pilot studies[145-150] in *Crohn's disease* suggest that oral doses
of Sandimmun® ranging from 5 to 15 mg kg^{-1}day^{-1} are effective in most,
but not all[147] patients with active disease, but a rapid relapse is seen after
stopping therapy. These promising early data have led to the initiation of
placebo-controlled studies for induction of remission in therapy-resistant
patients with chronic active disease. In one such study 5 mg kg^{-1}day^{-1} SIM
was significantly superior to placebo (Brynskov, J., personal communication).
A multi-centre, placebo-controlled study has recently started for prophylaxis
of relapses on long-term therapy.

Positive results have been published in a small number of patients with
ulcerative colitis[151,152]. Two case histories of *autoimmune chronic hepatitis* with
relevant improvements have been reported[153,154].

Considerably more clinical research is ongoing in *primary biliary cirrhosis.*
As early as 1980, Routhier *et al.*[155] reported on the effects of 5–10 mg kg^{-1}
day^{-1} in six patients. Liver function improved, but substantial toxicity
occurred. Results in several other series of patients have confirmed that
liver enzymes improve on a lower dose of Sandimmun® alone (3–
5 mg kg^{-1}day^{-1})[156-159], or with Sandimmun® in combination with low-dose
prednisone[157]. Large placebo-controlled long-term studies are ongoing with
the aim of evaluating if disease progression can be influenced[159,160]. The results
of the European placebo-controlled, double-blind study[160] in over 300 patients
treated for several years, will be available in 1989.

Neurology

Two double-blind, randomized studies have been completed in *multiple
sclerosis.* In the first, Sandimmun® was compared to placebo in 81 patients
treated for 2 years[161]. Dose of Sandimmun® was 10 mg kg^{-1}day^{-1} during
the first 2 months, then 8 mg kg^{-1}day^{-1}. There was only a slight trend
(not significant) for retardation of progression of neurological deficit and for

a longer time till first relapse in Sandimmun®-treated patients.

The German two-centre study[162] compared Sandimmun® (5 mg kg^{-1} day^{-1}) with azathioprine in 194 patients treated for 2 years. No significant differences could be detected between the two treatment groups on clinical parameters. The incidence of side-effects was more frequent on Sandimmun® than on azathioprine.

A further placebo-controlled study in chronic-progressive MS is still ongoing in the USA.

The results in *myasthenia gravis* (MG) are more encouraging. Several pilot studies[163-165] have been performed with 5–10 mg kg^{-1} day^{-1} of Sandimmun® in severe, generalized MG. Most patients entered into these studies were either resistant to corticosteroids or had experienced relevant toxicity, and usually already had received azathioprine without success. Relevant improvement in muscle strength occurred in 75% of patients. The onset of effect was quite variable (1–3 months) with a maximum after about 3–6 months. When Sandimmun® was used in combination with prednisone, the dose of prednisone could be reduced substantially. On long-term therapy (up to 37 months) the favourable effect could be maintained[164]. After stopping Sandimmun®, however, patients usually relapsed within a few weeks[164]. A placebo-controlled study in patients with progressively worsening generalized MG, who had not yet been treated with thymectomy, steroids or other immunosuppressants, showed that patients on Sandimmun® (6 mg kg^{-1} day^{-1}) had significantly greater improvement in strength after 6 months of therapy, than patients on placebo[166]. More studies are needed and ongoing to define more clearly the potential of Sandimmun® in MG, and to define its place in relation to corticosteroids and azathioprine. It is of interest that in most responders the titres of anti-acetylcholine receptor antibodies did not fall, and that if they eventually did, the clinical benefit preceded this by far. This suggests that cellularly mediated effector mechanisms may operate in MG[166].

Haematology

Several patient series have been published using Sandimmun® in *severe aplastic anaemia*[167-183]. Most patients either had no suitable donor or had contraindications to bone-marrow transplantation. Virtually all were failures to corticosteroids, and about 25% of the patients had not responded to either anti-lymphocyte globulin (ALG) or anti-thymocyte globulin (ATG). Usually Sandimmun® monotherapy was used, but in some studies Sandimmun® was combined with prednisone[171] and/or ALG[182,183] or ATG[175]. Doses of Sandimmun® ranged between 5 and 20 mg kg^{-1} day^{-1}, and treatment duration was also very variable. Complete or partial remissions were achieved in 53/109 patients (49%). Thus, response rate on Sandimmun® seems to be similar to that reported with ATG[184]. It is interesting that some non-responders to ALG or ATG went into remission on Sandimmun®[167,170,177,180,181]. Leonard et al.[177] reported this to have happened in five of 15 patients. On the other hand, of four non-responders to Sandimmun®, ATG was effective in three[177], and Jacobs et al.[182] reported no effect in 12 patients randomized to either Sandimmun® alone or Sandimmun® plus ALG. A further randomized study is comparing the combination of Sandimmun® and ALG to ALG alone[183]. After 3 months, 7/15 (47%) responded to ALG, and 15/20 (75%) to Sandimmun® plus ALG. A randomized study comparing monotherapy of Sandimmun® vs. ALG is ongoing in France and Belgium. No results have yet been reported. These need to be awaited before one can estimate the comparative efficacy of Sandimmun® vs. ALG or ATG.

Usually, platelet and reticulocyte responses occurred rapidly, mostly within the first 2–4 weeks. Full efficacy was mostly obtained within the first 3 months. Relapses occurred frequently within 3 months of stopping Sandimmun®.

Remissions have been reported in 13 of 21 (62%) patients treated with Sandimmun® for *pure red cell aplasia*, either congenital (Blackfan–Diamond syndrome)[177,185,186], idiopathic[186,189,190,191], or in patients with chronic lymphatic leukaemia[187,188,190]. Finally, case reports have been published describing positive results in patients with *idiopathic thrombocytopenia*[192–195], *amegakaryocytic, thrombocytopenic purpura*[196,197], *Felty's syndrome*[198], *cyclic neutropenia*[199] and two cases of *acquired haemophilia* (factor VIII inhibitor)[200,201], whereas a further patient with this disease did not respond[202].

Systemic lupus erythematosus (SLE)

As early as 1981, Isenberg et al.[203] reported improvement of arthralgia in two of five patients treated with $10 \, \text{mg} \, \text{kg}^{-1} \text{day}^{-1}$ Sandimmun®. Substantial toxicity occurred with this dose which, retrospectively judged, was too high. Feutren et al.[204] treated 13 patients with severe steroid-resistant or steroid-dependent SLE with $5 \, \text{mg} \, \text{kg}^{-1} \text{day}^{-1}$ Sandimmun® for 12 months. The main effect was the possibility of substantially reducing the steroid dosage needed to control disease. No relevant changes were found in antibody titres. Hypertension and reversible renal dysfunction were the most serious side-effects[204,205].

The largest experience with Sandimmun® in SLE has been gained by Miescher et al.[206,207] with 41 patients reported. Sandimmun® was prescribed initially at the dose of $5 \, \text{mg} \, \text{kg}^{-1} \text{day}^{-1}$ and was combined with fluocortolone. Standard activity score decreased in most patients[207]. This effect was maintained over a period up to 24 months of therapy despite significant reduction in steroid dosage. The effect on proteinuria was striking. Renal biopsies in 26 patients after 12–18 months of Sandimmun® therapy did not show signs of Sandimmun® nephrotoxicity.

The presently available experience with Sandimmun® in SLE is still quite limited. However, it seems that steroid-sparing is an important benefit of Sandimmun® therapy in this disease.

Varia

In addition to psoriasis (see above), pilot studies have been conducted in further dermatological autoimmune diseases, mostly with positive results:

atopic dermatitis[208], dermatomyositis[209,210], scleroderma[211,212], bullous pemphigoid[213,214], pemphigus[213] and pyoderma gangrenosum[215].

In Sjögren's disease 5 mg kg^{-1} day^{-1} Sandimmun® did not exert relevant clinical effects in a placebo-controlled study[216]. No change was seen in Schirmer's test or stimulated parotid flow rate. Histopathological lesions remained unchanged in patients treated with Sandimmun®, while in the placebo-treated group the lesions worsened slightly.

Several investigators have studied Sandimmun® in severe, mostly therapy-resistant cases of *Graves' ophthalmopathy*. The published results are quite varied, with some reporting excellent subjective and objective improvements[217-219], and some without apparent effect[220,221]. Randomized studies comparing Sandimmun® with prednisone are ongoing.

Case reports have been published in *Wegener's granulomatosis*[222], *pulmonary sarcoidosis*[223], *male autoimmune infertility*[224], *relapsing polychondritis*[225], *giant cell arteritis*[226], *myocarditis*[227] and *Hodgkin's disease*[228].

SIDE-EFFECTS

The side-effect profile of Sandimmun® in autoimmune diseases is similar to the one extensively reported in transplant patients[229] (Tables 11.9 and 11.10).

Table 11.9 Sandimmun® in autoimmune diseases–frequent adverse events

Renal dysfunction with increase in serum creatinine, urea, potassium, uric acid and decrease in serum magnesium. All these changes occur often within normal range
Gastrointestinal symptoms (nausea, loss of appetite, vomiting)
Tremor, paraesthesia, headache
Hypertrichosis
Gingiva hyperplasia
Hypertension
Anaemia, normochrom (reduction of HB by about 1 g/dl)
Transient increases in bilirubin and liver enzymes

Table 11.10 Sandimmun® in autoimmune diseases – serious adverse events, status June 1988

Hemolytic-uraemic syndrome (3)
Myocardial infarction (5)
Epileptic seizures (5)
Thrombocytopenia (3)
Septicemia (3)
Viral meningitis (3)
Pulmonary abcess (1)
B-cell lymphoma (2)
T-cell lymphoma (1)
Hodgkin lymphoma (1)
Mycosis fungoides (1)

Figures in parentheses show no. of patients with side-effect out of approximately 5000 exposed

The frequency with which the common side-effects listed in Table 11.9 have been reported is very variable between different studies. In 634 patients of various clinical trials in insulin-dependent diabetes, multiple sclerosis and uveitis, paraesthesia was reported in 48%, hypertrichosis in 46%, gastrointestinal complaints in 39%, gingiva hyperplasia in 35%, headache in 24% and tremor in 13% (data on file, Sandoz). In most patients the intensity of these side-effects was only slight or moderate. Of 938 patients included in various studies the withdrawal rates because of side-effects were 4% in diabetes, 6% in multiple sclerosis, 12% in uveitis and 22% in rheumatoid arthritis. By far the most frequent reasons for withdrawal were gastrointestinal symptoms. Renal side-effects were the reason for drug withdrawal in only 27/938 patients (3%).

In 11% of 321 treated patients, mild to moderate hypertension developed within the first 6 months of Sandimmun® therapy[230]. If therapy was required, conventional treatment of various kinds was successful. There was a significant association between the extent of renal dysfunction and hypertension[230].

The cause of the frequently observed hypertrichosis is unknown; there is no clinical or laboratory evidence for an endocrine origin[231]. Gingival hyperplasia is due to fibrous hyperplasia[232]. It has been suggested that Sandimmun®-induced hypomagnesaemia, a quite frequent finding[233], is responsible for some of the neurological side-effects[234]. Tremor and paraesthesia (often expressed as feeling of heat) are frequent during the first weeks of treatment, and very often disappear thereafter without change of dose. The same is true for slight increases in serum bilirubin and liver enzymes. Only rarely did this side-effect require discontinuation of treatment. A mild normochromic, normocytic anaemia with a reduction in haemoglobin of about 1 g/dl has been observed in several studies[59,61]. This effect may be due to the inhibition of lymphokines regulating erythropoiesis.

Infectious complications have been surprisingly infrequent and followed an unremarkable course. In long-term controlled studies in diabetes and multiple sclerosis the frequency of urinary, skin and respiratory tract infections was not significantly higher in Sandimmun®-treated patients than in those on placebo[59,61] or azathioprine[162].

By June 1988, five out of about 5000 patients treated for autoimmune diseases have developed lymphomas (data on file, Sandoz). B-cell lymphomas occurred after 2½ years of Sandimmun® therapy in a 69-year-old female with pure red cell anaemia, and in a 36-year-old male with polychondritis after 8 months of therapy. A T cell lymphoma was detected in a 50-year-old male after 5 months of Sandimmun® treatment for aplastic anaemia. The patient had been previously treated with cytotoxic agents for thymoma. At least in this case a causal relation with Sandimmun® is unlikely, since aplastic anaemia is known to be an early symptom of lymphomas, and the T cell type is unusual for lymphomas occurring on immunosuppression[235]. Hodgkin's disease was detected after 22 months of Sandimmun® treatment in a 23-year-old male with idiopathic nephrotic syndrome. Associations of this kind have been reported in patients not treated with Sandimmun®[236]. Finally, mycosis fungoides-like lesions were detected in a 59-year-old male patient with psoriasis after 6 weeks of therapy. The lesion regressed spontaneously within

2 months after stopping SIM. Recently, a benign nodular cutaneous T lymphocyte infiltrate has been described in a patient treated for 2 weeks with high-dose Sandimmun® (14 mg kg⁻¹ day⁻¹) for psoriasis with rapid regression after stopping therapy[140]. The Sandoz Postmarketing Surveillance Study in over 4000 prospectively followed transplant patients has shown that the incidence of lymphomas developing on Sandimmun® is the same as that in patients treated with other forms of immunosuppression[237].

The renal side-effects are those which limit most the therapeutic potential of Sandimmun®. It is useful to distinguish between functional and structural changes. Renal dysfunction is characterized by a reduction in glomerular filtration rate and disturbances of tubular function[233]. The main laboratory abnormalities are increases in serum creatinine, urea, potassium and uric acid, and decreases in serum levels of magnesium. Often, however, the changes remain within the normal range.

Renal dysfunction has been analysed in large numbers of autoimmune patients[230,238]. Within the first 2 weeks after starting Sandimmun® therapy renal function starts to drop and reaches a nadir around month 6. At this time the mean decrease of calculated creatinine clearance was 17% from baseline. There was no significant further decline, indicating that functional impairment is not progressive up to 2 years of continuous therapy[230]. At all time points, mean values of serum creatinine remained within the normal range. Nevertheless, 19% of patients had creatinine values above 130 μmol/l at month 6.

Impairment of renal function is dependent on dose and blood levels[230,238,239]. Multivariate analyses have confirmed these factors as the most important ones determining the extent of renal dysfunction[230]. Further enhancing factors are high patient age[240] and concomitant medication with nephrotoxic compounds, including non-steroidal anti-inflammatory drugs[241]. Renal dysfunction is reversible. It is the general experience that serum creatinine drops within 1–2 weeks after dose reduction or termination of therapy. In 139 patients with various autoimmune diseases, serum creatinine was within 5% of baseline values, 8 weeks after stopping Sandimmun®[230]. In most patients complete recovery is attained within 12 weeks[238], but in a minority, baseline values are not reached completely[31,33,230,238]. The more pronounced renal dysfunction was, the less probable was a complete return to baseline values. This clearly indicates that one should attempt to avoid large creatinine increases. This can be achieved with initial doses of not more than 5 mg kg⁻¹ day⁻¹, and reduction of dose by 25–50% if serum creatinine increases by more than 30% over baseline, even if still within the normal range. More relevant than acute and reversible functional changes are histological lesions which have been found in renal biopsies of Sandimmun®-treated autoimmune patients. Chronic Sandimmun®-associated nephropathy has been described as a combination of arteriolopathy, interstitial fibrosis (striped form) and tubular atrophy[242]. Results of over 200 renal biopsies are available in insulin-dependent diabetes mellitus[67,68], SLE and rheumatoid arthritis[26,113,243], uveitis[54,244], nephrotic syndrome[88,89,92,96,113] and various other diseases[113,245]. More than 'minimal' or 'slight' lesions (which cannot be attributed with certainty to Sandimmun®) were found in 47/210 (22%)

patients with reported frequencies ranging from 0 to 100% (Table 11.11). The reason for this large variation is most likely due to the quite different treatment schedules used. When analysing the entire data it appears that the risk of developing structural renal changes is low if Sandimmun® is used in such a way as to avoid pronounced functional impairment, i.e. to avoid increases of serum creatinine above 50% over baseline. In uveitis patients a significant correlation was found between severity of the lesions and the duration during which serum creatinine was increased by more than 50% over baseline[54]. Mihatsch et al.[113] showed that only those patients developed nephropathy who were treated with initial doses of 7.5 mg kg^{-1}day^{-1} or more, leading to substantial creatinine increases. Feutren[68] has analysed the data of 90 biopsied diabetic patients. In the group of patients with moderate lesions, maximal creatinine increase was 95% ± 10 (mean ± SEM), whereas it was 45% ± 4 in the group with normal histology (p < 0.01). In patients in whom the maximal creatinine on Sandimmun® was more than double the baseline value, lesions were found in 8/19 (42%), whereas this was the case in only 2/38 (5%) patients in whom creatinine never increased by more than 50%. This is confirmed by the series of 43 patients with SLE and RA reported by Miescher et al.[26,243] treated with low doses (3–5 mg kg^{-1}day^{-1}) and only very discrete increases of creatinine, and in whom no Sandimmun®-induced renal lesions were found. From all these data it appears that Sandimmun® can be administered in such a way as to minimize the risk of irreversible functional or structural renal damage. Initial doses of Sandimmun® should not exceed 5 mg kg^{-1}day^{-1} (except in life-threatening emergency situations). Dose should be reduced whenever serum creatinine increases by more than 30% over baseline. If such 'conservative' dosages do not lead to an optimal therapeutic result, it might be better to consider combining Sandimmun® with other immunosuppressive agents, e.g. steroids, rather than increasing the dose.

CONCLUSIONS

This review demonstrates that Sandimmun® is efficacious in many autoimmune diseases, for induction as well as maintenance of remission. Efficacy has been established in randomized controlled studies in rheumatoid arthritis, uveitis, psoriasis, insulin-dependent diabetes mellitus, Crohn's disease and myasthenia gravis. Convincing evidence of efficacy was demonstrated in uncontrolled trials in nephrotic syndrome, SLE, and various haematological and dermatological autoimmune diseases, whereas no relevant effect was seen in the so-far-completed studies in multiple sclerosis.

Common features of the clinical effects of Sandimmun® are the relatively quick onset of effect (2–12 weeks, dependent on dose), and also that relapses occurred when treatment was stopped. These facts are presumably linked to the rapid onset and reversibility of the inhibitory effect of Sandimmun® on lymphokine secretion. The autoimmune reaction is temporarily 'frozen' without abrogation of the intrinsic autoimmune defect[246].

Although it is obvious that more studies are needed to define the true

239

Table 11.11 Sandimmun® – associated structural renal changes

Main author	Reference	Diagnosis	Patient no.	Patients with moderate lesions	Mean Sandimmun® dose $(mg\ kg^{-1}\ day^{-1})$		Duration of therapy (months)	Risk factors (details see text)
					Initial	Later		
Palestine	54	Uveitis	17	17 (100%)	10	10	11–37	Creatinine > 50%
Nahman	245	Various	2	2 (100%)	7.5, 10		4; 7	High dose
Mihatsch	113[a]	Various	19	5 (26%)	6.9	6.3	6–27	High dose
Feutren	68[b]	Diabetes	90	17 (19%)	9.1	6.0	8–30	Creatinine↑
Miescher	26,243	SLE, RA[c]	43	0	5	3.3	17–24	
Niaudet	92	NS[d]	22	5 (23%)	6		2–16	
Brodehl	88	NS	4	0	3–6			
Brandis	89	NS	8	1 (12%)	5–10			
Clasen	96	NS	5	0				
			210	47 (22%)				

[a]Includes also patients of ref. 244
[b]Includes also patients of ref. 67
[c]RA = rheumatoid arthritis
[d]NS = nephrotic syndrome

benefit of Sandimmun® in autoimmune diseases, and to position the drug among conventional therapies, it appears already that many patients who do not respond satisfactorily to conventional therapy, either in terms of efficacy or toxicity, may profit from Sandimmun®. The steroid-sparing properties of Sandimmun® are possibly one of its major contributions to the treatment of autoimmune diseases. In therapy-resistant, end-stage patients who present with substantial pathology which is irreversible, full potential cannot be obtained. Thus the use of the drug may eventually be extended to less advanced disease stages where risk/benefit of Sandimmun® requires careful, individual consideration and must be balanced against risk of the disease itself and the risk of alternative therapy. The future may lie in combinations of Sandimmun® with other immunosuppressants thereby profiting from synergistic mechanisms of action and reduced toxicity with application of lower doses.

One of the most important issues is safety on long-term treatment. As described in the section on 'side-effects', relevant renal side-effects and probably also complications of over-immunosuppression (infections, malignancies) seem to be avoidable if the following treatment guidelines are adhered to: initial dosage should not exceed $5\,mg\,kg^{-1}day^{-1}$; in situations where rapid onset of effect is not critical, one may consider initiating treatment with $2.5\,mg\,kg^{-1}day^{-1}$, with the option of increasing dose if after about 1 month no effect is apparent, and no relevant toxicity has developed. Sandimmun® should be reduced by 25–50% whenever serum creatinine has increased by more than 30% over baseline, even if this remains within the normal range. Dosage of Sandimmun® should also be reduced if trough (= pre-dose) whole-blood Sandimmun® levels are consistently above 500 ng/ml (RIA, polyconal Abs) or above 200 ng/ml (RIA, specific monoclonal or HPLC). Patients with hypertension and those with pre-existing renal disease must be regarded as high-risk patients. If long-term therapy is indicated for maintenance of remission or prevention of chronic progression of disease, the lowest effective dose should be determined individually where parameters of disease activity are available. If this is not the case, the highest dose that does not induce relevant increases in creatinine or other side-effects should be sought.

REFERENCES

1. Hess, A. D. and Colombani, P. M. (1986) Mechanism of action of ciclosporin: *in vitro* studies. In Borel, J. F. (ed.) *Ciclosporin.* Prog. Allergy, 38 (Basel: Karger), pp. 198–221.
2. Wenger, R. M., Payne, T. G. and Schreier, M. H. (1986) Cyclosporine: chemistry, structure–activity relationships and mode of action. *Prog. Clin. Biochem. Med.* **3**, 176–191.
3. Greene, W. O. (1986). Cytokines: interleukin 2 and its receptor. In Gallin, J. I. *et al.* (eds) *Inflammation: Basic Principles and Clinical Correlates* (New York: Raven Press)
4. Halloran, P. F., Wadgymar, A. and Autenried, P. (1986) Inhibition of MHC product induction may contribute to the immunosuppressive action of ciclosporin. In Borel, J. F. (ed.), *Ciclosporin.* Prog. Allergy, 38 (Basel: Karger), pp. 258–268.
5. Borel, J. F. and Ryffel, B. (1986) The mechanism of action of ciclosporin: a continuing puzzle. In Schindler, R. (ed.) *Ciclosporin in Autoimmune Diseases* (Berlin: Springer), pp. 24–32.
6. Kronke, M., Leonard, W. J., Depper, J. M., Arya, S., Worg-Staal, F., Gallo, R. O., Waldmann, T. A. and Greene, W. O. (1984) Cyclosporin A inhibits T-cell growth factor

gene expression at the level of mRNA transcription. *Proc. Natl. Acad. Sci. USA*, **81**, 5214–5218.

7. Elliot, J. F., Lin, Y., Mizel, S. B., Bleackley, R. C., Harnisch, D. G. and Paetkan, V. (1984) Induction of Interleukin 2 messenger RNA inhibited by cyclosporin A. *Science*, **226**, 1439–1441.

8. Borel, J. F. and Gunn, H. (1986) Cyclosporine as a new approach to therapy. *Ann. NY Acad. Aci.*, **475**, 307–319.

9. NIH Conference (1984) Rheumatoid arthritis: evolving concepts of pathogenesis and treatment. *Ann. Intern. Med.*, **101**, 810–824.

10. Burmeister, G. R., Locher, P., Koch, B., Winchester, R. J., Dimitriu-Bona, A., Kalden, J. R. and Mohr, W. (1983) The tissue architecture of synovial membranes in inflammatory and non-inflammatory joint diseases. The localization of the major synovial populations as detected by monoclonal reagents directed towards Ia and monocyte/macrophage antigens. *Rheumatol. Int.*, **3**, 173–181.

11. Morrow, J. and Isenberg, D. (1987) *Autoimmune Rheumatic Disease: Rheumatoid Arthritis* (Oxford: Blackwell), pp. 148–207.

12. Harris, E. D. (1988) Pathogenesis of rheumatoid arthritis: A disorder associated with dysfunctional immunoregulation. In Gallin, J. I. *et al.* (eds.), *Inflammation: Basic Principles and Clinical Correlates* (New York: Raven Press).

13. Borel, J. F., Feurer, C., Gubler, H. U. and Stähelin, H. (1976) Biological effects of cyclosporin A: a new antilymphocyte agent. *Agents Actions*, **6**, 468–475.

14. Henderson, B., Staines, N. A., Burrai, I. and Cox, J. H. (1984) The anti-arthritic and immunosuppressive effects of cyclosporin on arthritis induced in the rat by type II collagen. *Clin. Exp. Immunol.*, **57**, 51–56.

15. Yocum, D., Allen, J. B. and Wahl, S. B. (1985) Inhibition by cyclosporin A of group A streptococcal cell wall-induced arthritis and hepatic granulomas in rats. *Arthritis Rheum.*, **28** (Suppl. 4), abstr. D40, p. S82.

16. Borel, J. F., Gubler, H. U., Hiestand, P. C. and Wenger, R. M. (1986) Immunological properties of cyclosporin (Sandimmun®) and (Val²) dihydro-cyclosporin and their prospect in chronic inflammation. *Adv. Inflam. Res.*, **11**, 277–291.

17. Herrmann, B. and Müller, W. (1979) Die Therapie der chronischen Polyarthritis mit Cyclosporin A, einem neuen Immunosuppressivum. *Akt. Rheumatol.*, **4**, 173–186.

18. Yocum, D., Wilder, R., Wahl, S., Gerber, L., Austin, H., Minor, J., Lesko, L., Dougherty, S., Yarboro, C., Berkebile, C. and Klippel, J. (1987) A double blind randomized trial of high dose and low dose cyclosporin A in rheumatoid arthritis. *Arthritis Rheum.*, **30**(4) (Suppl.), S58.

19. Bowles, C., Gabriel, S., Bunch, T. and Handwerger, B. S. (1987) Cyclosporin treatment for rheumatoid arthritis. *Arthritis Rheum.*, **30**(4) (Suppl.), S58.

20. Dougados, M. and Amor, B. (1985) Cyclosporin in rheumatoid arthritis. *Arthritis Rheum.*, **28** (Suppl. 4), S36 (abstract)

21. Weinblatt, M., Coblyn, J. S., Fraser, P. A., Anderson, R. J., Spragg, J., Trentham, D. E. and Austen, K. F. (1987) Cyclosporin A treatment of refractory rheumatoid arthritis. *Arthritis Rheum.*, **30**, 11–17.

22. Dougados, M. and Amor, B. (1987) Cyclosporine A in rheumatoid arthritis: preliminary results of an open trial. *Arthritis Rheum.*, **30**, 83–87.

23. Tugwell, P., Bombardier, C., Gent, M., Bennett, K., Ludwin, D., Grace, E., Buchanan, W. W., Bensen, W. G., Bellamy, N., Murphy, G. F. and von Graffenried, B. (1987) Low dose cyclosporon in rheumatoid arthritis: a pilot study. *J. Rheumatol.*, **14**, 1108–1114.

24. Weinblatt, M., Coblyn, J. S., Fraser, P. A., Spragg, J. and Austen, K. F. (1987) Cyclosporin A in refractory rheumatoid arthritis: extended observations at 3 mg/kg/day. *Arthritis Rheum.*, **30**(4) (Suppl.), S58.

25. Madhok, R. and Capell, H. (1988) Cyclosporin in rheumatoid arthritis: results at 30 months. *Transplant. Proc.*, **XX**(3) (Suppl. 4), 248–252.

26. Miescher, P. A., Favre, H., Mihatsch, M. J., Chatelenat, F., Huang, Y. P. and Zubler, R. (1988). The place of cyclosporin A in the treatment of connective tissue diseases. *Transplant. Proc.*, **XX**(3) (Suppl. 4), 224–237.

27. Yoshinoya, S., Yamamoto, K., Mitamura, T., Aikawa, T., Takeuchi, A., Takahashi, K. and Miyamoto, T. (1988) Successful treatment of rheumatoid arthritis with low-dose cyclosporin A. *Transplant. Proc.*, **XX**(3) (Suppl. 4), 243–247.

28. Forre, O., Bjerkjoel, F., Salversen, G. F., Berg, K. J., Rugstad, H. E., Saelid, G., Mellbye, O. J. and Käss, E. (1987) An open, controlled, randomized comparison of cyclosporine and azathioprine in the treatment of rheumatoid arthritis: a preliminary report. *Arthritis Rheum.*, **30**, 88–92.
29. Van Rijthoven, A. W. A. M., Dijkmans, B. A. C., GoeiThe, H. S., Hermans, J., Montnor-Beckers, Z. L. M. B., Jacobs, P. C. J. and Cats, A. (1986) Cyclosporin treatment for rheumatoid arthritis: a placebo controlled, double blind, multicentre study. *Ann. Rheum. Dis.*, **45**, 726–731.
30. Dougados, M., Awada, H. and Amor, B. (1988) Cyclosporin in rheumatoid arthritis: a double blind controlled study in 52 patients. *Ann. Rheum. Dis.*, **47**, 127–133.
31. Boers, M., van Rijthoven, A. W. A. M., GoeiThe, H. S., Dijkmans, B. A. C. and Cats, A. (1988) Serum creatinine levels two years later: follow-up of a placebo-controlled trial of cyclosporin in rheumatoid patients. *Transplant. Proc.*, **XX**(3) (Suppl. 4), 371–375.
32. Berg, K., Forre, O., Bjerkhoel, F., Amundsen, E., Djoseland, O., Rugstad, H. E. and Westre, B. (1986) Side effects of cyclosporin A treatment in patients with rheumatoid arthritis. *Kidney Int.*, **29**, 1180–1187.
33. Dijkmans, B. A. C., van Rijthoven, A. W. A. M., GoeiThe, H. S., Montnor-Beckers, Z. L. B. M., Jacobs, P. C. J. and Cats, A. (1987). Effect of cyclosporin on serum creatinine in patients with rheumatoid arthritis. *Eur. J. Clin. Pharmacol.*, **31**, 541–545.
34. BenEzra, D. (1980). Diseases of the choroid and anterior uvea. In Michaelson, I. C. (ed.), *Michaelson's Textbook of the Fundus of the Eye*, 3rd Edn. (Edinburgh: Churchill Livingstone).
35. Nussenblatt, R. B., Kuwabara, T., deMonasterio, F. M. and Wacker, W. B. (1981) Retinal S-antigen uveitis in primates. A new model for human disease. *Arch. Ophthalmol.*, **99**, 1090.
36. Chan, C. C., BenEzra, D., Rodrigues, M. M., Palestine, A. G., Hsu, S. M. and Nussenblatt, R. B. (1985) Immunohistochemistry and electron microscopy of choroidal infiltrates and Dalen–Fuchs nodules in sympathetic ophthalmia. *Ophthalmology*, **92**, 580.
37. Chan, C. C., Mochizuki, M., Nussenblatt, R. B., Palestine, A. G., McAllister, C., Gery, I. and BenEzra, D. (1985) T-lymphocyte subsets in experimental autoimmune uveitis. *Clin. Immunol. Immunopathol.*, **35**, 103.
38. Salinas-Carmona, M. C., Nussenblatt, R. B. and Gery, I. (1982) Experimental autoimmune uveitis in the Athymic nude rat. *Eur. J. Immunol.*, **12**, 480
39. BenEzra, D. and Pe'er, J. (1986) Interleukins in Behçet's disease. In: D'Ermo (ed.), *Proceedings of the XXV International Congress of Ophthalmology, Rome*, p. 68.
40. Mochizuki, M., Nussenblatt, R. B., Kuwabara, T. and Gery, I. (1983) Effects of cyclosporin on the efferent limb of the immune response. *Transplant Proc.*, **15**, 2364.
41. Nussenblatt, R. B., Salinas-Carmona, M. C., Gery, I., Cevario, S. and Wacker, W. B. (1982) Modulation of experimental autoimmune uveitis with cyclosporin A. *Arch. Ophthalmol.*, **100**, 1146.
42. BenEzra, D. (1986) Cyclosporin A in Behçet's disease – an overview. In Lehner, T. and Barnes, C. G. (eds.), *Recent Advances in Behçet's Disease*. (London: Royal Soc. of Med. Serv.), pp. 319–325.
43. Nussenblatt, R. B., Rook, A. H., Wacker, W. B., Palestine, A. G., Scher, I. and Gery, I. (1983) Treatment of intraocular inflammatory disease with cyclosporin A, *Lancet*, **2**, 235.
44. Nussenblatt, R. B., Palestine, A. G. and Chan, C. C. (1983) Cyclosporin A therapy in the treatment of intraocular inflammatory disease resistant to systemic corticosteroids and cytotoxic agents. *Am. J. Ophthalmol*, **96**, 275.
45. Nussenblatt, R. B., Palestine, A. G., Chan, C. C., Mochizuki, M. and Yancey, K. (1985) Effeciveness of cyclosporin therapy for Behçet's disease. *Arthritis Rheum.*, **28**, 671.
46. Nussenblatt, R. B. (1988). The use of cyclosporin in ocular inflammatory disorder. *Transplant. Proc.*, **XX**(3) (Suppl. 4), 114–121.
47. BenEzra, D., Cohen, E., Rakotomalala, M., de Courten, C., Harris, W., Chajek, T., Friedman, G. and Matamoros, N. (1988) Treatment of endogenous uveitis with cyclosporin A. *Transplant. Proc.*, **XX**(3) (Suppl. 4), 122–127.
48. Le Hoant, P., Girard, B., Deray, G., Le Minh, H., de Kozak, Y., Thillaye, B., Faure, J. P. and Rousselie, F. (1988) Cyclosporine in the treatment of birdshot retinochoroidopathy. *Transplant. Proc.*, **XX**(3) (Suppl. 4), 128–130'
49. Graham, E., Sanders, M. D., James, D. G., Hamblin, A., Grochowska, E. K. and Dumonde, D. (1985) Cyclosporin A in the treatment of posterior uveitis. *Trans. Ophthalmol. Soc.*

UK, **104,** 146.

50. BenEzra, D., Brodsky, M., Pe'er, J., Chajek, T., Pizanti, S., Vertman, E. and Sachs, U. (1985) Cyclosporin A(CyA) versus conventional therapy in Behçet's disease. Preliminary observations of a masked study. In Schindler, R. (ed.) *Cyclosporin in Autoimmune Diseases* (Berlin: Springer), pp. 158–161.

51. Masuda, K and Nakajiama, A. (1985) A double masked study of cyclosporin treatment in Behçet's disease. In Schindler, R. (ed.), *Cyclosporin in Autoimmune Diseases* (Berlin: Springer), pp. 162–164.

52. De Vries, J., Baarsma, G. S., Zaal, M. J. W., Boen-Tan, T. N., Rothova, A., Buitenhuis, H. J., Schweitzer, C. M. C., De Kaizer, R. J. W. and Kijlstra, A. (1987) Cyclosporine in the treatment of idiopathic posterior uveitis. *Second International Congress on Cyclosporine, Washington* (Abstract), p. 55.

53. BenEzra, D., Nussemblatt, R. B. and Timonen, P. (1988). *Optimal use of Sandimmun in endogenous uveitis* (Berlin: Springer).

54. Palestine, A. G., Austin, H. A., Balow, J. E., Antonovych, T. T., Sabnis, S. G., Preuss, H. G. and Nussenblatt, R. B. (1986) Renal histopathologic alterations in patients treated with cyclosporin for uveitis. *N. Engl. J. Med.,* **314,** 1293–1298.

55. Eisenbarth, G. S. (1986) Type 1 diabetes mellitus. A chronic autoimmune disease. *N. Engl. J. Med.,* **314,** 1360–1368.

56. Laupacis, A., Stiller, C. R., Gardell, C., Keown, P., Dupré, J., Wallace, A. C. and Thibert, P. (1983) Cyclosporin prevents diabetes in BB Wistar rats. *Lancet,* **1,** 10–12.

57. Mori, Y., Suko, M. and Okudaira, H. (1986) Preventive effect of cyclosporin in diabetes in NOD mice. *Diabetologia,* **29,** 244–247.

58. DCCT Research Group (1987) Are continuing studies of metabolic control and microvascular complications in insulin-dependent diabetes mellitus justified? *N. Engl. J. Med.,* **318,** 246–250.

59. Feutren, G., Papoz, L., Assan, R., Vialettes, B., Karsenty, G., Vexiau, P., Du Rostu, H., Rodier, M., Sirmai, J., Lallemand, A. and Bach, J. F. (1986). Cyclosporin increases the rate and length of remissions in insulin-dependent diabetes of recent onset. *Lancet,* **2,** 119–124.

60. Assan, R., Feutren, G. and Sirmai, J. (1988) Cyclosporin trials in diabetes: updated results of the French experience. *Transplant. Proc.,* **XX**(3) (Suppl. 4), 178–183.

61. Canadian–European Randomized Control Trial Group (1988) Cyclosporin-induced remission of IDDM after early intervention. Association of 1 yr. of cyclosporin treatment with enhanced insulin secretion. *Diabetes,* **37,** 1574–1582

62. Stiller, R., Laupacis, A., Dupré, J., Jenner, M. R., Keown, P. A., Rodger, W. and Wolfe, B. M. J. (1983) Cyclosporin for treatment of early type 1 diabetes: preliminary results. *N. Engl. J. Med.,* **308,** 1226–1227.

63. Stiller, R., Dupré, J., Gent, M., Jenner, M. R., Keown, P. A., Laupacis, A., Martell, R., Rodger, R., v. Graffenried, B. and Wolfe, B. M. J. (1984) Effects of cyclosporin immunosuppression in insulin-dependent diabetes mellitus of recent onset. *Science,* **223,** 1362–1367.

64. Assan, R., Feutren, G., Debray-Sachs, M., Quiniou-Debrie, M. C., Laborie, C., Thomas, G., Chatenoud, M. and Bach, J. F. (1985) Metabolic and immunological effects of cyclosporin in recently diagnosed type 1 diabetes mellitus. *Lancet,* **1,** 67–71.

65. Dupré, J., Stiller, C. R., Gent, M., Donner, A., v. Graffenried, B., Murphy, G., Heinrichs, D., Jenner, M. R., Keown, P. A., Laupacis, A., Mahon, J., Martell, R., Rodger, N. W. and Wolfe, B. W. (1988) Effects of immunosuppression with cyclosporin in insulin-dependent diabetes mellitus of recent onset: the Canadian open study at 44 months. *Transplant. Proc.,* **XX**(3) (Suppl. 4), 184–192.

66. Levy-Marchal, Cl., Tubiana-Rufi, N. and Czernichow, P. (1987) Efficacité de la ciclosporine A (CsA) dans le diabète insulino-dépendant de l'enfant et analyse des effets secondaires. *J. Ann. Diabétol. Hôtel-Dieu,* pp. 187–197.

67. Bougneres, P. F., Carel, J. C., Castano, L., Boitard, C., Gardin, J. P., Landais, P., Hors, P., Mihatsch, M. J., Paillard, F. M., Chaussain, J. L. and Bach, J. F. (1988), Factors determining early remission of type 1 diabetes in children treated with cyclosporin A. *N. Engl. J. Med.,* **318,** 663–670.

68. Feutren, G. (1988). Functional consequences and risk factors of chronic cyclosporin nephrotoxicity in type 1 diabetes trials. *Transplant. Proc.,* **XX**(3) (Suppl. 4), 356–366.

69. Rubenstein, A. H. and Pyke, D. (1987) Immunosuppression in the treatment of insulin-dependent (type 1) diabetes. *Lancet*, **1**, 436–437.
70. Barrett, T. M. and Geary, D. F. (1982). Steroids in renal disease. *Br. J. Hosp. Med.*, **27**, 349–356.
71. International Study of Kidney Disease in Children (1979) Nephrotic syndrome in children: a randomized trial comparing two prednisone regimens in steroid responsive patients who relapse early. *J. Pediatr.*, **95**, 239–243.
72. Churg, J., Habib, R. and White, R. H. R. (1970) Pathology of the nephrotic syndrome in children. A study for the International Study of Kidney Disease in Children. *Lancet*, **1**, 1299–1302
73. International Study of Kidney Disease in Children (1974) Prospective controlled study of cyclophosphamide therapy in children with the nephrotic syndrome. *Lancet*, **2**, 423–427.
74. International Study of Kidney Diseases in Children (1983) A controlled therapeutic trial of cyclophophamide plus prednisone vs. prednisone alone in children with focal segmental glomerulosclerosis. *Eur. J. Pediatr.* **140**, 149–154
75. Ponticelli, C. and Rivolta, E. (1988) Cyclosporine in nephrotic syndrome. *Transplant. Proc.*, **XX**(3) (Suppl. 4), 253–258.
76. Glassock, R. J., Adler, S. G., Ward, H. J. and Cohen, A. H. (1986) Primary glomerular diseases. In Brenner, B. M. and Rector, F. C. (eds.) *The Kidney*, 3rd edn. (Philadelphia: Saunders), pp. 929–1013.
77. Shalhoub, R. J. (1974) Pathogenesis of lipoid nephrosis: a disorder of T-cell function. *Lancet*, **2**, 556–559.
78. Meyrier, A. (1987) Treatment with cyclosporin of patients with idiopathic nephrotic syndrome. *Springer Semin. Immunopathol.*, **9**, 441–450.
79. Eyres, K. E., Mallick, N. P. and Taylor, G. (1976) Evidence for cell mediated immunity to renal antigens in minimal change nephrotic syndrome. *Lancet*, **1**, 1158–1159.
80. Lagrue, G., Branellec, A. and Blac, C. (1975) A vascular permeability factor in lymphocyte culture supernatants from patients with nephrotic syndrome. II. Pharmacological and physicochemical properties. *Biomedicine*, **23**, 73–75.
81. Moorthy, A. V., Zimmerman, S. W. and Burkholder, P. M. (1979) Inhibition of lymphocyte blastogenesis by plasma of patients with minimal change nephrotic syndrome. *Lancet*, **1**, 1160.
82. Schnaper, H. W. and Aune, T. M. (1985) Identification of the lymphokine soluble immune response suppressor in urine of nephrotic children. *J. Clin. Invest.*, **76**, 341–349.
83. Tejani, A., Butt, K. and Khawar, R. (1985) Cyclosporin induced remission of relapsing nephrotic syndrome in children. *Abstract, 18th Ann. Meet. Am. Soc. Nephrol. New Orleans.*
84. Gunn, H. C. and Ryffel, B. (1986) Glomerulonephritis in NZB/W mice, therapeutic effect of cyclosporin. *Clin. Nephrol.* **25** (Suppl. 1), 189–192.
85. Kojima, N., Nagamatsu, T., Ho, M. and Suzuki, Y. (1988) Effect of cyclosporin A on anti-GBM nephritis in rats. *Jpn J. Pharmacol.*, **46** (Suppl.), 87P.
86. Schrijver, G., Wezels, J. F. M., Assmann, K. J. M., Robben, J. C. M., Koene, R. A. P. and Berden, J. H. M. (1988) Reduction of proteinuria by cyclosporin in a passive model of anti-GBM nephritis in the mouse. *Kidney Int.*, **33**, 1039.
87. Shik, W., Hines, W. H. and Neilson, E. G. (1988) Effect of cyclosporin A on the development of immune-mediated interstitial nephritis. *Kidney Int.*, **33**, 1113–1188.
88. Brodehl, J., Hoyer, P. F., Oemar, B. S., Helmchen, U. and Wonigeit, K. (1988) Cyclosporin treatment of nephrotic syndrome in children. *Transplant. Proc.*, **XX**(3) (Suppl. 4), 269–274.
89. Brandis, M., Burghard, R., Leititis, J., Zimmerhackl, B., Hildebrandt, F. and Helmchen, U. (1988) Cyclosporin A for the treatment of nephrotic syndrome. *Transplant. Proc.*, **XX**(3) (Suppl. 4), 275–279.
90. Capodicasa, G., De Santo, N. G., Nuzzi, F. and Giordano, G. (1986) Cyclosporin A in nephrotic syndrome of childhood – a 14 months experience. *Int. J. Ped. Nephrology*, **7**, 69–72.
91. Mentser, M., Shaimon, B. and Mahan, J. D. (1988) Cyclosporin treatment of frequently relapsing minimal change nephrotic syndrome in children (abstract). *Kidney Int.*, **33**, 329.
92. Niaudet, P., Tete, M. J., Broyer, M. and Habib, R. (1988) Cyclosporin and childhood idiopathic nephrosis. *Transplant. Proc.*, **XX**(3) (Suppl. 4), 265–268.

93. Tejani, A., Butt, K. and Trachtman, H. (1988) Cyclosporin A induced remission of relapsing nephrotic syndrome in children. *Kidney Int.*, **33**, 729–734.
94. Balcke, P., Derfler, K. and Stockenhuber, F. (1987) Cyclosporin-Therapie bei minimal change nephritis. *Wien. Klin. Wochenschr.*, **99**, 242–245.
95. Chan, M. K. and Cheng, I. K. P. (1987) Cyclosporin A in steroidsensitive nephrotic syndrome with frequent relapses. *Postgrad. Med. J.*, **63**, 757–759.
96. Clasen, W., Kindler, J., Mihatsch, M. J., and Sieberth, H. G. (1988) Long-term treatment of minimal-change nephrotic syndrome with cyclosporin: a control biopsy study. *Nephrol. Dial. Transplant.* **3**, 733–737
97. Kindler, J., Clasen, W. and Sieberth, H. G. (1987). Cyclosporin A therapy in patients with focal glomerular sclerosis (abstract). *10th International Congress of Nephrology, London*, p. 70.
98. Gutierrez Millet, V., Bellow, I., Oliet, A. and Praga, M. (1987) Cyclosporin in minimal change nephrotic syndrome. (abstract). *Kidney Int.*, **32**, 614.
99. Lagrue, G., Laurent, J., Belghiti, D. and Robeva, R. (1986). Cyclosporin and idiopathic nephrotic syndrome. *Lancet*, **2**, 692–693.
100. Maher, E. R., Sweny, P. and Varghese, Z. (1988). Is cyclosporin A an alternative to cyclophosphamide for frequently relapsing minimal change nephropathy? (abstract). *Clin. Sci.* **74** (Suppl. 18), 47P.
101. Meyrier, A., Condamin, M. C. and Simon, P. (1988) Treatment with cyclosporin of adult idiopathic nephrotic syndrome resistant to corticosteroids and other immuno-suppressants. *Transplant. Proc.*, **XX**(3) (Suppl. 4), 259–261.
102. Waldo, F. B. and Kohant, E. C. (1987) Therapy of focal segmental glomerulosclerosis with cyclosporin. *Pediat. Nephrol.*, **1**, 180–182.
103. Confalonieri, R., Radaelli, L. and Civati, F. (1987) Cyclosporin A effect on refractory nephrotic syndrome in primary glomerulonephritis (abstract). *10th International Congress of Nephrology, London*, p. 57.
104. Van Hoof, J. P., Leunissen, K. M. L., Havenith, M. G. and Bosman, F. T. (1988) Cyclosporin and other therapy-resistant nephrotic syndrome. *Transplant. Proc.*, **XX**(3) (Suppl. 4), 293–296.
105. Sreepada Rao, T. K. and Friedman, E. (1987) Prospective trial of cyclosporin (CyA) in refractory nephrotic syndrome in adults, preliminary findings (abstract). *Kidney Int.*, **31**, 214.
106. Zietse, R., Wenting, G. J., Kramer, P., Schalekamp, M. A. D. H. and Weimar, W. (1988) Fractional excretion of protein: a marker of the efficacy of cyclosporin A treatment in nephrotic syndrome. *Transplant. Proc.*, **XX**(3) (Suppl. 4), 280–284.
107. Cattran, D. C., Dossetor, J. and Keown, P. (1986) Cyclosporin treatment of patients with glomerulonephritis. (abstract). *Kidney Int.*, **29**, 182.
108. DeSanto, N. G., Capodicasa, G. and Giordano, C. (1987) Treatment of idiopathic membranous nephropathy unresponsive to methylprednisolone and chlorambucil with cyclosporin. *Am. J. Nephrol.*, **7**, 74–76.
109. Erbay, B., Karaton, O., Duman, N. and Ertug, A. E. (1988) The effect of cyclosporin in idiopathic nephrotic syndrome resistant to immunosuppressive therapy. *Transplant. Proc.*, **XX**(3) (Suppl. 4), 289–292.
110. Macanovic, M., Verbic, D., Cengic, M. and Golemac, S. (1987) Treatment of refractory nephrotic syndrome with cyclosporin A (abstract). *10th International Congress on Nephrology, London*, p. 75
111. Tejani, A., Gonzalez, R., Rajpoort, D., Sharma, R. and Pomrantz, A. (1988) A randomized trial of cyclosporin with low-dose prednisone compared with high-dose prednisone in nephrotic syndrome. *Transplant. Proc.*, **XX**(3) (Suppl. 4), 262–264,
112. Lai, K. N., Lai, F. M., Li, P. K. T. and Owen, J. V. (1987) Cyclosporine treatment of IgA nephropathy: a short-term controlled trial. *Br. Med. J.*, **295**, 1165–1168.
113. Mihatsch, M. J., Bach, J. F., Coovadia, H. M., Forre, O., Moutsopoulos, H. M., Drosis, A. A., Siamopoulos, K. L., Noel, L. H., Ramsaroop, R., Hällgren, R., Svenson, K. and Bohman, S. O. (1988) Cyclosporin-associated nephropathy in patients with autoimmune diseases. *Klin. Wochenschr.*, **66**, 43–47.
114. Champion, R. H. (1986) Psoriasis. *Brit. Med. J.*, **292**, 1693–1696.
115. Valdimarsson, H., Baker, B. S., Jonsdottir, I. and Fry, L. (1986) Psoriasis, a disease of abnormal keratinocyte proliferation induced by T-lymphocytes. *Immunol. Today*, **7**(9),

256–259.
116. Brown, M. D., Gupta, A. K., Ellis, C. N., Cooper, K. D., Fisher, G. J. and Voorhees, J. J. (1988) Cyclosporin for the treatment of psoriasis. *Transplant. Proc.*, **XX**(3) (Suppl. 4), 26–31.
117 Kragballe, K., Desjarlais, L. and Voorhees, J. J. (1985) Leukotriens B4, C4 and D4 stimulate DNA synthesis in cultured human epidermal keratinocytes. *Br. J. Dermatol.*, **113**, 43–52.
118 Baker, B. S., Griffiths, C. E. M., Lambert, S., Powles, A. V., Leonard, J. N., Valdimarsson, H. and Fry, L. (1987) The effects of cyclosporin A on T-lymphocytes and dendritic cell sub-population in psoriasis. *Br. J. Dermatol.*, **116**, 503–510.
119. Bos, J. D. (1988) The pathomechanism of psoriasis; the skin immune system and cyclosporin. *Br. J. Dermatol.*, **118**, 141–158.
120. Mueller, W. and Herrmann, B. (1979). Cyclosporin A for psoriasis. *N. Engl. J. Med.*, **301**, 555.
121. Harper, J. I., Keat, A. C. S. and Straughton, R. C. D. (1984) Cyclosporin for psoriasis. *Lancet*, **2**, 981–982.
122. Van Hooff, J. P., Leunissen, K. M. L. and Staak, W. V. D. (1985) Cyclosporin and psoriasis. *Lancet*, **1**, 335.
123. Van Joost, T. H., Heule, F., Stolz, E. and Beukers, R. (1986) Short-term use of cyclosporin A in severe psoriasis. *Br. J. Dermatol.*, **114**, 615–620.
124. Wakeel, R. A. and Dick, D. V. (1986) Psoriasis. *Br. Med. J.*, **293**, 266.
125. Marks, J. (1986). Psoriasis. *Br. Med. J.*, **293**, 509.
126. Griffiths, C. E. M., Powles, A. V., Leonard, J. N., Fry, L., Baker, B. S. and Valdimarsson, H. (1986) Clearance of psoriasis with low dose cyclosporin. *Br. Med. J.*, **293**, 731–732.
127. Brookes, D. B. (1986) Clearance of psoriasis with low dose cyclosporin. *Br. Med. J.*, **293**, 1089–1099.
128. Ellis, C. N., Gorsulowsky, D. C., Hamilton, T. A., Billing, J. K., Brown, M. C., Headington, J. T., Cooper, K. D., Baadigaard, O., Duell, E. A., Annesley, T. M., Turcotte, J. G. and Voorhees, J. J. (1986) Cyclosporin improves psoriasis in a double-blind study. *J. Am. Med. Assoc.*, **256**, 3110–3116.
129. Wentzell, J. M., Boughman, R. D., O'Connor, G. T. and Bernier, G. M. (1987) Cyclosporin in the treatment of psoriasis. *Arch. Dermatol.*, **123**, 163–165.
130. Picascia, D. D., Garden, J. M., Freinkel, R. K. and Roenigk, H. H. (1987) Treatment of resistant severe psoriasis with systemic cyclosporin. *J. Am. Acad. Dermatol.*, **17**, 408–414.
131. Van Joost, T. H., Bos, J. D., Heule, F. and Meinardi, M. M. H. M. (1988) Low-dose cyclosporin A in severe psoriasis. A double-blind study. *Br. J. Dermatol.*, **118**, 183–190.
132. Fry, L., Griffiths, C. E. M., Powles, A. V., Valdimarsson, H. and Baker. B. S. (1988). Long-term cyclosporin in the management of psoriasis. *Transplant. Proc.*, **XX**(3) (Suppl. 4), 23–25.
133. Griffiths, C. E. M., Powles, A. V., Baker, B. S., Fry, L. and Valdimarsson, H. (1988). Combination of cyclosporin A and topical corticosteroids in the treatment of psoriasis. *Transplant. Proc.*, **XX**(3) (Suppl. 4), 50–52.
134. Picascia, D. D., Garden, J. M., Freinkel, R. K. and Roenigk, H. H. (1988) Resistant severe psoriasis controlled with systemic cyclosporin therapy. *Transplant. Proc.*, **XX**(3) (Suppl. 4), 58–62.
135. Harper, J. I., Zemelman, V., Keat, A. and Staughton, R. C. D. (1988) Cyclosporin for psoriasis: beneficial effect in refractory skin and joint disease. *Transplant. Proc.*, **XX**(3) (Suppl. 4), 63–67.
136. Marks, J. (1988) Low-dose cyclosporin A in severe psoriasis. *Transplant. Proc.*, **XX**(3) (Suppl. 4), 68–71.
137. Fredriksson, T. and Pettersson, V. (1978) Severe psoriasis – oral therapy with a new retinoid. *Dermatologia*, **157**, 238–244.
138. Schuster, S. (1988) Cyclosporine in dermatology. *Transplant. Proc.*, **XX**(3) (Suppl. 4), 19–22.
139. Cacon, G. P., Artru, L., Canesi, M., Koeger, A. C. and Camus, J. P. (1988) Life-threatening psoriasis relapse on withdrawal of cyclosporin. *Lancet*, **2**, 219–220.
140. Brown, M., Ellis, C., Billings, J., Cooper, K., Baadagaard, O., Headington, J., and Voorhees, J. (1988) Rapid occurrence of nodular cutaneous infiltrates with cyclosporin therapy. *Arch. Dermatol.*, **124**, 1097–1100.

141. Griffiths, C., Powles, A., Baker, B., Valdimarsson, H. and Fry, L. (1987) Topical cyclosporin and psoriasis. *Lancet*, **1**, 806.
142. Schauder, C. S. and Gorsulowsky, D. C. (1986) Topical cyclosporine A in the treatment of psoriasis. *Clin. Res.*, **34**, 1007A.
143. Schulze, H. J. and Mahrle, G. (1988) Absorption of topical ciclosporin and depression of neutrophils in psoriasis. *Skin Pharmacol.*, ,, **1**, 68.
144. Powles, A., Baker, B., McFadden, J., Rutman, A., Fry, L., Griffiths, C. and Valdimarsson, H. (1988) Intralesional injection of cyclosporin in psoriasis. *Lancet*, **1**, 537.
145. Allison, M. C. and Pounder, R. E. (1984) Cyclosporin for Crohn's disease. *Lancet*, **1**, 902–903.
146. Bianchi, P. A., Mondelli, M., Quarto di Palo, F. and Ranzi, T. (1984) Cyclosporin for Crohn's disease. *Lancet*, **1**, 1242.
147. Parrott, H. R., Taylor, R. M. R., Venables, C. W. and Record, C. O. (1986). Treatment of Crohn's disease with cyclosporin: a report of 11 cases. *Gut*, **27**, 1277–1278.
148. Allison, M. C. and Pounder, R. E. (1987). Early experience with cyclosporin for Crohn's disease. *Aliment. Pharmaccol.*, **1**, 39–43.
149. Brynskov, J., Binder, V., Riis, P., Schaffalitzky de Muckadell, O., Lauritsen, K., Freund, L., Falling org, J., Rasmussen, S. N., Matzen, P., Krag, E. and Tage-Jensen, U. (1987) Clinical experience with ciclosporin in chronically-active, therapy-resistant Crohn's disease. A pilot study. *Gastroenterology*, **92**, 1330.
150. Peltekian, K. M., Williams, C. N., MacDonald, A. S., Roy, P. and Czolpinska, E. (1988) Open trial of cyclosporine in patients with severe active Crohn's disease refractory to conventional therapy. *Can. J. Gastroenterol.*, **2**, 5–11.
151. Gupta, S., Keshavarzian, A. and Hodgson, H. J. F. (1984) Cyclosporin in ulcerative colitis. *Lancet*, **2**, 1277–1278.
152. Bianchi Porro, G., Panza, E. and Petrillo, M. (1987) Cyclosporin A in acute ulcerative colitis. *Ital. J. Gastroenterol.*, **9**, 40–41.
153. Hyams, J. S., Ballow, M. and Leichtner, A. M. (1987) Cyclosporin treatment for autoimmune chronic active hepatitis. *Gastroenterology*, **93**, 890–893.
154. Mistilis, S. P., Vicker, C. R., Darrock, M. H. and McCarthy, S. W. (1985) Cyclosporin, a new treatment for autoimmune chronic active hepatitis. *Med. J. Australia*, **143**, 463–464.
155. Routhier, G., Epstein, O., Janossy, G., Thomas, A. C. and Sherlock, S. (1980) Effects of cyclosporin A on suppressor and inducer T-lymphocytes in primary biliary cirrhosis. *Lancet*, **2**, 1223–1225.
156. Lucey, M. R., Neuberger, J. M., Alexander, G. J. M., Robson, S. and Williams, R. (1985) Treatment of primary biliary cirrhosis with cyclosporin: pilot study. In Schindler, R. (ed.), *Cyclosporin in Autoimmune Diseases* (Berlin: Springer), pp. 175–178.
157. Beukers, R. and Schalm, S. W. (1988) Effect of cyclosporin and cyclosporin plus prednisone in primary biliary cirrhosis. *Transplant. Proc.*, **XX**(3) (Suppl. 4), 340–343.
158. Parsons, H., Thirsk, J., Frohlich, J. and Minuk, G. (1988) Effect of cyclosporin A on serum lipid in primary biliary cirrhosis patients. *Gastroenterology*, **94**(5), Part 2, p. A580.
159. Wiesner, R. H., Dickson, E. R., Lindor, K. D., Jorgensen, R., LaRusso, N. F. and Baldus, W. (1987) A controlled clinical trial evaluating cyclosporin in the treatment of primary biliary cirrhosis: a preliminary report. *Hepatology*, **7**, 1025 (abstract No. 9).
160. Tygstrup, N., Ranek, L., Juhl, E., Keidnig, S., Christensen, E., Williams, R., Neuberger, J. and Rodes, J. (1985). Cyclosporin in primary biliary cirrhosis. A multicenter, double-blind, placebo-controlled longterm therapeutic study: the study design. In Schindler, R. (ed.), *Cyclosporin in Autoimmune Diseases* (Berlin: Springer), pp. 182–184.
161. Beyer, J., Koetsier, J., Rudge, P. and van Walbeek, double-blind controlled trial of cyclosporin in multiple sclerosis. *Second International Congress on Cyclosporin, Washington*, 4.–7.11.87, abstract 274.
162. Kappos, L., Patzold, U., Dommasch, D., Poser, S., Haas, J., Krauseneck, P., Malin, J. P., Fierz, W., v. Graffenried, B. and Gugerli, U. S. (1988) Cyclosporin vs. azathioprine in the longterm treatment of multiple sclerosis – results of the German multicenter study. *Ann. Neurol.*, **23**, 56–63.
163. Besinger, U. A., Mraz, W. and Fateh-Moghadam, A. (1985) Cyclosporin in myasthenia gravis. In Schindler, R. (ed.), *Cyclosporin in Autoimmune Diseases* (Berlin: Springer), pp. 100–109.

164. Nyberg-Hansen, R. and Gjerstad, L. (1988) Immunopharmacological treatment in myasthenia gravis. *Transplant. Proc.*, **XX**(3) (Suppl. 4), 201–210.
165. Goulon, M., Elkharrat, D., Lokiec, F. and Gajdos, P. (1988) Results of a one-year open trial of cyclosporin in ten patients with severe myasthenia gravis. *Transplant. Proc.*, **XX**(3) (Suppl. 4), 211–217.
16᠈. Tindall, R. S. A., Rollins, J. A., Phillips, J. T., Greenlee, R. G., Wells, L. and Belendiuk, G. (1987) Preliminary results of a double-blind, randomized, placebo-controlled trial of cyclosporin in myasthenia gravis. *N. Engl. J. Med.*, **316**, 719–724.
167. Stryckmans, P. A., Dumont, J. P., Velu, Th. and Debusscher, L. (1984) Cyclosporine in refractory severe aplastic anemia. *N. Engl. J. Med.*, **310**, 655–656.
168. Finlay, J. L., Toretsky, J., Hoffman, R., Bruno, E. and Shahidi, N. T. (1984) Cyclosporine A (CyA) in refractory aplastic anemia. *Blood*, **64**(5) (Suppl. 1), 104a.
169. Miescher, P. A. and Beris, Ph. (1984) Cyclosporin A. *Springer Semin. Immunopathol.*, **7**, 77–79.
170. Wisloff, F., Godal, H. C. (1985). Cyclosporine in refractory severe aplastic anemia. *N. Engl. J. Med.*, **312**, 1193.
171. Barreras, L. R., Ahn, Y. A., Temple, J. D. and Harrington, W. J. (1985). Successful use of cyclosporin A in severe aplastic anemia. *Blood*, **66**(5) (Suppl. 1), 119a (abstract).
172. Seip, M., Vidnes, J. (1985). Cyclosporine A in a case of refractory severe aplastic anemia. *Scand. J. Haematol.*, **34**, 228–230.
173. Shiobara, S., Harada, M., Odaka, K., Ootsuka, M., Kondo, K., Nakao, S., Ueda, M., Matsuda, T., Mori, T. and Hattori, K. (1986) Therapy for aplastic anemia with cyclosporine: a case report. *Acta Haematol. Jap.*, **49**, 1287–1290.
174. Vogt, H. G., Kaltwasser, J. P., Schalk, K. P. and Hoelzer, D. (1986) Successful treatment of aplastic anaemia with cyclosporin A after repeated relapses. *Blut*, **53**, 166 (abstract).
175. Frickhofen, N., Heit, W., Raghavachar, A., Porzsolt, F. and Heimpel, H. (1986) Treatment of aplastic anemia with cyclosporin A, methylprednisolone, and antithymocyte globulin. *Klin. Wochenschr.*, **64**, 1165–1170.
176. Tutschka, P. J. and Copelan, E. A. (1987) Cyclosporine as immunosuppression for severe aplastic anemia. *Blood*, **70** (Suppl. 1), 144a (abstract).
177. Leonard, E., Raefsky, E., Nienhuis, A. W., Griffith, P. and Young, N. (1987) Cyclosporin A therapy of aplastic anemia and pure red cell aplasia. *Blood*, **70** (Suppl. 1), 137a (abstract).
178. Seewan, H. L., Greinix, H. and Urban, Ch. (1987) Treatment of aplastic anemia with cyclosporin A. *Blut*, **55**, 305 (abstract).
179. Porwit, A., Panayotides, P., Mansson, E., Ösby, E., Hast, R. and Reizenstein, P. (1987) Cyclosporine A treatment in four cases of aplastic anemia. *Blut*, **54**, 73–78.
180. Bern, M. M., Roberts, M. S. and Yoburn, D. (1987) Cyclosporin treatment for aplastic anemia: a case report demonstrating a second response to second exposure to cyclosporin. *Am. J. Hematol.*, **24**, 307–309.
181. Bridges, R., Pineo, G. and Blahey, W. (1987) Cyclosporin A for the treatment of aplastic anemia refractory to antithymocyte globulin. *Am. J. Hematol.*, **26**, 83–87.
182. Jacobs, P., Wood, L. and Martell, R. W. (1985) Cyclosporin A in the treatment of severe acute aplastic anaemia. *Br. J. Haematol.*, **61**, 267–272.
183. Frickhofen, N. and Kaltwasser, J. P. (1988) Immunosuppressive treatment of aplastic anemia: a prospective, randomized multicenter trial evaluating antilymphocyte globulin (ALG) versus ALG and cyclosporin A. *Blut*, **56**, 191–192.
184. Champlin, R., Ho, W. and Gale, R. P. (1983) Antithymocyte globulin treatment in patients with aplastic anemia: a prospective randomized trial. *N. Engl. J. Med.*, **308**, 113–118.
185. Finlay, J. L. and Shahidi, N. T. (1984). Cyclosporine A (CyA) induced remission in Diamond–Blackfan anemia (DBA). *Blood*, **64**(5) (Suppl. 1), 104a (abstract).
186. Tötterman, T. H., Nisell, J., Killander, A., Gahrton, G. and Lönnqvist, B. (1984) Successful treatment of pure red-cell aplasia with cyclosporin. *Lancet*, **2**, 693.
187. Chikkappa, G., Pasquale, D., Phillips, P. G., Mangan, K. F. and Tsan, M. F. (1987) Cyclosporin A for the treatment of pure red cell aplasia in a patient with chronic lymphocytic leukemia. *Am. J. Hematol.*, **26**, 179–189.
188. Varet, B., Picard, F., Casadevall, N., Dreyfus, F., Muller, O. and Lacombe, C. (1987) Cyclosporin induced remission in two patients with B-C.L.L. associated P.R.C.A. who were resistant to other immunosuppressive drugs. *Blood*, **70** (Suppl. 1), 144a (abstract).

248

189. Williams, D. L., Mageed, A. S. A., Findley, H. and Ragab, A. H. (1987) Cyclosporine in the treatment of red cell aplasia. *Am. J. Pediat. Hematol. Oncol.*, **9**, 314–316.
190. Finelli, C., Bandini, G., Ricci, P., Giudice, V., Vianelli, N., Rabbi, C., Raspadori, D. and Tura, S. (1987) Ciclosporin A in idiopathic and CLL-associated pure red cell aplasia. *Haematologica*, **72**, 537–540.
191. Katakkar, S. E. (1988) Cyclosporine and pure red cell aplasia. *Transplant. Proc.*, **XX**(3) (Suppl. 4), 314–316.
192. Velu, Th., Dumont, J. P., Debusscher, L. snf Stryckmans, P. (1983) Successful treatment of refractory thrombocytopenia by cyclosporine A (CyA). *Blood*, **62**(5) (Suppl. 1), 248a (abstract).
193. Kelsey, P. R., Schofield, K. P. and Geary, C. G. (1985) Correspondence: Refractory idiopathic thrombocytopenic purpura ITP treated with cyclosporine. *Br. J. Haematol.*, **60**, 197–198.
194. Coiffier, B. and Dechavanne, M. (1985) Ciclosporine (CyA) in immunologic thrombocytopenias resistant to corticosteroids. *Blood*, **66**(5) (Suppl. 1), 287a (abstract).
195. Matsumura, O., Kawashima, Y., Kato, S., Sanaka, T., Teraoka, S., Kawai, T., Honda, H., Fichinoue, S., Takahashi, K., Toma, H., Ota, K. and Sugino, N. (1988) Therapeutic effect of cyclosporine in thrombocytopenia associated with autoimmune disease. *Transplant. Proc.*, **XX**(3) (Suppl. 4), 317–322.
196. Hill, W. and Landgraf, R. (1985) Successful treatment of amegakaryocytic thrombocytopenic purpura with cyclosporine. *N. Engl. J. Med.*, **312**, 1060–1061.
197. Schalk, K. P., Ganser, A., Kaltwasser, J. P., Frickhofen, N. and Hoelzer, D. (1986) Successful treatment of amegakaryocytic thrombocytopenic purpura with cyclosporin A. *Blut*, **53**, 182–183 (abstract).
198. Coiffier, B. (1986) Cyclosporine in Felty's syndrome. *N. Engl. J. Med.*, **314**, 184.
199. Selleri, C., Catalano, L., Alfinito, F., De Rosa, G., Vaglio, S. and Rotoli, B. (1988) Cyclosporin A in adult-onset cyclic neutropenia. *Br. J. Haematol.*, **68**, 137–138.
200. Boda, Z., Hársfalvi, J., Pecze, K. and Rak, K. (1987) Acquired haemophilia due to factor VIII inhibitor with severe haemorrhages in a 46 year old woman successfully treated with cyclosporin A. *Thrombos. Haemost.*, **58**(1), 552 (abstract).
201. Hart, H. C., Kraaijenhagen, R. J., Kerckhaert, J. A. M., Verdel, G., Freen, M. and van de Wiel, A. (1988) A patient with a spontaneous factor VIII:C autoantibody: successful treatment with cyclosporine. *Transplant. Proc.*, **XX**(3) (Suppl. 4), 323–328.
202. Bach, J. F. and Feutren, G. (1985) Contrasting effects of ciclosporin on humoral and cell-mediated immunity in patients with autoimmune diseases. In Schindler, R. (ed.), *Ciclosporin in Autoimmune Diseases* (Berlin: Springer), pp. 33–38.
203. Isenberg, D. A., Snaith, M. L., Morrow, W. J. W., Al-Khader, A. A., Cohen, S. L., Fisher, C. and Mowbray, J. (1981) Cyclosporin A for the treatment of systemic lupus erythematosus. *Int. J. Immunopharmacol.*, **3**, 163–165.
204. Feutren, G., Querin, S., Noel, L. H., Chatenoud, L., Beaurain, G., Rron, F., Lesavre, P. and Bach, J. F. (1987) Effects of cyclosporine in severe systemic lupus erythematosus. *J. Pediat.*, **111**, 1063–1068.
205. Ter Borg, E. J., Tegzess, A. M. and Kallenberg, C. G. M. (1988) Unexpected severe reversible cyclosporine A induced nephrotoxicity in a patient with systemic lupus erythematosus and tubulointerstinal renal disease. *Clin. Nephrol.*, **29**, 93–95.
206. Miescher, P. A. (1986) Treatment of systemic lupus erythematosus. *Springer Semin. Immunopathol.*, **9**, 271–282.
207. Miescher, P. A., Favre, H., Mihatsch, M. J., Chatelanat, F., Huang, Y. P. and Zubler, R. (1988) The place of cyclosporine A in the treatment of connective tissue diseases. *Transplant. Proc.*, **XX**(3) (Suppl. 4), 224–237.
208. Van Joost, T., Stolz, E. and Heule, F. (1987) Efficacy of low-dose cyclosporin in severe atopic skin disease. *Arch. Dermatol.*, **123**, 166–167.
209. Zabel, P., Leinenstoll, G. and Gross, W. (1984) Cyclosporin for acute dermatomyositis. *Lancet*, **1**, 343.
210. Bendtzen, K., Tvede, N., Andersen, V. and Bendixen, G. (1984) Cyclosporin for polymyositis. *Lancet*, **1**, 792–793.
211. Russell, M. and Schachter, R. (1988) Cyclosporin treatment of scleroderma (PSS). *Arthritis Rheum.*, **31** (Suppl. 4), s51 (abstract A79).
212. Zachariae, H. and Zachariae, E. (1987) Cyclosporine in severe progressive systemic

sclerosis. *Br. J. Dermatol.*, **116**, 741–742.
213. Thivolet, J., Barthelmy, H., Rigot-Müller, G. and Bendelac, A. (1985) Effects of cyclosporin on bullous pemphigoid and pemphigus. *Lancet*, **1**, 334–335.
214. Cunliffe, W. J. (1987) Bullous pemphigoid and response to cyclosporin. *Br. J. Dermatol.*, **117** (Suppl. 32), 113–114.
2 5. Curley, R. K., Macfarlane, A. W. and Vickers, C. F. H. (1985) Pyoderma gangraenosum treated with cyclosporin A. *Br. J. Dermatol.*, **113**, 601–604.
216. Drosos, A. A., Skopouli, F. N., Costopoulos, J. S., Papadimitriou, C. S. and Montsopoulos, H. M. (1986) Cyclosporin A in primary Sjoegren's syndrome: a double-blind study. *Ann. Rheum. Dis.*, **45**, 731–735.
217. Weetman, A. P., McGregor, A. M., Ludgate, M., Beck, L., Mills, P. V., Lazarus, J. H. and Hall, R. (1983) Cyclosporin improves Graves' ophthalmopathy. *Lancet*, **2**, 486–489.
218. Kahaly, G., Schrezenmeir, J., Krause, U., Schweikert, B., Meuer, S., Müller, W., Dennebaum, R. and Beyer, J. (1986) Ciclosporin and prednisone v. prednisone in treatment of Graves' ophthalmopathy: a controlled, randomized and prospective study. *Eur. J. Clin. Invest.*, **16**, 415–422.
219. Utech, C., Wulle, K. G., Kieffer, H. and Panit , N. (1985) Ciclosporin treatment in severe Graves' ophthalmopathy. In: Schindler, R. (ed.), *Ciclosporin in Autoimmune Diseases* (Berlin: Springer), pp. 247–252.
220. Howlett, T. A., Lawton, N. F. and Fells, P. (1984) Deterioration of severe Graves' ophthalmopathy during ciclosporin treatment. *Lancet*, **2**, 1101.
221. Brabant, G., Peter, H., Becker, H., Schwarzrock, R., Wonigeit, K. and Hesch, R. D. (1984) Cyclosporine in infiltrative eye disease. *Lancet*, **1**, 515–516.
222. Borleffs, J. C. C., Derksen, R. H. W. H. and Hesse, R. J. (1987) Treatment of Wegener's granulomatosis with cyclosporine A. *Ann. Rheum. Dis.*, **46**, 175.
223. Rebuck, A. S., Stiller, C. R., Brande, A. C., Laupacis, A., Cohen, R. D. and Chapman, K. R. (1984) Cyclosporin for pulmonary sarcoidosis. *Lancet*, **1**, 1174.
224. Bonloux, P. M. G., Wass, J. A. H., Parslow, J. M., Hendry, W. F. and Besser, G. M. (1986) Effect of cyclosporin A in male infertility. *Fertil. Steril.*, **46**, 81–85.
225. Svenson, K. L. G., Holmdahl, R., Klareskog, L., Wibell, L., Sjoeberg, O., Klintmalm, G. B. G. and Bostroem, H. (1984) Cyclosporin A treatment in a case of relapsing polychondritis. *Scand. J. Rheumatol.*, **13**, 329–333.
226. Wendling, D., Hory, B. and Blanc, D. (1985). Cyclosporine: a new adjurant therapy for giant cell arteritis? *Arthritis Rheum.*, **28**, 1078–1079.
227. Ettinger, J., Feucht, H., Gärtner, R., Kotzur, J., Schlag, R., Gokel, J. M. and Jahrmärker, H. (1986) Cyclosporine A for successful treatment of myocarditis. *Eur. Heart J.*, **7**, 452.
228. Zwitter, M., Drinovec, J., Dubravcic, M., Vodnik, A., Petric-Grabnar, J., Dolnicar, M., Konstantinivic, M. and Zemva, Z. (1987) Cyclosporin may alleviate B symptoms and induce a remission of heavily pre-treated Hodgkin disease: a preliminary report. *Ann. Intern. Med.*, **106**, 843–844.
229. von Graffenried, B. and Krupp, P. (1986) Side effects of cyclosporine (Sandimmun) in renal transplant recipients and in patients with autoimmune diseases. *Transplant. Proc.*, **18**, 876–883.
230. Dieterle, A., Abeywickrama, K. and von Graffenried, B. (1988) Nephrotoxicity and hypertension in patients with autoimmune diseases treated with cyclosporine. *Transplant. Proc.*, **XX**(3) (Suppl. 4), 349–355.
231. Schmidt, J. B., Gebhardt, W., Kopsa, H. and Spona, J. (1986) Does cyclosporine A influence sex hormone level? *Exp. Clin. Endocrinol.*, **88**, 207.
232. Wysocki, G. P., Gretzinger, H. A., Laupacis, A., Ulan, R. A. and Stiller, C. R. (1983) Fibrous hyperplasia of the gingiva: a side effect of cyclosporine A therapy. *Oral Surg.*, **55**, 274–278.
233. Palestine, A. G., Austin, H. A. and Nussenblatt, R. B. (1986) Renal tubular function in cyclosporine-treated patients. *Am. J. Med.*, **81**, 419–424.
234. Thompson, C. B., June, C. H., Sullivan, E. M. and Thomas, E. D. (1984) Association between cyclosporine neurotoxicity and hypomagnesemia. *Lancet*, **2**, 1116–1120.
235. Penn, I. and Brunson, (1988) Cancer after cyclosporine therapy. *Transplant Proc.*, **XX**(3) (Suppl. 3), 885–892.
236. Taube, D. and Williams, D. G. (1988) Pathogenesis of minimal change nephropathy. In Cameron, J. S. and Glanock, R. (eds), *The Nephrotic Syndrome* (Paris: Marcel Dekker).

237. Cockburn, I. (1987) Assessment of the risks of malignancy and lymphomas developing in patients using Sandimmun. *Transplant. Proc.*, **19**(1), 1804–1807.
238. von Graffenried, B. and Harrison, W. B. (1985) Renal function in patients with autoimmune diseases treated with cyclosporine. *Transplant. Proc.*, **XVIII**(4) (Suppl. 1), 215–231.
239. Berg, K. J., Forre, O., Mikkelsen, M., Narverud, J., Djoseland, O. and Rugstad, H. (1988) Side effects of high and low cyclosporine doses in patients with rheumatoid arthritis. *Kidney Int.*, **33**, 761.
240. Ludwin, D., Bennett, K. J., Grau, E. M., Buchanan, W. W., Bensen, W., Bombardier, C. and Tugwell, P. X. (1988) Nephrotoxicity in patients with rheumatoid arthritis treated with cyclosporine. *Transplant. Proc.*, **XX**(3) (Suppl. 4), 367–370.
241. Deray, G., Le Hoang, P., Aupetit, B., Achour, A., Rottembourg, J. and Baumelon, A. (1987) Enhancement of cyclosporine A nephrotoxicity by diclofenac. *Clin. Nephrol.*, **27**, 213–214.
242. Mihatsch, M. J. (1985) International workshop in cyclosporine nephropathy. *Clin. Nephrol.*, **24**, 107–119.
243. Miescher, P. A., Favre, H., Chatelenat, F. and Mihatsch, M. J. (1987) Combined steroid-cyclosporine treatment of chronic autoimmune diseases. Clinical results and assessment of nephrotoxicity by renal biopsy. *Klin. Wochenschr.*, **65**, 727–736.
244. Svenson, K., Bohman, S. O. and Hällgren, R. (1986) Renal interstitial fibrosis and vascular changes, occurrence in patients with autoimmune diseases treated with cyclosporine. *Arch. Intern. Med.*, **146**, 2007–2010.
245. Nahman, N. S., Cosio, F. G., Kolkin, S., Mendell, J. R. and Sharma, H. M. (1987) Cyclosporine nephrotoxicity without major organ transplantation. *Ann. Intern. Med.*, **106**, 400–402.
246. Bach, J. F. (1988). Cyclosporine in autoimmunity. *Transplant. Proc.*, **XX**(3) (Suppl. 4), 379–810.

12
Pharmacokinetics of cyclosporin A

Joachim Grevel and Barry D. Kahan

WHY ARE WE CONCERNED ABOUT THE PHARMACOKINETICS OF CYCLOSPORIN A?

What distinguishes cyclosporin A (CsA) from other medications (e.g. beta-blockers) whose pharmacokinetics are of interest only to a specialized group of clinical pharmacologists and not to the medical profession at large who prescribe these drugs on a daily basis? Why is it that one can claim rightfully that the proper therapeutic use of CsA requires an understanding and appreciation of its pharmacokinetics? The answer is simple: standard dosing regimens of CsA do not work because the therapeutic range of CsA is narrow and the variability of its dose–concentration relationship (i.e. pharmacokinetics) is large between different patients and within an individual patient. This predicament leaves the physician only two choices: (1) he uses standardized, but subtherapeutic, doses of CsA, and he substitutes with therapeutic doses of other conventional immunosuppressive medications (azathioprine, anti-lymphocyte globulin), thus exploiting a putatively synergistic effect of CsA; or (2) he individualizes the CsA dose for each patient by strictly monitoring CsA blood concentrations. The latter approach can be applied successfully only when the pharmacokinetic properties of CsA are taken into account. It is self-evident that this chapter will appeal only to those who try to exploit the uniquely selective effects of CsA by prescribing it in therapeutic doses as the cornerstone of their immunomodulating strategy.

Granted that monitoring is an essential part of CsA therapy, why should we monitor blood concentrations? Wouldn't it be more logical to monitor CsA concentration at the site of action, or, even better, to monitor directly the therapeutic or toxic effects? Attempts have been made to quantify the immunosuppressive effect of CsA[1], namely by using the ratio of T4 and T8 lymphocytes, a mixed lymphocyte proliferation assay, and the measurement by a dependent cell line or monoclonal antibodies of interleukin-2 (IL-2) produced during the mixed lymphocyte reaction. All these measurements are rather time-consuming and lack specificity for CsA. On the other hand, the

252

toxic effects of CsA are monitored more easily. While parameters describing renal and hepatic function as part of routine blood biochemistry provide a general indication of CsA toxicity, biopsies and isotope scanning techniques can afford more specific answers. In addition, hypertension and glucose intolerance are readily detected. In contrast, other observations such as rejection and infection can be classified as all-or-none responses. All pharmacodynamic measurements have in common the fact that they are related to the dose rate of CsA in some non-linear fashion which makes it practically impossible to decide dosage adjustments, e.g. how much to reduce the oral dose rate once an increase in bilirubin indicates hepatotoxicity.

Since it is quite likely that CsA obeys the rules of linear pharmacokinetics (evidence will be provided later in this chapter), concentrations measured at steady state should be directly proportional to the dose rate. If the site of action of CsA were known, and if samples could be obtained from it to measure concentrations, clearly these 'effect compartment' concentrations would be the focus of monitoring. At the present time, however, CsA concentrations in blood (this term will henceforth be used whenever a specification such as serum, plasma or whole blood is not necessary) is the only clinically useful feedback information on which dosing decisions can be based.

SOURCES OF PHARMACOKINETIC VARIABILITY

Before we can look at strategies to cope with the high degree of pharmacokinetic variability of CsA we have to learn about its sources. A general source of variability is the error associated with the method of measuring CsA concentrations in blood. Of all the available methods[2], high-performance liquid chromatography (HPLC) of whole-blood samples shows the highest degree of accuracy and precision, and was therefore selected as the standard[3] against which other methods are compared. Until recently a polyclonal radioimmunoassay was the most widely used test[4]. Its lack of specificity for unchanged CsA did not prevent its clinical acceptance. Now that this assay is no longer commercially available, many laboratories have had to switch to alternatives, and at the same time have had to adjust the therapeutic range of CsA concentrations. A recently published correlation[2] between five different assays in serum and whole blood may serve as a rough guideline.

Variability in absorption

The bioavailability of CsA (i.e. the fraction of the oral dose which reaches the central circulation intact) is highly variable and generally ranges between 10% and 70%[5]. The reason is not a high first-pass effect in the liver but is, instead, an incomplete absorption from the gut lumen into the portal blood.

An optimal and consistent absorption of CsA starts with the proper mixing of the oral formulation (Sandimmun®) with the drink. Though not conclusively studied, chocolate milk seems to be the optimal vehicle for the dispersion of the oral formulation which consists of 30 parts emulsifier

253

(peglicol-5-oleate), 60 parts olive oil, and 10 parts ethanol. Mixing with any other drink, however, still provides better absorption than direct ingestion of the formulation.

It was recently shown by Wadhwa and co-workers[6] that CsA is not absorbed in the stomach. The acceleration of gastric emptying by metoclopramide led to earlier absorption; also, the fraction of the oral dose which was absorbed was increased, probably due to simultaneous emptying of the gall bladder.

In general, sufficient bile flow into the small intestine seems to be a prerequisite for optimal absorption of CsA. In this respect extracorporal diversion of bile after liver transplantation causes poor absorption[7]. The negative correlation between bioavailability and alanine transaminase activity[8] can also be explained by impaired liver function which is accompanied by reduced bile flow. Furthermore, the increased area under the blood concentration–time curve (AUC), observed when CsA was given with food in a controlled study[9], indicates higher absorption in the presence of a bile release triggered by a solid meal. Even the circadian differences in CsA pharmacokinetics which were recently reported[10] are likely to be caused by oral dosing without (A.M.) and with (P.M.) solid food.

Bone marrow transplantation patients with intestinal dysfunction from various causes (e.g. chemoradiation, *Candida* enteritis, or acute graft-versus-host disease of the intestine) showed smaller AUC values than control patients[11]. Those patients with a diarrhoea volume greater than 500 ml/72 h had a significant reduction in AUC. This phenomenon can be explained by the fact that CsA seems to be absorbed only in the upper part of the small intestine[12] by a process of limited capacity[13]. Therefore, when the transit time is short, absorption is impaired. Second peaks in the pharmacokinetic profiles of CsA are quite frequent (Figure 12.1). They are not caused by enterohepatic recycling of CsA since only very small amounts of unchanged CsA are present in bile[14]. They are likely to be a combination of recycling metabolites and a delayed portion of the oral dose which was trapped in the stomach by incomplete emptying.

The role of lymphatic absorption of CsA was addressed in several animal experiments. Measurements of CsA in thoracic duct lymph are not conclusive since there is transfer of CsA from blood to lymph, at least in rats[15]. Determination of CsA concentrations in intestinal lymph of rats showed that lymphatic absorption is minimal compared with absorption into the systemic circulation[16]. High concentrations of CsA were found in thoracic duct lymph in dogs[12], but no calculations were performed regarding the fraction of the dose absorbed lymphatically. This finding was again validated in rats[17]; these investigators also studied the influence of the vehicle on thoracic duct CsA levels, and a high dispersion of CsA in mixed micelles proved to be optimal. Recently, the total amount of CsA in intestinal lymph of rats was recovered after intraduodenal dosing[18]; again, it was shown that, despite high concentrations, only around 1% of the administered dose was absorbed via this route. In transplant patients, intravenous dosing of CsA leads to considerably higher lymphatic concentrations than does oral dosing[19], yet it is known that both routes provide effective protection against graft rejection. Targeting CsA formulations towards the lymphatic system[20] therefore provides no therapeutic

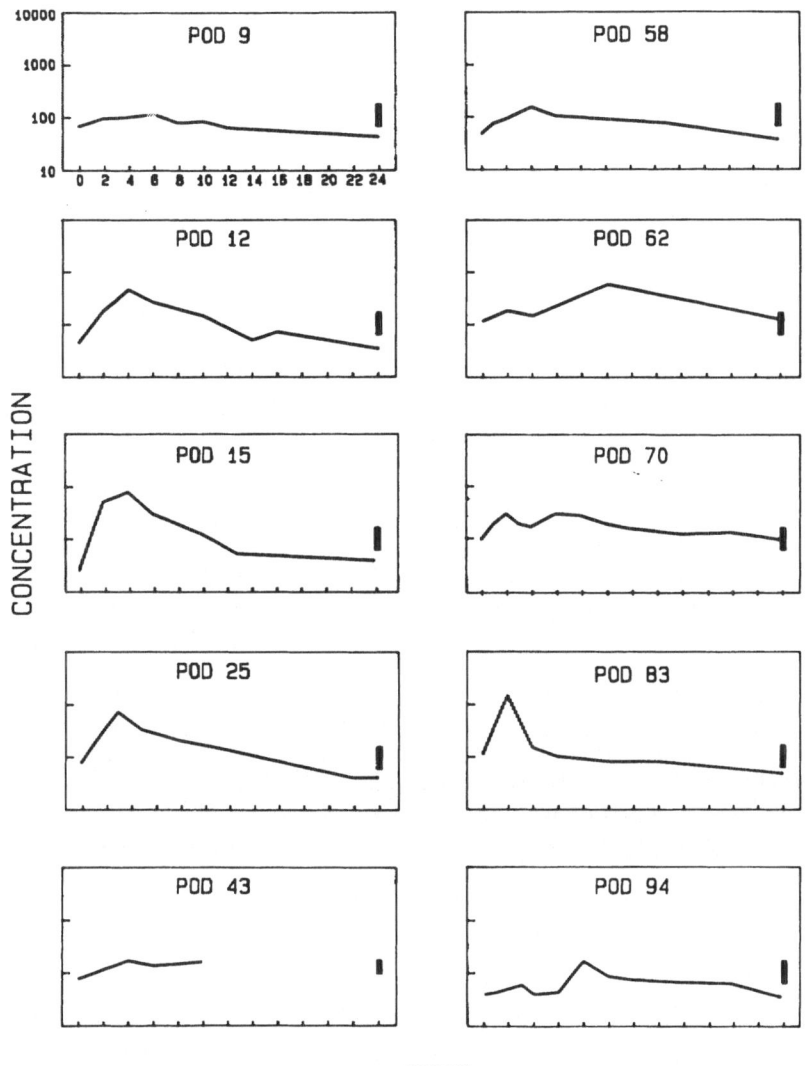

Figure 12.1 AUC monitoring in patient A.M. between postoperative day (POD) 9 and 94. The bar at the right end of each panel indicates the therapeutic range for 24-h trough levels (50–150 ng/ml)

advantage. However, formulations, which reduce the variability in CsA absorption would be very desirable.

The oral CsA dose rate required to achieve therapeutic blood concentrations declines with time after transplantation. This phenomenon has been demonstrated in several hundred pharmacokinetic profiles as an increase of the AUC per dose unit[21]. Either the absorption of CsA increases continuously with

255

time or the drug (or its metabolites) has the ability to impede its own elimination. It is interesting to note in this context that CsA was shown to interact directly with some types of cytochrome P-450 in a mouse model[22].

Variability in distribution

The volume of distribution of CsA at steady state in adult patients is several hundred litres. This is the volume in which the amount of CsA in the body would have to dissolve to reach a uniform concentration equal to the average concentration in blood at steady state. The size of this theoretical parameter indicates clearly that CsA does not uniformly distribute throughout the body. To the contrary, this agent is extensively bound within the blood compartment and even more to tissues. CsA is not only a very lipophilic compound but also a very large molecule (1202 dalton) by comparison with other drugs. The maximal solubility in pure water at 37°C is 3000 ng/ml, but such concentrations are never reached in the body where favourable binding partners are abundant. As a matter of fact, it is extremely difficult to determine exactly what fraction of CsA is unbound in plasma water. An ultracentrifugation method[23] produced highly variable results, and the free fraction varied between 4% and 12% within and between patients. Equilibrium dialysis in specifically designed steel chambers to reduce binding to the surface yielded more consistent results[24]: the free fraction ranged between 1.0% and 2.4% in plasma samples with a total CsA concentration ranging between 100 and 3000 ng/ml as determined by HPLC. Serial determinations of the unbound fraction in 66 renal transplant patients did not provide any correlation with clinical events[25], nor with selected lipoprotein markers in plasma[26].

Of the CsA bound in plasma at 37°C, 34% is associated with LDL, another 34% with HDL, 10% with VLDL, and the remaining 22% is bound to non-lipoproteins[27]. Non-covalent associative forces permit rapid exchange reactions between protein-bound fractions[28] and cell membranes, possibly via lipoprotein receptors. In this respect, it seems likely that in the case of CsA, contrary to the pharmacological models developed for smaller more hydrophilic compounds, the lipoprotein-bound fraction and not the free fraction is biologically active. This hypothesis is supported by the fact that 78% of the variability in CsA clearance (calculated from HPLC concentrations in plasma) could be explained by the triglyceride and cholesterol content of LDL, while the free fraction was not a determinant[29]. The distribution of CsA among the different lipoprotein classes is not affected by food intake[30], and one can infer that clearance also will be unaffected by meals.

About 50% of the CsA in whole blood is bound to erythrocytes[31] in a temperature-dependent[32] and saturable fashion[33]. Erythrocytes contain a CsA-binding protein[34] which is structurally different from haemoglobin, calmodulin and also from cyclophilin, a ubiquitous binding protein in other tissues[35]. While the ratio of CsA trough concentrations in whole blood over plasma increases with the haematocrit[36], the clearance of CsA is not correlated with it[8].

CsA concentrations in tissues are several times higher than blood concentrations. After dosing $10 \, mg \, kg^{-1} day^{-1}$ [^{3}H]cyclosporine for 21 days to rats, the following factors for tissue over blood were measured[37]: 5.4 for muscle, 16 for skin, 14 for fat, 1.1 for kidney, 9.5 for liver, and 0.02 for brain. CsA concentrations in tissues obtained at postmortem examinations[38] are probably not representative, since CsA therapy was discontinued while the patients were fighting the infections. Kidney needle biopsies performed routinely in renal transplant patients under CsA therapy contained concentrations (by polyclonal radioimmunoassay) 6 to 7 times higher than in plasma. During episodes of nephrotoxicity, kidney tissue levels were 19 times higher than plasma levels[39]. The pharmacodynamic relevance of tissue concentrations is still unclear; however, it is important to keep in mind that the body tissues constitute a large reservoir, which after cessation of CsA therapy is emptied slowly via the blood circulation over the course of several weeks.

Variability in elimination

Drugs can be eliminated from the body either by excretion of the unchanged compound in urine and/or bile or by metabolism. All routes of elimination contribute to the total body clearance of the drug. In the case of CsA, elimination occurs predominantly by metabolism in the liver[40] and only less than 1% of an oral dose is excreted unchanged in urine[40] or bile[41]. Therefore, total clearance and hepatic clearance are identical. The comparison of the average CsA clearance from whole blood (500 ml/min)[8] with the average hepatic blood flow (1400 ml/min) demonstrates that CsA does not have a high extraction ratio. The same conclusion was recently drawn from a pharmacokinetic experiment in rats[42]. Despite a 30% reduction in hepatic blood flow due to shunting the portal and caval vein CsA clearance did not change[42]. A similar independence from liver blood flow can be expected in transplant patients. On the other hand, changes in the intrinsic activity of the metabolizing enzymes and changes in binding of CsA in blood (see above) are prone to influence CsA clearance.

The strongest effect on the metabolizing enzymes is exerted by drugs which are known for pharmacokinetic interactions with CsA (see chapter 14). Several factors indicative of liver function were tested in 30 uraemic patients awaiting renal transplants. Only alanine transaminase activity, but not aspartate transaminase, lactate dehydrogenase, or alkaline phosphatase activity, nor the total bilirubin concentration, correlated with clearance[8]. Two other reports, however, found elevated serum bilirubin to be indicative of impaired liver function and reduced CsA clearance[21,43]. Reduced hepatic function is known to result in less bile production and an accumulation of CsA metabolites in blood[44]. The former effect may cause a reduced absorption, while the latter effect may result in a decreased clearance when measurements are made with a non-specific assay. The net effect on the oral clearance of CsA (clearance over bioavailability) is therefore not predictable.

Body size of adult patients seems to have no influence on the capacity of the liver to eliminate CsA. Neither body weight, surface area, nor the percentage of ideal weight correlated with CsA clearance determined by specific and non-specific assays. On the contrary, normalization of clearance by body weight introduced additional variability into the parameter estimate[8]. In that respect, the dosing of adult patients on a body-weight basis counteracts the implied intention: it increases pharmacokinetic variability.

One of the best-established determinants of CsA clearance is the patient's age. Children have generally higher clearances than adults[45,46] and the weight-normalized clearance is highest in very young paediatric patients. Indeed, patients under the age of 10 years had a clearance four times higher than patients older than 40 years[45]. But even this well-established relationship between the patient's age and CsA clearance is contaminated by so much intersubject variability, as are any of the above-mentioned relationships with other demographic factors, that it cannot be used to reliably predict an individual patient's clearance and dosing requirement.

HOW CAN WE USE PHARMACOKINETICS TO OPTIMIZE CsA THERAPY?

Of the host of pharmacokinetic parameters presented in the literature, only three are useful for the clinical management of patients on continuous CsA therapy. The bioavailability, F, is the fraction of the oral dose which reaches the central circulation intact. The clearance, CL, is the proportionality constant between dose rate (amount given per unit of time) and steady-state concentration. Finally, the half-life is the time which elapses while concentrations fall by 50% when no further dose is given. The half-life also determines how fast steady state is reached while the dose rate is kept constant. As a rule of thumb, steady state is reached after 2 days of continuously infusing CsA when the patient receives the drug for the first time. When infusion rates are changed, the new steady state is reached within 24 h. When CsA is given orally, steady state (no changes in peak and trough levels) can be assumed after giving three doses, provided the dosing interval is not shorter than 12 h.

Intravenous and oral dose linearity

A major prerequisite for using pharmacokinetics as a tool to optimize CsA therapy is a linear relationship between dose rate and steady-state concentrations (i.e. dose linearity). The intravenous dose linearity of CsA was tested immediately after renal transplantation in 30 patients who initially received a standard intravenous infusion of $2.5\ mg\ kg^{-1}\ day^{-1}$ for 3 days (J. Grevel et al., in preparation)[47]. At the end of the third day the steady-state concentration, C_{ss}, was measured as the mean of five hourly blood concentrations. Thereafter the infusion rate was deliberately changed by a factor ranging from 0.4 to 2.4. The new C_{ss} was determined 24–48 h later, and the error or deviation from the rule of proportionality was expressed as a percentage of the expected C_{ss}. The mean error was not significantly different from 0%; however, the spread was considerable, ranging from -60% to $+80\%$. C_{ss} measured in serum by the polyclonal radioimmunoassay lay within $\pm 20\%$ of expectation in only 10 of 30 cases. Measurements in whole blood by HPLC showed a better performance with 14 of 24 cases within $\pm 20\%$. The study demonstrated, on the one hand, intravenous dose linearity for CsA, but on the other hand it detected considerable intrasubject pharmacokinetic variability during the first days after transplantation.

The oral dose linearity of CsA in renal transplant patients was demonstrated by two approaches[48]. First, 71 AUCs at steady state were calculated for 36 patients up to 36 months after transplantation, and they were significantly correlated with the oral dose rate ($r = 0.538, p = 0.0001$). Second, the error in average steady-state concentrations, $C_{ss\,av}$, calculated by dividing the AUC at steady state by the dosing interval (24 h) associated with 38 dose changes in 25 patients during the first 3 months after transplantation, was not significantly different from 0%. The range -30 to $+44\%$, was narrower than after changes in intravenous dose rates. Both observations argue in favour of an oral dose linearity of CsA. These findings in a clinical setting contrast pharmacokinetic studies of CsA in the rabbit where non-linearity was observed[49].

Trough level monitoring

Dosage adjustments based on trough level monitoring have to follow a strict pattern when they intend to take advantage of the dose linearity of CsA. All trough concentrations have to be measured at the same time after the dose is given, e.g. at 24 h when the schedule is once-daily. The trough level on which a dose adjustment is based has to reflect clinical steady state, i.e. it has to be drawn after 3 days of unaltered dosing. The principle of linearity dictates that the oral dose rate has to be increased by the same factor by which the trough level deviates from the target. But intrasubject variability, especially during the first weeks after transplantation, demands a check on the new trough level after steady state is again reached.

Adjusting the dosing interval while leaving the dose rate unchanged results in a situation whose outcome cannot be easily predicted. A shortening of the dosing interval generally increases the trough concentration and decreases the peak concentration ($C_{ss\,av}$ remains the same). The increase in the trough level, however, cannot be predicted without modelling the complete pharmacokinetic profile of the individual patient. Furthermore, 12-h and 24-h trough concentrations are two different optimization criteria requiring different target ranges. The same also applies to a continuous infusion where the dosing interval is formally zero. Unless target ranges are defined for different dosing intervals, changes in the intervals cannot be rationally justified as an attempt to optimize CsA therapy.

Trough level monitoring of CsA is unlikely to benefit from traditional Bayesian forecasting techniques[50]. A simulated application[51] was restricted to intravenous infusions leading to steady state, and no strategies are included to deal with the most common and most serious complication after oral dosing: intrasubject variability in oral clearance (CL/F). A detailed argumentation in that respect was recently published[52].

ADVANTAGES OF AUC MONITORING OVER TROUGH LEVEL MONITORING

The practical problems of monitoring trough levels are illustrated in Figure 12.1 The patient suffered from rejection on postoperative day (POD) 9, which was correctly indicated by a trough level below the target of 50–150 ng/ml for serum concentrations measured by polyclonal radioimmunoassay. However, trough levels below target on POD 12, 15 and 25 were measured while there was no rejection. During a subsequent period of severe chronic nephrotoxicity trough levels were either within (POD 43, 62 and 70) or below target (POD 58 and 83). Again on POD 94 the trough level was below target while there was no rejection. It is evident that the shapes, peaks, and AUCs of the curves varied considerably while the trough levels fluctuated only within a rather narrow range.

While 71 AUCs of 36 patients significantly correlated with the oral dose rate ($r = 0.538, p = 0.0001$), the corresponding trough levels (the 24-h time points of the AUCs) did not ($r = 0.136, p = 0.26$). Also the absolute error associated with 38 dose changes in 25 patients was significantly larger ($p = 0.0005$) when the new steady state was monitored as a trough level (mean = 30.6%) compared with an AUC (mean = 13.6%). Already, other investigators have noted the lack of correlation between steady-state trough concentration and oral dose rate[53] and have subsequently dismissed all monitoring as useless[54].

We believe that the response to the dissatisfying performance of trough level monitoring should not be 'no monitoring' but rather 'more monitoring'. AUC monitoring offers not only better performance in reaching the therapeutic range, but also one consistent target for any oral dosing interval and for continuous intravenous infusions.

AUC monitoring

The basic element of this strategy is a series of seven blood concentrations drawn during a 24-h dosing interval (0, 2, 4, 6, 10, 14, and 24 h), or five blood samples during a 12-h dosing interval (0, 2, 4, 8, and 12 h). These series are drawn only at clinical steady state. The AUC is calculated by the trapezoidal rule, and the C_{ssav} is obtained by dividing the AUC by the dosing interval.

An identical target concentration of 200 ng/ml applies for C_{ss} during intravenous infusion and for C_{ssav} during oral dosing. This target was identified when, in a group of 250 patients receiving steady-state infusions initially after renal transplantation, the incidence of rejection and nephrotoxicity was associated with $C_{ss} < 150$ ng/ml and $C_{ss} > 250$ ng/ml, respectively[55].

The initial intravenous (i.v.) and oral (p.o.) dose rates for a patient after renal transplantation are calculated using the following equations:

$$\text{i.v. dose rate} = CL \cdot C_{ss} \tag{1}$$

$$\text{p.o. dose rate} = CL/F \cdot C_{ssav} \tag{2}$$

where C_{ss} and C_{ssav} are 200 ng/ml and CL and F are the individual kinetic parameters of the patient. These parameters cannot be calculated by knowing the patient's demographic factors, since the relationships between pharmacokinetic parameters and patient demographics are afflicted with too much variability (see above). The parameters must be obtained from pre-transplant pharmacokinetic studies. For that purpose patients on the transplant waiting list receive 3.0 mg/kg CsA as a 1 h infusion and 14 mg/kg as a single oral dose 2 days later. Both doses are followed by serial blood sampling (15 samples for i.v. and 12 samples for p.o.) for 24 h. The Cl and F are calculated from the two AUCs. Table 12.1 lists a comparison of paired pharmacokinetic parameters before and after transplantation. The significantly increased CL after transplantation caused 23 of 35 C_{ss} to be below 150 ng/ml. This situation prompted us to increase the calculated i.v. infusion rate by 50%. Subsequently only one of nine C_{ss} was below 150 ng/ml, and the rest fell within the acceptable range of 150–250 ng/ml. The pre-transplant infusion reached very high concentrations in all patients (> 2000 ng/ml) which had the potential of causing non-linear effects. After the pre-transplant infusion was prolonged to 2 h and the high concentrations were avoided, the discrepancy between pre- and post-transplant CL was reduced (Table 12.2) and, using equation (1)

Table 12.1 Comparison of pharmacokinetic parameter values before and after transplantation[a]

Parameter	Pre-transplant	Post-transplant	p
CL (ml min^{-1} kg^{-1})	10.7 ± 5.1	15.3 ± 8.8	<0.01[b]
F (%)	38.6 ± 17.6	49.3 ± 24.2	0.03[c]

[a]Measurements were made in serum by the polyclonal radioimmunoassay. The time between the pre-transplant pharmacokinetic study and the transplant operation ranged from 1 to 24 weeks. Post-transplant pharmacokinetic parameters (CL and F) were measured during the first 5 days
[b]Level of statistical significance comparing pre- and post-transplant CL values, using the Wilcoxon sign rank test on 30 paired observations
[c]Level of significance comparing pre- and post-transplant F values, using Student's t-test on 27 paired observations

Table 12.2 Comparison of pre- and post-transplant pharmacokinetic parameters[a]

	Pre-transplant		Post-transplant	
Patient no.	CL (ml min^{-1} kg^{-1})	F (%)	CL (ml min^{-1} kg^{-1})	F (%)
39	7.1	34	5.4	22
44	11.7	32	14.4	90
57	8.4	37	28.9	43
58	10.8	44	14.3	54
59	5.9	36	7.5	70
60	16.8	52	14.3	43
62	7.3	40	10.0	100
64	4.8	37	6.2	88
Mean[b]	9.1	39	12.6	64
	3.9	6	7.6	27

[a]Conditions are identical to Table 12.1, except the pre-transplant infusion ran for 2 h, and no more than 12 weeks elapsed between the pre- and post-transplant determinations.
[b]The numbers are too small for meaningful statistical tests.

without correction, C_{ss} was below 150 ng/ml in only two of eight cases. The prediction of the post-transplant F from pre-transplant determinations is almost impossible because the variability in this parameter, especially after transplantation, is too high. Therefore we perform an absorption test post-transplant (see below) in every patient while the infusion of CsA is still running.

After the initial dose rates are established, the AUC monitoring strategy is executed as outlined in Figure 12.2. In living related transplant patients, the calculated intravenous infusion rate can be tested immediately before the scheduled transplant, and an adjusted rate can be used after transplantation if C_{ss} is outside the range of 150–250 ng/ml. During the first postoperative day (POD) the infusion starts 6 h after the end of surgery at 25% of the calculated rate. After 2, 4, and 6 h the rate is increased to 50%, 75%, and 100%, respectively. On POD 2 C_{ss} is tested with a series of five blood samples between approximately 40 and 48 h after start of the infusion.

Concentrations of CsA in serum measured by the polyclonal radioimmunoassay, RIA, and by the fluorescent polarization immunoassay, TDX, are equivalent once steady state is reached (for C_{ss}: TDX $= 0.97 \cdot$ RIA $- 13.78$, $r = 0.857$, $p = 0.0001$, $n = 35$; for C_{ssav}: TDX $= 1.06 \cdot$ RIA $+ 20.67$, $r = 0.810$, $p = 0.0001$, $n = 173$). Thereafter during POD 3, the continuous infusion is still running, and an oral dose calculated for 24 h is given simultaneously to test the absorption. Blood samples are drawn 1, 2, 3, 4, 6, and 8 h after the oral dose. The five concentrations describing C_{ss} are averaged, and the difference to the highest concentration after the oral dose is calculated. The patient passes the absorption test and continues on oral dosing without infusion when the difference is > 400 ng/ml. Otherwise, the infusion continues, if necessary at an adjusted rate, when C_{ss} is outside the 150–250 ng/ml range, and the absorption test is repeated once C_{ss} is again established. After the first oral dose without infusion (ideally on POD 4) blood samples are drawn 10, 11, and 12 h after dosing. All three concentrations have to be larger than 100 ng/ml in order to continue with once-a-day dosing. Otherwise, CsA is given as half the calculated daily dose every 12 h. The third oral dose without infusion (ideally on POD 6) is accompanied by seven blood samples at 0, 2, 4, 6, 10, 14, and 24 h for the calculation of C_{ssav}. If the dosing interval is 12 h the C_{ssav} is calculated from five concentrations at 0, 2, 4, 8, and 12 h. The oral dose rate is adjusted proportionally if C_{ssav} deviates more than $\pm 20\%$ from the target of 200 ng/ml. No earlier than after three doses is the C_{ssav} tested again. Even if no adjustment is necessary, the C_{ssav} is measured after 1–2 weeks and then once monthly for 6 months and occasionally thereafter.

Between January and October 1988, 60 renal transplant patients were followed by the AUC monitoring strategy. Thirty-one patients were evaluated at 3–4 months after transplantation. Of a total of nine rejection episodes which were accompanied by a C_{ss} or a C_{ssav} between POD 1 and 15, five occurred in patients who had C_{ss} or C_{ssav} below 150 ng/ml during this period. There were also five episodes of nephrotoxicity, three of which occurred in patients with C_{ss} or C_{ssav} above 250 ng/ml. The numbers are still too small to draw statistical conclusions, but the overall experience is encouraging. It may seem that the analytical burden of AUC monitoring is considerable, but one

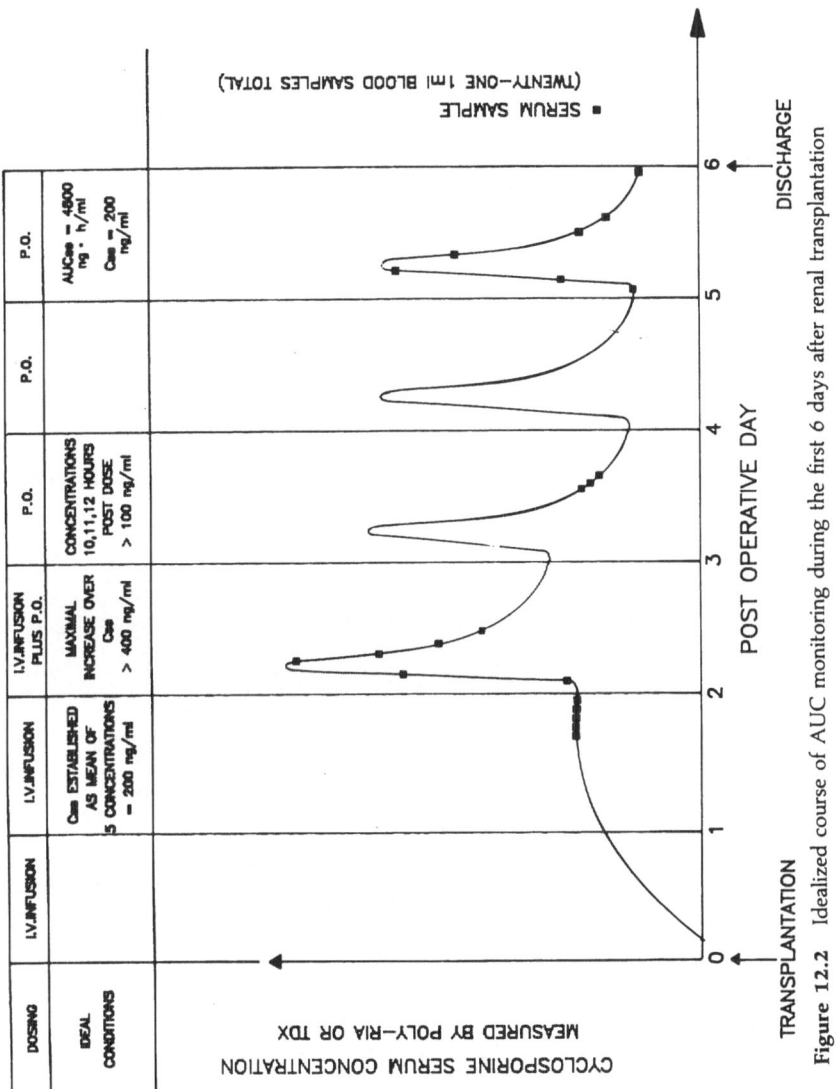

Figure 12.2 Idealized course of AUC monitoring during the first 6 days after renal transplantation

has to take into account that the target concentration is reached with more precision, and that less dosage adjustments are necessary than with conventional trough level monitoring. The target of 200 ng/ml for C_{ssav} requires oral starting doses of 400 mg/24 h, or 6 mg/kg per 24 h on average. This is about half of the dose previously used in our centre, and is roughly equivalent to doses used in multiple-drug protocols of immunosuppression. Furthermore, the hospital stay of patients with initial graft function and without early rejection is only 6 days. The AUC monitoring strategy is presently based on serum concentrations measured by RIA or TDX. Whole blood samples have been drawn in all patients, and the measurements by HPLC and monoclonal RIA will be analysed retrospectively to determine the therapeutic target for those methods.

ACKNOWLEDGEMENTS

Our research presented in this chapter was supported by a grant (DK 38016) of the National Institute of Diabetes, Digestive, and Kidney Disease.

REFERENCES

1. Kahan, B. D. (1985) Individualization of cyclosporine therapy using pharmacokinetic and pharmacodynamic parameters. *Transplantation*, **40**, 457–476.
2. Gibbons, S., Grevel, J., Reynolds, K., Ried, M., Rutzky, L. P. and Kahan, B. D. (1988) Comparison and correlation of assays for monitoring cyclosporine drug levels in renal transplant recipients. *Transplant. Proc.*, **20** (Suppl. 2), 339–344.
3. Shaw, L. M., Bowers, L., Demers, L., Freeman, D., Moyer, T., Sanghvi, A., Seltman, H. and Venkataramanan, R. (1987) Report of the task force on cyclosporine monitoring. *Clin. Chem.*, **33**, 1269–1288.
4. Donatsch, P., Abisch, E., Homberger, M., Traber, R., Trapp, M. and Voges, R. (1981) A radioimmunoassay to measure cyclosporin A in plasma and serum samples. *J. Immunoassay*, **2**, 19–32.
5. Grevel, J. (1986) Absorption of cyclosporine A after oral dosing. *Transplant. Proc.*, **18** (Suppl. 5), 9–15.
6. Wadhwa, N. K., Schroeder, T. J., O'Flaherty, E., Pesce, A. J., Myre, S. A. and First, M. R. (1987) The effect of oral metoclopramide on the absorption of cyclosporine. *Transplantation*, **43**, 211–213.
7. Tredger, J. M., Naomov, N. V., Steward, C. M., O'Grady, J. G., Grevel, J., Niven, A. A., Kelmann, A. W., Whiting, B. and Williams, R. (1988). Influence of biliary T tube clamping on cyclosporine pharmacokinetics in liver transplant recipients. *Transplant. Proc.*, **20** (Suppl. 2), 512–515.
8. Grevel, J., Reynolds, K. L., Rutzky, L. P. and Kahan, B. D. (1989) Influence of demographic factors on cyclosporine pharmacokinetics in adult uremic patients. *J. Clin. Pharmacol.*, **29**, 261–266.
9. Ptachcinski, R. J., Venkataramanan, R., Rosenthal, J. T., Burckart, G. J., Taylor, R. J. and Hakala, T. R. (1985) The effect of food on cyclosporine absorption. *Transplantation*, **40**, 174–176.
10. Canafax, D. M., Cipolle, R. J., Hrushesky, W. J. M., Rabatin, J. T., Min, D. I., Graves, N. M., Sutherland, D. E. R. and Bowers, L. D. (1988) The chronopharmacokinetics of cyclosporine and its metabolites in recipients of pancreas allografts. *Transplant. Proc.*, **20** (Suppl. 2), 471–477.
11. Atkinson, K., Britton, K., Paull, P., Farrell, C., Concannon, A., Dodds, A. and Biggs, J. (1983) Detrimental effect of intestinal disease on absorption administered cyclosporine. *Transplant. Proc.*, **15**, 2446–2449.

12. Wassef, R., Cohen, Z., Nordgren, S. and Langer, B. (1985) Cyclosporine absorption in intestinal transplantation. *Transplantation*, **39**, 496–499.
13. Grevel, J., Nuesch, E., Abisch, E. and Kutz, K. (1986) Pharmacokinetics of oral cyclosporine A (Sandimmun) in healthy subjects. *Eur. J. Clin. Pharmacol.*, **31**, 211–216.
14. Venkataramanan, R., Starzl, T. E., Yang, S., Burckart, G. J., Ptachcinski, R. J., Shaw, B. W. and Iwatsuki, S. (1985) Biliary excretion of cyclosporine in liver transplantation patients. *Transplant. Proc.*, **17**, 286–289
15. Ueda, C. T., Lemaire, M. and Misslin, P. (1983) Pharmacokinetic evaluation of the blood-to-lymph transfer of cyclosporine A in rats. *Biopharm. Drug Dispos.*, **4**, 83–94.
16. Ueda, C. T., Lemaire, M., Gsell, G. and Nussbaumer, K. (1983) Intestinal lymphatic absorption of cyclosporine A following oral administration in an olive oil solution in rats. *Biopharm. Drug Dispos.*, **4**, 113–124.
17. Takada, K., Shibata, N., Yoshimura, H., Masuda, Y., Yoshikawa, H., Muranishi, S. and Oka, T. (1985) Promotion of the selective lymphatic delivery of cyclosporin A by lipid-surfactant mixed micelles. *J. Pharmacobiodyn.*, **8**, 320–323.
18. Albrechtsen, D., Helgerud, P., Rugstad, H. E. and Dueland, S. (1985) Very high concentration in intestinal lymph after oral but not after intravenous cyclosporine in the rat. *Transplantation*, **40**, 220–222.
19. Ono, Y., Ohshima, S., Yamada, S., Hattori, R. and Hasegawa, S. (1988) Cyclosporine level of lymph in the thoracic duct and the lymph node. *Transplant. Proc.*, **20** (Suppl. 1), 167–169.
20. Takada, K., Yoshimura, H., Yoshikawa, H., Muranishi, S., Yasumura, T. and Oka, T. (1986) Enhanced selective lymphatic delivery of cyclosporin A by solubilizers and intensified immunosuppressive activity against mice skin allograft. *Pharm. Res.*, **3**, 48–51.
21. Kahan, B. D., Kramer, W. G., Wideman, C., Flechner, S. M., Lorber, M. I. and Van Buren, C. T. (1986) Demographic factors affecting the pharmacokinetics of cyclosporine estimated by radioimmunoassay. *Transplantation*, **41**, 459–464.
22. Moochhala, S. M. and Renton, K. W. (1986) Inhibition of hepatic microsomal drug metabolism by the immunosuppressive agent cyclosporin A. *Biochem. Pharmacol.*, **35**, 1499–1503.
23. Legg, B. and Rowland, M. (1987) Cyclosporin measurement of fraction unbound in plasma. *J. Pharm. Pharmacol.*, **39**, 599–603.
24. Henricsson, S. (1987) A new method for measuring the free fraction of cyclosporin in plasma by equilibrium dialysis. *J. Pharm. Pharmacol.*, **39**, 384–385.
25. Lindholm, A., Henricsson, S. and Gang, P. (1988) The free fraction of cyclosporine in plasma: clinical findings with a new method. *Transplant. Proc.*, **20** (Suppl. 2), 377–381.
26. Lindholm, A., Henricsson, S., Lind, M. and Dahlquist, R. (1988) Intraindividual variability in the relative systemic availability of cyclosporine after oral dosing. *Eur. J. Clin. Pharmacol.*, **34**, 461–464.
27. Gurecki, J., Warty, V. and Sanghvi, A. (1985) The transport of cyclosporine in association with plasma lipoproteins in heart and liver transplant patients. *Transplant. Proc.*, **17**(4), 1997–2002.
28. Mraz, W., Zink, R. A., Graf, A., Preis, D., Illner, W. D., Land, W., Siebert, W. and Zottlein, H. (1983) Distribution and transfer of cyclosporine among the various human lipoprotein classes. *Transplant. Proc.*, **15** (Suppl. 1), 2426–2429.
29. Lithell, H., Odlind, B., Selinus, I., Lindberg, A., Lindstrom, B. and Frodin, L. (1986) Is the plasma lipoprotein pattern of importance for treatment with cyclosporine? *Transplant. Proc.*, **18**, 50–51.
30. Sgoutas, D., MacMohon, W., Love, A. and Jerkunica, I. (1986) Interaction of cyclosporin A with human lipoproteins. *J. Pharm. Pharmacol.*, **38**, 583–588.
31. Lemaire, M. and Tillement, J. P. (1982) Role of lipoproteins and erythrocytes in the *in vitro* binding and distribution of cyclosporin A in the blood. *J. Pharm. Pharmacol.*, **34**, 715–718.
32. Wenk, M., Follath, F. and Abisch, E. (1983) Temperature dependency of apparent cyclosporin A concentrations in plasma. *Clin. Chem.*, **29**, 1865.
33. Legg, 5B. and Rowland, M. (1988) Saturable binding of cyclosporin A to erythrocytes: estimation of binding parameters in renal transplant patients and implications for bioavailability assessment. *Pharm. Res.*, **5**, 80–85.
34. Agarwal, R. P., McPherson, R. A. and Threatte, G. A. (1986). Evidence of a cyclosporine-

binding protein in human erythrocytes. *Transplantation*, **42**, 627–632.

35. Handschumacher, R. E., Harding, M. W., Rice, J., Drugger, R. J. and Speicher, D. (1984) Cyclophilin: a specific cytosolic binding protein for cyclosporin A. *Science*, **226**, 544–547.

36. Rosano, T. G. (1985) Effect of hematocrit on cyclosporine in whole blood and plasma of renal transplant patients. *Clin. Chem.*, **31**, 410–412.

37 Wagner, O., Schreier, E., Heitz, F. and Maurer, G. (1987) Tissue distribution, disposition and metabolism of cyclosporine in rats. *Drug Metab. Dispos.*, **15**, 377–383.

38. Ried, M., Gibbons, S., Kwok, D., Van Buren, C. T., Flechner, S. and Kahan, B. D. (1983) Cyclosporine levels in human tissues of patients treated for one week to one year. *Transplant. Proc.*, **15** (Suppl. I), 2434–2437.

39. Totterman, T. H., Lindgren, P. G., Frondin, L., Sjoberg, O., Wahlberg, J. and Tufveson, G. (1985) Cyclosporine determinations in kidney needle biopsies: method and clinical results. *Transplant. Proc.*, **17**, 2730–2731.

40. Maurer, G. and Lemaire, M. (1986) Biotransformation and distribution in blood of cyclosporine and its metabolites. *Transplant. Proc.*, **18** (Suppl. 5), 25–34.

41. Venkataramanan, R., Starzl, T. E., Yang, S., Burckart, G. J., Ptachcinski, R. J., Shaw, B. W., Iwatsuki, S., van Thiel, D. H., Sanghvi, A. and Seltman, H. (1985). Biliary excretion of cyclosporine in liver transplant patients. *Transplant. Proc.*, **17**, 286–289.

42. Grevel, J., Rigotti, P., Citterio, F., Plebani, M. and Kahan, B. D. (1989) The effect of end-to-side portacaval shunt on cyclosporine pharmacokinetics in rats. *Pharm. Res.*, **6**, 255–257.

43. Yee, G. C., Kennedy, M. S., Storb, R. and Thomas, E. D. (1984) Pharmacokinetics of intravenous cyclosporine in bone marrow transplant patients: comparison of two assay methods. *Transplantation*, **38**, 511–513.

44. Venkataramanan, R., Burckart, G. J. and Ptachcinski, R. J. (1985) Pharmacokinetics and monitoring of cyclosporine following orthotopic liver transplantation. *Semin. Liver Dis.*, **5**, 357–368.

45. Yee, G. C., Lennon, T. P., Gmur, D. J., Kennedy, M. S. and Deeg, H. J. (1986) Age-dependent cyclosporine pharmacokinetics in marrow transplant recipients. *Clin. Pharmacol. Ther.*, **40**, 438–443.

46. Lokiec, F., Fischer, A. and Gluckman, E. (1986) A safer approach to the clinical use of cyclosporine: the predose calculations. *Transplant. Proc.*, **18** (Suppl. 5), 194–199.

47. Grevel, J., Welsh, M. and Kahan, B. D. (1988) Linear cyclosporine pharmacokinetics. *Clin. Pharmacol. Ther.*, **43**, 175 (abstract).

48. Grevel, J., Welsh, M. and Kahan, B. D. (1980) Cyclosporine monitoring in renal transplantation: AUC monitoring is superior to trough level monitoring. *Ther. Drug Monit.* (In press).

49. Awni, W. M. and Sawchuk, R. J. (1985) The pharmacokinetics of cyclosporine. II. Blood plasma distribution and binding sites. *Drug Metab. Dispos.*, **13**, 133–138.

50. Sheiner, L. B., Beal, S. L., Rosenberg, B. and Marathe, V. V. (1979) Forecasting individual pharmacokinetics. *Clin. Pharmacol. Ther.*, **26**, 294–305.

51. Mentre, F., Mallet, A., Steimer, J.-L. and Lokiec, F. (1988) An application of population pharmacokinetics to the clinical use of cyclosporine in bone patients. *Transplant. Proc.*, **20** (Suppl. 2), 466–470.

52. Grevel, J. (1988). Significance of cyclosporine pharmacokinetics. *Transplant. Proc.*, **20** (Suppl. 2), 428–434.

53. Ferguson, R. M., Canafax, D. M., Sawchuk, R. T. and Simmons, R. L. (1986) Cyclosporine blood level monitoring: the early posttransplant period. *Transplant. Proc.*, **18** (Suppl. 1), 113–116.

54. Henry, M. L., Bowers, V. D., Fanning, W. J., Sommer, B. G. and Ferguson, R. M. (1988) Cyclosporine levels are not helpful. *Transplant. Proc.*, **20** (Suppl. 2), 419–421.

55. Dunn, J., Grevel, J., Napoli, K., Lewis, R. M., Van Buren, C. T. and Kahan, B. D. (1989) Impact of steady state cyclosporine concentrations on renal allograft outcome. *Transplant Proc.* (submitted).

13
Cyclosporin A Metabolism and Drug Interactions

M. Danny Burke, Fiona Macintyre, D. Cameron and Paul H. Whiting

ABBREVIATIONS

BNF, β-naphthoflavone; CsA, cyclosporin A; GT, glucuronyltransferase; HPLC, high performance (or pressure) liquid chromatography; PB, phenobarbitone; PCN, pregnenolone 16α-carbonitrile; RIA, radioimmunoassay; 3MC, 3-methylcholanthrene.

Cyclosporin A (CsA) has revolutionized post-transplantation immunosuppressive therapy, due to its potent selective immunological properties, and also has potential advantages over conventional treatments in the area of autoimmune diseases. However, the side-effects of CsA, of which nephrotoxicity and hepatotoxicity are the most clinically important, are still poorly understood, as also is the relationship between CsA metabolism and the induction and maintenance of immunosuppression and the mechanisms underlying its adverse effects. The purpose of this chapter is to review the metabolism and clinically important drug interactions of CsA in the context of its immunosuppressive and toxic properties. The reader is also referred to a recent review of various aspects of the pharmacokinetics, metabolism and analysis of CsA in patients, including the effects of disease and drug interactions[1].

CsA DISPOSITION*

Tissue localization

The absorption, distribution and elimination of CsA following its oral administration have been extensively studied in several experimental species,

*In the studies summarized in this section, unchanged CsA was not distinguished from its metabolites.

including rats, mice and dogs[2-4]. Between 4 and 24 h after its administration, CsA accumulates in most tissues, including skin, adipose tissue, liver and kidney, at concentrations 3−14 times those found in serum. In rats the highest concentrations were found in liver and kidney, followed by adipose tissue, endocrine organs (adrenals, pancreas, thymus and thyroid), lymph nodes, spleen and bone marrow, with lowest levels in skeletal muscle and brain. CsA uptake was particularly high in lymphomyeloid tissue, with a marked long-term retention of upto 10 days in liver, bone marrow and the cortical areas of lymph nodes[4]. Uptake into the kidney was restricted to the outer zone of the medulla, corresponding to proximal tubular epithelium and/or the thick ascending limb of Henle[4].

Although tissue distribution studies in man are less extensive, analysis of postmortem samples inicated a tissue distribution similar to that found in animals[5], with the highest levels following chronic dosage being found in fat, and low levels occurring in the brain and cerebrospinal fluid, which suggests that CsA does not cross the blood−brain barrier. Conversely, significant CsA levels have been observed in the cerebellum[6]. Although CsA was detected in all postmortem tissue samples tested up to 16 days following the cessation of drug treatment[7], other studies demonstrated that only body fat contained significant CsA levels 20 days following withdrawal of treatment[5]. Adipose tissue may, in fact, be a primary reservoir for CsA[8]. During pregnancy CsA is also present in amniotic fluid, while low levels are found in breast milk and also in the neonate's peripheral blood for up to 48 h after birth[9].

Subcellular localization

CsA is found in large cytosolic lipid droplets within lymphocytes and macrophages, due possibly to either endocytosis of plasma membrane containing CsA or a disturbance in lipid metabolism[10]. It has also been shown that cytosolic CsA is bound to the low molecular weight protein, cyclophilin[11]. A recent study demonstrated that the subcellular distribution of CsA in rat whole kidney was 60%, 20%, 10% and 7% in the soluble, mitochondrial/lysosomal, microsomal and nuclear fractions respectively[12]. In the same study[12] it was concluded, however, that from the distribution profiles of various marker enzymes, and taking into account histological considerations, the high CsA content of the soluble fraction was probably due to the disruption of lysosomes during homogenization of the kidney cortex.

Although no specific receptors for CsA were demonstrated on the surface of lymphocytes, and binding appeared to be the result of non-specific partitioning of CsA into membrane lipids[13], recent studies have suggested that CsA immunosuppression may be due, in part, to a specific blockade of the T-lymphocyte prolactin receptor[14,15].

CsA METABOLISM

Metabolite structures

The structures of 12 CsA metabolites and the pathways of CsA metabolism were described initially by Maurer et al.[16] and expanded subsequently[17,18].

Only a limited number of reactions are involved in CsA metabolism, which results in the structural modification of only four of the 11 amino acids, and the intact cyclic oligopeptide structure is retained in all identified metabolites (Figure 13.1). Biotransformation involves hydroxylation at the terminal carbons of the side-chains of amino acids 1, 4, 6 and 9, further oxidation of amino acid 1 to a carboxylic acid, N-demethylation of the methylated peptide-bond nitrogen of amino acid 4 and the formation of a cyclic ether on the side-chain of amino acid 1. Unfortunately, a rather confusing numerical nomenclature is generally used to designate the metabolites, which does not relate directly to the numbering of the atoms in the CsA structure[16]. There are two monohydroxy metabolites (M1 and M17), three dihydroxy metabolites (M8, M10 and M16), one N-desmethyl metabolite (M21), two hydroxy-N-desmethyl metabolites (M13 and M25), a dihydroxy-N-desmethyl metabolite (M9), a carboxylic acid metabolite (originally reported by Hartman et al.[17], but referred to as M203–M218 by Maurer and Lemaire[18]) and two metabolites, M18 and M26, which contain a cyclic ether moiety and are monohydroxylated and dihydroxylated respectively. It is generally accepted that the metabolites which incorporate more than one structural modification are 'secondary' metabolites formed by further metabolism of the 'primary' metabolites, M1, M17 and M21[18,19]: their structures and interrelationships are shown in Figure 13.2. The positions of metabolic substitution in the monohydroxy-N-desmethyl metabolite M13 have not yet been determined[18]. Several additional, incompletely identified CsA metabolites have recently been described[8,20,21]. The metabolism pathways for CsA are similar in mouse, rat, rabbit, dog, cat and human[18,28] and no glucuronide or sulphate conjugates of CsA have yet been discovered[16]. The hydroxylation, oxidation and N-demethylation reactions are considered to be enzymatic[18] (and see below), but the ether cyclization is thought to be spontaneous[16]. Differing opinions have been expressed as to whether the tritium in the radiolabelled CsA supplied by Sandoz for metabolism studies is stable[19,32].

The analysis of CsA and its metabolites is one of the more challenging assays in the fields of drug metabolism and therapeutic drug monitoring, and has been recently reviewed[1]. Virtually all of the CsA-derived compounds in combined rat, dog and human blood, bile and urine are soluble in methanol; 70% of these compounds, including all of the metabolites described above, are extractable into ether from water, while the 30% remaining in the aqueous phase include two additional, unidentified metabolites[16]. The carboxylic acid metabolite, M203–218, however, is soluble in ethyl acetate but not in ether[1]. If a protein precipitation step is used at the beginning of an analytical procedure, for example with blood or microsomal incubations, there is a danger that, due to their high lipophilicity, CsA and many of its metabolites will remain bound to the protein. Acetonitrile is currently favoured as a protein precipitant in CsA assays, since it is water-miscible and gives an aqueous solution of sufficiently high organic strength to strip most CsA-derived material from proteins, without dissolving excessive amounts of lipid, which could interfere at later stages of the assay. Most studies of CsA metabolism identify the metabolites by a comparison of HPLC retention times with those of authentic standards, but there are difficulties with this, primarily

CYCLOSPORIN

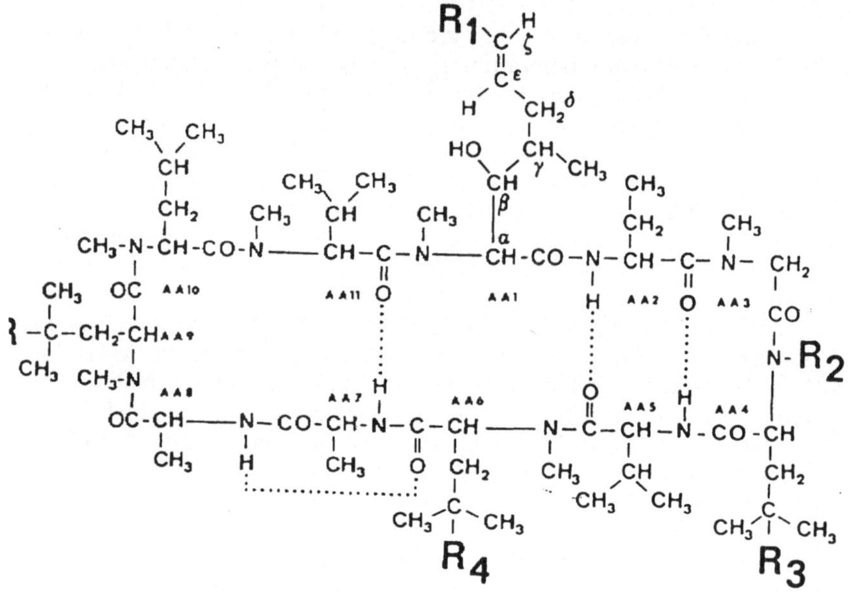

R$_1$

CH$_3$ CH$_3$
CH
CH$_2$
CH$_3$-N-CH-CO-N — CH-C-N — CH-CO-N-CH-C-N-CH$_2$
CH$_3$ OC AA10   AA11 O   AA1 H AA2 O AA3 CO
}-C-CH$_2$-CH AA9   N-R$_2$
CH$_3$ CH$_3$-N AA8   AA7 H   AA6 O AA5 H AA4
OC-CH — N-CO-CH-N-C-CH — N-C-CH-N-CO-CH
CH$_3$ H CH$_3$ O CH$_2$ CH$_3$ CH CH$_2$
R$_4$ R$_3$

Figure 13.1 structure (R$_1$–R$_4$ substituents shown)

Metabolite No.	R	R$_1$	R$_2$	R$_3$	R$_4$	Other modification	Molecular weigh'
Cyclosporine	H	CH$_3$	CH$_3$	H	H		1202.64
1	OH	CH$_3$	CH$_3$	H	H		1218.54
8	OH	CH$_2$OH	CH$_3$	H	H		1234.64
9	OH	CH$_3$	H	H	OH		1220.62
10	OH	CH$_3$	CH$_3$	OH	H		1234.64
13	hydroxylated and N-demethylated derivative of cyclosporine						1204.62
16	OH	CH$_3$	CH$_3$	H	OH		1234.64
17	H	CH$_2$OH	CH$_3$	H	H		1218.64
18	H	CH$_2$OH	CH$_3$	H	H	$\overset{O}{CH}\ CH-CH_2$ of AA1 $\beta\ \epsilon\ \zeta$	1218.64
21	H	CH$_3$	H	H	H		1188.62
25	H	CH$_2$OH	H	H	H		1202.64
26	OH	CH$_2$OH	CH$_3$	H	H	$\overset{O}{CH}\ CH-CH_2$ of AA1 $\beta\ \epsilon\ \zeta$	1204.62
203–218	H	COOH	CH$_3$	H	H		1234.64

Figure 13.1 CsA metabolite structures. Reproduced from reference 18 with permission

270

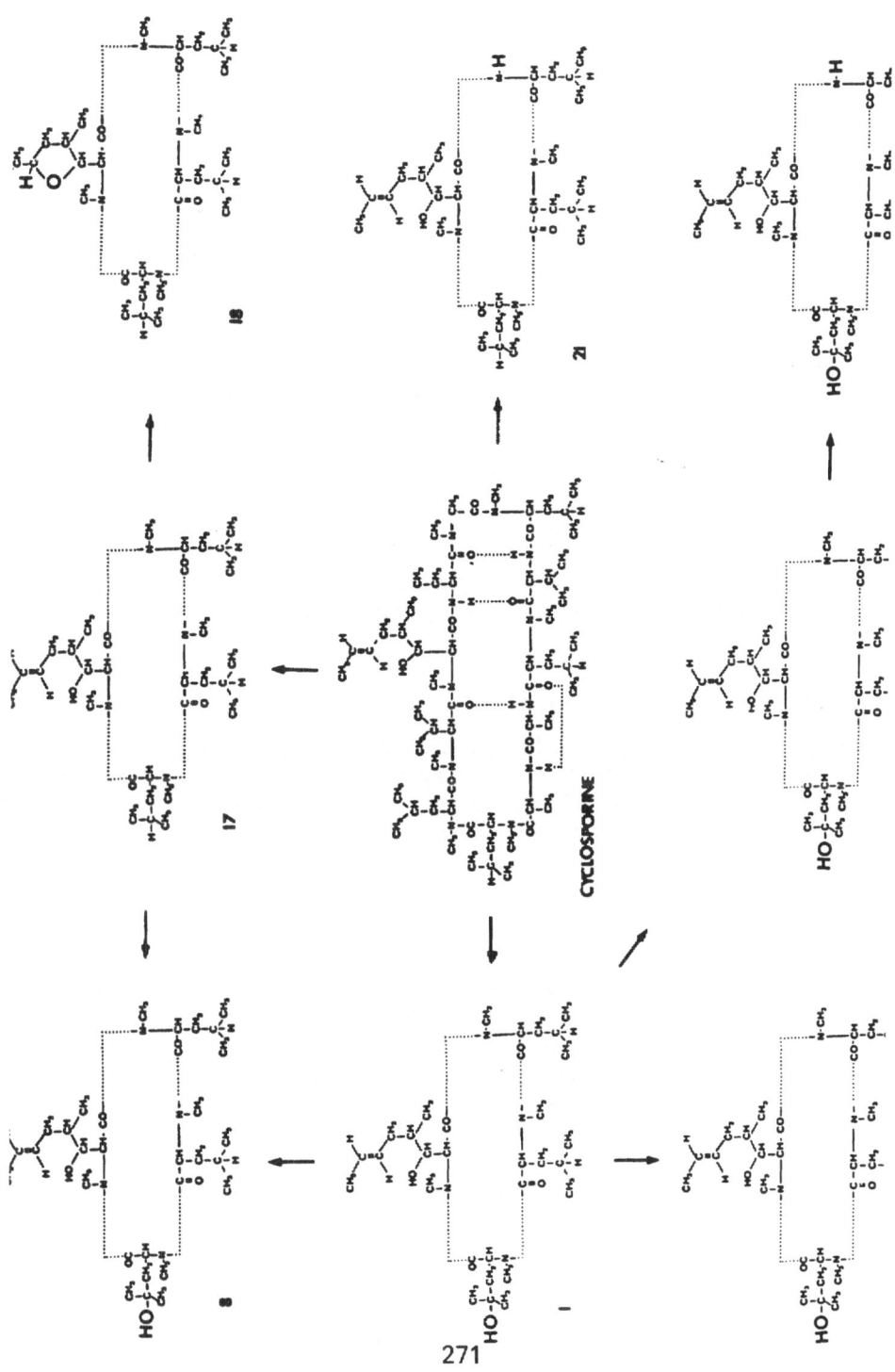

271

due to the large number of metabolites, the generally poor HPLC resolution achieved for many of them and, perhaps the greatest problem of all, the scarcity of authentic metabolites for use as standards. Several groups have recently addressed this problem by analysing HPLC peaks using fast atom bombardment ionization (FAB) and tandem mass spectrometry (FABMS and MS/MS)[20–22], but as yet these can hardly be viewed as routine procedures. Many clinical studies rely on radioimmunoassays (RIA). The original polyclonal antibodies used for this are now known to recognize CsA metabolites in addition to the parent compound, showing 32% cross-reactivity with M17 and 7–12% cross-reactivity with M1, M8, M18 and M21[23]. However, two new monoclonal antibodies are available for RIA, a 'non-specific' antibody, which measures CsA parent compound and its metabolites, and a 'specific' antibody, which measures almost exclusively the parent compound. Whereas the specific-RIA gives measurements that are virtually identical with CsA parent compound levels measured by HPLC[23], some 50–74% of the concentration determined in patients' blood by polyclonal and nonspecific RIA is CsA metabolites, with 95–98% of the nonspecific RIA measurement in blood of patients or rats being accounted for by CsA, M1 and M17 combined[24–26]. HPLC assay with UV detection and RIA have similar lower limits of detection: 20–30 ng/ml of blood[23,27–29]. It is considered that all CsA metabolites in patients' blood other than M17, M1 and M21 are below the current detection limit for routine clinical therapeutic drug monitoring[29].

CsA METABOLISM *IN VIVO*

CsA metabolites have been detected in blood, bile, urine, faeces and many tissues of man, rats and some other species. Whilst structures have been described only for the 12 metabolites referred to above, a total of 17 metabolites have been reported in human urine[20]. The liver is the organ primarily responsible for CsA metabolism, which is catalysed mainly by the cytochrome P-450-dependent microsomal mono-oxygenase enzyme system, in particular by members of the P-450III gene family[30,31,55] (and see below). The metabolism of CsA by cytochrome P-450 is doubly interesting in that peptides are uncommon substrates for this enzyme, and peptide nitrogen is a most unexpected site for its reaction. CsA is extensively metabolized in man and rats, with metabolites accounting for 50–70% of the total CsA-derived material in whole blood measured several hours after oral dosing with CsA[8,18,32]. CsA metabolites are absorbed more poorly but eliminated more rapidly than CsA itself[33,34]. In man and rats CsA is eliminated predominantly as a result of its metabolism in the liver, being excreted almost entirely as metabolites, which comprise greater than 95% of the total CsA-derived compounds in bile and urine[1,8,18,32,35]. There is evidence for enterohepatic recirculation of CsA in humans, which involves almost exclusively CsA metabolites rather than the parent compound[36,37]. In this respect the enterohepatic recirculation of CsA is unusual, since with most drugs recirculation involves the biliary excretion of conjugated metabolites, which are then hydrolysed by bacterial enzymes in the gut and reabsorbed as the parent compound, but the biliary CsA metabolites are not conjugates and are probably not reconverted back to CsA. A further consequence is that blood levels of CsA are unlikely to be affected by the administration of antibiotics which decrease intestinal bacteria. CsA metabolite profiles are similar in blood, bile and urine, but there is a significant species difference, with M17 and M1 being the major metabolites in man and rats respectively and M21 being far more prevalent in cats and dogs than in man or rats[8,18,24,27,28,30,32,38-40]. The hepatic extraction ratio is a measure of the relative rate of hepatic drug metabolism *in vivo*, with a maximum theoretical value $= 1$ indicating that those molecules of a drug passing through the liver are completely metabolized during this passage. The hepatic extraction ratio for CsA has been estimated at 0.4 in man[35,36] and 0.03 in rats[32]; this large species difference warrants further investigation, implying as it does a much slower metabolism of CsA in rats than in man, which is reflected in the almost 7-fold higher ratio of CsA:total metabolites in the blood of rats than humans (see below).

Blood

The analysis of patients' blood for CsA and its metabolites is usually carried out around 12 h after administration of CsA and immediately preceding the next dose, the concentrations measured being known as trough levels[1]. In contrast, most reported studies of CsA metabolites in rat blood have measured the levels 16−24 h following a CsA dose. However, these schedules ensure that in both species, provided there is no renal failure, the blood is sampled at a time corresponding to approximately 1−2 CsA half-lives after CsA administration[1,28,36]. In human blood the main metabolites are M17 and M1, of which M17 is predominant, with much less M8, M10, M13, M18 and M21[8,18,27,38,39]. Following a single 300 mg oral dose of [^{3}H]CsA in six healthy volunteers, the 24-h AUC (area under the concentration versus time curve measured during the 24 h period following dosing) for CsA-derived radioactivity in whole blood showed the following approximate percentage composition: CsA (40%), M17 (28%), M1 (14%), M8 (5%), M21 (3%), M13 (2%), M18 (1%) and M10 (0.5%)[18]. A remarkably similar percentage composition was seen in the 12 h trough levels of CsA-derived material in the blood of liver and kidney allograft recipients: CsA (33%), M17 (34%), M1 (10%), M8 (23%), M21 (0.2%) and M18 (9%)[8]. In nine separate studies analysing blood from a total of 151 individuals, including healthy volunteers and recipients of kidney, liver, heart, bone marrow and pancreas allografts, the mean blood 12 h trough concentrations (ng/ml) were: CsA $= 264$, M17 $= 289$ and M1 $= 161$ (ranges CsA $= 112-426$, M17 $= 217-714$ and M1 $= 69-278$) and the mean ratios for the trough levels of CsA metabolites in blood were: CsA:M17:M1:M21:M18 $= 1.0:1.5:0.6:0.2:0.1$[8,26-29,38,39,41,42]. In one of the studies a mean ratio of 1:0.7 for CsA:M8 was reported[8]. (In the report of Freeman et al.[27], summarized above, an HPLC peak was identified as M18, but after a comparison with the other studies, and in view of the poor resolution of M1 and M18 on HPLC, we have presumed that the peak was, in fact, M1).

273

In renal transplant recipients CsA attains peak blood levels 1–3 h after oral dosing, while the peak for CsA metabolites occurs 1–3 h later still[25–27,43]. The blood CsA:metabolite ratio is at its highest during the first hour after oral dosing but subsequently the pattern of CsA and metabolites changes only slightly during the 24 h post-dose period[25–27,42,43]. The pattern of CsA and metabolites in blood does not show a noticeable diurnal variation[29,43,44]. A consensus of 10 different studies shows that, between 4 and 24 h after oral dosing, human blood has a 2.2-fold higher concentration of total CsA metabolites than of parent compound (range 1.3–3.3 fold)[8,18,26–29,38,39,43,44].

Although the studies summarized above each described similar average CsA metabolite patterns in patients' blood, there was, nevertheless, a large interindividual variation in circulating CsA metabolite profiles. The metabolite profile may be influenced by the route of administration of CsA[42] and by the particular type of organ received[38]. The cytochrome P-450-dependent metabolism of several drugs in vivo exhibits a genetic polymorphism, characterized by two populations, one of which shows a genetic defect in the ability to metabolize the drug; the archetypal example is the hydroxylation of debrisoquine[60]. A study of 300 patients showed no evidence, however, for two separate populations characterized by high and low blood CsA levels respectively[45], suggesting that CsA metabolism probably does not exhibit a genetic polymorphism. During 3 months of treatment of renal transplant recipients there was a marked increase in the dose-adjusted blood levels of CsA and its major metabolites, but the pattern of metabolites and parent compound in blood did not change[33], whereas there was a marked increase in the metabolite:CsA ratio in the blood of bone marrow recipients during 5 months of treatment[38]. The metabolite:CsA ratio in the blood of a renal allograft recipient increased during a nephrotoxic episode, with a preferential rise in the level of dihydroxylated metabolites[26].

Drug metabolism in rats is markedly affected by the strain and sex of the animal, in addition to considerations of the effects of route of administration. Although each of the published studies on CsA metabolism in rats unfortunately encompasses a different combination of these factors, thus making comparisons difficult, the overall pattern of CsA and its metabolites in whole blood is very similar in each case. In rat whole blood, M1 is the predominant metabolite, with up to 3-fold lower levels of M17 and M18 and lesser or undetectable amounts of other metabolites[24,28,32,46]. From these studies, which used between them male and female Sprague-Dawley, Wistar-Furth and Lewis rats and oral, subcutaneous and intravenous routes of CsA administration, the mean ratios of CsA and its major metabolites in blood were: CsA:M1:M17:M21 = 1.0:0.2:0.1:0.02 (ranges M1 = 0.1–0.4, M17 = 0.06–0.1 and M21 = 0.004–0.05). Following oral dosing at 10–15 mg/kg, in male Sprague-Dawley rats CsA and M1 constituted approximately 50% and 30% respectively of the 24-h AUC for whole blood CsA-derived radioactivity[32], while in male Wistar-Furth rats CsA, M1 and M17 accounted for 98% of the CsA-derived compounds in 24 h post-dose blood, their levels being 1677, 359 and 163 ng/ml respectively[24]. These studies in various strains and sexes show that rat blood contains, on average, a 3.4-fold higher concentration of CsA than of its total metabolites[24,28,32,46].

The ratio of CsA:M1 + M17 in rat blood appears to be influenced by the route of CsA administration and possibly by the dose also. Thus, in male Wistar-Furth rats, subcutaneous dosing gave higher blood levels of CsA, M1 and M17 than did oral dosing (4750, 702 and 296 ng/ml respectively at 24 h after subcutaneous dosing) and resulted in a higher ratio of CsA:M1 + M17, this being 5:1 and 3:1 for subcutaneous and oral administration respectively[24,46]. Compared to oral dosing in male Wistar-Furth rats (15 mg/kg), intravenous dosing at a lower level in male Lewis rats (5 mg/kg) resulted in a lower ratio of CsA:M1 + M17 in blood (3:1 and 1.7:1 for oral and i.v. dosing respectively), although there was no appreciable difference in the M1:M17 ratio[24,28]. Following an oral dose of CsA, the ratio of CsA: M1:M17 in blood did not alter greatly with time after dosing, being similar at 4 h and 24 h post-dose in Sprague-Dawley and Wistar-Furth rats respectively[24,32]. In female Wistar-Furth rats dosed subcutaneously, the 24 h post-dose blood levels of both CsA and M1 were approximately 50% of the levels in males, whereas M17 levels were similar in both sexes: consequently, M17 was a more major metabolite in females than in males[46]. CsA and M1 have a long residence time in male Sprague-Dawley rats, being detectable in blood 10 days after the last of 21 consecutive daily doses of CsA[32].

It is clear from the studies summarized above that several different patterns of CsA and metabolites have been observed in the blood of any one species. Nevertheless, a species difference in the general pattern is apparent, with M17 and M1 being the major metabolite in man and rat respectively and the ratio of CsA:total metabolites being much higher in rats (3:1) than in man (1:0.5). Much less work has been carried out in other experimental species, but M17 is the major metabolite in rabbits and M21 is a much more pre-eminent metabolite in cats and dogs than in rats, rabbits or man[28]. These species differences in metabolism should be taken into consideration when evaluating CsA toxicology and pharmacology in animals, especially since some of the metabolites may show immunosuppressive and toxic activity (see below).

CsA and several of its metabolites are preferentially distributed in blood cells compared to plasma, such that under physiological conditions around 60% of CsA is associated with erythrocytes[47]. The erythrocyte may provide a rapidly accessible pool of CsA and the relationship between whole blood and plasma CsA concentrations is dependent on the haematocrit value, which itself may vary after transplantation[48,49,148]. Blood cells show a pattern of parent drug and metabolites similar to whole blood, but plasma does not[18]. In freshly fractionated blood the concentrations of M1, M8, M17 and unchanged CsA were each many-fold higher in the cellular fraction than in plasma, whereas levels of M13 and M21 were approximately equal in plasma and cells and M10 and M18 were distributed preferentially in plasma[18,25,27,39]. In whole blood left standing for an unknown period of time at 37°C *in vitro*, CsA, M1, M8, M10 and M17 were strongly (more than 70%) taken up from whole blood into the cellular fraction, while M13 and M21 were 40% and 25% taken up respectively[18]. The partitioning of CsA into erythrocytes is complete after 90 min and remains stable for 24 h (standard clinical practice is to let whole blood stand for 120 min at ambient temperature before analysis of serum or plasma for CsA)[23]. The partitioning of CsA and its metabolites between plasma and blood cells *in vitro* is temperature-dependent, with a lowering from 37°C to 22°C favouring association with erythrocytes: this must be an important consideration during analysis[39,50]. CsA, M1, M17 and M21 are more than 70% bound to plasma proteins *in vitro*, while M13, M10 and M8 are approximately 60%, 35% and 25% bound respectively[18]. CsA is also associated with leukocytes (10–20%) and is extensively bound to plasma lipoproteins, especially HDL and LDL, and to intracellular erythrocyte proteins[47,51,52]. The intracellular CsA-binding protein, cyclophilin, binds M1, M8, M17 and CsA almost equally well, but M18, M21, M26 and the acid metabolite are bound only poorly[34]. It has not yet been reported whether the uptake into blood cells is an active or a passive process, but CsA is bound within erythrocytes rather than to cell membranes[47]. Values for the binding constants of CsA and its metabolites to proteins are needed urgently.

Bile and urine

In man and rats CsA is eliminated virtually entirely as metabolites and mainly in the bile, where less than 3% of the total CsA-derived material is parent compound[8,18,32,40]. At least 17 CsA metabolites have been detected in human urine and 10 in human bile[20,21]. Human bile was originally reported to contain predominantly M8 and M17[30], with a more complete pattern being given as M8 > M17 > M21 > M18 > M13 > CsA > M1[40]. More recent reports indicate that M17 is present in human bile mainly as its carboxylic acid derivative (M203–218), with a biliary metabolite profile given as M203–218 > M8 > M17 > 'undefined metabolites' > M26 > M25 > M18 > M21 > CsA > M1, plus a claim that several additional, unidentified metabolites are also present[8,21]. In bile collected from a total of 10 kidney or liver transplant recipients, M203–218, M8, M17 and M1 respectively comprised 26%, 22%, 14% and <1% of the CsA-derived compounds present[8]. A contradictory report states that M1 is also a major human biliary metabolite[20].

The metabolite profile in rat bile collected during the 48 h following an oral dose was: 'polar and unidentified metabolites' > M8 > M1 > M10 = M13 > M17 > M18 > M9 = M21[32]. In this study the 'polar and unidentified metabolites', M8 and M1 accounted for 24%, 17% and 11% of the CsA-derived biliary radioactivity respectively, the other metabolites comprised 2–11% each, and unchanged CsA represented less than 1%. From a comparison of the HPLC retention times[21,32], it appears that the 'polar and unidentified metabolites', also called 'peak 1' after their HPLC elution characteristics, did not include the carboxylic acid metabolite of M17.

In man and rats less than 15% of an oral or intravenous dose of CsA is excreted in the urine during the first 72 h, with less than 3% of the CsA dose being excreted in the urine as the parent compound[18,28,32]. Only approximately 60% of the CsA metabolites in 96 h urine from healthy volunteers could be identified: M17 and M18 were the major metabolites, accounting for 1% and 0.5% of an oral dose respectively, while M1, M8, M10, M13, M21 and unchanged CsA each represented 0.1–0.2% of the dose[18]. In urine collected from a total of 10 kidney or liver allograft recipients, M17 was the major metabolite, accounting for 36% of the CsA-derived compounds, followed by M18 and M8 (14–15% each), whereas unchanged CsA comprised less than 8% and M1 and M21 were each less than 3%[8]. An average human urinary metabolite profile was given as M17 > M18 > M8 > CsA > M1 > M21, but the pattern showed a marked interindividual variation[8,20]. Human urinary profiles containing many unidentified CsA metabolites were reported recently[20,21].

In urine collected over a 24 h period from male Sprague-Dawley rats the two major metabolites were 'polar and unidentified metabolites' (peak 1) and M1, accounting for 32% and 22% of CsA-derived radioactivity respectively, followed by M17 and M8, representing 12% and 10% respectively, whereas M9, M13, M18, M21 and unchanged CsA each accounted for only 1–2%[32]. M1 and M17 were also the major metabolites in 72 h urine from male Lewis rats, accounting for 3% and 1% of the dose respectively, with lesser amounts of M18, M21 and unchanged CsA (<0.5% of the dose each)[28]. A urine/bile mixture from dogs yielded the CsA metabolite profile: M21 > M1 > M18 > M17 > CsA[28].

The relative pre-eminence of M17 in human bile and urine, M1 in rat bile and urine and M21 in dog urine/bile mixture broadly reflects the species differences in the relative levels of these metabolites in blood. In rats the 'polar and unidentified metabolites' are minimal in blood but major in bile and urine[32], which suggests a selective excretion process for these metabolites of CsA.

Tissues

In kidneys removed from two transplant recipients due to rejection, the renal cortical concentration of metabolite M17 was 2–3-fold that of CsA[39]. In this same study M1 was at the same level as CsA in one of these patients but was not detectable in the other, while M21 was not detectable in either individual, and there was no difference between renal cortex and medulla in levels of CsA and metabolites. In various tissues of five other CsA-treated patients the concentrations of CsA and metabolites were up to 53-fold higher than in blood: the major metabolite was M17, followed by M8[8]. In liver, kidney and several other tissues the concentration of CsA was less than its total metabolites, but adipose tissue contained mainly unchanged CsA and may constitute a significant depot tissue for the drug[8].

In rats dosed with [³H]CsA the highest concentrations of radioactivity were found in the liver, kidneys, lymph nodes, adipose tissue and skin[30]. In these tissues, measured 24 h after CsA dosing, the predominant CsA compound was unchanged parent drug, accounting for approximately 90% of the radioactivity in fat, 75% in lymph nodes and 40–60% in liver, kidney and skin. The most abundant metabolite was M1, followed by 'polar and unidentified metabolites' (peak 1), which jointly constituted up to 36% of the radioactivity in liver, kidneys and skin (peak 1 was largely restricted to the liver and kidneys)[32]. Concentrations of CsA and metabolites were many-fold higher in rat liver and kidney than in rat blood, but the pattern of metabolites and parent compound was similar in blood and the tissues: CsA > M1 > M17[24]. In another study M17, M1 and eight other unidentified CsA metabolites were extracted from livers of CsA-treated rats[53]. CsA accumulates rapidly in rabbit hepatocytes *in vitro*, where it is apparently bound to a specific cytosolic protein, from which, however, it is displaced by its metabolites[19].

Thus, as with bile and urine, the same metabolite appears to predominate in tissues and blood: M17 in man but M1 in rats.

CsA METABOLISM *IN VITRO*

CsA is metabolized by human, rat and rabbit liver microsomes and the resulting metabolite profiles broadly reflect those seen in blood, bile and urine. With human liver microsomes, 3.5 mmol/l CsA incubated for 60 min gave rise to M1, M17 and 'unidentified polar metabolites' (peak 1) as the major metabolites, plus smaller quantities of M8, M21, M10 and M18[30], while a lower CsA concentration incubated for less time (25 μmol/l for 10 min) produced M1 as the main metabolite with somewhat smaller amounts of M17 and M21[157]. We have recently studied the metabolism of [^{3}H]CsA by rat and human liver microsomes. The incubation of 50 μmol/l CsA for 60 min with human liver microsomes from renal transplant *donors* generated up to eight metabolites, including dihydroxy compounds (Figure 13.3). M1 and M17 combined (they were not resolved in our HPLC system) were the predominant metabolites with microsomes from six different individuals, but there was a marked interindividual variation in both the metabolite profile and the rate of CsA metabolism, with the rate varying 11-fold from 4 to 44 pmol min^{-1} (mg protein)$^{-1}$ (Figure 13.4). Kronbach *et al.*[157] found a similar range of hepatic microsomal CsA metabolism activities among 15 individuals.

Liver microsomes from erythromycin-treated rabbits metabolized 5 μmol/l CsA to three incompletely identified groups of metabolites: (i) M21, (ii) a single HPLC peak representing a mixture of the monohydroxy compounds M1, M17 and M18 in unknown proportions, and (iii) two HPLC peaks representing dihydroxy/dihydroxy-*N*-desmethyl compounds[31]. The mono-hydroxylated metabolites and M21 predominated during the early period of the incubation, but subsequently the dihydroxylated metabolites became preponderant. Maximum rates of formation of all the metabolites occurred at 10 μmol/l CsA, with substrate inhibition occurring at higher concentrations, which particularly reduced the amount of dihydroxy metabolites. The microsomal CsA metabolism was induced 30–50-fold by pretreatment of the rabbits with rifampicin, erythromycin or triacetyloleandomycin *in vivo*, but was not induced by phenobarbitone (PB) or β-naphthoflavone (BNF). The incubation of 0.3 μmol/l CsA for 16 h with the post-nuclear fraction of liver from untreated rabbits yielded M21 and six unidentified CsA metabolites, but neither M1 nor M17[53]. The *N*-demethylation of CsA by liver microsomes of PB-induced rats and untreated mice has also been detected by measurement of the formaldehyde released as co-metabolite[54,59]. It has been suggested that

278

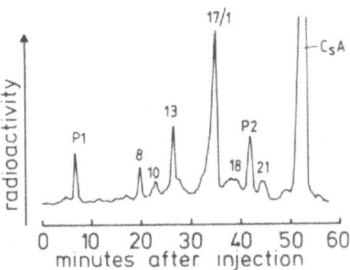

Figure 13.3 HPLC chromatogram of CsA metabolites generated with human hepatic microsomes *in vitro*. [³H]CsA (50 μmol/l, 39 μCi/μmol) was incubated aerobically with hepatic microsomes (6 mg protein) from a renal transplant donor (individual no. 11) for 45 min at 37°C in the presence of an NADPH-generating mixture (total reaction volume = 6 ml). The reaction was stopped by the addition of 4 ml ice-cold acetonitrile and the microsomal protein precipitated by centrifugation (3500 g × 20 min). CsA and metabolites were extracted from the supernatant into 10 ml glass-distilled ether in a glass tube by continuous re-inversion for 15 min. A 10 ml aliquot of the 13.5 ml organic layer was removed, filtered at 0.45 μm into a fresh, ether-washed glass tube and evaporated to dryness under nitrogen. The residue was redissolved in 50 μl acetonitrile (far UV grade) and a 10 μl aliquot analysed by HPLC, using a C1 column (5 μm Hypersil SAS) developed at 70°C with a linear mobile phase gradient of water/acetonitrile (far UV grade) (60:40 changing over 60 min to 40:60 v/v) at 1 ml/min. Radioactive CsA and metabolites were measured using an on-line radioisotope detector (Reeve Analytical, Glasgow). Metabolite identities (M1, M8, M10, M13, M17, M18 and M21, shown by numbers above the HPLC trace) were assigned by a comparison of their retention times with those of authentic metabolites supplied by Sandoz (Basel). Metabolites M1 and M17 were not resolved using this system. Peak P1 was probably identical with the 'peak 1' reported by Wagner *et al.*[32], while the identity of metabolite peak P2 is not known

a useful way of obtaining CsA metabolites for further study is either to extract them from the livers of rats pretreated with CsA *in vivo* or to generate them by incubating CsA with rabbit liver *in vitro*: 60 μg of metabolites were extracted from 100 mg of liver obtained from rats treated *in vivo* with approximately 5.5 mg CsA per 250 g rat, whilst 30 μg of metabolites were generated from 100 μg CsA incubated with 50 ml of post-nuclear fraction obtained from 250 g of rabbit liver[53].

Metabolite profiles, in the form of HPLC chromatograms, resulting from the metabolism of 12.5 μmol/l CsA by rat liver microsomes in our own recent studies are shown in Figure 13.5. The major metabolite was M1, while M17, M18 and M21 were also formed, plus several small metabolites that could not be identified. 3-Methylcholanthrene (3MC) did not induce CsA metabolism, whereas PB and pregnenolone 16α-carbonitrile (PCN) selectively induced the formation of M1 and M21, whilst having little effect on M17 and M18. In fact, M21 was detected only with the PB- and PCN-induced microsomes. The group of monohydroxy metabolites (M1 + M17 + M18) constituted 36–47% of the total CsA metabolites, depending on the type of induction of the microsomes, while M21 comprised approximately 7% of the total metabolites with PB- and PCN-induced microsomes. In contrast to Bertault-Peres' published study with rabbit liver microsomes[31], in our experiments dihydroxylated, dihydroxy-N-demethylated or 'more polar' metabolites

279

CYCLOSPORIN

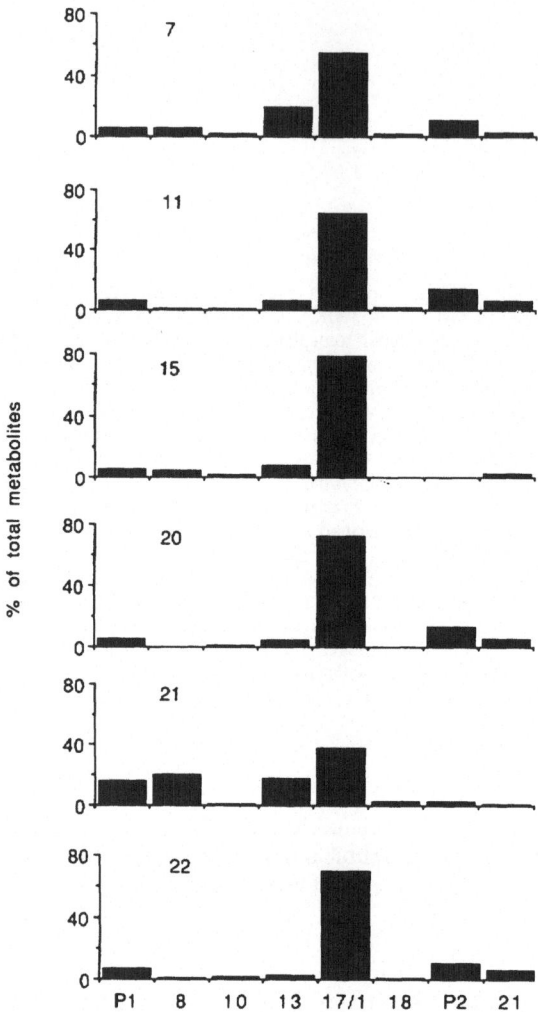

Figure 13.4 CsA metabolite profiles produced by human hepatic microsomes from six different individuals. [³H]CsA was incubated with human liver microsomes from six renal transplant donors and analysed by HPLC as in Figure 13.3. The metabolite identities are shown below the bars (M1 and M17 were measured jointly); see Figure 13.3 for details. The abundance of each metabolite is expressed as a percentage of the total metabolites. The identification number of each individual is shown above the bar for M8. The total rates of CsA metabolism *in vitro* by individuals 7, 11, 15, 20, 21 and 22 were 44, 19, 4, 23, 26 and 15 pmol min⁻¹ (mg microsomal protein)⁻¹, respectively

appeared not to be formed with any of the rat microsomes. This discrepancy may have arisen because, whilst in the rabbit study[31] the dihydroxy metabolites were formed in major amounts only after CsA had been largely consumed in the incubation, and then only with microsomes from rabbits induced with erythromycin and similar types of inducer, in contrast less than 12% of the

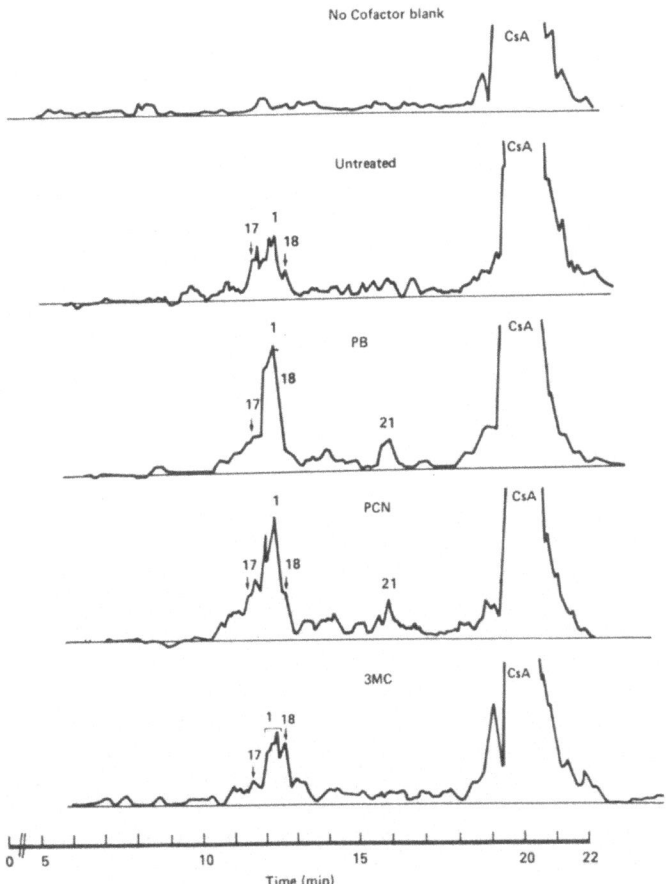

Figure 13.5 HPLC chromatograms of CsA metabolites generated with rat hepatic microsomes *in vitro.* [³H]CsA (25 μmol/l, 14C μCi/μmol) was incubated as in Figure 13.3 for 15 min with liver microsomes (5 mg protein) from untreated or phenobarbitone (PB)-, pregnenolone 16α-carbonitrile (PCN)- or 3-methylcholanthrene (3MC)-induced adult, male Sprague-Dawley rats. A 'no co-factor blank' incubation contained CsA and PB-induced microsomes but lacked the NADPH-generating system. Extraction, HPLC assay and metabolite identification was as for Figure 13.3, except that the mobile phase was: water/acetonitrile (42:58) isocratically for 10 min, followed by a linear gradient changing to water/acetonitrile (30:70) over 5 min, which was then maintained isocratically for 10 min

CsA was consumed in our incubations. Liver microsomes from rats pretreated for 14 days with CsA (50 mg/kg orally) did not metabolize CsA at all (data not shown), although whether this was due to selective suppression *in vivo* of cytochrome P450 or to direct inhibition *in vitro* by residual CsA is not yet known. It will be important to discover whether CsA pretreatment diminishes its own metabolism in patients.

The hepatic microsomal metabolism of CsA, measured either by the amount of substrate consumed or the quantity of total metabolites produced, has K_m

281

values that are similar ($6-30\,\mu$mol/l) in man[30,55] and control, PB-induced and 3MC-induced rats[55], while V_{max} values (pmol min^{-1} (mg microsomal proteins)$^{-1}$) range from 50 to 733 in man[30,55] and 70 to 170 in control, PB-induced and 3MC-induced rats[55] (Table 13.1). PCN-induced rat liver microsomes gave biphasic kinetics for CsA metabolism[55]: $K_{m1} = \mu$mol/l, $V_{max1} = 20$ pmol min^{-1} (mg protein)$^{-1}$ $K_{m2} = 109\,\mu$mol/l, $V_{max2} = 440$ pmol min^{-1} (mg protein)$^{-1}$. These results show that hepatic microsomal CsA metabolism is apparently induced in man by anticonvulsant drugs and in rats by PCN and, to a lesser extent, by PB but not by 3MC. Erythromycin-induced rabbit liver gave the highest of all measured rates of CsA metabolism, 1.1 nmol min^{-1} at 7 μmol/l CsA[31]. K_m and V_{max} values for CsA N-demethylation by control mouse liver microsomes, measured by the formaldehyde co-metabolite, were 808 μmol/l and 1 nmol min^{-1} (mg protein)$^{-1}$ respectively[59].

CsA metabolism by human and rat liver microsomes is NADPH-dependent and can be inhibited by carbon monoxide and by the experimental drug SKF-525A (β-diethylaminoethyl diphenylpropylacetate) and the antifungal agent ketoconazole, which indicates that CsA oxidation is catalysed by the cytochrome P-450-dependent mono-oxygenase system[30,55]. Cytochrome P-450 is a genetic superfamily of many different forms, which respond differently to different inducing agents[56,60]. The effects of inducers on CsA metabolism by human, rabbit and rat liver microsomes (see above) point to the metabolism being catalysed preferentially by P-450 forms belonging to the PCN-, erythromycin- and anticonvulsant-inducible family of cytochrome P-450 (the P-450III family). This was confirmed by the demonstration that the purified rabbit P-450III form, P-450 3c, metabolized CsA and that antibodies against P-450 3c inhibited rabbit liver microsomal CsA metabolism, whereas purified rabbit P-450 forms 2, 3b and 4 did not appreciably metabolize CsA and antibodies against rabbit P-450 forms 2, 3b, 4 and 6 did not inhibit CsA metabolism[31]. The human P-450III form, P-450$_{NF}$, is stimulated by cytochrome b$_5$[57], but cytochrome b$_5$ did not stimulate CsA oxidation by rabbit P-450 3c[31].

Table 13.1 K_m and V_{max} values for CsA metabolism by liver microsomes from induced and non-induced humans and rats

Species	Sex	Age (years)	Inducing agent	K_m (μmol/l)	V_{max} (pmol min^{-1} (mg protein)$^{-1}$)
Human	?	?	?	6[a]	50[a]
	M	33	Anticonvulsants[b]	15	733
	M	51	None	30	66
Rat (Sprague–Dawley)	M	Adult	None	15	83
	M	Adult	PB	17	170
	M	Adult	3MC	13	70
	M	Adult	PCN (i)[c]	4	20
			(ii)[c]	109	440

[a]Data from reference 30, all other data from reference 55
[b]Long-term therapy with phenobarbitone, phenytoin, carbamazepine and valproate. Evidence of induced cytochrome P-450 was provided by raised microsomal alkoxyresorufin O-dealkylase activities and P-450hA7 levels
[c]Biphasic kinetics, giving a pair of K_m and V_{max} values, (i) and (ii)

Human hepatic microsomal CsA metabolism activity correlated with the microsomal level of P450$_{NF}$[157] and was inhibited by an antibody against a PCN-induced rat P-450III form[157] and by an antibody against a human P-450III form recently purified by us, P-450hA7[58], which is closely related to P-450$_{NF}$ (Figure 13.6). These results indicate that P-450hA7, and probably also P-450$_{NF}$, has a dominant role in human hepatic CsA metabolism. Human liver microsomes contain forms of cytochrome P-450 belonging to different gene families from P-450$_{NF}$, including two forms known respectively as bufuralol (or debrisoquine) hydroxylase and mephenytoin hydroxylase[56,60]. However, a lack of correlation between CsA, bufuralol and mephenytoin metabolism activities *in vitro* suggests that these other two cytochrome P-450 forms play no major role in CsA metabolism in human hepatic microsomes[157].

Substrate binding to cytochrome P-450 can be measured by perturbations in the absorption spectrum of the enzyme's haem group. Three different

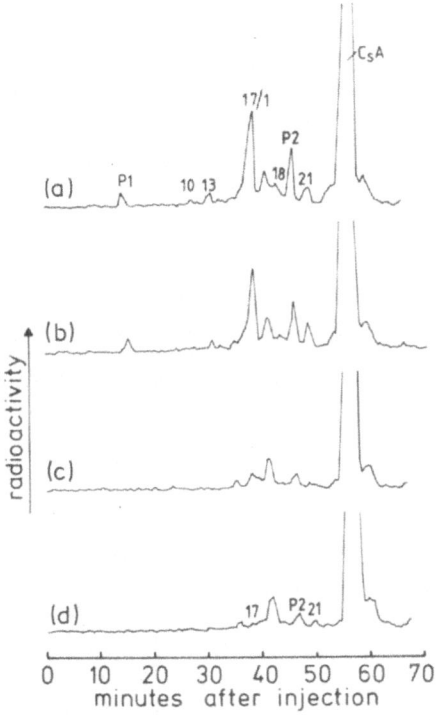

Figure 13.6 Inhibition of human hepatic microsomal CsA metabolism by an antibody against human cytochrome P-450hA7. Trace (a): [³H]CsA was incubated with human liver microsomes from a renal transplant donor (individual no. 11) and analysed by HPLC as in Figure 13.3. The metabolite identities (M10, M13, M17, M1, M18 and M21) of the HPLC peaks are shown by numbers above trace (a); peak 'p' is probably the 'peak 1' reported by Wagner *et al.*[32]. Trace (d) is a blank incubation, as (a) but lacking the NADPH-generating system. For traces (b) and (c) the microsomes were preincubated for 10 min at 0°C with either non-immune IgG (trace b) or a polyclonal antibody against P-450hA7 (trace c) at a ratio of 20 mg IgG per mg microsomal protein, prior to starting the reaction

modes of binding are distinguishable by different types of spectral perturbation: type I binding reflects a hydrophobic interaction between the hydrocarbon moieties of the substrate and the protein forming the haem pocket and active site of cytochrome P-450, while type II and modified type II binding reflect direct ligand interactions between the cytochrome P-450 haem and substrate nitrogen and oxygen atoms respectively. There are conflicting reports as to the type of CsA binding to cytochrome P-450: type I binding was reported with liver microsomes from PB-induced rats[54] and erythromycin-induced rabbits and with purified rabbit P-450 3c[31], but modified type II binding occurred with control mouse liver microsomes[59]. CsA binding to cytochrome P-450 could not be detected with control, PB- or BNF-induced rabbit liver microsomes[31]. The apparent dissociation constant (K_s) for type I cytochrome P-450 binding in rabbits was $1-2 \, \mu mol/l$, which was similar to the K_m for CsA metabolism[31], whereas a much higher K_s, $407 \, \mu mol/l$, characterized the modified type II P-450 binding in mice[59]. This accords with the concept that type 1 binding reflects true enzyme-substrate binding, whereas modified type II binding reflects a non-productive, inhibitory interaction. Certain drugs form long-lived product—adduct complexes between their metabolites and cytochrome P-450, and these complexes are important because they usually inhibit the metabolism of other substrates. Although CsA added to liver microsomes *in vitro* directly inhibits the cytochrome P-450 metabolism of other substrates (see below), it did not form product—adduct complexes with mouse microsomal cytochrome P-450[59]; this experiment needs repeating, however, with microsome species that bind CsA in a type I fashion and are known to metabolize it.

Isolated rabbit hepatocytes rapidly take up CsA and metabolize it to mono- and dihydroxylated metabolites but not M21[19]. As with rabbit liver microsomes, monohydroxylated metabolites appeared to be formed first and then to disappear as they were further metabolized to dihydroxylated compounds. CsA and its metabolites accumulated in hepatocytes relative to the extracellular medium, possibly due to their binding to an intracellular hepatocyte protein. An important observation in this study was that RIA seriously underestimated the CsA metabolites.

The results summarized here indicate that in human, rat and rabbit liver microsomes CsA is metabolized primarily by members of the PCN-inducible, P-450III family of cytochrome P-450, including the form P-450hA7 in man. Two observations lead us to believe that the most studied rat P-450III form, $P-450_{PCN-E}$ or P-450p, may not be the main CsA-oxidase in this species. First, $P-450_{PCN-E}$ is present at a much lower level in female compared to male rats[60], yet CsA is reportedly metabolized *in vivo* at least as extensively in females as in males[46]. Secondly, whilst rifampicin apparently induces CsA metabolism in rats[61], it notably fails to induce P-450p in this species[62]. The hepatic extraction ratio for CsA metabolism *in vivo* is much larger in man than in rats[32,35,36] (see above): it is important to elucidate whether this is because the particular P-450III form(s) involved in CsA metabolism are more abundant in human than rat liver, or whether it reflects an intrinsic functional difference in human and rat P-450 forms that are structurally similar. Since the specific activities and K_m and V_{max} values for *in vitro* hepatic microsomal CsA metabolism are not greatly dissimilar in humans and rats (Table 13.1 and see above), however, this suggests that non-enzymatic factors may be influential in determining the rate of hepatic CsA metabolism *in vivo*. It is also possible that extrahepatic metabolism of CsA in man contributes significantly to the much higher metabolites:CsA ratio seen in human than in rat blood *in vivo* (see above). In this context it may be significant that P-450hA7, which is the cytochrome P-450 form predominantly responsible for CsA metabolism in human liver microsomes[55] (see above), is abundant in human small intestinal epithelium but present at only a low level in human kidney[158]. This suggests that CsA may undergo significant intestinal first-pass metabolism following oral administration in man, but may not be appreciably metabolized in the kidney.

THE EFFECTS OF CsA ON HEPATIC DRUG METABOLISM

Experiments in rats suggest that CsA, which is metabolized by mono-oxygenation, including *N*-demethylation (see above), causes a decrease in hepatic mono-oxygenase activity and thereby limits its own metabolism *in vivo*[63]. During the administration of CsA to male Sprague-Dawley rats for 7 weeks *in vivo* there were oscillatory changes in circulating CsA levels, which showed an inverse temporal relationship to decreases in the hepatic microsomal mono-oxygenase activities, aminopyrine *N*-demethylation and NADPH–cytochrome P-450 reductase, although there was no change in cytochrome P-450 levels[64]. We have recently also found that the hepatic microsomal metabolism of CsA itself is abolished by prior treatment of the rats with CsA *in vivo*[55]. Our recent observations on the effects of 2 weeks of CsA treatment in rats on a wider range of hepatic phase I and phase II drug metabolism activities are shown in Figures 13.7 and 13.8. There were significant oscillatory decreases, reaching up to 66%, in all the mono-oxygenase components and activities measured, but the various activities differed considerably in both the extent of the decrease and the time course of the oscillatory changes. The content of total microsomal protein per gram of liver did not change. The non-uniformity in the responses of the various mono-oxygenase activities may reflect differences in the behaviour of various P-450 forms. In general, the cytochrome P-450 and cytochrome b_5 levels, and the activities of their reductases, were less affected than the mono-oxygenase activities. In contrast, microsomal epoxide hydrolase underwent a transient 40% increase in activity. 1-Naphthol-glucuronyltransferase (naphthol-GT) was decreased but bilirubin-GT was not There was a transient decrease in the cytosolic glutathione concentration but cytosolic glutathione transferase activity was not affected. Microsomal aryl esterase and glucose-6-phosphatase activities were also decreased. In contrast to its effects on liver, CsA administration did not alter male rat kidney cytochrome P-450, NADPH–cytochrome P-450 reductase or glutathione levels. Whereas CsA administration caused selective decreases in hepatic microsomal drug metabolizing enzymes in male rats, in female rats it caused an approximate 63% increase in microsomal ethoxy- and benzyloxy-resorufin *O*-dealkylases after 14 days treatment (no change on day 7) and an

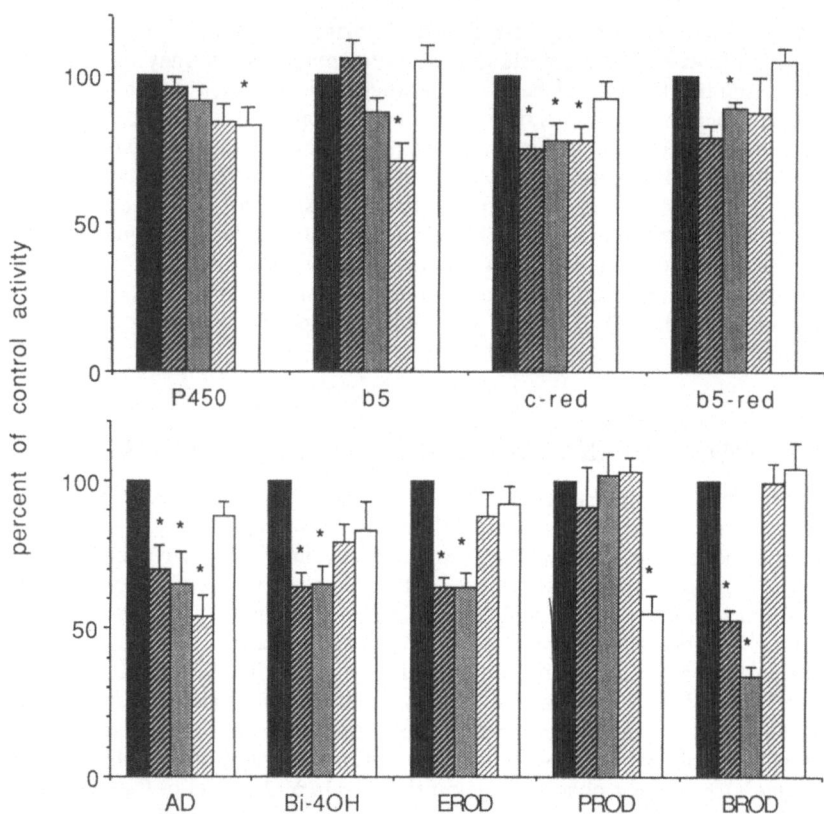

Figure 13.7 The effect of CsA treatment *in vivo* on rat hepatic microsomal drug metabolizing enzyme activities. Male Sprague-Dawley rats were administered CsA (50 mg/kg, orally) once daily for 4 ▨, 7 ▨, 10 ▨ or 14 ☐ days. Control rats ■ received an equal volume of drug vehicle (10% ethanol in olive oil). Liver microsomes were prepared 24 h following the final dose. The results are means ± SE for four rats measured individually, showing the activity in the microsomes of CsA-treated rats as a percentage of the mean activity in microsomes of control rats treated for the same number of days. *Significantly different from control ($p \leq 0.05$). The concentrations of cytochromes P-450 and b_5 were measured and the following activities: c-red, NADPH–cytochrome c (P-450) reductase; b_5-red, NADH–cytochrome b_5 reductase; AD, aminopyrine N-demethylase; Bi-4OH, biphenyl 4-hydroxylase; EROD, PROD and BROD, ethoxy-, pentoxy- and benzyloxyresorufin O-dealkylases. Biphenyl 2-hydroxylase activity was not detectable.

approximate 41% decrease in glucose-6-phosphatase after 7 and 14 days, with no effect on cytochrome P-450, NADPH–cytochrome P-450 reductase, aminopyrine N-demethylase or aryl esterase.

A similar effect of CsA on drug metabolizing enzymes has been reported by other groups. Pigs treated with CsA showed a transient decrease in hepatic glutathione levels but no change in glutathione transferase[30]. CsA treatment of male rats caused dose-dependent, approximate 24% decreases in hepatic microsomal cytochrome P-450, NADPH–cytochrome P-450 reductase, naphthol-GT and testosterone-GT, and 60% decreases in ethylmorphine N-

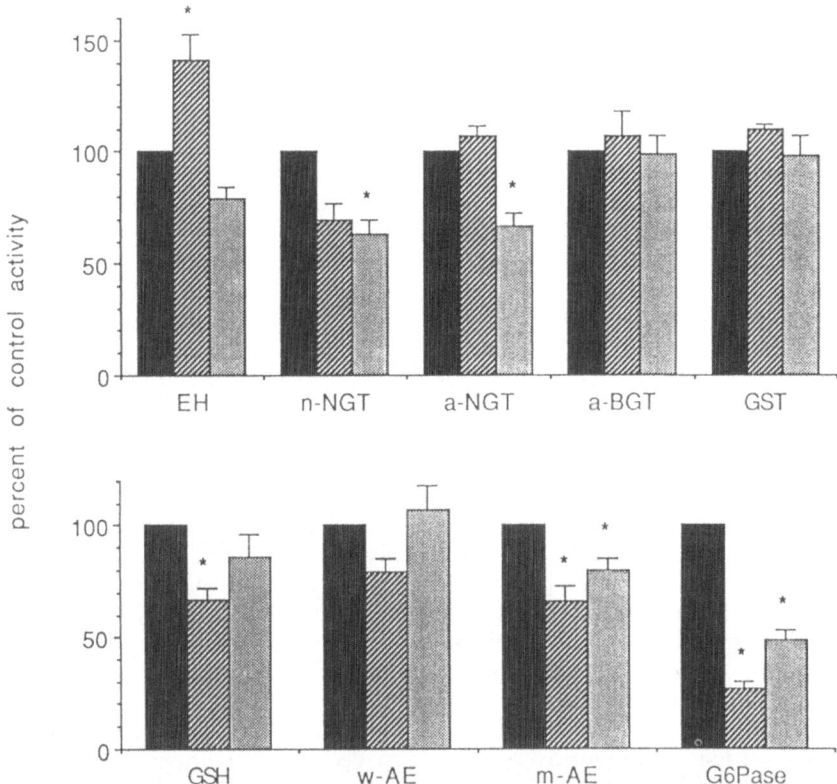

Figure 13.8 The effect of CsA treatment *in vivo* on rat hepatic microsomal and cytosolic enzyme activities and glutathione. Male Sprague-Dawley rats were administered CsA (50 mg/kg, orally) once daily for 7 or 14 days. Control rats received an equal volume of drug vehicle (10% ethanol in olive oil). Liver microsomes and cytosol were prepared 24 h following the final dose. The results are means ± SE for four rats measured individually, showing the activity in the preparations of CsA-treated rats as a percentage of the mean activity in preparations of control rats treated for the same number of days. *Significantly different from control ($p \leqslant 0.05$). The concentration of cytosolic reduced glutathione (GST) was measured and the following activities: EH, microsomal phenanthrene 9,10-epoxide hydrolase; n-NGT and a-NGT, native and detergent-activated microsomal 1-naphthol glucuronyltransferase; a-BGT, detergent-activated microsomal bilirubin glucuronyltransferase; GST, cytosolic chlorodinitrobenzene glutathione transferase; w-AE and m-AE, whole homogenate and microsomal aryl esterase; G6Pase, microsomal glucose-6-phosphatase.

demethylase and aniline hydroxylase, together with decreases in both the K_m and V_{max} for the two mono-oxygenase reactions, but there was no change in microsomal total protein content, cytochrome b_5, *p*-nitroanisole *O*-demethylase, morphine-GT or oestrone-GT, or in cytosolic glutathione transferase or sulphotransferase[54,65]. CsA treatment in rats and mice also selectively inhibited drug metabolism *in vivo*, causing a decrease in the clearance of theophylline but no change in the clearance of antipyrine or in the clearance of sulphate and glucuronide conjugation of paracetamol *in vivo*[59,65].

CsA added *in vitro* to hepatic microsomes from untreated mice competitively inhibited microsomal mono-oxygenation, but here also the effect was selective, with benzo(a)pyrene hydroxylase (AHH) being inhibited more strongly ($I_{50} = 1.2$ mmol/l) than aminopyrine N-demethylase ($I_{50} > 5$ mmol/l)[59]. In view of these I_{50} values it is perhaps not surprising that rat liver microsomal ethylmorphine N-demethylase and aniline hydroxylase were not inhibited by 0.1 mmol/l CsA *in vitro*[54].

The results summarized here indicate that CsA inhibits metabolism in a highly selective fashion. Microsomal glucuronyltransferases and cytochrome P-450-dependent mono-oxygenases are affected but cytosolic glutathione transferase and sulphotransferase are not, while microsomal epoxide hydrolase is initially increased. The effect on microsomal proteins is further selective, in that there is no overall decrease in total microsomal protein per gram of liver, but it is not confined to drug metabolizing enzymes, since aryl esterase and glucose-6-phosphatase are also decreased. Moreover, CsA has recently been shown to cause a general decrease in the synthesis of many hepatic proteins[66,67]. The fact that the oxidation and glucuronidation of different drugs are inhibited to differing extents, suggests that only certain forms of cytochrome P-450 and GT are affected. Since all the cytochromes and enzymes discussed here were measured by either ligand-binding or a catalytic activity, we do not know whether the changes caused by CsA treatment were due to decreases in the amounts of the enzymes or to a direct inhibition of their function by residual CsA. It will be important to resolve this question and, if enzyme expression is indeed altered, to ascertain whether this is a selective effect on only certain forms of the enzymes.

An increase in serum bilirubin, routinely interpreted as an indication of liver damage, could equally result from a decrease in bilirubin-GT activity: our results indicate that the increase in serum bilirubin, which is frequently seen following the administration of a toxic dose of CsA, is not due to decreased bilirubin-GT activity. The clinical consequences implied by the results discussed here are that CsA will inhibit the clearance of certain co-administered drugs, with the possibility of an alteration in their efficacy and toxicity. Since glutathione is an important cellular defence against toxic chemicals, its depletion by CsA could, on the one hand, be part of the mechanism of CsA cytotoxicity and, on the other hand, render tissues more susceptible to damage by other drugs.

IMMUNOSUPPRESSIVE PROPERTIES OF CsA METABOLITES

Earlier studies from this laboratory demonstrated that CsA-induced immuno-suppression in rats was maintained despite an increased rate of drug metabolism[68,69]. However, the relative immunosuppressive activities of indi-vidual CsA metabolites have not yet been clearly defined. One authoritative view, based on observations that M1, M8, M17 and M21 were less than 10% as potent as CsA in a variety of immunosuppression tests *in vivo* and *in vitro*, is that metabolites make only a minor contribution to the overall immunosuppressive effect of CsA[34]. Conversely, other workers reported that, in the mixed lymphocyte reaction test *in vitro*, M1 and M17 were almost as immunosuppressive as CsA and that M21 was 50% as potent[70]. Resolution of this discrepancy is complicated by the fact that the relative immunosuppressive potencies of CsA metabolites vary greatly depending on the particular *in vitro* test used[20,34,71]. However, a variety of *in vitro* tests, including inhibition of mixed lymphocyte reactions, alloreactive cell proliferation, Concanavalin A-induced mitogenesis and interleukin-2 production, indicate that, whilst M1, M8, M13, M17, M18, M21 and several unidentified metabolites do have immunosuppressive activity, their potency is generally less than 50% that of CsA, while M8 and the carboxylic acid metabolite possess little activity[17,20,70-73]. However, since in patients' blood the concentration of CsA is generally exceeded by its metabolites in total, and often equalled by M17 alone, the contribution of CsA metabolites to immunosuppression warrants further consideration and investigation.

TOXIC PROPERTIES OF CsA METABOLITES

Temporal relationships in rats between the severity of CsA renal tubular damage, trough circulating CsA levels and hepatic microsomal mono-oxygenase drug metabolizing enzyme activities suggest that kidney damage occurs when circulating drug levels exceed a threshold value[63,64]. However, since in these studies the circulating drug levels were measured using polyclonal antibody RIA, we do not know whether the renal damage caused by supra-threshold circulating drug levels was due to parent drug or to its metabolites. However, observations that CsA renal toxicity and circulating CsA levels in rats are both decreased by phenobarbitone induction of drug metabolism, but are increased by the drug metabolism inhibitors, ketoconazole and cimetidine, suggest that the toxicity is mainly due to CsA itself[63,68,74,75]. This is also the opinion of Ryffel *et al.*[34], who showed that neither M17 nor a pooled bile metabolite extract caused renal or hepatic toxicity after 4 weeks of parenteral administration to rats, whereas similar dosing with CsA caused damage to both organs. Results of biliary ligation and cannulation experiments in rats also support this view[140]. Moreover, circulating levels of unchanged CsA, measured by specific monoclonal antibody-RIA, were higher in patients showing nephrotoxicity compared to those who did not[76]. There is still a suspicion, though, that clinical CsA nephrotoxicity can be attributed, at least in part, to its metabolites. Renal clearance in kidney recipients correlated with the patients' creatinine clearance[33], while CsA-related nephrotoxic episodes were accompanied either by raised trough blood levels of both M17 and unchanged CsA or by an increase in circulating levels of CsA metabolites relative to parent compound[26,29,77]. However, since urinary excretion is a major route of elimination for CsA metabolites, although not for the parent compound, it is arguable whether the increases in CsA metabolites were the cause or the consequence of diminished renal function. Nevertheless, since M17 and other metabolites appear to accumulate preferentially relative to CsA in human kidney tissue[8,26], their toxic properties need to be thoroughly investigated.

DRUG INTERACTIONS WITH CsA

There is a large potential for drug interactions involving CsA, which relates to several of its properties: (1) its metabolism by hepatic (and also possibly small intestinal) cytochrome P-450-dependent mono-oxygenases; (2) its many toxic effects; and (3) its excellent immunosuppressive qualities. Moreover, due to the complex treatment and management of all transplant patients, CsA is commonly administered in combination with several other drugs, notably glucocorticoids, antibiotics, antifungal, antiviral and alkylating agents, calcium channel antagonists and diuretics. In the clinical context, any interaction which either increases or decreases circulating CsA concentrations, or which may lead to an enhancement of nephro- and/or hepatotoxicity, is extremely important and may have serious consequences for the patient.

Drug interactions with CsA can be divided broadly into three categories: (1) those which lead directly to an alteration in the pharmaco- and toxico-dynamics of CsA; (2) those which cause initially a change in the pharmaco-kinetics and/or metabolism of CsA; and (3) those which lead to a change in the actions, pharmacokinetics or metabolism of the co-administered drug. The usual consequence of an interaction involving CsA is either a decrease in immunosuppression, with the accompanying danger of graft rejection, or the appearance of toxicity, which is characteristic either of CsA, in which case it is usually nephrotoxicity, or of the co-administered drug.

Although there are many reports of drug interactions with CsA, many of these are anecdotal and involve only small numbers of patients – frequently a single patient. A list of confirmed drug interactions with CsA is given in Table 13.2. Selected examples of these are discussed below. It should be remembered that suggested mechanisms for these drug interactions are almost entirely based upon observations in experimental animals[78]: the assumption that the same mechanism will operate in man may or may not be true, and in almost all cases is untried. For more information relating to interactions not considered here the reader is referred to the booklet *Drug Interactions*, published by the Medical Information Services of Sandoz Pharmaceuticals Ltd.

Direct pharmacodynamic interactions

CsA is nephrotoxic and the most notable pharmacological interactions with CsA are those which occur after the co-administration of other potentially nephrotoxic agents, for example the aminoglycoside antibiotic, gentamicin, amphotericin B and trimethoprim/cotrimoxazole[79–81]. In experimental animals the enhanced renal proximal straight and convoluted tubular damage observed following the co-administration of gentamicin and CsA was dose-dependent[82] and in patients receiving this drug combination regular drug level monitoring is essential to reduce the risk of this interaction. Cephalosporin antibiotics showing a similar spectrum of antimicrobial activity to gentamicin, but which do not potentiate CsA nephrotoxicity to the same extent[85], are now available and might be preferable to aminoglycosides in co-therapy with CsA. The mechanism of CsA renal toxicity may include a diminution of renal

Table 13.2 Reported drug interactions with CsA in animals and man

Drug	Proposed mechanisms	References
Those increasing CsA levels		
Erythromycin	Inhibition/activation of cytochrome P-450, competition for biliary excretion.	105–107, 111
Ketoconazole	Inhibition/inactivation of cytochrome P-450, competition for biliary excretion.	78, 111, 115, 116
Diltiazem	Inhibition of cytochrome P-450	117–119
Nicardipine	—	120
Cimetidine*	Inhibition of cytochrome P-450	108–110
Frusemide	Inhibition of cytochrome P-450/sodium depletion	149
Methylprednisolone (maintenance dose)	Inhibition of cytochrome P-450	90, 181, 150
Methyltestosterone	Inhibition of CsA elimination	112
Danazol	Inhibition of cytochrome P-450	122, 123
Norethisterone	Inhibition of cytochrome P-450	123
Marvelon	—	30
Nordette	Inhibition of cytochrome P-450	124

*No effect of cimetidine on CsA levels either in *vivo*[112] or in *vitro*[127]

Those decreasing CsA levels		
Rifampicin (+ isoniazid)	Induction of cytochrome P-450	91–93
Phenytoin	Induction of cytochrome P-450	95–97
Phenobarbitone	Induction of cytochrome P-450	98, 99
Carbamazepine	Induction of cytochrome P-450	100
Methylprednisolone	Induction of cytochrome P-450	89
Sulphadimidine i.v. (+ trimethoprim)	—	151, 152
Hydergine	—	153

prostaglandin production[78], and in the light of this it may be significant that the antiarthritic agent and prostaglandin synthetase inhibitor, indomethacin, in a dose which was not itself toxic, exacerbated CsA renal toxicity in rats[83].

Pharmacokinetic and metabolic interactions

The majority of drug interactions with CsA are probably those with a primary effect on its pharmacokinetics and/or metabolism. The site of interaction can be the absorption, tissue distribution, protein binding, metabolism or excretion of CsA, and although in most instances the primary mechanism is believed to be an effect on CsA metabolism, in few cases has this been proven.

As discussed above, hepatic metabolism by cytochrome P-450-dependent mono-oxygenases is the primary means of elimination of CsA. Consequently, the co-administration of any drug possessing the ability to alter the activity of the mono-oxygenases has the potential to alter circulating levels of CsA, with the attendant clinical risks. Since liver contains many different forms of cytochrome P-450[56,60], and since these differ to a lesser or greater extent in their substrate specificities, it is probable that drug interactions due to changes in CsA metabolism will selectively involve mainly those drugs that increase or decrease the acticity of those particular cytochrome P-450 forms which metabolize CsA. Increased CsA metabolism would probably lead to decreased circulating CsA levels and a danger of transplant rejection, whereas decreased CsA metabolism would tend to result in increased circulating CsA levels and a danger of renal toxicity[41]. Conversely, in experimental animals CsA decreases the activity of certain of the hepatic mono-oxygenases and glucuronyltransferases responsible for the metabolism of the other drugs, and therefore has the potential to cause a decrease in the metabolism of co-administered drugs in patients. In experimental animals the effect of CsA on the metabolism of other drugs is selective, decreasing the clearance of theophylline but not that of antipyrine and paracetamol[59,65]. CsA inhibits prednisolone metabolism by isolated perfused rat liver[86], while in patients CsA decreases the clearance of prednisolone[87-89] and symptoms of steroid toxicity have occurred during combined CsA-methylprednisolone therapy[87,90].

There is ample evidence in experimental animals that inducers of cytochrome P-450 increase CsA metabolism, both *in vivo* and *in vitro*, and that *in vivo* this interaction diminishes the nephrotoxicity of CsA[31,46,55,68,69] (and see above). It is noteworthy that, of the inducers tested, barbiturate and rifampicin-type inducers (inducers of forms of cytochrome P-450 belonging to the P-450II and P-450III gene families[60,62,84]) did increase CsA metabolism, whereas polycyclic aromatic hydrocarbon carcinogen-type inducers (inducers of cytochrome P-450 forms belonging to the P-450 family) did not. If this distinction extends also to man, it will help to predict which drugs will undergo this type of metabolic interaction with CsA in patients and which drugs will not. Thus, in patients the co-administration of phenobarbitone, phenytoin or rifampicin, which induce P-450III forms in man (see above) or of carbamazepine, which induces a P-450III form in rats (unpublished observations), results in increased CsA clearance and large reductions in circulating CsA levels[91-103]. These observations can be rationalized by the discovery that CsA is metabolized primarily by forms of cytochrome P-450 belonging to the P-450III family (see above). The co-administration of rifampicin resulted in trough circulating CsA falling to negligible levels within 2 days, whereas they took 11 days to return to pre-rifampicin levels upon withdrawal of this drug[91]: this is an appropriate chronology for rifampicin induction of drug metabolism[101,102].

An increase in circulating levels of CsA is caused by co-treatment with a number of drugs that are known or suspected inhibitors of cytochrome P-450-dependent mono-oxygenases, for example erythromycin, ketoconazole, diltiazem, nicardipine and steroids[41,78,104-126]. Clinical renal toxicity is a frequent consequence of the erythromycin interaction. A biochemical basis for these interactions has been established in recent studies, which have shown that ketoconazole, diltiazem, erythromycin and verapamil each inhibit the metabolism of CsA by human hepatic microsomes *in vitro*[30,127]. This also raises the possibility that experiments based on the hepatic microsomal metabolism of CsA, particularly if human microsomes are used, may be an effective means of demonstrating and predicting certain types of potentially dangerous drug interactions with CsA. Most of the drugs that inhibit CsA metabolism will do so probably because they are themselves substrates for the same fo m(s) of cytochrome P-450 and will compete with CsA. Such inhibition is likely to be readily reversible and the interaction is likely to be short-lived once the interacting drug is removed from the regimen. In contrast, ketoconazole inhibits cytochrome P-450 through a direct ligand interaction between its imidazole nitrogens and the haem group of cytochrome P-450[128,129], which results in a non-competitive inhibition of microsomal CsA metabolism *in vitro*[30], although ketoconazole inhibition of drug metabolism is not necessarily of a non-competitive type[78,128,129]. This type of inhibition, which can arise with any drug possessing suitable nitrogen atoms, e.g. sterically unhindered imidazole, pyridine or primary amine nitrogens, is also reversible but may be more persistent. Cimetidine is also an imidazole drug, but is a relatively weak inhibitor of cytochrome P-450, probably because its imidazole nitrogens are both sterically hindered[108,130–132], and whilst there are several reports of cimetidine co-treatment causing an increase in circulating CsA levels[75,108,109], other studies failed to demonstrate any inhibiton of CsA metabolism either *in vivo* or *in vitro*[110,127]. A third mode of inhibition of cytochrome P-450 is restricted to a small number of drugs which form a stable, inhibitory 'product-adduct' between one of their metabolites and cytochrome P-450: sometimes the same form of cytochrome P-450 that is inhibited by the drug metabolite is responsible for generating it in the first place, and in these instances the effect is generally known as suicide inactivation. Erythromycin, triacetyloleandomycin and other macrolide antibiotics inhibit cytochrome P-450 by this mechanism[133,134]. This type of inhibition is likely to be long-lasting after withdrawal of the inhibitory drug: it is therefore significant that in patients where trough blood CsA levels doubled within 2 days of initiating erythromycin co-administration, they took 1–2 weeks to return to normal levels following withdrawal of erythromycin[105,106].

There is enzymological evidence to support a theory that induction of CsA metabolism is the mechanism underlying the interaction with phenobarbitone, phenytoin and rifampicin and that inhibition of CsA metabolism is the mechanism of the erythromycin interaction. As discussed above, in human and animal hepatic microsomes CsA is metabolized primarily by a form or forms of cytochrome P-450 belonging to the P-450III gene family. Phenobarbitone and phenytoin induce in human liver microsomes the same P-450III form, P-450hA7, that metabolizes CsA[135] and in rats these drugs induce both a related P-450III form[135] and the metabolism of CsA (see above), while in rabbits rifampicin induces another related P-450III form, P-450 3c, which also metabolizes CsA[31]. Conversely, a related P-450III form in rats, P-450p, is especially sensitive to suicide inactivation by erythromycin[134]. Furthermore, since erythromycin is also a substrate for the human P-450hA7[58], it could be expected to compete with CsA for it. Moreover, the chronology of these interactions in patients also fits this theory, as discussed above. However, alternative explanations have been put forward, notably an inhibition by erythromycin of the biliary excretion of CsA[107] and a decrease and increase of CsA absorption by phenytoin and erythromycin respectively[136–138]. Vereerstraeten et al.[139], however, explicitly discounted an increase in CsA absorption as the cause of the erythromycin interaction. In support of a non-inductive mechanism for the interaction of rifampicin with CsA is a report tha⁻ rifampicin causes a large decrease in circulating CsA levels in rats[61], despite its failure to induce P-450III forms in this species[62]. However, in the same study[61] rifampicin accelerated the reversal of kidney damage after the withdrawal of CsA – suggesting that rifampicin increased either the metabolism or the excretion of CsA. A further anomaly, militating against a simple inhibition of CsA metabolism by calcium antagonists, is the observation that circulating CsA levels in patients are increased by co-treatment with verapamil, diltiazem and nicardipine, but not by nifedipine[41,126,127] – yet nifedipine and CsA are alternative substrates for the same form of human cytochrome P-450, P-450hA[55,58].

The difficulty of predicting the consequences and mechanisms of drug interactions is illustrated by prednisolone and CsA. CsA decreases prednisolone clearance in patients[87–89], yet prednisolone may well increase the clearance of CsA, since it appears to induce human cytochrome P-450hA7[135], which metabolizes CsA (see above). In patients receiving combined prednisolone–CsA therapy, is an improvement in renal function due to prednisolone ameliorating CsA toxicity by inducing CsA metabolism, or is it because the prednisolone helps to prevent graft rejection by contributing to immunosuppression?

Although many drug interactions with CsA are adverse, leading to an increased risk of either graft rejection or nephrotoxicity, there are a number of interactions that can be considered beneficial, leading to a decrease in CsA nephrotoxicity while maintaining or even enhancing immunosuppression. Drugs entering into beneficial interactions with CsA can be divided into four categories:

1. Potent immunosuppressive agents: FK506, a recently discovered macrolide antibiotic, can act synergistically with CsA to suppress T-cell responses in vitro[141] and also graft rejection[142]. Smaller doses of each agent would be required to produce the appropriate degree of immunosuppression, with consequently less toxicity.
2. Drugs which modulate arachidonic acid metabolism may correct the alterations in prostaglandin levels that are seen following CsA administration, and which are suggested as being responsible for the attendant renal toxicity by affecting the intrarenal control of the glomerular filtration rate (GFR). For example, increased urinary excretion of thromboxane B_2, the stable breakdown product of thromboxane A_2, but not of 6-keto-prostaglandin $F_{1\alpha}$ or prostaglandin E_2, has been observed following CsA administration in animals[143,144]. The co-administration of thromboxane B_2 synthetase inhibitors with CsA produces an improvement in GFR which correlates with a reduction in thromboxane B_2 excretion[78,143]. The current development of thromboxane A_2 receptor antagonists offers additional exciting prospects for the alleviation of CsA nephrotoxicity.
3. Prostaglandins and their synthetic analogues or fish oil, a rich source of

eicosanoid precursors, protect against CsA nephrotoxicity in experimental animals[83,145-147]. This effect of prostaglandins may be due to a direct cytoprotection of renal cells, but an alternative mechanism may be to correct the abnormal ratio between vasoconstrictory and vasodilatory eicosanoids which results from CsA administration.

4. The calcium channel antagonist diltiazem, appears to protect against CsA nephrotoxicity despite causing an increase in circulating CsA levels[41]. The mechanism of this protection may involve the maintenance of renal circulation, or alternatively a direct action in tubule cells.

CONCLUSIONS

CsA is eliminated primarily through biotransformation by the hepatic cytochrome P-450-dependent mono-oxygenase enzyme system to an extensive series of metabolites. A particular group of related forms of cytochrome P-450, belonging to the P-450III gene family, appear to have prime responsibility for CsA metabolism in both man and experimental animals, yet despite this there are marked species differences in both the pattern and the overall rate of formation of CsA metabolites. It seems prudent in clinical practice to give due consideration to the drugs co-administered with CsA as to their own metabolism and toxicity. If a compound is given which is itself metabolized by or inhibits or induces cytochrome P-450, especially if it affects P-450III forms, there is a good chance that it will alter the metabolism of CsA and lead to an increase or a decrease in circulating CsA levels. Indeed, the majority of recognized CsA–drug interactions involve agents that come into this category, leading most frequently to either an increased risk of graft rejection as a result of decreased blood CsA levels, or an increased risk of renal toxicity as a result of increased circulating CsA levels. Conversely, CsA can inhibit the metabolism of the co-administered drugs and cause their circulating concentration to rise to toxic levels. Furthermore, if an agent is administered which is toxic to the same target organs as CsA, in particular if it is nephrotoxic, there is a good chance that it will exacerbate CsA toxicity. In any event it is important where any interaction is suspected to monitor the blood levels of CsA daily. It is also important to monitor the interacting drug itself, if this is one for which it is known that an alteration in its metabolism gives rise to toxicity or a serious loss of efficacy.

ACKNOWLEDGEMENTS

We are grateful to Sandoz Ltd, Basel, and in particular to Dr G. Maurer and Dr J. F. Borel, for gifts of CsA, [³H]CsA and authentic CsA metabolites, and for helpful discussions. Our own studies into the human microsomal metabolism of CsA could not have taken place but for the help of our colleagues, Mr J. Engeset (Department of Surgery) and Professor J. C. Petrie (Department of Medicine and Therapeutics), to whom we are most grateful. Our work was supported by grants from the Medical Research Council, the

Scottish Home and Health Department, Grampian Health Board and Tenovus (Aberdeen).

REFERENCES

1. Critical Issues in Cyclosporine Monitoring: Report of the Task Force on Cyclosporine Monitoring (1988) *Clin. Chem.*, **33**, 1269–1288.
2. Ryffel, B. (1983) Experimental toxicological studies with cyclosporin A. In White, D. J. G. (ed.), *Cyclosporin A*. (Elsevier Biomedical Press, Amsterdam), pp. 45–76.
3. Bellitsky, P., Ghose, T., Givner, M., Rowden, G. and Pope, B. (1985) Tissue distribution of cyclosporine A in the mouse: a clue to toxicity? *Clin. Nephrol.*, **25** (Suppl. 1), S27–S29.
4. Backman, L., Brandt, I., Dallner, G. and Ringden, O. (1988) Tissue distribution of (^{3}H)cyclosporine in mice. *Transpl. Proc.* **20** (Suppl. 2), 684–691.
5. Newberger, J. and Kahan, B. D. (1983) Cyclosporine pharmacokinetics in man. *Transplant. Proc.*, **15** (Suppl. 1), 2413–2415.
6. Reid, M., Gibbons, S., Kwok, D., Van Buren, C. T., Flechner, S. and Kahan, B. D. (1983). Cyclosporine levels in human tissues of patients treated for one week to one year. *Transplant. Proc.*, **15** (Suppl. 1), 2435–2437.
7. Atkinson, K., Boland, J., Britton, K. and Biggs, J. (1983) Blood and tissue distribution of cyclosporine in humans and mice. *Transplant. Proc.*, **15**, 2430–2449.
8. Lensmeyer, G., Wiebe, D. and Carlson, I. (1988) Deposition of nine metabolites of cyclosporine in human tissues, bile, urine and whole blood. *Transplant. Proc.*, **20** (Suppl. 2), 614–622.
9. Ptachcinski, R. J., Venkataramanan, R. and Burckart, G. J. (1986) Clinical pharmacokinetics of cyclosporin. *Clin. Pharmacokinetics*, **II**, 107–132.
10. Koponen, M. and Loor, F. (1983) Cytoplasmic lipid droplets as the possible eventual cellular fate of active forms of cyclosporine. *Exp. Cell. Res.*, **149**, 499–512.
11. Hanschumaker, R. E., Harding, M. W., Rice, J., Drugge, R. J. and Speicher, D. W. (1984) Cyclophilin: a specific cytosolic binding protein for CsA. *Science*, **22**, 544–547.
12. Dabrota, M. and Louis, J. (1989) Intracellular localisation of Cyclosporin A in the rat kidney. In Bach, P. H. and Lock, E. A. (eds.), *Nephrotoxicity: Extrapolation from in vitro to in vivo, and Animals to Man*, pp. 325–330. (London: Plenum Press).
13. LeGrue, S. J., Friedman, A. W. and Kahan, B. D. (1983) Lack of evidence for a cyclosporine receptor on human lymphocyte membranes. *Transplant. Proc.*, **15** (Suppl 1), 2259–2264.
14. Larson, D. F. (1986) Mechanism of action: antagonism of the prolactin receptor. In Borel, J. F. (ed.), *Ciclosporin* (New York: Karger), pp. 222–238.
15. Hiestand, P. C. and Meckler, P. (1986) Mechanism of action: ciclosporin- and prolactin-mediated control of immunity. In Borel, J. F. (ed.), *Ciclosporin* (New York: Karger), pp. 239–256.
16. Maurer, G., Loosli, H. R., Schreier, E. and Keller, B. (1984) Disposition of cyclosporine in several animal species. *Drug Metab. Disp.*, **12**, 120–126.
17. Hartman, N. R., Trimble, L. A., Vederas, J. C. and Jardine, I. (1985) An acid metabolite of cyclosporine. *Biochem. Biophys. Res. Commun.*, **133**, 964–971.
18. Maurer, G. and Lemaire, M. (1986) Biotransformation and distribution in blood of cyclosporine and its metabolites. *Transplant. Proc.*, **18** (Suppl. 5), 25–34.
19. Fabre, G., Berthault-Peres, P., Fabre, I., Maurel, P., Just, S. and Cano, J-P. (1987) Metabolism of cyclosporin A. I. Study in freshly isolated rabbit hepatocytes. *Drug Metab. Dispos.*, **15**, 384–390.
20. Cheung, F., Wong, P. Y., Loo, J., Cole, E. H. and Levy, G. A. (1988) Identification of cyclosporine metabolites in human bile, blood, and urine by high-performance liquid chromatography/radioimmunoassay/fast atomic bombardment mass spectroscopy. *Transplant. Proc.*, **20** (Suppl. 2), 602–608.
21. Christians, U., Schlitt, H. J., Bleck, J. S., Schiebel, H. M., Kownatzki, R., Maurer, G., Strohmeyer, S. S., Schottmann, R., Wonigeit, K., Pichlmayr, R. and Sewing, K-F. (1988) Measurement of cyclosporine and 18 metabolites in blood, bile, and urine by high-performance liquid chromatography. *Transplant. Proc.*, **20** (Suppl. 2), 609–613.

22. Bowers, L. D., Norman, D. D. and Henion, J. D. (1988) Isolation and characterization of cyclosporine metabolites using high-performance liquid chromatography and tandem mass spectrometry. *Transplant. Proc.*, **20**(Suppl. 2), 597–601.

23. Keown, P. A. (1988) Optimizing cyclosporine therapy: dose, levels and monitoring. *Transplant. Proc.*, **20** (Suppl. 2), 382–389.

24. Pell, M. /.., Rosano, T., Brayman, K. and Shaw, L. (1988) Predominance of native cyclosporine over metabolites in rat blood and tissue. *Transplant. Proc.*, **20** (Suppl. 2), 674–679.

25. Alexander, D. P., Horning, L. and Bowers, L. D. (1988) Cyclosporine metabolite disposition after oral administration in pretransplant end-stage renal disease patients. *Transplant. Proc.*, **20** (Suppl. 2), 499–508.

26. Rosano, T. G., Pell, M. A., Freed, B. M., Dybas, M. T. and Lempert, N. (1988) Cyclosporine and metabolites in blood from renal allograft recipients with nephrotoxicity, rejection, or good renal function: comparative high-performance liquid chromatography and monoclonal radioimmunoassay studies. *Transplant. Proc.*, **20** (Suppl. 2), 330–338.

27. Freeman, D. J., Laupacis, A., Keown, P. A., Stiller, C. R. and Carruthers, S. G. (1984) Evaluation of cyclosporin-phenytoin interaction with observations on cyclosporine metabolites. *Br. J. Clin. Pharmacol.*, **18**, 886–893.

28. Venkataraman, R., Wang, C., Burckart, G., Ptachcinski, R., Todo, S., Koneru, B. and Starzl, T. (1988). Species-specific cyclosporine metabolism. *Transplant. Proc.*, **20** (Suppl. 2), 680–683.

29. Roberts, N. B., Lane, C., Scott, M. H. and Sells, R. A. (1988) The measurement of cyclosporine A and metabolite M17 in whole blood by high-performance liquid chromatography. *Transplant. Proc.*, **20** (Suppl. 2), 625–632.

30. Maurer, G. (1985) Metabolism of cyclosporine. *Transplant. Proc.*, **17** (Suppl. 1), 19–26.

31. Berthault-Peres, P., Bonfils, C., Fabre, G., Just, S., Cano, J-P. and Maurel, P. (1987) Metabolism of cyclosporin A. II. Implication of the macrolide antibiotic inducible cytochrome P-450 3c from rabbit liver microsomes. *Drug Metab. Dispos.*, **15**, 391–398.

32. Wagner, O., Schreier, E., Heitz, F. and Maurer, G. (1987) Tissue distribution, disposition, and metabolism of cyclosporine in rats. *Drug Metab. Dispos.*, **15**, 377–383.

33. Awni, W., Heim-Duthoy, K., Rose, M., Kasiske, B., Rao, V., Bloom, P., Ney, A., Andrisevic, J., Odland, M. and Anderson, R. (1988) Changes in the pharmacokinetics of cyclosporine and three of its metabolites in renal transplant patients early in the posttransplant. period. *Transplant. Proc.*, **20** (Suppl. 2), 623–624.

34. Ryffel, B., Foxwell, B. M. J., Mihatsch, M. J., Donatsch, P. and Maurer, G. (1988) Biologic significance of cyclosporine metabolites. *Transplant. Proc.*, **20**, (Suppl. 2), 575–584.

35. Greval, J. (1988) Significance of cyclosporine pharmacokinetics. *Transplant. Proc.*, **20** (Suppl. 2), 428–434.

36. Kahan, B. D. (1985). Individualization of cyclosporine therapy using pharmacokinetic and pharmacodynamic parameters. *Transplantation*, **40**, 457–476.

37. Lokiec, F., Vernillet, L., Le Bigot, J. F., Ricour, C. and Goulet, O. (1988). Small intestinal transplantation and cyclosporine predose calculation. *Transplant. Proc.*, **20** (Suppl. 2), 491–493.

38. Wang, C., Burckart, G., Ptachcinski, R., Venkataramanan, R., Schwinghammer, T., Hakala, T., Griffith, B., Hardesty, R., Shadduck, R. and Starzl, T. (1988) Cyclosporine metabolite concentrations in the blood of liver, heart, kidney and bone marrow transplant patients. *Transplant. Proc.*, **20** (Suppl. 2), 591–596.

39. Rosano, T. G., Freed, B. M., Pell, M. A. and Lempert, N. (1986) Cyclosporine metabolites in human blood and renal tissue. *Transplant. Proc.*, **18** (Suppl. 5), 35–40.

40. Burckart, G. J., Starzl, T. E., Venkataramanan, R., Hashim, H., Wong, L., Wang, P., Makowka, L., Zeevi, A., Ptachcinski, R. J., Knapp, J. E., Iwatsuki, S., Esquivel, C., Sanghvi, A. and Van Thiel, D. H. (1986) Excretion of cyclosporine and its metabolites in human bile. *Transplant. Proc.*, **18**, (Suppl. 5), 46–49.

41. Wagner, K., Henkel, M., Heinemeyer, G. and Neumayer, H-H. (1988) Interaction of calcium blockers and cyclosporine. *Transplant. Proc.*, **20** (Suppl. 2), 561–568.

42. Yee, G. C., Gmur, D. J. and Meier, P. (1988) Measurement of blood cyclosporine metabolite concentrations with a new column-switching high-performance liquid chromatographic assay. *Transplant. Proc.*, **20** (Suppl. 2), 585–590.

43. Albano, J. D. M., Lawes, L. and Raman, G. V. (1988) Monitoring of blood cyclosporine

concentrations by a finger stab method and its applications. *Transplant. Proc.*, **20** (Suppl. 2), 451–456.

44. Canafax, D. M., Cipolle, R. J., Hrushesky, W. J. M., Rabatin, J. T., Min, D. I., Graves, N. M., Sutherland, D. E. R. and Bowers, L. D. (1988) The chronopharmacokinetics of cyclosporine and its metabolites in recipients of pancreas allografts. *Transplant. Proc.*, **20** (Suppl. 2), 471–477.

45. Vine, W., Olson, K. N. and Bowers, L. D. (1988) Therapeutic drug monitoring of cyclosporine by high-performance liquid chromatography in high volume. *Transplant. Proc.*, **20** (Suppl. 2), 354–356.

46. Brayman, K. L., Nakamura, J., Naji, A., Barker, C. F., Choti, M. A. and Shaw, L. M. (1988) The effect of phenobarbital and methylprednisolone on the biotransformation of cyclosporine in the rat. *Transplant. Proc.*, **20** (Suppl. 2), 553–556.

47. Lemaire, M. and Tillement, J. P. (1982) Role of lipoproteins and erythrocytes in the *in vitro* binding and distribution of cyclosporine. *J. Pharm. Pharmacol.*, **34**, 715–718.

48. Rosano, T. G. (1985) Effect of hematocrit on cyclosporine in whole blood and plasma of renal transplant patients. *Clin. Chem.*, **31**, 410–412.

49. Yatscoff, R. W., Rush, D. N. and Jeffrey, J. R. (1984) Effects of sample preparation on the concentration of cyclosporin A measured in plasma. *Clin. Chem.*, **30**, 1812–1814.

50. Van den Berg, J. W. O., Verhoef, M. I., de Boer, A. J. H. and Schalm, S. W. (1985) Cyclosporin A assay: conditions for sampling and processing of blood. *Clin. Chim. Acta*, **147**, 291–297.

51. Mraz, W., Zink, R. A. and Graf, A. (1983) Distribution and transfer of cyclosporine among the various lipoprotein classes. *Transplant. Proc.*, **15** (Suppl. 1), 2426–2429.

52. Gurecke, J., Warty, V. and Sanghvi, A. (1985) The transport of cyclosporine in association with plasma lipoproteins in heart and liver transplant patients. *Transplant. Proc.*, **17**, 1997–2002.

53. Cheung, F., Wong, P., Cole, E., Cohen, Z. and Levy, G. (1988) Generation and characterisation of cyclosporine metabolites produced in a hepatic microsomal system. *Transplant. Proc.*, **20** (Suppl. 2), 633–636.

54. Augustine, J. A. and Zemaitis, M. A. (1986) The effects of cyclosporin A (CsA) on hepatic microsomal drug metabolism in the rat. *Drug. Metab. Dispos.*, **14**, 73–78.

55. Burke, M. D., MacIntyre, F., Cameron, D. and Whiting, P. H. Unpublished observations.

56. Nebert, D. W. and Gonzalez, F. J. (1987). P450 Genes: structure, evolution and regulation. *Ann. Rev. Biochem.*, **56**, 945–993.

57. Guengerich, F. P., Martin, M. V., Beaune, P. H., Kremers, P., Wolff, T. and Waxman, D. J. (1986) Characterization of rat and human liver microsomal cytochrome P-450 forms involved in nifedipine oxidation, a prototype for genetic polymorphism in oxidative drug metabolism. *J. Biol. Chem.*, **261**, 5051–5060.

58. Shaw, P. M. (1987). PhD thesis, University of Aberdeen.

59. Moochala, S. M. and Renton, K. W. (1986) Inhibition of hepatic microsomal drug metabolism by the immunosuppressive agent cyclosporin A. *Biochem. Pharmacol.*, **35**, 1499–1503.

60. Guengerich, F. P. (1987). Cytochrome P-450 enzymes and drug metabolism. In Bridges, J. W., Chasseaud, L. F. and Gibson, G. G. (eds), *Progress in Drug Metabolism*, vol. 10 (London: Taylor and Francis).

61. Hopps, V., Galione, A., Biondi, F., Vaccaro, F., Sorrentino, M. C., Vetri, P. and Leone, F. (1988) Rifampicin reduces nephrotoxicity of cyclosporine A in rats: studies of renal enzyme excretion. *Trans. Proc.*, **20** (Suppl. 2), 557–560.

62. Wrighton, S. A., Schuetz, E. G., Watkins, P. B., Maurel, P., Barwick, J., Bailey, B. S., Hartle, H. T., Young, B. and Guzelian, P. (1985) Demonstration in multiple species of inducible hepatic cytochromes P-450 and their mRNAs related to the glucocorticoid-inducible cytochrome P-450 of the rat. *Mol. Pharmacol.*, **28**, 312–321.

63. Burke, M. D. and Whiting, P. H. (1986) The role of drug metabolism in cyclosporine A nephrotoxicity. *Clin. Nephrol.*, **25**(Suppl. 1), S111–S116.

64. Cunningham, C., Gavin, M. P., Whiting, P. H., Burke, M. D., Macintyre, F., Thomson, A. W. and Simpson, J. G. (1984) Serum cyclosporin levels, hepatic drug metabolism and renal tubulotoxicity. *Biochem. Pharmacol.*, **33**, 2857–2861.

65. Galinsky, R. E., Alexander, D. P. and Franklin, M. R. (1987) Effect of cyclosporine on hepatic oxidative and conjugative metabolism. *Drug Metab. Dispos.*, **15**, 731–733.

66. Backman, L., AppelKwist, E-L., Ringden, O. and Dallner, G. (1988) Effects of cyclosporine on hepatic protein synthesis. *Transplant. Proc.*, **20**(Suppl. 3), 853–858.
67. Buss, W., Stepanek, J. and Bennett, W. (1988) Proposed mechanism of cyclosporine toxicity: inhibition of protein synthesis. *Transplant. Proc.*, **20** (Suppl. 3), 863–867.
68. Cunningham, C., Burke, M. D., Wheatley, D. N., Thomson, A. W., Simpson, J. G. and Whiting, P H. (1985) Amelioration of cyclosporin-induced nephrotoxicity in rats by induction of hepatic drug metabolism. *Biochem. Parmacol.*, **34**, 573–578.
69. Duncan, J. I., Whiting, P. H., Simpson, J. G. and Thomson, A. W. (1986) Alleviation of cyclosporine-mediated nephrotoxicity by phenobarbitone, during the suppression of graft-versus-host reactivity. *Transplant. Proc.*, **18**, 645–649.
70. Freed, B. M., Rosano, T. G. and Lempert, N. (1987) *In vitro* immunosuppressive properties of cyclosporine metabolites. *Transplantation*, **43**, 123–127.
71. Zeevi, A., Eiras, G., Burckart, G., Makowka, L., Venkataramanan, R., Wang, C., Van Thiel, D. H., Murase, N., Starzl, T. and Duquesnoy, R. (1988) Immunosuppressive effect of cyclosporine metabolites from human bile on alloreactive T cells. *Transplant. Proc.*, **20** (Suppl. 2), 115–121.
72. Rosano, T. G., Freed, B. M., Cerilli, J. and Lempert, N. (1986) Immunosuppressive metabolites of cyclosporine in the blood of renal allograft recipients. *Transplantation*, **42**, 262–266.
73. Freed, B. M., Rosano, T. G., Quick, C. and Lempert, N. (1987) Effects of cyclosporine metabolites M17 and M18 on proliferation and IL-2 production in the mixed lymphocyte culture. *Transplant. Proc.*, **19**, 1223–1226.
74. Gumbleton, M., Brown, J. E., Hawksworth, G. and Whiting, P. H. (1985) The possible relationship between hepatic drug metabolism and ketoconazole enhancement of cyclosporine A-nephrotoxicity. *Transplantation*, **46**, 454–456.
75. Schwass, D. E., Sasaki, A. W., Houghton, D. C., Benner, K. E. and Bennett, W. M. (1985) Effect of phenobarbital and cimetidine on experimental cyclosporine nephrotoxicity: preliminary observations. *Clin. Nephrol.*, **25** (Suppl. 1), S117–S120.
76. Gunson, B. K., Jones, S. R., Maclean, S., Neuberger, J. and McMaster, P. (1988) Is the new specific monoclonal radioimmunoassay for cyclosporine of value in liver transplantation? *Transplant. Proc.*, **20** (Suppl. 2), 323–329.
77. Leunissen, K., Bosman, F., Beuman, G. and van Hoof, J. (1988) The nephrotoxic effects of cyclosporine metabolites. *Transplant. Proc.*, **20** (Suppl. 3), 738–739.
78. Whiting, P. H., Burke, M. D. and Thomson, A. W. (1985) Drug interactions with cyclosporine: implications from animal studies. *Transparant. Proc.*, **18**, 56–70.
79. Hows, J. M., Smith, J. M., Baughan, A. and Gordon-Smith, E. C. (1983) Nephrotoxicity in marrow graft recipients treated with cyclosporine. *Transplant. Proc.*, **15** (Suppl. 1), 2708–2711.
80. Kennedy, M. S., Deeg, H. J., Siegel, M., Crowley, J. J. and Storb, R. (1983) Acute renal toxicity with combined use of amphotericin B and cyclosporine after marrow transplantation. *Transplantation*, **35**, 211–215.
81. Thompson, J. F., Chalmers, D. H. K., Hunnisett, A. G. W., Wood, R. F. M. and Morris, P. J. (1983) Nephrotoxicity of trimethoprim and cotrimoxazole in renal allograft recipients treated with cyclosporine. *Transplantation*, **36**, 204–205.
82. Whiting, P. H. and Simpson, J. G. (1983). The enhancement of cyclosporin A-induced nephrotoxicity by gentamicin. *Biochem. Pharmacol.*, **32**, 2025–2058.
83. Whiting, P. H., Barnard, N., Neilsch, A., Simpson, J. G., and Burke, M. D. (1988) Interactions between cyclosporin A, indomethacin and 16,16-dimethyl prostaglandin E_2: effects on renal, hepatic and gastrointestinal toxicity in the rat. *Br. J. Exp. Pathol.*, **68**, 777–786.
84. Ryffel, B., Donatsch, P., Hiestand, P. and Mihatsch, M. J. (1985) PGE_2 reduces nephrotoxicity and immunosuppression of cyclosporine in rats. *Clin. Nephrol.*, **25** (Suppl. 1), S34–S37.
85. Whiting, P. H., Thomson, A. W. and Simpson, J. G. (1983) Renal and hepatic function in rats treated with cyclosporin A in combination with gentamicin or cephalosporin antibiotics. *Br. J. Exp. Pathol.*, **64**, 693–701.
86. Egfjord, M., Daugaard, H. and Olgaard, K. (1988) The effect of cyclosporine A on the hepatic clearance rate of prednisone in isolated perfused livers of normal and uremic rats. *Transplant. Proc.*, **20** (Suppl. 2), 549–552.

87. Ost, L. (1984) Effects of cyclosporine on prednisolone metabolism. *Lancet*, **1**, 451.
88. Ost, L., Klintmalm, G. and Ringden, O. (1985) Mutual interaction between prednisolone and cyclosporine in renal transplant patients. *Transplant. Proc.*, **17**, 1252–1255.
89. Langhoff, E., Madsen, S., Flachs, H., Olgaard, K., Ladeforged, J. and Hvidberg, E. F. (1985) Inhibition of prednisolone metabolism by cyclosporine in kidney transplant patients. *Transplantation*, **39**, 107–109.
90. Boogaerts, M. A., Zachee, P. and Verwilghen, R. L. (1982). Cyclosporine, methyl-prednisolone and convulsions. *Lancet*, **2**, 1217.
91. Daniels, N. J., Dover, J. S. and Schachter, R. K. (1984) Interaction between cyclosporin and rifampicin. *Lancet*, **2**, 639.
92. Allen, R. D., Hunnisett, A. G. and Morris, P. J. (1985) Cyclosporin and rifampicin in renal transplantation. *Lancet*, **1**, 980.
93. Langhoff, E. and Madsen, S. (1983). Rapid metabolism of cyclosporin and prednisone in kidney transplant patient receiving tuberculostatic treatment. *Lancet*, **2**, 1031.
94. Modry, D. L., Stinson, E. B., Oyer, P. E., Jamieson, S. W., Baldwin, J. C. and Shumway, N. E. (1985) Acute rejection and massive cyclosporine requirements in heart transplant recipients treated with rifampicin. *Transplantation*, **39**, 313–314.
95. Keown, P. A., Laupacis, A., Carruthers, G., Stawecki, M., Koegler, J., McKenzie, F. N., Wall, W. and Stiller, C. R. (1984) Interaction between phenytoin and cyclosporine following organ transplantation. *Transplantation*, **38**, 304–305.
96. Freeman, D. J., Laupacis, A., Keown, P. A., Stiller, C. and Carruthers, S. G. (1984) Evaluation of cyclosporin–phenytoin interaction with observations on cyclosporin metabolites. *Br. J. Clin. Pharmacol.*, **18**, 887–893.
97. Wood, A. J., Maurer, G., Niederberger, W. and Beveridge, T. (1983) Cyclosporine: pharmacokinetics, metabolism and drug interactions. *Transplant. Proc.*, **15** (Suppl. 1), 2409–2412.
98. Burckart, G. J., Venkataramanan, R., Starzl, T. E., Ptachcinski, R. J., Gartner, C. J. and Rosenthal, T. (1984) Cyclosporine clearance in children following organ transplantation. *J. Clin. Pharmacol.*, **24**, 412–416.
99. Carstensen, H. and Jacobsen, N. (1986). Interaction between cyclosporin A and phenobarbitone. *Br. J. Clin. Pharmacol.*, **21**, 550–551.
100. Lele, P., Peterson, P., Yang, S., Jarrell, B. and Burke, J. F. (1985) Cyclosporine and tegretol – another drug interaction. *Kidney Int.*, **27**, 344.
101. Miguet, J. P., Mavier, P., Soussy, C. J. and Dhumeaux, D. (1987) Induction of hepatic microsomal enzymes after brief administration of rifampicin in man. *Gastroenterology*, **72**, 924–6.
102. Buffington, G. A., Dominquez, J. H., Piering, W. F., Herbert, L. E., Kauffman, H. M. and Lemann, J. (1986) Interaction of rifampicin and glucocorticoids. *J. Am. Med. Assoc.*, **236**, 1958–1960.
103. Van Buren, D., Wideman, C. A., Reid, M., Gibbons, S., Van Buren, C. T., Janowenko, M., Flechner, S. M., Frazier, O. H., Cooley, D. A. and Kahan, B. D. (1984) The antagonistic effect of rifampicin upon Cyclosporine bioavailability. *Transplant. Proc.*, **16**, 1642–1645.
104. Wong, Y. Y., Ludden, T. M. and Bell, R. D. (1983). Effect of erythromycin on carbamazepine kinetics. *Clin. Pharmacol. Ther.*, **33**, 460–464.
105. Ptachcinski, R. J., Carpenter, B. J., Burckart, G. J., Venkataramanan, R. and Rosenthal, J. T. (1985) Effect of erythromycin on cyclosporine levels. *N. Engl. J. Med.*, **313**, 1416–1417.
106. Martell, R., Heinrichs, D., Stiller, C. R., Jenner, M., Keown, P. A. and Dupre, J. (1986) The effects of erythromycin in patients treated with Cyclosporine. *Ann. Intern. Med.*, **104**, 660–661.
107. Hourmant, M., Le Bigot, J. F., Vernillet, L., Sagniez, G., Remi, J. P. and Soulillou, J. P. (1985) Coadministration of erythromycin results in an increase of blood cyclosporine to toxic levels. *Transplant. Proc.*, **17**, 2723–2727.
108. D'Souza, M. J., Pollock, S. H. and Solomon, H. M. (1988) Cyclosporine–cimetidine interaction. *Drug Metab. Dispos.*, **16**, 57–59.
109. Babany, G., Morris, R. E., Babany, I., Shepherd, S. and Kates, R. E. (1988) Effects of the administration of cimetidine or phenobarbital on the immunosuppression of cyclosporine in mice *in vivo*. *Transplant. Proc.* (In press).
110. Freeman, D. J., Laupacis, A., Keown, P., Stiller, C. and Carruthers, G. (1984) The effect

of agents that alter drug metabolising anzyme activity on the pharmacokinetics of cyclosporine. *Ann. R. Coll. Phys. Surg., Canada,* **17**, 301.

111. White, D. J. G., Blatchford, N. R. and Cauwenbergh, G. (1984) Cyclosporine and ketoconazole. *Transplantation,* **37**, 214–215.

112. Moller, B. P. and Ekelund, B. (1985) Toxicity of cyclosporine during treatment with androgens. *J. Engl. J. Med.,* **313**, 1416.

113. Field, B., Lu, C. and Hepner, G. W. (1979) Inhibition of hepatic drug metabolism by norethindrone. *Clin. Pharmacol. Ther.,* **25**, 196–198.

114. Kohan, D. E. (1986) Possible interaction between cyclosporine and erythromycin. *N. Engl. J. Med.,* **314**, 448.

115. Dieperink, H. and Moller, J. (1982) Ketoconazole and cyclosporin. *Lancet,* **2**, 1217.

116. Ferguson, R. M., Sutherland, D. F. R., Simmons, R. L. and Najarian, J. S. (1982). Ketoconazole, cyclosporine metabolism and renal transplantation. *Lancet,* **2**, 882–883.

117. Grino, J. M., Sabate, I., Castelao, A. M. and Alsina, J. (1986). Influence of diltiazem on cyclosporin clearance. *Lancet,* **1**, 1387.

118. Pochet, J. M. and Pirson, Y. (1986) Cyclosporin–diltiazem interaction. *Lancet,* **1**, 979.

119. Neumayer, H. H. and Wagner, K. (1986). Diltiazem and economic use of cyclosporin. *Lancet,* **2**, 523.

120. Bourbigot, B., Guiserix, J., Airiau, J., Bressollette, L., Morin, J. F. and Cledes, J. (1986) Nicardipine increases cyclosporin blood levels. *Lancet,* **1**, 1447.

121. Klintmalm, G. and Sawe, J. (1984) High dose methylprednisolone increases plasma cyclosporine levels in renal transplant recipients. *Lancet,* **1**, 731.

122. Ross, W. B., Roberts, D., Griffin, P. J. A. and Salaman, J. R. (1986) Cyclosporin interaction with danazol and norethisterone. *Lancet,* **1**, 330.

123. Schroder, O., Schmitz, N., Kayser, W., Euler, H. H. and Loffler, H. (1986) Erhohte Ciclosporin-A-spiegel bei gleichzeitiger therapie mit danazol. *D. Med. Wochenschr.,* **111**, 602–603.

124. Deray, G., Le Hoang, P., Cacoub, P., Assogba, U., Grippon, P. and Baumelou, A. (1987) Oral contraceptive interactions with cyclosporin. *Lancet,* **1**, 158–9.

125. Morgernstern, G. R., Powles, R., Robinson, B. and McElwain, T. J. (1982) Cyclosporin interaction with ketoconazole and melphalan. *Lancet,* **2**, 1342.

126. Robson, R. A., Miners, J. O. and Birkett, D. J. (1988) Selective inhibitory effects of nifedipine and verapamil on oxidative metabolism: effects on theophylline. *Br. J. Clin. Pharmacol.,* **25**, 397–400.

127. Henricsson, S. and Lindholm, A. (1988). Inhibition of cyclosporine metabolism by other drugs *in vitro. Transplant. Proc.,* **20** (Suppl. 2), 569–571.

128. Meredith, C. G., Maldonado, A. L. and Spegg, K. V. (1985) The effect of ketoconazole on hepatic oxidative drug metabolism in the rat *in vivo* and *in vitro. Drug Metab. Dispos.,* **13**, 156–162.

129. Sheets, J. J., Mason, J. I., Wise, C. A. and Estabrook, R. W. (1986) Inhibition of rat liver microsomal cytochrome P-450 steroid hydroxylase reactions by imidazole antimycotic agents. *Biochem. Pharmacol.,* **35**, 487–491.

130. Somogyi, A. and Guglar, R. (1982) Drug interactions with cimetidine. *Clin. Pharmacokinet.,* **7**, 23–41.

131. Grassela, D. M. and Rocci, M. L. (1984) Inhibition of carbamazepine metabolism by cimetidine. *Drug Metab. Dispos.,* **12**, 204–208.

132. Knadell, R. G., Holtzman, J. L., Crankshaw, D., Steele, N. M. and Stanley, L. M. (1982) Drug metabolism by rat and human microsomes in response to interaction with H2-receptor antagonists. *Gastroenterology,* **82**, 84–88.

133. Delaforge, M., Jaouen, M. and Mansuy, D. (1983) Dual effects of macrolide antibiotics on rat liver cytochrome P-450. *Biochem. Pharmacol.,* **32**, 2309–2318.

134. Wrighton, S. A., Maurel, P., Scheutz, E. G., Watkins, P. B., Young, B. and Guzelian, P. S. (1985) Identification of the cytochrome P-450 induced by macrolide antibiotics in rat liver as the glucocorticoid responsive P-450p. *Biochemistry,* **24**, 2171–2178.

135. Shaw, P. M., Barnes, T. S., Melvin, W. T. and Burke, M. D. Unpublished observations.

136. Rowland, M. and Gupta, S. K. (1987) Cyclosporin–phenytoin interaction: Re-evaluation using metabolite data. *Br. J. Clin. Pharmacol.,* **24**, 329–334.

137. Gupta, S. K., Bakran, A., Johnson, R. W. G., and Rowland, M. (1988) Erythromycin enhances the absorption of cyclosporin. *Br. J. Clin. Pharmacol.,* **25**, 401–402.

138. Lysz, K., Rosenberg, J. C., Kaplan, M. P., Migdal, S. and Sillix, D. (1988) Interaction of Erythromycin with Cyclosporine. *Transplant. Proc.*, **20** (Suppl. 2), 543–548.
139. Vereerstraeten, P., Thiry, P., Kinnaert, P., Toussaint, C. (1987) Influence of erythromycin on cyclosporine pharmacokinetics. *Transplantation*, **44**, 155–156.
140. Whiting, P. H., Duncan, J. I. and Heys, S. D. (1988) The effect of biliary cannulation or ligation on cyclosporine nephrotoxicity in the rat. *Transplant. Proc.*, **20** (Suppl. 3), 845–849.
141. Zeevi, A., Duquesnoy, R. and Eiras, G. (1987) Immunosuppressive effect of FK-506 on *in vitro* lymphocyte alloactivation: synergism with cyclosporin A. *Transplant. Proc.*, **19** (Suppl. 5), 40–43.
142. Murase, N., Todo, S. and Lee, P-H. (1987) Heterotopic heart transplantation in the rat receiving FK-506 alone or in combination with cyclosporine. *Transplant. Proc.*, **19** (Suppl. 5), 71–74.
143. Perico, N., Benigni, A., Zoja, C., Delaini, F. and Remuzzi, G. (1986) Functional significance of exaggerated renal thromboxane A_2 synthesis induced by cyclosporin A. *Am. J. Physiol.*, **251**, F581–F587.
144. Kawaguchi, A., Goldman, M. H., Shapiro, R., Foegh, M. L., Ramwell, P. W. and Lower, R. R. (1985) Increase in urinary thromboxane B_2 in rats caused by cyclosporine. *Transplantation*, **40**, 214–216.
145. Paller, M. S. (1988) Effects of the prostaglandin E_1 analog misoprostol on cyclosporine nephrotoxicity. *Transplantation*, **45**, 1126–1131
146. Makowka, L., Lopatin, W., Gilas, T., Falk, J., Phillips, M. J. and Falk, R. (1985) Prevention of cyclosporine (CyA) nephrotoxicity by synthetic prostaglandins. *Clin. Nephrol.*, **25** (Suppl. 1), S89–S94.
147. Bennett, W. (1988) Pathophysiology of cyclosporine nephrotoxicity: role of eicosanoids. *Transplant. Proc.*, **20** (Suppl. 3), 628–633.
148. Robson, S., Neuberger, J., Alexander, G. and Williams, R. (1984) Cyclosporin A nephrotoxicity related to changes in haemoglobin concentration. *Br. Med. J.* **228**, 1417–1481.
149. Whiting, P. H., Cunningham, C., Thomson, A. W. and Simpson, J. G. (1984) Enhancement of high dose cyclosporin A toxicity by frusemide. *Biochem. Pharmacol.*, **33**, 1075–1079.
150. Durrant, S., Chipping, P. M., Palmer, S. and Gordon-Smith, E. C. (1982) Cyclosporin A, methylprednisolone and convulsions. *Lancet*, **2**, 829–830.
151. Wallwork, J., McGregor, C. G. A., Wells, F. C., Cory-Pearce, R. and English, T. A. H. (1983) Cyclosporin and intravenous sulphadimidine and trimethoprim therapy. *Lancet*, **1**, 366–7.
152. Jones, D. K., Hakim, M., Wallwork, J., Higenbottam, T. W. and White, D. J. G. (1986) Serious interaction between cyclosporin A and sulphadimidine. *Br. Med. J.*, **292**, 728–729.
153. Benditzen, K., Nissen, C., Tvede, N. and Anderson, V. (1985) Ciclosporin treatment of autoimmune inflammatory disorders of the eye. In Schindler, R. (ed.), *Ciclosporin in Autoimmune Diseases* (Berlin: Springer), pp. 143–146.
154. Berg, K. J., Nordby, G., Rootwell, K., Djöseland, O. Z., Fanchauld, P., Mehl, A., Naverud, J. and Talseth, J. (1988) Effects on renal function of combined treatment with trimethoprim and cyclosporine A in kidney transplant patients. *Transplant Proc.*, **20**, (Suppl. 3), 413–415
155. Dale, B. M., Sage, R. E., Norman, J. E., Barber, S. and Kotasek, D. (1985) Bone marrow transplantation following treatment with high dose melphalan. *Transplant. Proc.*, **17**, 1711–1713.
156. Petric, R., Freeman, D., Wallace, A., McDonald, J., Stiller, C. and Keown, P. (1988) Effect of cyclosporine on urinary prostanoid excretion, renal blood flow and glomerillotubular function. *Transplantation*, **45**, 883–889
157. Kronbach, T., Fischer, V. and Meyer, U. A. (1988) Cyclosporine metabolism in human liver: identification of a cytochrome P-450III gene family as the major cyclosporine-metabolizing enzyme explains interactions of cyclosporine with other drugs. *Clin. Pharmacol. Ther.*, **43**, 630–635.
158. Murray, G. I., Barnes, T. S., Sewell, H. F., Ewen, S. W. B., Melvin, W. T. and Burke, M. D. (1988) The immunocytochemical localisation and distribution of cytochrome P-450 in normal human hepatic and extrahepatic tissues with a monoclonal antibody to human cytochrome P-450. *Br. J. Clin. Pharmacol.*, **25**, 465–475.

14
Pathological effects of cyclosporin A in experimental models

Paul H. Whiting and Angus W. Thompson

Cyclosporin A (CsA), administered either alone or in combination with steroids or azathioprine, is now the immunotherapeutic agent of choice in the management of organ allograft rejection. The prospective value of CsA in the treatment of certain autoimmune diseases is presently being evaluated in numerous clinical trials. However, it has been demonstrated both in animals and man that CsA possesses many adverse side-effects, which include renal and hepatic dysfunction, hypertension, mild tremors, hirsutism, abnormal glucose homeostasis and gingival hypertrophy. Some degree of renal impairment is observed in virtually all patients receiving CsA, and it is this attendant nephrotoxicity which limits its clinical use.

Although CsA has been used clinically for over 10 years, the mechanisms underlying its potent immunoefficacy have not been fully elucidated. Similarly, those mechanisms responsible for the development of the toxic side-effects observed following CsA administration, particularly nephrotoxicity, are also as yet poorly understood. It is in this context that animal models have an important role to play, both in the elucidation of these mechanisms and in the development of effective countermeasures which may ultimately improve graft survival and renal function in these patients. The principal side-effects of CsA which have been documented in man and laboratory animals are listed in Table 14.1. It is clear that a similar spectrum of pathological effects to those encountered in clinical practice can be reproduced in animals, in particular the rat, which has been the subject of most CsA toxicology investigations. In contrast to the use of CsA in man, however, doses of the drug in excess of those required for adequate immunosuppression are needed to produce pathological effects in the rat and other species. In this review we shall focus attention principally on the nephrotoxic and hepatotoxic properties of CsA, and on the influence of the drug on glucose homeostasis – the most important problems usually encountered in the management of patients receiving the drug.

Table 14.1 Pathological effects of CsA in humans and animals

Organ/system	Humans	Animals*
Kidney	Increased serum creatinine levels and enzymuria; tubular damage; arterial and glomerular thrombosis; interstitial nephritis	*Acute* Reduced GFR; enzymuria; proximal and distal tubular damage *Chronic* Reduced GFR; polyuria; tubular dilatation or atrophy; striped interstitial fibrosis
Liver	Jaundice; altered serum enzymes	Hyperbilirubinaemia; altered serum enzymes; hypoproteinaemia and albuminaemia; fatty change; focal hepatocyte necrosis
Alimentary system	Diarrhoea, gingival hypertrophy	Gingivitis; periodontitis (dog); failure to digest food (rabbit); diarrhoea
Skin	Hirsutism	Hair loss/growth (nude mice); papillomatosis (dog)
Vascular system	Hypertension	Hypertension
Lymphoid	Increased incidence of lymphoma†	Lymphoproliferation in gut-associated lymphoid tissue; reduced cellularity of thymic cortex and medulla, splenic periarteriolar sheaths and marginal zones, paracortex of lymph nodes
Haemopoietic system	Non-myelotoxic	Lymphopenia; atypical mononuclear cells; monocytosis; granulocytosis; eosinophilia; hypochromic anaemia
Glucose homeostasis	Reduced glucose tolerance	Reduced glucose tolerance; pancreatic β cell damage; peripheral insulin resistance
Other	Tremor; convulsions; epileptic fits	Irritability; epileptic-like fits; fetotoxicity

* Many of these changes found only at levels above the immunotherapeutic range in animals, and relate mainly to studies conducted in rats
† Early clinical reports only; associated with excessive immunosuppression

NEPHROTOXICITY

Clinically, there appear to be three main types of renal structural damage associated with CsA administration[1,2]. None of these is specific, but all are present more commonly following CsA administration than in other situations. First, in patients with prolonged oliguria or anuria following renal transplantation, the kidneys may show diffuse interstitial fibrosis ('interactive toxicity'). Second, acute toxicity, which is dose-related and less common now that lower initial doses of CsA and drug tapering are employed, may be accompanied by structural abnormalities; if changes are present, they comprise a toxic proximal tubulopathy. The third type of CsA-induced renal lesion is chronic toxicity, associated with either striped (i.e. radial) interstitial fibrosis and/or an arteriolopathy.

Nearly all patients on CsA demonstrate some degree of renal impairment, which in the most severe cases has lead to renal failure, necessitating renal transplantation in certain CsA-treated heart transplant patients[3]. The functional correlate most commonly used to describe CsA nephrotoxicity is an increase in serum creatinine concentration and, less commonly, the demonstration of a reduced glomerular filtration rate (GFR)[3-7].

Acute nephrotoxicity

Early animal studies were most often performed in the rat, and included work on normotensive and spontaneously hypertensive animals and also on animals having undergone either unilateral or 5/6 nephrectomy, renal denervation or experimental renal transplantation[8]. These investigations were performed using relatively high doses of CsA (≥ 25 mg/kg body weight per day) usually administered over a 2–4 week period. Over this short time, only acute nephrotoxicity was usually encountered. The renal dysfunction was characterized, functionally, by reductions in GFR (and enhanced tubular enzymuria, including the activities of N-acetyl-β-D-glucosaminidase, γ-glutamyl transferase, glutathione S-transferase, pyruvate kinase, and fructose-1,6-bisphosphatase)[8-11]. The concomitant renal structural abnormalities observed in rats were focal, convoluted proximal tubular cell vacuolation and necrosis, and the presence of basal lipid droplets, clearly evident on light microscopy (Figure 14.1). Ultrastructurally, the tubular epithelial dilatation and vesiculation of the smooth endoplasmic reticulum, together with increased lysosome production and the presence of myeloid figures. This acute renal injury, related to the dose administered and to circulating drug levels, is reversible on drug withdrawal or dose reduction (similar to the acute nephrotoxicity experienced in clinical practice)[8,12,13] and is apparently non-progressive. The short-term administration of CsA in animals is also associated with altered renal tubular and glomerulotubular function, including reduced lithium clearance and deficient urinary acidification and diluting capacity[14-19].

Although most studies of short-term CsA nephrotoxicity in animals have failed to demonstrate any structural defects in either glomeruli or distal tubules, a recent elegant ultrastructural study[20] has revealed CsA-induced glomerular afferent arteriole constriction in the rat (Figure 14.2). It has also been demonstrated that granular juxtaglomerular cell hyperplasia is associated with CsA administration in the rabbit[21]. Furthermore, other studies have demonstrated that altered distal tubular function may play a role in the reduction in GFR caused by CsA[22-24]. An isolated report has also demonstrated structural alterations to the distal nephron, but only at high CsA dose[25].

Modification of acute nephrotoxicity

There is now extensive evidence that interference with hepatic CsA metabolism in rats affects the extent of renal functional and structural impairment. Thus, co-treatment with known inducers (e.g. phenobarbitone) or inhibitors (e.g. ketoconazole) of hepatic cytochrome P-450-dependent mono-oxygenase

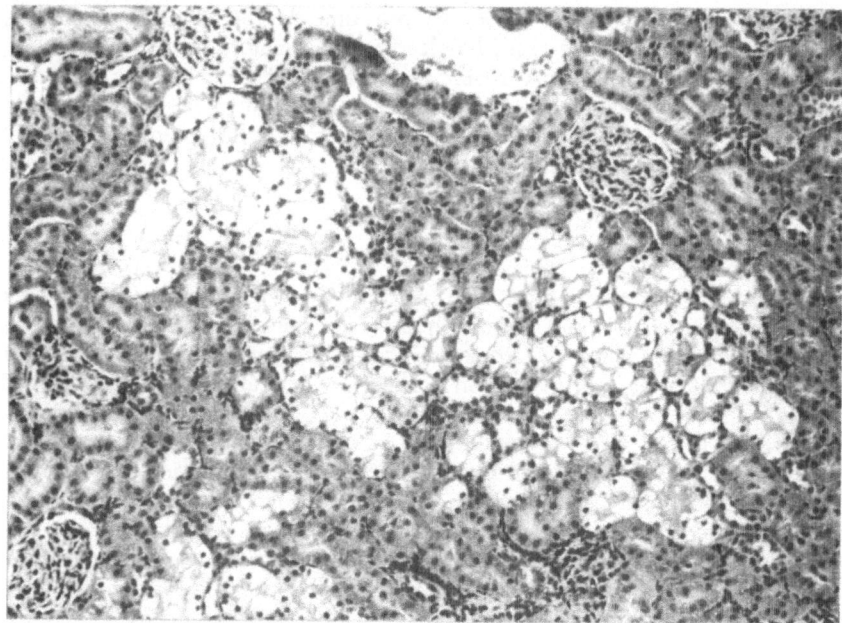

Figure 14.1 Acute CsA renal damage in the rat. Proximal straight tubular vacuolation in the deep cortex, from an animal treated with CsA (50 mg kg^{-1} day^{-1}) for 7 days. (H&E × 140)

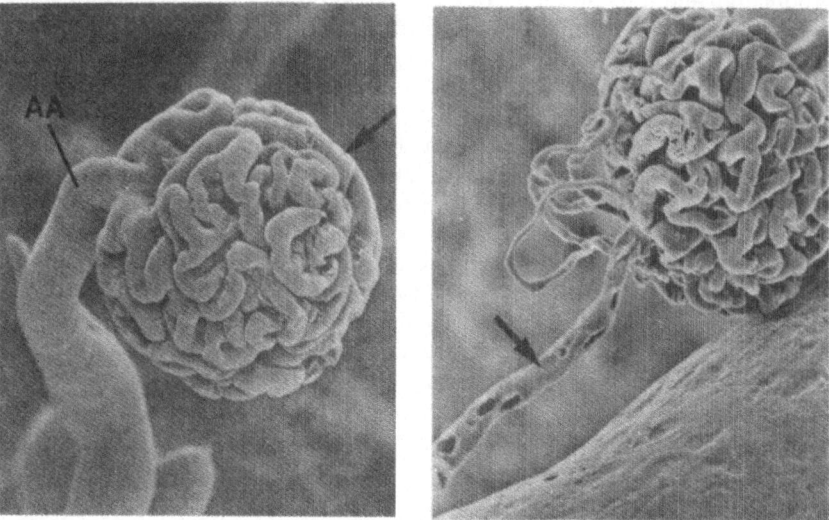

Figure 14.2 Scanning electron micrograph (right) of a vascular cast from a rat treated with CsA (50 mg kg^{-1} day^{-1}) for 14 days. An afferent glomerular arteriole (AA) shows obvious narrowing (arrow) near the glomerular tuft (× 500). Reproduced with permission from English et al.[20]. Compare with drug vehicle-treated control (left)

activity results in lower circulating CsA levels and diminished nephrotoxicity or higher circulating drug concentrations and enhanced nephrotoxicity, respectively[26-32]. Paradoxically, however, a recent study[33] has demonstrated the induction of a cytochrome P-450 isozyme, immunochemically similar to the phenobarbitone-inducible form in liver, in the kidneys of CsA-treated rats. These workers concluded that increased CsA metabolism in kidney may be involved in the development of the attendant nephrotoxicity, perhaps through the generation of a toxic metabolite. For further detailed discussion on CsA metabolism in relation to drug toxicity the reader is referred to Chapter 13 of this volume.

The severity of acute CsA nephrotoxicity in rats is also increased by co-treatment with other nephrotoxic agents, including the aminoglycoside antibiotic gentamicin and amphotericin B[34-36], and also by concomitant administration of the diuretic agents frusemide[37,38] and mannitol[39]. Partial protection against CsA nephrotoxicity in the rat is observed when either the angiotensin-converting enzyme inhibitor enalapril or the distal tubular antagonist of aldosterone, spironolactone, are co-administered[23,24].

CsA and vascular injury

There is evidence that relatively high doses of CsA in patients may be associated with vascular injury. Thus, glomerular thrombosis associated with a haemolytic uraemic syndrome may occur, and glomerular thrombosis has also been reported in renal allografts with high levels of CsA. Damage to arteries and arterioles also occurs[40], leading to the ischaemic injury linked with chronic CsA nephrotoxicity in man.

In an experimental model of acute serum sickness in the rabbit, CsA treatment ($25 \, mg \, kg^{-1} day^{-1}$) was associated with glomerular thrombosis and infarction[41] and with severe, diffuse necrosis of the splanchnic arteries[42]. In contrast, however, no evidence of either glomerular thrombi or necrotizing arteries was observed in CsA-treated rats with chronic serum sickness[43]. Based on their experimental findings, Neild et al.[44] have postulated that endothelial cell injury occurring in the presence of reduced production or release of prostacyclin-stimulating factor by endothelial cells (and consequently impaired vasodilatory prostaglandin production) could predispose to platelet aggregation and thrombosis in the capillary circulation. However, in the rat the acute, haemodynamically mediated CsA nephrotoxicity may be related either to inhibition of vasodilatory prostaglandins or to a lack of response to vasodilators, but not mediated via endothelium-derived relaxant factor[45]. The apparent reduction of CsA nephrotoxicity by PGE_2 administration in spontaneously hypertensive rats observed by Ryffel et al.[46] could, however, be attributed to reduced bioavailability of the immunosuppressant.

Chronic renal damage

There are, to date, few studies which describe the pathological effects of chronic administration of CsA ($\geqslant 6$ weeks) on renal structure and function in animal models. Such information is particularly important as most clinicians suspect that it is this form of CsA nephrotoxicity, apparently neither dose-related nor responsive to dose reduction, which may restrict the potential of CsA in clinical practice.

Mild chronic tubular and glomerular lesions in the rat, developing after 3 months treatment with CsA at 40 mg/kg per 48 h have been described[12,47]. In these studies no vascular abnormalities were observed, even when CsA administration was continued for 5 months. Although CsA-induced reductions in GFR were not related to proximal tubular abnormalities, the development of polyuria and increased sodium excretion was associated with the distal tubular accumulation of glycogen. Furthermore, after treatment with CsA for 3 months, withdrawal of the drug resulted in reversal of the morphological and functional abnormalities within 2 months.

Recent studies performed in this laboratory have also demonstrated increased urine flow and chronic renal tubular damage in rats treated daily with oral CsA at 10 or 20 mg/kg body weight for up to 12 weeks. However, only at the higher dose was acute renal toxicity noted, and distal tubular accumulation of glycogen was not observed. Chronic tubular damage developed from day 7 and 10 onwards in the high- and low-dose groups respectively, and was progressive in nature. In the early stages the abnormality was noticed only in the superficial cortex, especially in the immediate subcapsular area (Figure 14.3). Affected proximal tubules were either dilated or

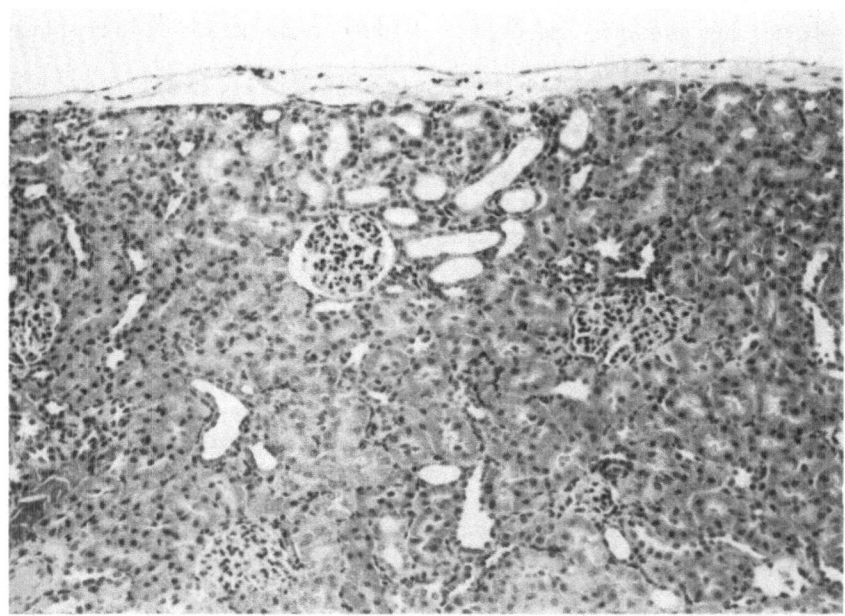

Figure 14.3   Early chronic CsA renal damage in the rat. Cortex, showing early subcapsular proximal tubular dilatation from an animal treated with 20 mg kg^{-1}day^{-1} for 21 days. The adjacent periglomerular space is also dilated. (H&E × 140)

narrowed, and demonstrated epithelial simplification and basement membrane thickening and there was often an associated interstitial infiltrate of mature lymphocytes. The severity of this lesion increased with time and was well established by 4 weeks in the higher-dose group. By 4 weeks, foci of tubular atrophy had also appeared deeper in the cortex (but never below the corticomedullary junction) and joined to the subcapsular lesions in a radial fashion: the degree of tubular dilatation or atrophy, even as far as tubular collapse, had increased, although the intervening cortex was normal. Radial stripes of tubular atrophy increased in number and thickness, the latter due to interstitial nephritis, with the length of CsA administration, particularly at the higher dose (Figure 14.4).

Glomeruli caught up in the radial lesions demonstrated periglomerular fibrosis, but no intrinsic abnormality, and the arteries, arterioles and pelvical-cyeal system were all normal. The chronic tubular damage was, however, associated with striking calcification at the corticomedullary junction.

The chronic tubular damage present in animals treated with the lower dose for 28 days was not reversed by CsA withdrawal, although GFR returned to control values, as did urine enzyme activities. Similar structural changes to those described above have also been observed in the rat, by Dieperink et al.[48]. In addition, in this latter study, although the interstitial fibrosis was irreversible on drug withdrawal, only a partial normalization of GFR was noted.

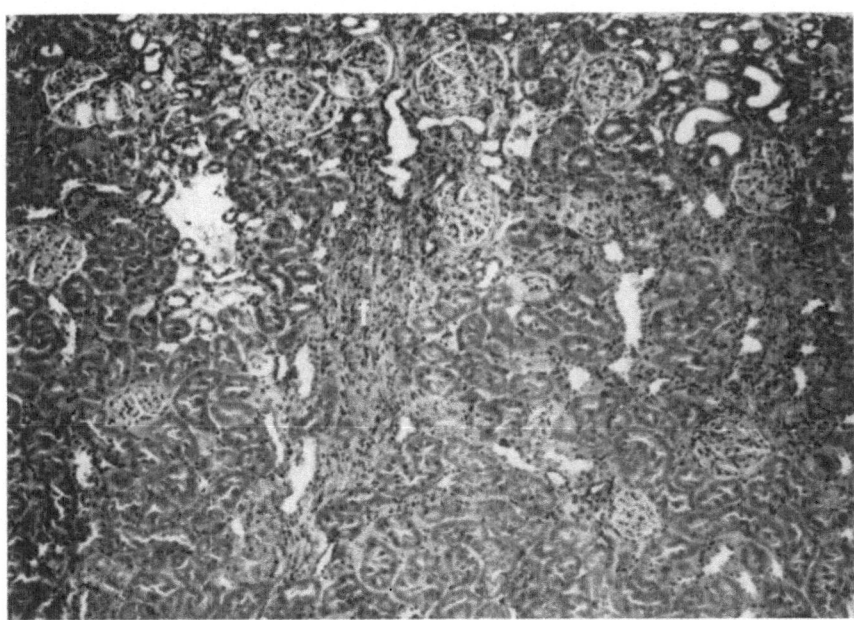

Figure 14.4 Chronic CsA renal damage in the rat. Cortex, showing a stripe of interstitial fibrosis running perpendicular to the cortical surface from an animal treated with 20 mg kg^{-1} day^{-1} for 56 days. (H&E × 89)

HEPATOTOXICITY

In patient studies[49,50], abnormal liver function tests have been observed, and in many of these investigations increased serum bilirubin concentration has been the most notable abnormality. However, there have been recent reports that many serum enzyme activities, including those of aspartate transaminase (AST), lactate dehydrogenase, alkaline phosphatase and γ-glutamyl transpeptidase (γGT) are increased in renal transplant recipients treated with CsA[50]. The most reliable indication of CsA hepatotoxicity in this study was found to be increased serum activity of γGT.

A dose-related impairment of liver function, with attendant light microscopic and ultrastructural abnormalities, has also been observed in rats treated with CsA for 3–15 weeks[51-55]. At CsA doses exceeding 25 mg kg^{-1}day^{-1}, hyperbilirubinaemia and hypoalbuminaemia, decreased serum activity of aspartate transaminase but with increased circulating alkaline phosphatase activities, have been observed[56]. These biochemical abnormalities, usually reversible on drug withdrawal, are associated with centrilobar hepatic fatty change and with dilatation of the endoplasmic reticulum, together with loss of ribosomes[51]. Individual hepatocyte necrosis has also been reported[51] and in long-term studies hepatic granulomas have also been observed[56]. These structural alterations, along with serum biochemical changes, are consistent with an effect on hepatic protein synthesis[57]. Dose-dependent CsA toxicity has also been demonstrated using hepatocytes in culture, and may provide a convenient method for investigating the underlying cytopathic mechanisms[58].

CsA has no effect on either the rate of hepatic regeneration or mitochondrial phosphorylation following partial hepatectomy[59-61], but reduced hepatic arterial perfusion has been demonstrated in both animal and patient studies[62]. In addition, CsA inhibits both bile acid-dependent and -independent flow in the rat[63], which may explain the attendant cholestasis observed in many animal and clinical studies[49,50].

MECHANISMS UNDERLYING CsA TOXICITY

Since the introduction of CsA into clinical practice it has become clear that it is the attendant nephrotoxicity that presents the most serious clinical problems, not only in diagnosis but in the differentiation between nephrotoxicity and rejection in renal transplant recipients. Consequently, most attention has been directed towards understanding the pathogenesis of CsA-induced renal dysfunction, in particular acute nephrotoxicity. It is only recently, with the development of appropriate animal models, that the study of chronic CsA renal dysfunction has begun.

To date the mechanisms underlying CsA-induced renal dysfunction remain unclear and the literature contains many anecdotal and conflicting reports. Altered renal haemodynamics mediated via either stimulation of the renin-angiotensin-aldosterone-system (RAAS)[23,24,64,65], altered renal prostaglandin metabolism[66-69], α-adrenergic stimulation[70], tubuloglomerular feedback mechanisms stimulated by renal tubular damage and/or dysfunction[22-24,69], or altered intrarenal control of GFR[71] caused, perhaps, by hyperplasia of the juxtaglomerular apparatus[21], have all been suggested from the results of animal studies. Considering the structural and functional abnormalities associated with CsA administration, it seems likely that the underlying overall mechanism will involve a combination of several processes, including those mentioned above and summarized in Table 14.2. Neither is it clear whether native CsA or its metabolites initiates the toxic response, although most information favours the former (for more details see Chapter 13). Furthermore, the development of toxicity in an individual organ or organ system may be temporally unrelated to that developing in other systems and also unrelated to its immunological mode of action[72]. Although many underlying pathophysiological processes have been suggested, it is not clear whether one CsA-induced abnormality alone, or a combination of one or more effects, is the primary signal for the development of toxicity.

Although a role for the RAAS has not been confirmed in patient studies, it is worth recording that many of the patients studied were receiving drugs which themselves affected the intrarenal control of GFR[3,73]. However, evidence of a pre-renal element in the development of CsA nephrotoxicity, a reduced fractional clearance of lithium, explained by renal arteriole vasoconstriction, has been obtained in both patient and animal studies[17-19,74,75]. Conversely, other animal studies have observed increased enzymuria and urinary flow rate suggesting additional mild renal proximal tubule damage[16]. In addition, the increased excretion of thromboxane B_2 caused by CsA and prevented by cotreatment with either thromboxane A_2 synthetase inhibitors or p-aminobenzoid acid-N-D-mannoside[67,68,76,77], also supports the view that GFR reduction is caused by renal arteriole vasoconstriction[20].

GLUCOSE TOLERANCE

Conflicting results have been obtained in patient studies with regard to the effect of CsA on glucose homeostasis in general, and pancreatic endocrine

Table 14.2 Proposed pathogenetic mechanisms of CsA nephrotoxicity (dose-dependent cell damage)

Tubule: high levels	Small vessels	
	Low levels	High levels
Giant mitochondria, vacuoles, microcalcification	Vasoconstriction, possibly caused by:	Endothelial and smooth muscle cell damage
↓	Direct effect	↓
Minor functional disturbance	Sympathetic nerve activity RAAS	Platelet aggregation
	Prostaglandins	↓
		Local i.v. coagulation
		↓
		CsA arteriolopathy
↓	↓	↓
		Interstitial fibrosis
Unknown	GFR↓, RPF↓, hypertension	

Reproduced with permission from Ryffel *et al.*[72]

function in particular. Several studies have demonstrated either improved pancreatic metabolic function following organ transplantation and CsA treatment or a reduction in insulin requirement in newly diagnosed insulin-dependent diabetic patients receiving CsA[78-81]. However, other studies of CsA-treated patients have revealed deterioration in graft function following pancreatic transplantation[82], improved glucose tolerance following CsA dose reduction or withdrawal in renal transplant recipients[83], or even the development of insulin-dependent diabetes mellitus in renal transplant recipients[84].

All animal studies to date, using either rodent or canine models, have confirmed the adverse effect of CsA, given at doses from 10 to 50 mg/kg for up to 12 weeks, on glucose homeostasis[85]. Pancreatic β cell vacuolation (Figure 14.5), with reduced islet insulin content and impaired glucose tolerance, were observed[86] in rats at $15 \, \mathrm{mg \, kg^{-1} day^{-1}}$. When the CsA dose was increased to $50 \, \mathrm{mg \, kg^{-1} day^{-1}}$ in the rat, β cell degranulation and hydropic degeneration, with overt hyperglycaemia and both hyperglucagonaemia and hypoinsulinaemia, but with normal pancreatic glucagon content, were noted[87]. These studies suggested that abnormal glucose homeostasis would be precipitated by the combination of hyperglucagonaemia and hypoinsulinaemia

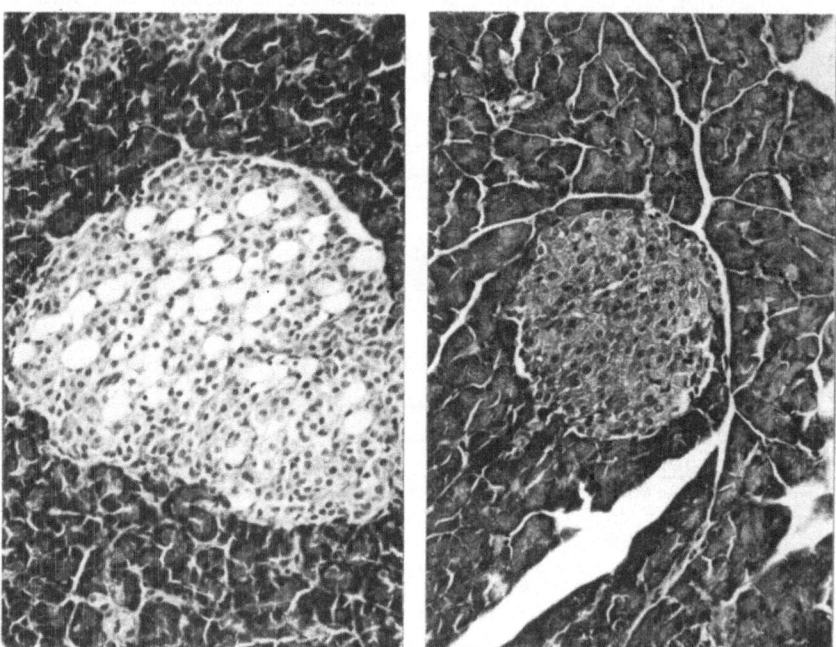

Figure 14.5 Pancreatic islet damage in the rat. Normal islet from a drug–vehicle treated animal (right) showing a regular profile and uniform, homogeneous contents compared with CsA-treated animal (left: $25 \, \mathrm{mg \, kg^{-1} day^{-1}}$ for 7 days), in which 'ballooning vacuolation' is observed. This lesion tends to occur centrally, with peripheral cells rarely being involved. (H&E × 250)

on hepatic glycogen synthesis. It has also recently been demonstrated, in rats, that CsA treatment reduced basal hepatic glycogen synthesis to 40% of control values, with no increase in synthetic capacity following insulin administration. Paradoxically, a 60% increase in the number of glucagon binding sites was also noted, although administered glucagon was without effect on glycogen synthesis[88]. Consequently, altered hepatic glycogen synthetic capability will enhance the diabetogenic effects of CsA.

Other studies, however, using low-dose CsA in the rat or dog[89,90] have demonstrated reversible glucose intolerance and augmentation of the abnormality with increasing CsA dose due to inhibition of insulin secretion and/or synthesis. CsA has also been shown to inhibit glucose but not somatostatin-dependent insulin secretion in the rat[91]. Regardless of direct effects on the endocrine pancreas, in rats the effects of CsA on the liver may precipitate altered glycogen metabolism[51]. Yale and colleagues[92] have also suggested that the regulation of hepatic glycogen is altered, due initially to peripheral insulin resistance in the presence of a mild insulin secretory insufficiency which then worsens. In their studies, following CsA withdrawal, insulin resistance disappeared first, leaving hypoinsulinaemia with almost normal glucose tolerance.

OTHER METABOLIC/BIOCHEMICAL STUDIES

Early animal studies[8,51,57] demonstrated that CsA treatment caused a disproportionate increase in serum urea concentration, compared to that of creatinine, with hypoalbuminaemia and, ultrastructurally, a reduction in the number of ribosomes within hepatocytes, all of which suggested an adverse effect on protein synthesis. Recent studies have confirmed that CsA inhibits hepatic protein synthesis[93,94]. Furthermore, it has been postulated that it is this inhibitory effect on protein synthesis in general which may be the underlying mechanism responsible for CsA toxicity. CsA has also recently been shown to inhibit the renal cortical synthesis of both DNA and RNA and also to lower the activity of Na^+/K^+-ATPase[95], a membrane-bound enzyme. Other studies have demonstrated that CsA increases the mobility of lipids in the inner membrane, with a potential for altered membrane properties, and also directly inhibits nuclear function in human lymphocytes[96,97]. CsA also inhibits the Na^+/glucose co-transporter in LLC-PK1 cells in culture; altered renal glucose uptake associated with cell membrane damage and increased lipid peroxidation has also been demonstrated, and a role for O_2 free radicals suggested[98,99].

Clinical studies of renal transplant recipients have demonstrated that CsA nephrotoxicity was more pronounced in patients receiving kidneys with long warm or cold ischaemic times[100,101], suggesting an effect on renal energy metabolism. In experimental studies CsA nephrotoxicity is also enhanced by surgical stress and renal ischaemia[102-104]. The presence of giant mitochondria in the proximal renal tubule of both animals and patients treated with CsA is also suggestive of an effect on energy metabolism. Other animal studies have demonstrated that CsA administration is associated with a decreased level of β subunit antigen of mitochondrial F_1-ATPase, predominantly in the renal medulla, and also that pre-existing hypertension or renal ischaemia may predispose to nephrotoxicity[105]. One possible explanation for the increased susceptibility is that CsA prevents the adaptive increase in mitochondrial respiration and Ca^{2+} extrusion, particularly in the renal cortex, following an ischaemic insult[106]. It has been demonstrated that CsA inhibits renal mitochondrial electron transfer *in vitro*[107], and that the drug also decreases state 3 respiration and the uncoupled respiration of succinate and glutamate/-malate *in vivo*[108] without, however, adversely effecting renal cortical ATP concentrations[95].

OTHER ASPECTS OF TOXICITY IN ANIMALS

Two additional aspects of CsA toxicity which have been studied in animal models include evaluation of its possible influence on fetal growth and tumour development.

Fetotoxicity

Considerable caution continues to be exercised with respect to the use of CsA in women of childbearing age, and during gestation. Information concerning the distribution and transfer of CsA across the placenta in women or in animals is scant, although a recent pharmacokinetic study[109] demonstrated considerable levels of CsA in the placenta and mammary glands of pregnant rabbits receiving $5\,mg\,kg^{-1}day^{-1}$ intravenously. Fetal blood CsA concentration was, however, only around 6% of the maternal blood drug level. Whilst successful pregnancies have been reported in women treated with CsA during gestation[110-112], fetal growth retardation has been reported in one renal transplant recipient receiving the drug[113].

Ryffel[52] reported embryotoxicity and fetotoxicity of CsA in rats given 30 and $300\,mg\,kg^{-1}day^{-1}$ and in rabbits given $> 100\,mg/kg$ from days 6 to 20 post-coitus, but no teratogenic effects were observed. In addition, fertility of the F_1 generation was normal. Zschauer and Hodel[114], however, reported inhibition of meiosis in rats after prolonged high-dosage CsA. Using standard protocols, Matter et al.[115] confirmed that the drug did not have any mutagenic potential.

We have shown that, in the rat, administration of CsA throughout gestation causes a dose-dependent fetotoxic effect (Figure 14.6), which is independent of major histocompatibility differences between parental strains (Table 14.3). Fetal kidneys that could be examined, showed evidence of CsA-induced proximal tubular cell damage[116]. Subsequent studies in rats revealed a very striking increase in the incidence of fetal mortality when CsA ($25\,mg\,kg^{-1} day^{-1}$) was administered throughout the second week of gestation. In surviving fetuses, the presence of focal decidual necrosis (Figure 14.7) was more frequent in mothers receiving CsA, compared with vehicle-treated controls, suggesting a possible mechanism whereby CsA might mediate its

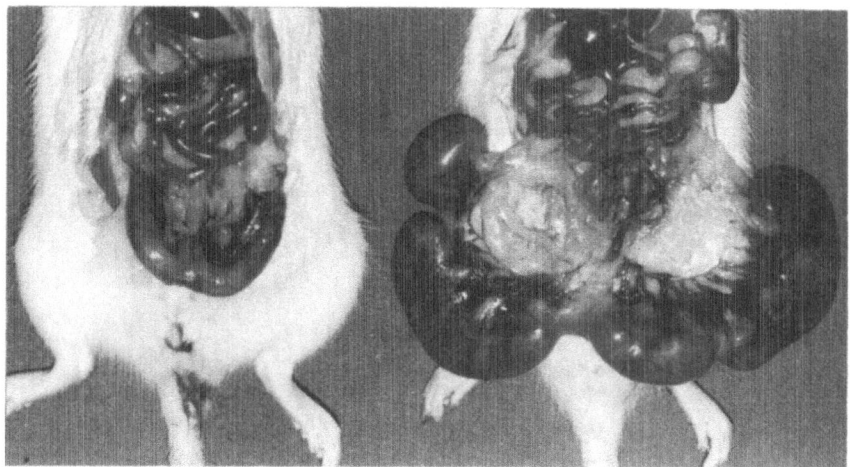

Figure 14.6 Normal gravid uterus 20 days post-coitus in a drug–vehicle-treated rat (right) compared with CsA-treated animal (left: 25 mg kg^{-1} day^{-1} throughout gestation), in which the uterus contains numerous resorptions

Table 14.3 Numbers of placentae and fetuses 20 days post-coitus in allogeneically and syngeneically mated CsA-treated Lewis rats

Mating: treatment	No. mothers	No. placentae (mean ± SD)	Fetuses		
			No./uterus	Weight (g)	Percentage viable
Lew × DA:					
Vehicle	6	9.5 ± 2.9	8.8 ± 3.9	3.3 ± 1.1	100(53/53)
CsA					
25 mg/kg	15*	8.1 ± 3.0	0.8 ± 3.0†	1.7 ± 0.1†	75(9/12)
10 mg/kg	7	7.6 ± 3.5	7.7 ± 3.7	3.0 ± 0.8	98(52/53)
Lew × Lew:					
Vehicle	4	9.5 ± 1.3	9.0 ± 1.7	3.1 ± 0.6	100(36/36)
CsA 25 mg/kg	4	11.5 ± 2.6	2.7 ± 2.1†	3.6 ± 0.4	82(9/11)

* Two experiments
† $p < 0.01$ compared with vehicle controls
Reproduced from Mason et al.[116].

fetotoxic effects[117]. Further animal studies are required to elucidate the mechanism(s) underlying CsA-induced fetotoxicity.

Tumour growth

No tumorigenic effect of CsA has been detected in mice given 8 mg kg^{-1} day^{-1} for 78 weeks[52] or in rats given this dose for 104 weeks: the frequency of tumours was similar to that in untreated controls. However, up to 24% of cynomolgus monkeys given CsA in combination with other immune

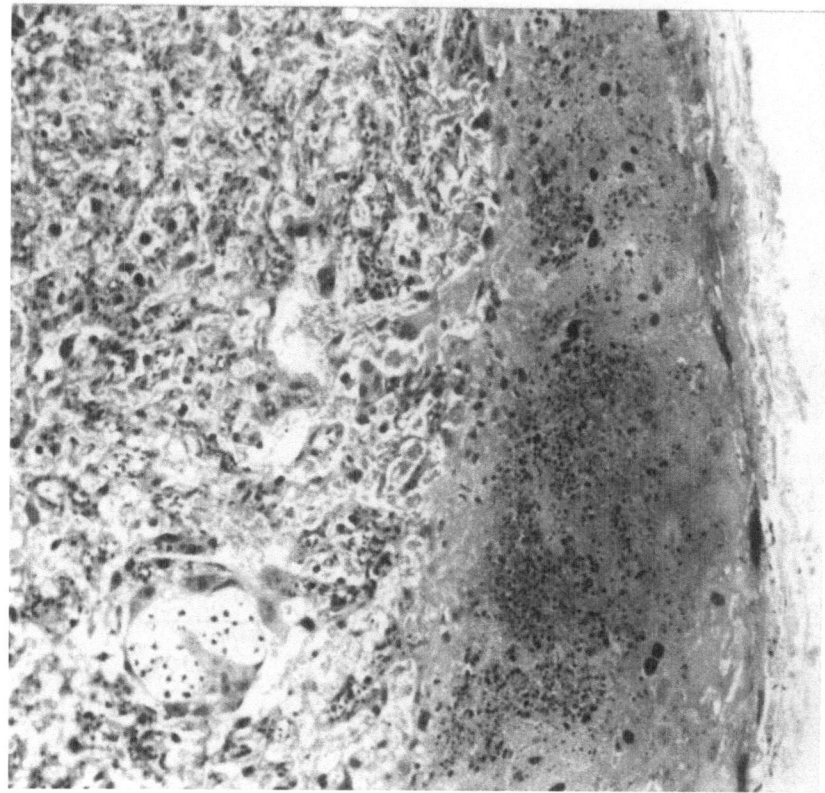

Figure 14.7 Placenta (left) and necrotic decidua basalis (right) from a CsA-treated rat mother (25 mg kg^{-1} day^{-1} from days 8 to 14, inclusive) on day 19 of gestation. (H&E × 65)

suppressants developed histiocytic lymphomas[118,119], which may have been associated with Epstein–Barr virus (EBV)-like infections. In contrast, Borleffs et al.[120] found no lymphomas up to 160 days in rhesus monkeys receiving CsA in combination with initial short-term treatment with azathioprine and prednisolone. In dogs, Deeg et al.[121] found that CsA permitted the engraftment of spontaneously arising allogeneic tumours which showed only minimal evidence of inflammatory cell infiltration. Some anti-tumour activity of CsA has been demonstrated for certain murine ascites tumours[122], and an anti-leukaemic effect has been demonstrated in rats bearing a syngeneic acute T cell leukaemia/lymphoma[123]. In the latter study, however, survival was not prolonged. On the other hand, accelerated development of spontaneous thymic lymphomas[124] and an increased incidence of chemically induced thymomas[125] have been reported in CsA-treated mice.

Other studies have shown CsA to have no effect on the growth of primary syngeneic implants of various sarcomas, carcinomas or a T cell-derived

316

lymphoma[126]. In contrast, both sarcomas and lymphomas of rodents showed greatly increased metastatic potential after treatment with CsA[126,127]. Since this latter property was a feature exhibited by immunogenic tumours, it was not considered of any clinical importance in view of the poor immunogenicity of many human malignancies.

Prospects for further study

Experimental studies will continue to play a major role in elucidation of the pathogenetic mechanisms underlying CsA toxicity, and in the design of improved treatment protocols, including the further evaluation of CsA analogues/derivatives and drug combination therapies aimed at improving the therapeutic index of this valuable immunosuppressive agent.

ACKNOWLEDGEMENTS

We acknowledge the financial assistance of the Medical Research Council and the Grampian Health Board. These investigations would not have been possible without the expert assistance of all the staff of the University Animal Department, Foresterhill, Aberdeen. The contribution of Dr J. G. Simpson to the histological investigations is also gratefully acknowledged.

REFERENCES

1. Mihatsch, M. J., Thiel, G. and Ryffel, B. (1986) Morphology of ciclosporin nephropathy. *Prog. Allergy*, **38**, 447–457.
2. Mihatsch, M. J., Ryffel, B., Hermle, M., Brunner, F. P. and Thiel, G. (1986) Morphology of cyclosporine nephrotoxicity in the rat. *Clin. Nephrol.*, **25** (Suppl. 1), S2–S8.
3. Myers, B. D., Ross, J., Newton, L., Leutscher, J. and Perlroth, M. (1984) Cyclosporine-associated chronic nephropathy. *N. Engl. J. Med.*, **311**, 699–705
4. Kahan, B. D. (1985) Clinical summation: an algorithm for the management of patients with cyclosporine-induced renal dysfunction. *Transplant. Proc.*, **17** (Suppl. 4), 303–308.
5. Klintmalm, G. B. G., Iwatsuki, I. and Starzl, T. (1981) Nephrotoxicity of cyclosporin A in liver and kidney transplant patients. *Lancet*, **1**, 470–471.
6. Calne, R. Y., White, D. J. G., Evans, D. B., Thiru, S., Henderson, R. G., Hamilton, D. V., Rolles, K., McMaster, P., Duffy, T. J., MacDougall, B. R. D. and Williams, R. (1981) Cyclosporin A in cadaveric organ transplantation. *Br. Med. J.*, **282**, 934–936.
7. Hows, J. M., Palmer, S., Want, S., Dearden, C. and Gordon-Smith, E. C. (1981) Serum levels of cyclosporin A and nephrotoxicity in bone marrow transplant patients. *Lancet*, **2**, 145–146.
8. Thomson, A. W., Whiting, P. H. and Simpson, J. G. (1984) Cyclosporine: Immunology, toxicity and pharmacology in experimental animals. *Agents Actions*, **15**, 306–327.
9. McAuley, F. T., Simpson, J. G., Thomson, A. W. and Whiting, P. H. (1986) The predictive value of enzymuria in cyclosporin A-induced renal toxicity in the rat. *Toxicol. Lett.* **32**, 163–169.
10. Whiting, P. H., Thomson, A. W. and Simpson, J. G. (1986) Cyclosporine and renal enzyme excretion. *Clin. Nephrol.*, **25** (Suppl. 1), S100–S104.
11. Pfaller, W., Kotanko, P. and Bazzanella, A. (1986) Morphological and biochemical observations in rat nephron epithelia following cyclosporine A (CsA) treatment. *Clin. Nephrol.*, **25** (Suppl. 1), S105–S110.
12. Bertani, T., Perico, N., Abbate, M., Battaglia, C. and Remuzzi, G. (1987) Renal injury

induced by long-term administration of cyclosporin A to rats. *Am. J. Pathol.*, **127**, 569–579.

13. Simpson, J. G., Saunders, N. J., Thomson, K. J. and Whiting, P. H. (1988) Chronic renal damage caused by cyclosporine. *Transplant. Proc.*, **20**, (Suppl. 3), 792–799.

1 . Battle, D. C., Gutterman, C., Tarka, J. and Prassad, R. (1986) Effect of short-term cyclosporine A administration on urinary acidification. *Clin. Nephrol.*, **25** (Suppl. 1), S62–S69.

15. Gnutzmann, K. H., Hering, K. and Gutsche, H-U. (1986) Effect of cyclosporine on the diluting capacity of the kidney. *Clin. Nephrol.*, **25** (Suppl. 1), S51–S56.

16. Whiting, P. H. and Simpson, J. G. (1988) Lithium clearance measurements as an indicator of cyclosporin A nephrotoxicity in the rat. *Clin. Sci.*, **74**, 173–178.

17. Dieperink, H., Leyssac, P. P., Kemp, E., Steinbruckl, D. and Starklint, H. (1986). Glomerulotubular function in cyclosporin A treated rats. *Clin. Nephrol.*, **25** (Suppl. 1), S70–S74.

18. Dieperink, H., Kemp, E., Leyssac, P. P. and Starklint, H. (1986) Cyclosporine A: effectiveness and toxicity in a rat model. *Clin. Nephrol.*, **25** (Suppl. 1), S46–S50.

19. Dieperink, H., Starklint, H. and Leyssac, P. P. (1983) Nephrotoxicity of cyclosporin – an animal model: study of the nephrotoxic effect of cyclosporine on overall renal and tubular function in conscious rats. *Transplant. Proc.*, **15**, (Suppl. 15), 2736–2741.

20. English, J., Evan, A., Houghton, D. C. and Bennett, W. M. (1987) Cyclosporine-induced acute renal dysfunction in the rat. *Transplantation*, **44**, 135–141.

21. Nitta, K., Friedman, A. L., Nicastri, D., Soonmyoung Paik and Friedman, E. A. (1987) Granular juxtaglomerular cell hyperplasia caused by cyclosporine. *Transplantation*, **44**, 417–421.

22. Gerkens, J. F., Bhagwandeen, S. B., Dosen, P. J. and Smith, A. J. (1984) The effect of salt intake on cyclosporine-induced impairment of renal function in rats. *Transplantation*, **38**, 412–417.

23. McAuley, F. T., Simpson, J. G., Thomson, A. W. and Whiting, P. H. (1986) Cyclosporin A induced nephrotoxicity in the rat: relationship to increased plasma renin activity. *Agents Actions*, **23**, 676–680.

24. McAuley, F. T., Whiting, P. H., Thomson, A. W. and Simpson, J. G. (1987) The influence of enalapril or spironolactone on experimental cyclosporin nephrotoxicity. *Biochem. Pharmacol.*, **36**, 699–703.

25. Nemlander, A., Soots, A., Von Willebrand, E., Tallqvist, G. and Häyry, P. (1982) Effect of cyclosporin A on the *in situ* inflammatory response of rat renal allograft rejection. *Scand. J. Immunol.*, **16**, 91–102.

26. Duncan, J. I., Whiting, P. H., Simpson, J. G., and Thomson, A. W. (1986) Alleviation of cyclosporine-mediated nephrotoxicity by phenobarbitone, during the suppression of Graft-Versus-Host reactivity. *Transplant. Proc.*, **18**, 645–649.

27. Duncan, J. I., Heys, S. D., Thomson, A. W., Simpson, J. G. and Whiting, P. H. (1988) Influence of the hepatic drug-metabolizing enzyme inducer phenobarbitone on cyclosporine nephrotoxicity and hepatotoxicity in renal-allografted rats. *Transplantation*, **45**, 693–697.

28. Whiting, P. H. and Burke, M. D. (1986) The role of drug metabolism in cyclosporine A nephrotoxicity. *Clin. Nephrol.*, **25** (Suppl. 1), S111–S115.

29. Gumbleton, M., Brown, J. E., Hawksworth, G. and Whiting, P. H. (1985) The possible relationship between hepatic drug metabolism and ketoconazole enhancement of cyclosporin A nephrotoxicity. *Transplantation*, **46**, 545–455.

30. Cunningham, C., Gavin, M. P., Whiting, P. H., Burke, M. D., Macintyre, F., Thomson, A. W. and Simpson, J. G. (1984) Serum cyclosporin levels, hepatic drug metabolism and renal tubulotoxicity. *Biochem. Pharmacol.*, **33**, 2857–2861.

31. Cunningham, C., Burke, M. D., Wheatley, D. N., Thomson, A. W., Simpson, J. G. and Whiting, P. H. (1985) Amelioration of cyclosporin-induced nephrotoxicity in rats by induction of hepatic drug metabolism. *Biochem. Pharmacol.*, **34**, 573–578.

32. Schwass, D. E., Sasaki, A. W., Houghton, D. C., Benner, K. E. and Bennett, W. M. (1986) Effect of phenobarbital and cimetidine on experimental cyclosporine nephrotoxicity: preliminary observations. *Clin. Nephrol.*, **25** (Suppl. 1), S117–S120.

33. Yoshimura, R., Yoshimura, N., Kusunose, E., Kituta, T., Matsui, S., Hamashima, T., Kishimoto, T., Oka, T., Kusunose, M. and Maekawa, M. (1989) Role of kidney microsomal

318

cytochrome P-450 in cyclosporine-induced nephropathy. *Transplant. Proc.*, **21**, 934–936.
34. Whiting, P. H. and Simpson, J. G. (1983) The enhancement of cyclosporin A induced nephrotoxicity by gentamicin. *Biochem. Pharmacol.*, **32**, 2025–2028.
35. Whiting, P. H., Thomson, A. W. and Simpson, J. G. (1983) Renal and hepatic function in rats treated with cyclosporin A in combination with gentamicin or cephalosporin antibiotics. *Br. J. Exp. Pathol.*, **64**, 693–701.
36. Ryffel, B., Müller, A. M. and Mihatsch, M. J. (1986) Experimental cyclosporine nephrotoxicity: risk of concomitant chemotherapy. *Clin. Nephrol.*, **25** (Suppl. 1), S121–S125.
37. Whiting, P. H., Cunningham, C., Thomson, A. W. and Simpson, A. W. (1984) Enhancement of high dose cyclosporin A toxicity by frusemide. *Biochem. Pharmacol.*, **33**, 1075–1079.
38. Racusen, L. C., McGraw, D. J. and Solez, K. (1985) Cyclosporine nephrotoxicity: effect of clonidine and furosemide. *Monogr. Appl. Toxicol.*, **2**, 419–428.
39. Brunner, F. P., Hermle, M., Mihatsch, M. J. and Thiel, G. (1986) Mannitol potentiates cyclosporine nephrotoxicity. *Clin. Nephrol.*, **25** (Suppl. 1), S130–S136.
40. Mihatsch, M. J., Thiel, G., Spichtin, H. P., Oberholzer, M., Brunner, F. P., Harder, E., Olivieri, V., Bremer, R., Ryffel, B., Stöcklin, E., Torhorst, J., Gudat, F., Zollinger, H. U. and Loertscher, R. (1983) Morphological findings in kidney transplants after treatment with cyclosporine. *Transplant. Proc.*, **15** (Suppl. 1), 2821–2836.
41. Nield, G. H., Ivory, K. and Williams, D. G. (1984) Glomerular thrombosis and cortical infarction in cyclosporin-treated rabbits with acute serum sickness. *Br. J. Exp. Pathol.*, **65**, 133–144.
42. Neild, G. H., Ivory, K. and Williams, D. G. (1984) Severe systemic vascular necrosis in cyclosporin-treated rabbits with acute serum sickness. *Br. J. Exp. Pathol.*, **65**, 731–743.
43. Neild, G. H., Ivory, K. and Williams, D. G. (1984) Effects of cyclosporine on proteinuria in chronic serum sickness in rats. *Clin. Nephrol.*, **25** (Suppl. 1), S186–S188.
44. Neild, G. H., Rocchi, G., Imberti, L., Fumagalli, F., Brown, Z., Remuzzi, G. and Williams, D. G. (1983) Effect of cyclosporin A on prostacyclin synthesis by vascular tissue. *Thrombosis Res.*, **32**, 373–379.
45. Fairchilds, L., Cairns, H. S., Westwick, J. and Neild, G. H. (1989) Endothelium derived relaxant factor (EDRF) and cyclosporin (CS) nephrotoxicity. *Transplant. Proc.* (In press).
46. Ryffel, B., Donatsch, P., Hiestand, P. and Mihatsch, M. J. (1986) PGE_2 reduces nephrotoxicity and immunosuppression of cyclosporine in rats. *Clin. Nephrol.*, **25** (Suppl. 1), S95–S99.
47. Whiting, P. H., Thomson, K. J., Saunders, N. J. and Simpson, J. G. (1989) Cyclosporin A nephrotoxicity in streptozotocin-diabetic rats. *Transplant. Proc.*, **21**, 946–947.
48. Dieperink, H., Starklint, H., Kemp, E. and Leyssac, P. P. (1989) Mechanisms of cyclosporin A nephrotoxicity – rat to man. In: Bach, P. H. and Lock, E. A. (eds.) *Nephrotoxicity: Extrapolation from in vitro to in vivo, and Animals to Man*, pp. 277–284. (London: Plenum Press).
49. Critical issues in cyclosporine monitoring: report of the task force on cyclosporine monitoring. (1988) *Clin. Chem.*, **33**, 1269–1288.
50. Jones, M. C., Whiting, P. H., Innes, A., Propper, D. J., Edward, N. and Catto, G. R. D. (1989) Biochemical abnormalities in serum and urine from renal transplant recipients receiving cyclosporine. *Transplant. Proc.*, **21**, 1487–1489.
51. Blair, J. T., Thomson, A. W., Whiting, P. H., Davidson, R. J. L. and Simpson, J. G. (1982) Toxicity of the immunosuppressive agent cyclosporin A in the rat. *J. Pathol.*, **138**, 163–178.
52. Ryffel, B. (1982) Experimental toxicological studies with cyclosporin A. In: White, D. J. G. (ed.), *Cyclosporin A*, (Amsterdam: Elsevier), pp. 45–75.
53. Ryffel, B., Donatsch, P., Madörin, B. E., Matter, G., Rüttiman, G., Schön, H., Stoll, R. and Wilson, J. (1983) Toxicological evaluation of cyclosporin A. *Arch. Toxicol.*, **53**, 107–141.
54. Thomson, A. W., Whiting, P. H., Cameron, I. D., Lessels, S. E. and Simpson, J. G. (1981) A toxicological study in rats receiving immunotherapeutic doses of cyclosporin A. *Transplantation*, **31**, 121–124.
55. Heys, S. D., Duncan, J. I. and Whiting, P. H. (1988) Experimental cyclosporine nephrotoxicity in the rat: effect of biliary ligation and cannulation. *Transplant. Proc.*, **20** (Suppl. 3), 845–849.

56. Whiting, P. H., Simpson, J. G., Davidson, R. J. L. and Thomson, A. W. (1983). Pathological changes in rats receiving cyclosporin A at immunotherapeutic dosage for 7 weeks. *Br. J. Exp. Pathol.*, **64**, 437–444.

57. Farthing, M. J. G., Clark, M. L., Pendry, A., Sloane, J. and Alexander, P. (1981). Nature of the toxicity of cyclosporin A in the rat. *Biochem. Pharmacol.*, **30**, 3311–3316.

58. Vine, W., Billiar, T., Simmons, R. and Bowers, L. (1988) Cyclosporine-induced hepatotoxicity: a microassay by hepatocytes in tissue culture. *Transplant. Proc.*, **20** (Suppl. 3), 859–862.

59. Uemoto, S., Tanaka, K., Asonuma, K., Kitakado, Y., Katayama, T., Tanaka, M., Inomata, Y. and Ozawa, K. (1989) Effects of cyclosporine on oxidative phosphorylation and adenylate energy charge of regenerating rat liver. *Transplant. Proc.*, **21**, 924–925.

60. Grant, D., Black, R., Zhong, R., Watt, W. and Duff, C. (1988) The effect of cyclosporine on liver regeneration. *Transplant. Proc.*, **20**, 877–879.

61. Kahn, D., Lai, H. S., Romovacek, H., Makowka, I., Van Theil, D. and Starzl, T. (1988) Cyclosporine augments the regenerative response after partial hepatectomy in the rat. *Transplant. Proc.*, **20**, 850–852.

62. Leunissen, K., Teule, J., Degenaar, C. and van Hooff, J. (1988) The effect of cyclosporine on liver perfusion and liver synthetic function. *Transplant. Proc.*, (In press).

63. Stone, B., Warty, V., Dindzans, V., and Van Thiel, D. (1988) The mechanism for cyclosporine-induced cholestasis in the rat. *Transplant. Proc.*, **20**, 841–844.

64. Siegl, H., Petric, R. and Ryffel, B. (1983) Effects of cyclosporine on the renin–angiotensin–aldosterone system. *Transplant. Proc.*, **15** (Suppl. 1), 2719–2725.

65. Baxter, C. R., Duggin, G. G., Hall, B. M., Horvath, J. S. and Tiller, D. J. (1984) Stimulation of renin release from rat renal cortical slices by cyclosporin A. *Res. Commun. Chem. Pathol. Pharmacol.*, **43**, 417–423.

66. Stahl, R. A. K. and Kudelka, S. (1986) Chronic cyclosporin A treatment reduces prostaglandin E_2 formation in isolated glomeruli and papilla of rat kidneys. *Clin. Nephrol.*, **25** (Suppl. 1), S78–S82.

67. Kawaguchi, A., Goldman, M. H., Shapiro, R., Foegh, M. L., Ramwell, P. W. and Lower, R. R. (1985) Increase in urinary thromboxane B_2 in rats caused by cyclosporine. *Transplantation*, **40**, 214–216.

68. Perico, N., Benigni, A., Zoja, C., Delaini, F. and Remuzzi, G. (1986) Functional significance of exaggerated renal thromboxane A_2 synthesis induced by cyclosporin A. *Am. J. Physiol.*, **251**, F581–F587.

69. Whiting, P. H., Barnard, N., Neilsch, A., Simpson, J. G. and Burke, M. D. (1988) Interactions between cyclosporin A, indomethacin and 16,16-dimethyl prostaglandin E_2: effects on renal, hepatic and gastrointestinal toxicity in the rat. *Br. J. Exp. Pathol.*, **68**, 777–786.

70. Murray, B. M. and Paller, M. S. (1986). Beneficial effects of renal denervation and prazosin on GFR and renal blood flow after cyclosporine in rats. *Clin. Nephrol.*, **25** (Suppl. 1), S37–S39.

71. Duggin, G. G., Baxter, C., Hall, B. M., Horvath, J. S. and Tiller, D. J. (1986) Influence of cyclosporine A (CSA) on intrarenal control of GFR. *Clin. Nephrol.*, **25** (Suppl. 1), S43–S45.

72. Ryffel, B., Foxwell, B. M., Gee, A., Greiner, B., Woerly, G. and Mihatsch, M. J. (1988) Cyclosporine – relationship of side effects to mode of action. *Transplantation*, **46**, 90S–96S.

73. Bantle, J. P., Nath, K. A., Sutherland, D. E. R., Najarian, J. S. and Ferris, T. F. (1985) Effects of cyclosporine on the renin-angiotensin-aldosterone system and potassium excretion in renal transplant recipients. *Arch. Intern. Med.*, **145**, 505–508.

74. Dieperink, H., Leyssac, P. P., Starklint, H. and Kemp, E. (1986) Nephrotoxicity of cyclosporin A. A lithium clearance and micropuncture study in rats. *Eur. J. Clin. Invest.*, **16**, 69–77.

75. Vincent, H., Wenting, G. J., Schalenkamp, M. A., Jeekel, J. and Weimar, W. (1988) Impaired fractional excretion of lithium: a very early marker of cyclosporine nephrotoxicity. *Transplant. Proc.*, **19**, 4147–4148.

76. Whiting, P. H., Burke, M. D. and Thomson, A. W. (1986) Drug interactions with cyclosporine: implications from animal studies. *Transplant. Proc.*, **18**, 56–70.

77. Teraoka, S., Sanaka, T., Takahashi, K., Toma, H., Yamaguchi, Y., Yagisawa, T., Tanake,

K., Sato, H., Matsumura, O. and Nakajima, I. (1988) Stimulation of intrinsic prostacyclin synthesis and inhibition of thromboxane production to minimize cyclosporine nephrotoxicity. *Transplant. Proc.,* **20**, 638–645.

78. Skyler, J. S. (1988) Cyclosporine in insulin-dependent diabetes mellitus: effects on islet beta cell f unction. *Transplant. Proc.,* (In press).

79. Traeger, J. Dubernard, J. M., Pozza, G. (1983) Influence of immunosuppressive therapy on the endocrine function of segmental pancreatic allografts. *Transplant. Proc.,* **15**, 1326–1329.

80. Stiller, C. R., Dupre, J. and Gent, M. (1984) Effects of cyclosporine immunosuppression in insulin-dependent diabetes mellitus of recent onset. *Science,* **223**, 1362–1367.

81. Assan, R., Feutren, G., Debray-Sachs, M., Quiniou-Debrie, M. C., Laborie, C., Thomas, G., Chatenoud, L. and Bach, J. F. (1985) Metabolic and immunological effects of cyclosporin in recently diagnosed type 1 diabetes mellitus. *Lancet,* **1**, 67–71.

82. Gunnarson, R., Klintmalm, R., Lundgren, G., Wilczec, H., Östman, J. and Groth, C. G. (1983) Deterioration in glucose metabolism in pancreatic transplant recipients given cyclosporin. *Lancet,* **2**, 571–572.

83. Harris, K. P. G., Russell, G. I., Parvin, S. D., Veitch, P. S. and Walls, J. (1986) Alterations in lipid and carbohydrate metabolism attributable to cyclosporin A in renal transplant recipients. *Br. Med. J.,* **292**, 16.

84. Nakai, I., Omori, Y., Aikawa, I., Yasumura, T., Suzuki, S., Yashimura, N., Arakawa, K., Matsui, S. and Oka, T. (1988) Effect of cyclosporine on glucose metabolism in kidney transplant recipients. *Transplant. Proc.,* **20**, 969–978.

85. Whiting, P. H., Thomson, K. J., Saunders, N. J. and Simpson, J. G. (1987) The effect of cyclosporin A on glucose tolerance and renal function in the normal rat. *Diabetic Med.* **4**, 352.

86. Hahn, H. J., Laube, F., Lucke, S., Klötting, I., Kohnert, K. D. and Warzock, R. (1986) Toxic effects of cyclosporine on the endocrine pancreas of Wistar rats. *Transplantation,* **41**, 44–47.

87. Helmchen, U., Schmidt, W. E., Siegel, E. G. and Creutzfeldt, W. (1984) Morphological and functional changes of pancreatic β-cells in cyclosporine-A-treated rats. *Diabetologia,* **27**, 416–418.

88. Betschart, J., Virji, M. and Shinozuka, H. (1988) Cyclosporine-induced alterations in rat hepatic glycogen metabolism. *Transplant. Proc.* **20** (Suppl. 3), 880–884.

89. Yale, J. F., Roy, R. D., Grose, M., Seemayer, T. A., Murphy, G. F. and Marliss, E. B. (1985) Effects of cyclosporine on glucose tolerance in the rat. *Diabetes,* **34**, 1309–131.

90. Garvin, P. J., Niehoff, M. and Staggenborg, J. (1988) Cyclosporine's effect on canine pancreatic endocrine function. *Transplantation,* **45**, 1027–1031.

91. Müller, M. K., Bergmann, K., Degenhardt, H., Klöppel, G., Löhr, M., Coone, H. J. and Goebell, H. (1988) Differential sensitivity of rat exocrine and endocrine pancreas to cyclosporine. *Transplantation,* **45**, 698–700.

92. Yale, J-F., Chamellian, M., Courchesne, S. and Vigeant, C. (1988) Peripheral insulin resistance and decreased insulin secretion after cyclosporine A treatment. *Transplant. Proc.,* **20** (Suppl. 3), 955–958.

93. Buss, W., Stepanek, J. and Bennett, W. M. (1988) Proposed mechanism of cyclosporine toxicity: inhibition of protein synthesis. *Transplant. Proc.,* **20** (Suppl. 3), 863–867.

94. Backman, L., AppelKwist, E-L., Ringden, O. and Dallner, G. (1988) Effects of cyclosporine on hepatic protein synthesis. *Transplant. Proc.,* **20** (Suppl. 3), 853–858.

95. Suzuki, S., Oka, T., Ohkuma, S. and Kuriyama, K. (1987) Biochemical mechanisms underlying cyclosporine-induced nephrotoxicity. *Transplantation,* **44**, 363–368.

96. Rossaro, L., Dowd, S., Ho, C. and Van Thiel, D. (1988) ^{19}F nuclear magnetic resonance studies of cyclosporine and model unilamellar vesicles: where does the drug sit within the membrane? *Transplant. Proc.,* **20** (Suppl. 3), 41–45.

97. Citterio, F. and Kahan, B. D. (1988) Effects of cyclosporine on the nuclear function. *Transplant. Proc.,* **20**, 75–79.

98. Chan, P., Scoble, J. E., Senior, J. C. M., Sweny, P., Varghese, Z. and Moorhead, J. F. (1989) Cyclosporin inhibition of glucose transport in a renal proximal tubular cell line. *Transplant. Proc.,* **21**, 922–923.

99. Kumano, K., Yoshida, K., Iwamura, M., Endo, T., Sakai, T., Nakamura, K. and Kuwao, T. (1989) Oxygen free radical scavengers reduce cyclosporine A nephrotoxicity in the rat.

Transplant. Proc., **21**, 941–942.

100. Hall, B. M., Tiller, D. J., Duggin, G. G., Horvath, J. S., Farnsworth, A., May, J., Johnson, J. R. and Sheil, A. G. R. (1985) Post-transplant acute renal failure in cadaver renal recipients treated with cyclosporine. *Kidney Int.*, **28**, 178–186.

101 Pichlmayer, R., Wonigeit, K., Ringe, B., Block, T., Raab, R., Heigel, B. and Neubaus, P. (1984) Rejection and nephrotoxicity, diagnostic problems with cyclosporine in renal transplantation. *Proc. EDTA-ERA*, **21**, 947–960.

102. Whiting, P. H., Duncan, J. I., Gavin, M. P., Heys, S. D., Simpson, J. G., Asfar, S. K. and Thomson, A. W. (1985) Renal function in rats treated with cyclosporin following unilateral nephrectomy. *Br. J. Exp. Pathol.*, **66**, 535–542.

103. Thiel, G., Brunner, F. P., Hermle, M., Stahl, R. A. K. and Mihatsch, M. J. (1986) Effect of cyclosporine A on ischaemic renal failure in the rat. *Clin. Nephrol.*, **25** (Suppl. 1), S155–S161.

104. Iaina, A., Herzog, D., Cohen, D., Gavendo, S., Kapuler, S., Serban, I., Schiby, G. and Eliahou, H. E. (1986) Calcium entry-blockade with verapamil in cyclosporine A plus ischemia-induced acute renal failure in rats. *Clin. Nephrol.*, **25** (Suppl. 1), S168–S170.

105. Hay, R., Tammi, K., Ryffel, B. and Mihatsch, M. J. (1986) Alterations in molecular structure of renal mitochondria associated with cyclosporine A treatment. *Clin. Nephrol.*, **25** (Suppl. 1), S23–S26.

106. Khauli, R., Strzelecki, T., Stoff, J. and Menon, M. (1988) Cyclosporine-ischemia effects in the rat kidney: further biochemical observations with emphasis on calcium handling. *Transplant. Proc.*, **20**, 551–555.

107. Jung, K. and Pergande, M. (1985) Influence of cyclosporin A on the respiration of isolated rat kidney. *FEBS Lett.*, **183**, 167.

108. Jung, K., Reinholdt, C., and Scholz, D. (1987). Inhibited efficiency of kidney mitochondria isolated from rats treated with cyclosporin A. *Nephron*, **45**, 43–47.

109. Sangalli, L., Bortolotti, A., Passerini, F. and Bonati, M. (1989) Placental transfer, tissue distribution, and pharmacokinetics of cyclosporine in the pregnant rabbit. *Transplantation* (In press).

110. Deeg, H. J., Kennedy, M. S., Sanders, J. E., Thomas, E. D. and Storb, R. (1983) Successful pregnancy after marrow transplantation for severe aplastic anemia and immunosuppression with cyclosporine. *J. Am. Med. Assoc.*, **250**, 647.

111. Lewis, G. J., Lamont, C. A. R., Leel, H. A. and Slapak, M. (1983) Successful pregnancy in a renal transplant recipient taking cyclosporin A. *Br. Med. J.*, **286**, 603–604.

112. Klintmalm, G., Althoff, P., Appleby, G. and Segerbrandt, E. (1984) Renal function in a newborn baby delivered of a renal transplant patient taking cyclosporine. *Transplantation*, **38**, 198–199.

113. Pickerell, M. D., Sawers, R. and Michael, J. (1988) Pregnancy after renal transplantation: severe intra-uterine growth retardation during treatment with cyclosporin A. *Br. Med. J.*, **296**, 825.

114. Zschauer, A. and Hodel, Ch. (1980) Drug-induced changes in rat seminiferous tubular epithelium. *Arch. Toxicol.*, Suppl. 4, 466–470.

115. Matter, B. E., Donatsch, P., Rocine, R. R., Schmid, B. and Suter, W. (1982) Genotoxicity evaluation of cyclosporin A, a new immunosuppressive agent. *Mutation Res.*, **105**, 257–264.

116. Mason, R. J., Thomson, A. W., Whiting, P. H., Gray, E. S., Brown, P. A. J., Catto, G. R. D. and Simpson, J. G. (1985) Cyclosporine-induced fetotoxicity in the rat. *Transplantation*, **39**, 9–12.

117. Brown, P. A. J., Gray, E. S., Whiting, P. H., Simpson, J. G. and Thomson, A. W. (1985) Effects of cyclosporin A on fetal development in the rat. *Biol. Neonate*, **48**, 172–180.

118. Pennock, J. L., Reitz, B. A., Bieber, C. P., Jamieson, S. W., Burton, N. A., Raney, A. A., Oyer, P. E. and Stinson, E. B. (1980) Lethal complications due to cyclosporin A immune suppression with combination drug and combined heart and lung transplantation. *Surg. Forum*, **31**, 375–378.

119. Reitz, B. A., Bieber, C. P. and Pennock, J. L. (1982) Cyclosporin A and lymphoma in non-human primates. In White, D. J. G. (ed.), (Amsterdam: Elsevier), pp. 317–328.

120. Borleffs, J. C. C., Neuhaus, P., Marquet, R. L., Zurcher, C. and Balmer, H. (1982) Cyclosporin A and kidney transplantation in rhesus monkeys. In White, D. J. G. (ed.), *Cyclosporin A* (Amsterdam: Elsevier), pp. 329–342.

121. Deeg, H. J., Hackman, R. C., Weiden, P. L. and Storb, R. (1982) Growth of canine tumours transplanted into normal adult dogs immunosuppressed by cyclosporin A. *Immunol. Immunother.*, **12**, 147–152.
122. Kreis, W. and Soricelli, A. (1979) Cyclosporins: immunosuppressive agents with antitumour activity. *Experimentia*, **35**, 1506–1508.
123. Thomson, A. W., Forrest, E. M., Smart, L. M., Sewell, H. F., Whiting, P. H. and Davidson, R. J. L. (1988) Influence of cyclosporin A on growth of an acute T-cell leukaemia in PVG rats. *Int. J. Cancer*, **41**, 473–479.
124. Hattori, A., Perera, M. I. R., Witkowski, L. A., Kunl, H. W., Gill, T. J. and Shinozuka, H. (1986) Accelerated development of spontaneous thymic lymphomas in male AKR mice receiving cyclosporine. *Transplantation*, **41**, 784–786.
125. Shinozuka, H., Gill, T. J., Kunz, H. W., Witkowski, L. A., Dimitris, A. J. and Perera, M. I. R. (1988) Enhancement of the induction of murine thymic lymphomas by cyclosporine. *Transplantation*, **41**, 377–380.
126. Eccles, S. A., Hedeford, S. E. and Alexander, P. (1980) Effect of cyclosporin A on the growth and spontaneous metastasis of syngeneic animal tumours. *Br. J. Cancer*, **42**, 252–259.
127. Alexander, P. (1982) Cyclosporin A and the growth, dissemination and induction of tumours. In White, D. J. G. (ed.), (Amsterdam: Elsevier), pp. 299–305.

15
Pathological effects of cyclosporin A in clinical practice

Sathia Thiru

INTRODUCTION

In the first report on the efficacy of cyclosporin A (CsA) in clinical renal transplantation three side-effects were observed: hirsutism, hepatotoxicity and nephrotoxicity[1]. Two female patients were reported to have slight increase in facial and limb hair, all seven patients had elevated levels of serum bilirubin and alkaline phosphatase, and serum creatinine was elevated in all, with four having unexplained primary oligo-anuria. The authors stated that nephrotoxicity had made management of the patients very difficult – still true a decade later – and that they had probably persisted with too high a dose of CsA and were hampered by the inability to measure blood levels. Since then a list of other, less serious, adverse effects of CsA therapy have been reported[2]. In the succeeding paragraphs an attempt will be made to elucidate these complications of CsA with particular attention given to nephrotoxicity.

TOXIC EFFECTS OF CsA

The toxic effects of CsA therapy can be due to the drug alone, to its interaction with other drugs, or to CsA enhancing and exacerbating pathological injury caused by unrelated factors such as preservation injury in grafts, hypertension, infections, rejection, etc. The reported side-effects of CsA have included: nephrotoxicity, hypertension, hepatotoxicity, infections, malignancy, in particular lymphomas, gingival hyperplasia, dermatological toxicity, neurological toxicity, capillary leak syndrome, and minor miscellaneous problems. In spite of this long list the usage of CsA is not seriously affected, as many of the side-effects are quite mild and almost all are reversible by reduction of drug dose.

NEPHROTOXICITY

In their original report Calne *et al.*[1] stated: 'It seems likely that Cyclosporin A has direct toxic effect on renal tubules or on the blood supply of the tubules and that patients vary in their susceptibility to these toxic reactions although nephrotoxicity is probably dose dependent.' Even though a vast amount of experimental and clinical work has been done since then to elucidate the nephrotoxicity of CsA, and the published literature is phenomenal, the exact mechanism by which the drug injures the kidney is still poorly understood. Nephrotoxicity is manifest not only as acute dose-dependent reversible toxicity in the early period after renal transplantation, but also as chronic and permanent damage in the years following successful transplantation. Moreover, kidney function is altered in almost all patients treated with CsA. This includes native kidneys of cardiac, hepatic and bone marrow graft recipients and patients receiving the drug for autoimmune disorders.

Clinical features

Clinical use of CsA is associated with reversible, dose-related increases in serum creatinine, depression of creatinine clearance, disproportionate increase of blood urea nitrogen relative to serum creatinine, hyperkalaemia, metabolic acidosis and hyperuricaemia. There are no characteristic changes in the urinary sediment. Nephrotoxicity may be acute or chronic with one form imperceptibly merging into the other.

Acute toxicity

Acute renal insufficiency occurs in the first weeks following initiation of therapy, and can occur not only in allograft kidneys but also in previously healthy native kidneys. This acute injury can be brief and rapidly reversible with reduction of CsA dose, or on the other hand manifest as prolonged delayed function.

Acute reversible injury. In these cases the patient has initial good function following initiation of therapy, followed by abrupt renal dysfunction with elevation of serum creatinine, fall in GFR, impaired urinary concentrating ability and sodium retention. Clinically in renal allograft recipients it can be almost impossible to differentiate from acute rejection. Histologically the diagnosis is made by the absence of evidence for rejection rather than by any specific features of CsA toxicity. CsA trough levels may be within the so-called therapeutic range of 200–800 μg/ml, or may be high. Reduction in drug dose produces improvement in function by 24 h, thereby giving further retrospective proof of toxicity. The incidence of this type of renal dysfunction can vary from 20% to up to 40% depending on drug regime and other 'centre variables'.

Prolonged delayed function. This is seen almost exclusively in recipients of cadaveric renal allografts, especially where the quality of the donor organ has been compromised by donor hypotension, prolonged ischaemia time,

325

preservation problems, age-related ischaemic disease of donor kidney and operative technical problems in the recipient. Other factors include postoperative infections, in particular urinary tract infections, and use of nephrotoxic drugs such as the antibiotics gentamicin and amphotericin B. Such primary non-function of renal transplants is seen frequently in centres that have organs transported from long distances, and in places where absence of brain death legislation permits cadaveric kidneys to be harvested only after the donor's heart has stopped beating. The incidence of prolonged anuria requiring dialysis can vary between 30 and 50% at such centres. In one centre allograft functions recovered by an average of 2 weeks in patients treated with azathioprine and prednisolone, but took 3–14 weeks in 72% of the patients treated with CsA[3]. Reduction in drug dose, or even complete withdrawal, may be necessary for renal function to be restored, but it seldom reaches the normal range. Graft failure requiring nephrectomy occurs in approximately 2% of these patients. In primary graft anuria of patients treated with azathioprine and prednisolone, on the other hand, there is usually no compromising of long-term graft function. Less commonly, prolonged renal dysfunction can occur after initial good function has been complicated by episodes of acute rejection, presumably the vascular compromisation and ischaemia of rejection enhancing the toxic effects of CsA.

Chronic toxicity
Chronic nephrotoxicity may manifest either as residual damage from previous episodes of rejection and/or toxicity, or as spontaneous, insidious and progessive renal dysfunction after an initial honeymoon of good function. Reports of 'recovery' from acute nephrotoxicity seldom indicate resolution to normal function, and even in patients who do not have acute episodes of nephrotoxicity the renal function is often not completely normal. It is likely that all kidneys, grafts and native organs are subjected to some degree of background nephrotoxicity which is mild and compatible with sufficient or even normal renal function in the initial phase. With time, this may progress to more severe, permanent and irreversible dysfunction. Once renal function has stabilized at this lower level most centres report no further progress in deterioration of function[4-6]. In a report of 5 years experience with CsA in cadaveric renal transplants Merion and co-workers[4] reported serum creatinine levels of 221 ± 10 μmol/l in CsA patients and 198 ± 28 μmol/l in azathioprine and prednisolone patients at time of discharge, and levels of 213 ± 13 μmol/l and 157 ± 21 μmol/l respectively at the most recent follow-up. Follow-up was more than 1 year in 80% and more than 2 years in 55% of the patients. In an attempt to circumvent chronic nephrotoxicity, Morris *et al.*[7] conducted a randomized prospective trial of CsA for 3 months with conversion to azathioprine and prednisolone compared with conventional therapy of azathiopine and prednisolone throughout. In the 64 CsA patients survival was 92%, and graft survival was 72% and 67% at 1 and 4 years after transplantation. In the alternative group of 65 patients survival was 94% and graft survival was 59% and 47% at 1 and 4 years. Although serum creatinine was significantly higher at 90 days in patients on CsA there was a fall in serum creatinine by 45% within 1–2 weeks of conversion. Good renal function

was maintained as assessed by serum creatinine, and at 3 years these patients had a lower mean creatinine level, 119 µmol/l, than those who were treated with azathioprine and prednisolone throughout, 164 µmol/l. Those patients who remained on CsA after 90 days had the highest mean level of serum creatinine, 207 µmol/l. The drawback in this protocol was that, after conversion, 32% of the patients had acute rejection, generally within 30 days, with two grafts being lost.

Nephrotoxicity in native kidneys

It is clearly apparent that it can be extremely difficult, both clinically and histologically, to study the nature and degree of CsA-induced nephrotoxicity in renal transplants, as matters can be complicated by coexisting rejection. Liver and cardiac transplant recipients, and patients treated for autoimmune disorders such as uveitis, on the other hand, have no such dual pathology.

Liver. In eleven liver transplant patients followed for periods of 6–12 months the GFR and effective renal plasma flow fell by 60% postoperatively and subsequently improved and stabilized at 45–60% of normal despite continued drug administration[8]. All patients had good renal function before surgery. Renal biopsies on six patients showed the histopathological changes were mild to moderate in severity with arteriolar sclerosis, non-specific ischaemic changes in up to 4% glomeruli, some patchy interstitial fibrosis and tubular atrophy. There was strikingly poor correlation between morphology and the corresponding renal function. These findings indicated that while CsA nephrotoxicity was associated with both functional and morphological changes, the former played a more dominant role as the cause of renal dysfunction. In another series of 56 liver allograft patients treated with CsA and dosage-adjusted to keep trough levels in the therapeutic range of 200–800 ng/ml (mainly between 300 and 400 ng/ml) eight patients developed substantial renal impairment[9]. Patients had been on CsA for a period of 1.5–4.5 years. Serum creatinine before therapy was 76–114 µmol/l and at time of biopsy 93–256 µmol/l with creatinine clearance 57–122 ml/min and 23–86 ml/min respectively. Four developed hypertension requiring treatment. In the group as a whole mean serum creatinines rose from 88 µmol/l before CsA to 150 µmol/l in 72% of cases. Sixty-six per cent had become hypertensive and DTPA scanning revealed impaired perfusion in every patient on CsA for more than 2 months. Ischaemic changes in glomeruli were found to be greater than in controls, and there was focal tubular atrophy but no significant vascular lesions were demonstrated. The exact pathogenesis of the ischaemia was uncertain, but a primary vasomotor mechanism causing functional decrease of renal blood flow and GFR without permanent arterial narrowing was postulated.

Cardiac transplants. The Stanford University group published a report of cardiac transplant patients treated with CsA and prednisolone compared to a historical control group of azathioprine- and prednisolone-treated patients[10]. The serum creatinine at 12 months post-transplant was above 126.0 µmol/l in the patients receiving CsA and below 126.0 µmol/l in the majority not receiving it. Mean serum creatinine was 189.0 μmol/l in the CsA group and 108.0 μmol/l in the azathioprine group. Approximately a third of each group was selected at random for more detailed renal function tests, and the GFR in the CsA group was 53 $\pm$ 4 versus 91 $\pm$ 4 ml/min per 1.73 m^2 in the azathioprine group. The glomerular hypofiltration associated with chronic CsA therapy was due in large part to a decrease in renal plasma flow and intrinsic loss of ultrafiltration capacity. Neither of these findings could be attributed to impaired performance of the cardiac allograft. Other features of chronic nephropathy included mild proteinuria, tubular dysfunction and severe arterial hypertension. Some of these patients had progressive renal dysfunction terminating in end-stage renal failure despite lowering of CsA dose. Five CsA patients with moderate to severe impairment of function were biopsied[11] and were reported to have the following: mild to moderate global—segmental glomerular sclerosis, focal arteriolar hyalinosis, patchy tubular atrophy and loss, degenerative changes in tubular epithelium and increase in interstitial fibrous tissue. Tubulo-interstitial damage was observed to be greater than glomerular.

Diabetes. In eleven Type I diabetic patients who underwent pancreatic transplantation without renal transplants and treated with CsA and maintenance trough levels of 200 ng/ml the serum creatinine was 91.8 μmol/l and creatinine clearance 96.8 $\pm$ 10.31 ml/min before transplantation, and the respective values 134 μmol/l and 52.6 $\pm$ 6.57 ml/min 1 month post-transplantation[12]. But unlike the report of Myers *et al.*[10] there was no continuous decrease in renal function, the mean serum creatinine being 125.1 μmol/l and creatinine clearance 59.3 ml/min at 6—23 months post-transplant.

Uveitis. In a series of 40 patients who had received CsA alone for severe uveitis none had pre-existing renal disease or hypertension. Serum creatinine before CsA therapy was 106 μmol/l, after 6 weeks 114, and at 6 months and 1 year[13] 132.6 μmol/l. CsA dose was adjusted on the basis of ocular inflammation and degree of renal dysfunction to keep the serum creatinine below 180 μmol/l and CsA trough levels were generally around 102 ng/ml. Five patients developed hypertension requiring treatment with lasix, methyldopa and propranolol. Seventeen patients agreed to renal biopsy at 1 year. There was a variable amount of tubular atrophy and interstitial fibrosis, which was band-like in some cases and corresponded to the distribution of vascular channels. Compared to controls there was no significant abnormality of glomeruli or vessels, although 13 patients had variable numbers of completely sclerosed glomeruli, and small arteries and arterioles were thickened in 15. Severity of renal abnormalities did *not* correlate with the average or cumulative doses of CsA or with GFR at the time of biopsy.

Autoimmune disorders. In another study of 21 patients treated with CsA and steroids for autoimmune disorders, such as systemic lupus, rheumatoid arthritis and Sjögren's syndrome, all patients tolerated the drug well and renal biospy showed no significant abnormality of CsA toxicity in any patient[14].

328

Pathogenesis of CsA nephrotoxicity

Acute and chronic nephrotoxicity are dose-dependent, and toxicity, especially in the acute phase, is reversible by reduction of the dose. There is no doubt that factors in addition to dose level may contribute to nephrotoxicity; concomitant use of other drugs which act synergistically to increase the toxic effects of CsA, infections, hypertension, and in the case of renal transplantation, pre-transplant graft ischaemia related to harvesting and preservation problems, age of donor and concomitant rejection episodes. The controversey over the exact mechanism of nephrotoxicity is unresolved and many questions remain unanswered:

1. Is there a therapeutic window between adequate immunosuppression and renal toxicity?
2. Are blood levels of CsA of any use? The wide range of accepted therapeutic levels, and the lack of close relationship between these and changes in renal function, indicate renal effects of CsA appear to vary widely in individual patients. Nephrotoxicity can occur with CsA in therapeutic levels or even low levels.
3. Should CsA be used in the initial phase, especially in patients with initial oligo-anuria and/or acute tubular necrosis?
4. Is chronic toxicity due to initial damage to the kidney in the early post-transplantation period, or is it due to insidious cumulative toxic effects or both?
5. Is nephrotoxicity progressive?
6. Is there any way of distinguishing nephrotoxicity from rejection as the cause of impaired renal function? CsA-treated recipients undergoing rejection often lack the classic signs of fever and graft tenderness, and acute rejection may occur despite high CsA blood levels.

Although nephrotoxicity of CsA is readily observed in clinical practice there is no equivalent experimental animal model. The precise pathogenesis of the nephrotoxicity therefore remains speculative. Two theories, which may not be mutually exclusive, have been offered so far: a tubular toxic effect and a vasoconstrictive effect.

Tubular toxicity theory

This suggests that CsA causes tubular damage leading to functional impairment[15, 16]. Back pressure along nephrons blocked by damaged tubules caused a feedback mechanism whereby angiotensin lowered the glomerular flow. The mechanism of the tubular injury is uncertain and it may be due to[17]:

1. A direct effect of increased serum CsA levels with deposition in proximal tubular cells as seen in gentamicin toxicity;
2. Local generation of toxic metabolites;
3. Adverse effects of other tubular toxins, enhancing CsA toxicity, e.g. amphotericin B, aminoglycosides.

In liver transplant patients treated with CsA nephrotoxic effects on renal tubular function have been documented[8]. Despite a lower GFR and filtered sodium load, there is a significantly greater decrease in tubular sodium reabsorption with a resulting increase in urinary sodium excretion. That the decrease in tubular sodium reabsorption is absolute, and not just the result of the decreased GFR, is shown by the decrease in functional sodium reabsorption as well. This suggests that the proximal tubule is a major site of CsA nephrotoxicity. Activation of glomerular feedback mechanism through increased delivery of filtrate to the distal tubule stimulates the macula densa, thereby increasing renin secretion.

Myers et al.[11] in their report of CsA-associated chronic nephropathy suggested the tubule as the primary site of injury with subsequent nephron destruction leading to loss of filtration surface area and adaptive increase in glomerular capillary hydraulic pressure. This would enhance further development of glomerulosclerosis, and a vicious circle would be set up with progressive decrease in functioning nephrons, development of hypertension and acceleration of glomerulosclerosis.

Connecting the tubular toxicity theory with the vasoconstrictive theory is the proposal[18] that CsA alters renal haemodynamics thereby causing proximal tubular hypoxia and a fall in GFR.

Vasoconstrictive theory
Many clinical and experimental studies have demonstrated that CsA reduces effective renal plasma flow[8,10,11,19-22]. Moreover the rapid improvement in renal function following the reduction of CsA is further corroborative evidence of involvement of a vasomotor mechanism in producing nephrotoxicity. Myers has modified the earlier concept of the tubule being the primary site of injury[11] and put forward the following hypothesis for the pathogenesis of CsA toxicity[10]. Low-dose 'non-toxic' administration of CsA is associated from the outset with persistent renal vasoconstriction causing reduction in renal plasma flow and fall in GFR. This would cause the mild increase in serum creatinine seen almost universally in all CsA-treated patients. Superimposed on this 'background toxicity' there could be episodes of dose-associated further falls in renal blood flow leading to reversible episodes of acute renal failure. Vasoconstriction in the early phase, perhaps the first few months, is reversible, as evidenced by the return to normal renal function when CsA is withdrawn. With continued therapy, however, there is development of irreversible renal injury with further reduction of GFR and low filtration fraction, probably secondary to nephron loss and vascular morphological damage. There is in addition coexistent hypertension, due to primary effect of CsA and/or secondary to chronic renal injury, which further adds to the viscious circle. There may also be chronic rejection further enhancing the renal damage. Although most reports[4-6] state patients remain on a 'stable level' of chronic azotaemia after 2–5 years of therapy it is plausible that once the functional reserve capacity has been dissipated they will progress to end-stage renal failure.

How does CsA decrease renal blood flow, increase vascular tone and produce vasoconstriction? A variety of haemodynamic mechanisms have been proposed and include:

1. Activation of the renin–angiotensin system;
2. Inhibition of prostaglandin mediated vasodilatation;
3. Stimulation of the sympathetic nervous system.

The arguments for and against each of these mechanisms will be reviewed briefly.

Renin activity. The association between increased plasma renin activity and reduced renal function has not been firmly established. Plasma renin acitivity has been found to be elevated in some studies and depressed in others. Paller et al.[23] found, in animal models, that despite an elevation in plasma renin activity following CsA infusion, inhibition of angiotensin II formation by captopril failed to prevent the CsA-induced decrease in renal blood flow. Myers et al.[24] have recently reported that CsA therapy is associated with elevation of renal vascular resistance, proteinuria, arterial hypertension and impaired intrarenal conversion of inactive prorenin to active renin.

Prostaglandins. The evidence for prostaglandin involvement in CsA nephrotoxicity is again conflicting. Several studies have suggested a decrease in prostaglandin synthesis following CsA administration[25,26]. Others have found renal prostaglandin stimulation[21], while inhibition of prostaglandin synthesis enhanced CsA-induced renal vasoconstriction. Neild et al.[27] have reported that decreased synthesis of prostacyclin (prostaglandin I2—PGI2) stimulating factor (PSF) leads to decreased prostacyclin production. In the presence of increased renal vasoconstriction, synthesis of prostaglandin is normally elevated in order to produce adequate perfusion. CsA therapy, on the other hand, causes increased vasoconstriction and impairs prostacyclin productions, thereby giving rise to reduced renal blood flow. Rossi et al.[28] have shown that interleukin 1, the production of which is depressed by CsA, induces the synthesis of prostacyclin by endothelial cells. The prostaglandins and their effects on the vascular system can vary in different specifies, and as most of the work on the association between CsA and the prostaglandins has been done on animals, it should not be automatically assumed that these effects are operative in clinical practice as well.

However, recently Voss et al.[29] have examined the direct effects of CsA on prostacyclin (PGI1) production by cultured human umbilical vein endothelial cells and found it to be decreased. This effect is reversible when CsA is withdrawn for 24 h. As normal endothelium maintains vasodilatation and thromboresistance partly through production of PGI2, its reduction causes endothelial dysfunction leading to increase in vascular tone and predisposition to platelet aggregation. This would lead to decline in renal blood flow and GFR, and in addition produce the vascular lesions that have been described in association with CsA toxicity. Furthermore it must be remembered that vascular damage from harvest injury, and preservation ischaemia, and hypotension, all lead to impairment of endothelial cell integrity, as do many systemic infections; these are additional factors which may enhance or trigger the inhibitory effect of CsA on PGI2 synthesis.

Finally, during allograft rejection and graft-versus-host disease there is damage to vascular endothelium by the effector mechanisms of the rejection reaction, increased procoagulant activity[30] and involvement of the coagulation cascade. CsA can therefore act synergistically with a variety of unrelated vascular injuries to cause protracted renal damage.

Sympathetic nervous system. Several recent studies have suggested a role for sympathetic stimulation in CsA-induced renal vasoconstriction[21,25]. Renal denervation, or the administration of phenoxy benzamine reduced CsA-induced renal vasoconstriciton. Sympathetic nervous system-mediated renal vasoconstriction could explain many of the effects of CsA on renal function, including a decrease in GFR and an increase in plasma renin activity.

It is important to remember that these proposed mechanisms are not mutually exclusive, and could well be operating synergistically with each other.

Renal histopathology in patients treated with CsA

In the initial report of seven patients treated with CsA, six had been biopsied because of poor function[1]. One patient had evidence of humoral rejection, which improved with antirejection therapy, and the rest had mild non-specific features of proximal tubular epithelial vacuolization and degeneration, acute tubular necrosis, interstitial oedema and mild to moderate cellular infiltration. The authors state that the degree of cellular infiltration was not very severe, and that similar degrees of cellular infiltration can be found in allografts with normal function. Features specific or diagnostic of CsA toxicity were not identified, and the diagnosis of nephrotoxicity was made purely on the absence of significant rejection. In a subsequent paper the Cambridge group[31] reported that in early toxicity histological changes on biospy were generally minimal in comparison to the degree of renal impairment purported to be due to the drug. In six patients who had received CsA for more than 1 year, foci of interstitial fibrosis and tubular atrophy were noted in absence of evidence for chronic vascular rejection. Glomerular and vascular abnormalities were not seen. The authors were of the opinion that the changes of 'interstitial nephritis' were non-specific and may reflect chronic low-grade rejection and/or CsA nephrotoxicity.

Since then there have been numerous seemingly contradictory reports, some claiming specific diagnostic features of CsA toxicity, other reporting features that are associated more often with CsA toxicity but not specific for it, and yet others reporting no morphological differences between CsA patients and those treated with azathioprine and prednisolone[15,32,42].

In renal allografts the major difficulty in defining the pathological abnormalities that could be associated with CsA toxicity is the problem of sorting out concomitant changes of rejection. No such problems are encountered in patients with healthy kidneys receiving the drug for autoimmune disorders or recipients of other organ grafts such as heart and liver. Biopsies from such cases have gone a long way in sorting out some of the problems of CsA-associated morphological abnormalities, although there are still many unanswered questions. It must be stated at the very outset that there are *no* specific diagnostic pathological features that can be attributed to CsA nephrotoxicity. All the abnormalities that have been described in the literature so far are entirely non-specific and can be seen in the kidney of transplant recipients and other patients who have never received CsA. These lesions can be caused by a variety of injurious agents such as ischaemia, hypertension, infection, other drugs and the rejection reaction itself. However, though non-specific, there are certain morphological features that are seen more frequently in CsA-treated patients, and therefore by inference are associated with CsA nephrotoxicity. Furthermore it is not certain if even these abnormalities are caused by CsA on its own, or by the drug triggering and enhancing the damaging effect of the other injurious agents named above. Finally, it must be mentioned that, in the presence of profound clinical nephrotoxicity, especially in the acute phase, the allograft biopsy can on occasion be entirely 'within normal limits' by light microscopy.

Rejection
It has been reported that, compared to classically treated patients, the incidence of rejection episodes was not reduced in CsA patients[4], although the severity of rejection was reduced[43]. There are many other reports confirming the efficacy of CsA in reducing the severity of the rejection reaction[42,44]. However, grade for grade, the morphological pattern of rejection in CsA-treated renal allografts is essentially similar to those treated with azathioprine and prednisolone[35-37,40,41]. As in classically treated patients rejection in CsA patients may be cellular or humoral, or both types may be present with one more dominant than the other. In cellular rejection there is a combination of features including interstitial oedema, diffuse or focal interstitial cellular infiltrate of activated mononuclear cells, endovasculitis with infiltration of cells in the intima, glomerulitis and tubulitis (Figures 15.1 and 15.2). Humoral rejection is characterized by fibrinoid necrotizing vasculitis and interstitial haemorrhage (Figures 15.3 and 15.4).

Rejection or nephrotoxicity?
When there is renal dysfunction in the early post-transplant period the all-important problem is differentiating rejection from nephrotoxicity. Clinically this can be extremely difficult, as patients often do not have the characteristic features of pyrexia, graft enlargement and tenderness associated with classical rejection. Moreover, although high trough levels of serum CsA are more likely to cause toxicity, nephrotoxicity can occur with CsA in therapeutic levels or even low levels. Perhaps the only reliable clinical criterion is the retrospective evidence of rapid improvement – within 24 h – in renal function when the dose of CsA is reduced. Renal allograft biopsy during acute dysfunction does not, unfortunately, always answer the question. In the absence of morphological evidence of rejection dysfunction can be ascribed to CsA toxicity. But what is the situation when there is histological evidence of cellular and/or humoral rejection? Is it possible to have both rejection and nephrotoxicity at the same time? It is the author's opinion that rejection and nephrotoxicity are *not* mutually exclusive. Although impossible to prove

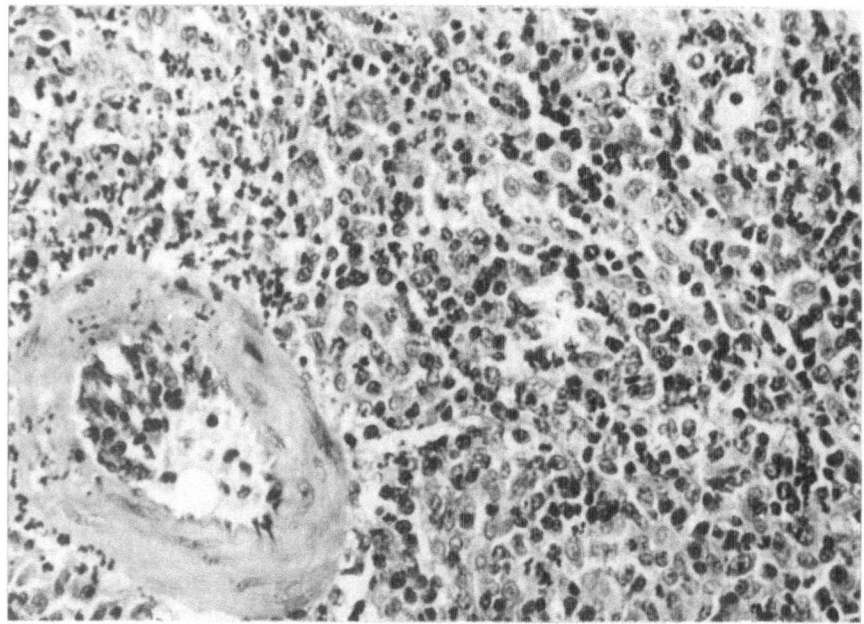

Figure 15.1 Severe cellular rejection. Diffuse cellular infiltration of renal parenchyma. Endovasculitis of small artery with cells infiltrating the intima. × 335

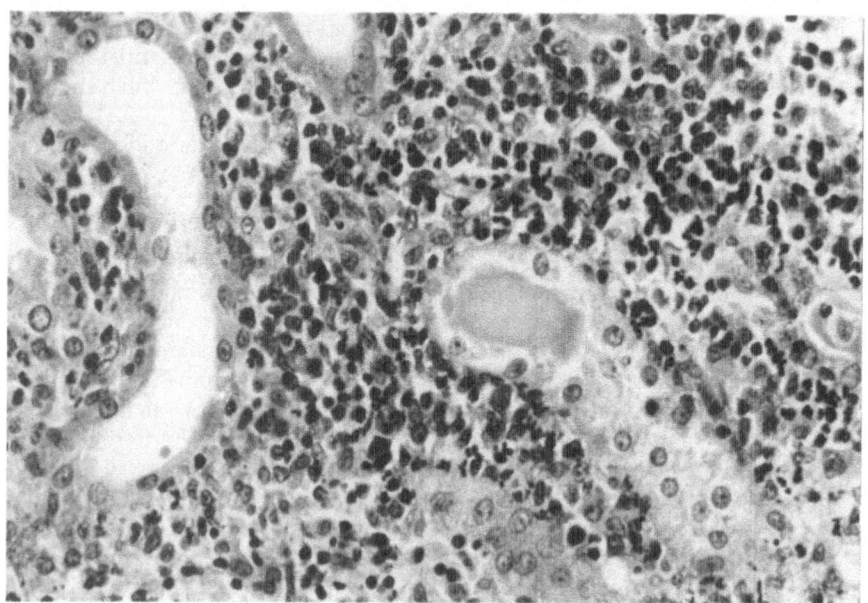

Figure 15.2 Cellular rejection. Interstitial infiltrate and tubulitis. × 335

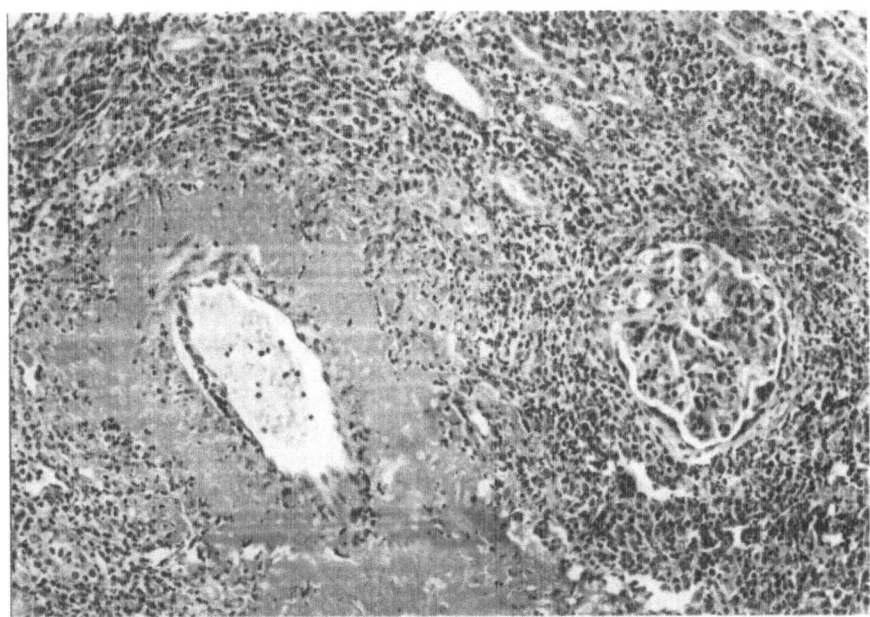

Figure 15.3 Humoral and cellular rejection. Fibrinoid necrosis of wall of artery and diffuse cellular infiltration of parenchyma. Note hypercellularity of glomerulus. × 134

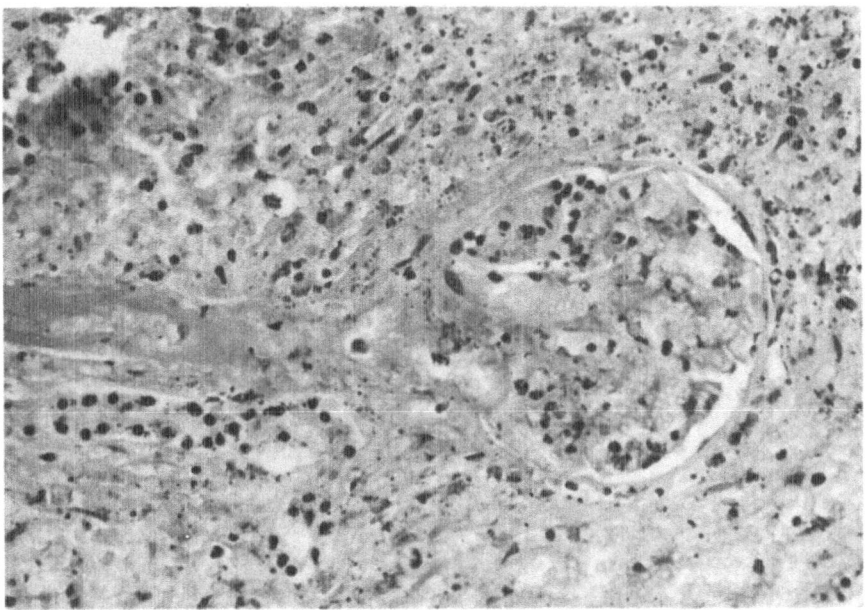

Figure 15.4 Severe humoral rejection. Necrosis of parenchyma with interstitial haemorrhage. × 335

there is sufficient circumstantial evidence to support this theory:

1. Nephrotoxicity can occur with CsA levels being within the therapeutic range or even below the therapeutic range.
2. Reduction of CsA dose, though improving function, does not always restore it to normal; the patient requires additional anti-rejection therapy.
3. The vascular endothelial damage caused by rejection can be enhanced by the effects of CsA on prostacyclin synthesis and vasomotor tone (see above).

Sibley et al.[35] reported a detailed morphological study of 132 biopsies from 54 patients treated with CsA. There were 105 episodes of increase in serum creatinine and some patients had two or more biopsies. Nine parameters were examined, including vasculitis, interstitial oedema, glomerulitis, tubular ectasia, tubular necrosis, tubulitis, distribution and intensity of mononuclear cell interstitial infiltrate and ratio of mononuclear cells in interstitium and peritubular capillaries (1/C ratio). Acute rejection was defined as steroid-responsive tubulo-interstitial nephritis in which the steroid therapy resulted in return of serum creatinine to normal levels. CsA nephrotoxicity was defined as failure to respond to steroid therapy and fall in serum creatinine level following subsequent decrease of CsA dose. In CsA nephrotoxicity there was mild cellular infiltrate in 85% and moderate to severe in 15%. In rejection there was a severe infiltrate in 70%. However, the overlap led to unreliable diagnostic criteria. The same applied with tubular ectasia and necrosis. Glomerulitis was present in 27% of nephrotoxicity and 77% of acute rejection, and with tubulitis the figures were 35.8% and 77% respectively. Oedema was present in 34.6% of nephrotoxicity and 80% of acute rejection cases. Endovasculitis was almost exclusively present in acute rejection. Finally the I/C ratio was $\geqslant 3:1$ in rejection and $\leqslant 1:3$ in nephrotoxicity. This study showed quote clearly that although vasculitis, glomerulitis, oedema and I/C ratio were useful criteria even these features are not absolutely reliable in differentiating rejection from nephrotoxicity. Mononuclear cells were found in almost all the biopsies, and it is important to remember that tubulo-interstitial infiltration does not automatically mean rejection. Marker studies with monoclonal antibodies were again not specific, although T cytotoxic/suppressor cells were markedly increased in acute rejection with the T cytoxic to T helper ratio usually less than $2:1$ in CsA nephrotoxicity.

Clearly, the presence or absence of rejection can be easily ascertained on most biopsies. Nephrotoxicity, on the other hand, is not so straightforward; it can be diagnosed quite easily on biopsy when rejection is *not* present, but when rejection is present it can be almost impossible to assess histological evidence of CsA toxicity. The only reliable criterion for differentiating acute rejection from nephrotoxicity is the retrospective one of patients' response to increased steroids or reduction in CsA dose.

Histopathological changes associated with nephrotoxicity
A number of morphological abnormalities have been reported to be associated with CsA nephrotoxicity and these could be divided into two broad groups – tubulo-interstitial and glomerular–arteriolar changes[15,33–40,45].

Tubulo-interstitial abnormalities associated with CsA are:

giant mitochrondria;
Isometric vacuolization;
microcalcincation;
peritubular capillary congestion;
tubular atrophy and interstitial fibrosis – focal or diffuse.

Giant mitochrondria. These occur predominantly in the proximal convoluted tubular cells. They are difficult to identify by light microscopy, often requiring special stains. Identification by electron microscopy is much easier, but this is not useful for routine diagnostic purposes. Moreover, giant mitochondria are not specific for CsA toxicity and can be seen in a number of conditions of native kidneys and also in renal grafts not treated with CsA[46].

Isometric vacuolizaton. Isometric vacuolization of tubular epithelial cells was noted in the first report of nephrotoxicity reported from Cambridge[1]. Mihatsch *et al.*[33] introduced the term to describe the formation of numerous fine, uniform, small vacuoles within the epithelial cells. The vacuolization involves the entire circumference of the tubule and tends to occur predominantly in the descending straight portion of the proximal tubule (Figure 15.5). Under electron microscopy the vacuoles are empty and probably represent dilated endoplasmic retriculum. The abnormality is very similar to the changes seen

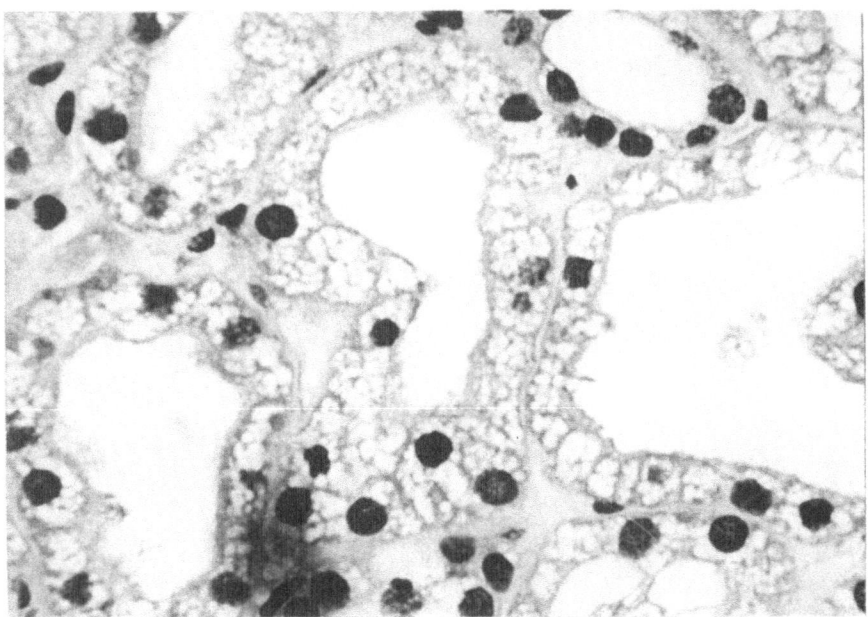

Figure 15.5 Isometric vacuolization. Uniform, small vacuoles involving the entire cirumference of descending proximal tubules. × 335

in osmotic nephrosis secondary to infusion of hyperosmolar solutions, though in that situation the fine vacuolization is present in almost all the cortical tubules. Isometric vacuolization should not be confused with coarse irregular vacuolization which can be seen with ischaemic renal damage (Figure 15.6). Isometric vacuolization can be produced in experimental animals by administering large doses of CsA[47]. This is a reversible lesion and can be seen as early as 1 week, or as late as 1 year, post-transplant. It is an indicator of acute toxicity and there tends to be a good correlation between the presence of this change, renal dysfunction and high trough levels of CsA. However, as it is not specific for CsA and can also occur with other causes of ischaemic tubular damage such as poor preservation and rejection, it is not a helpful feature in diagnosis of nephrotoxicity.

Microcalcification. This is secondary to dystrophic calcification of degenerate and necrotic tubular damage from any cause (Figure 15.7).

Peritubular capillary congestion. This implies numerous mononuclear cells in dilated capillaries. It is identified in most cases of ATN; therefore it is not surprising that it is found in allografts with CsA-associated tubular toxicity[35]. Mononuclear cells within peritubular capillaries are also a morphological feature of early rejection in both CsA and non-CsA-treated allografts, and is therefore not a diagnostic characteristic of CsA toxicity.

Tubular atrophy and interstitial fibrosis. Focal collections of atrophic tubules

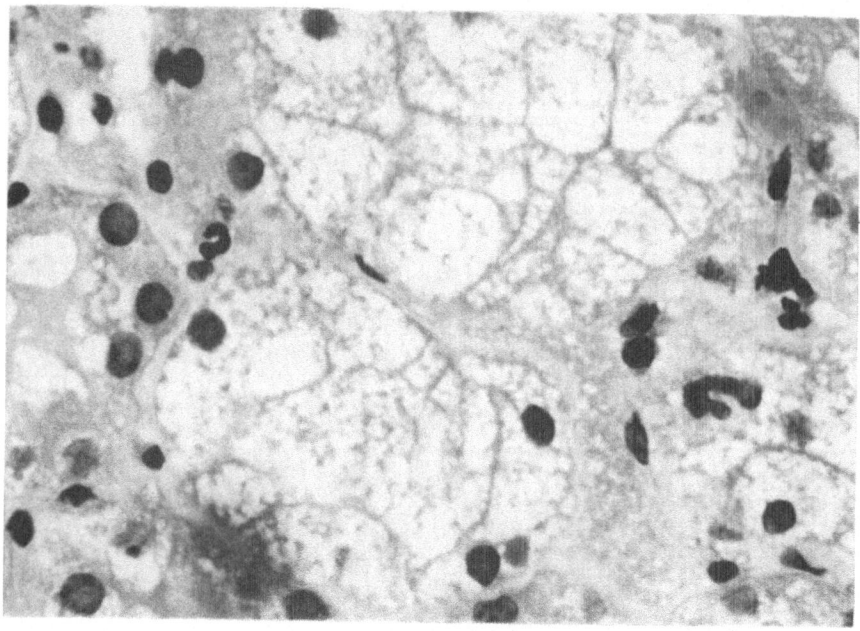

Figure 15.6 Coarse vacuolization. Tubular epithelial cells with irregular vacuoles of different sizes. × 335

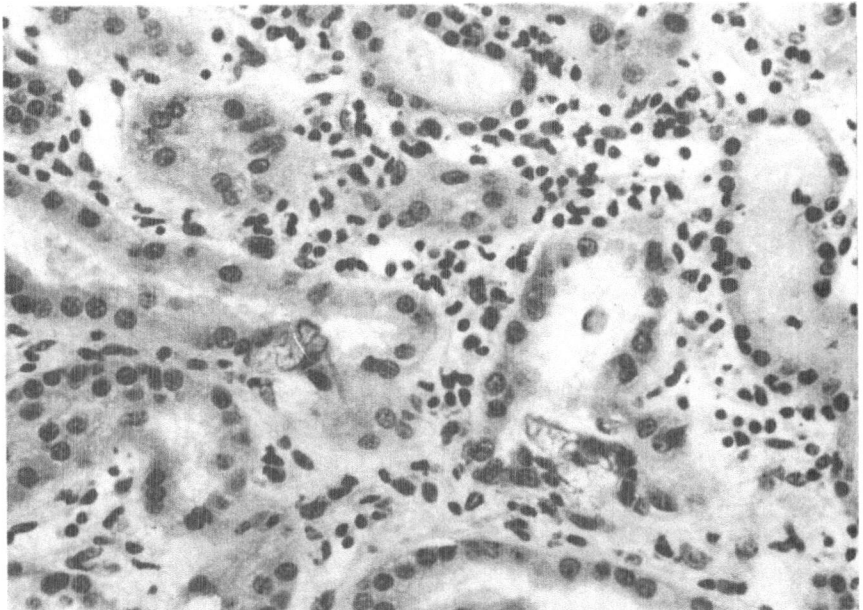

Figure 15.7 Microcalcification. Two foci of dystrophic calcification (↑). Mild cellular infiltrate in interstitium. × 335

with accompanying interstitial fibrosis are found in the cortex with the surrounding cortical tubules and medulla appearing quite unremarkable (Figure 15.8 and 15.9). On biopsy these foci may have a linear appearance, but in nephrectomy specimens the linear effect is not so clear. This abnormality is usually seen in patients who have had CsA therapy for longer than 6 months. The pathogenesis of this tubulo-interstitial scarring may be:

1. Progressive irreversible tubular damage with ongoing nephrotoxicity;
2. Secondary to CsA-associated vascular lesions;
3. Secondary to non-CsA-associated factors such as rejection;
4. Due to a combination of the above factors.

Foci of tubular atrophy and interstitial fibrosis, so-called 'chronic interstitial nephritis', in CsA-treated renal allografts was first reported by the Cambridge group[31,32]. The reports stated that these findings were not specific for CsA nephrotoxicity and reflected 'CsA toxicity and/or low-grade rejection'. In a subsequent report of a morphometric study comparing CsA-treated renal allografts with non-CsA-treated grafts, the authors reported significant differences in tubular atrophy, but not interstitial fibrosis, between the two groups[15]. The numbers in the study, however, were small and ideally tubular atrophy and interstitial fibrosis should be considered as a unit because with time fibrous tissue shrinks and occupies less volume, thereby giving a false impression of its significance. In a study of 38 renal allograft biopsies from 28 patients treated with CsA tubular atrophy and interstitial fibrosis was

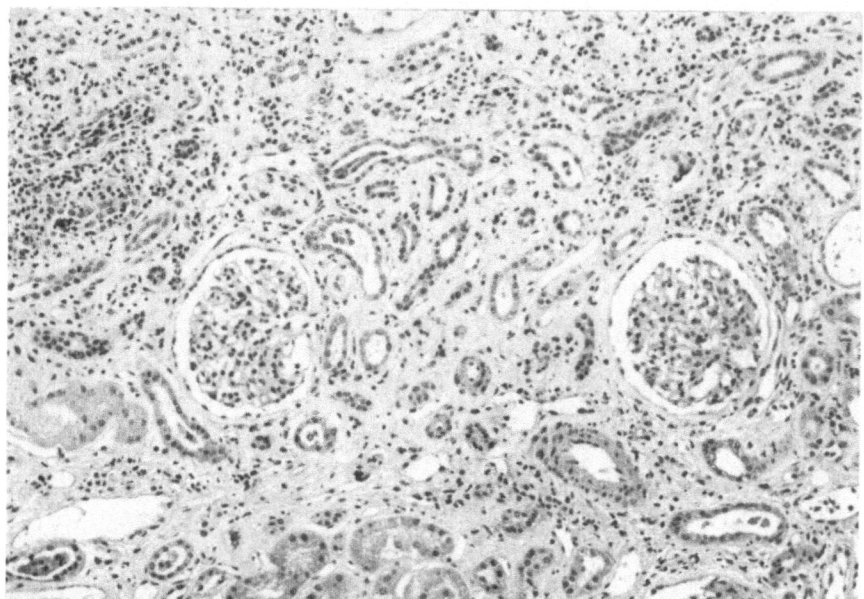

Figure 15.8 Tubulo-interstitial atrophy. An area of small atrophic tubules separated by an increased, fibrous interstitium containing a mild cellular infiltrate. Glomeruli unremarkable. × 134

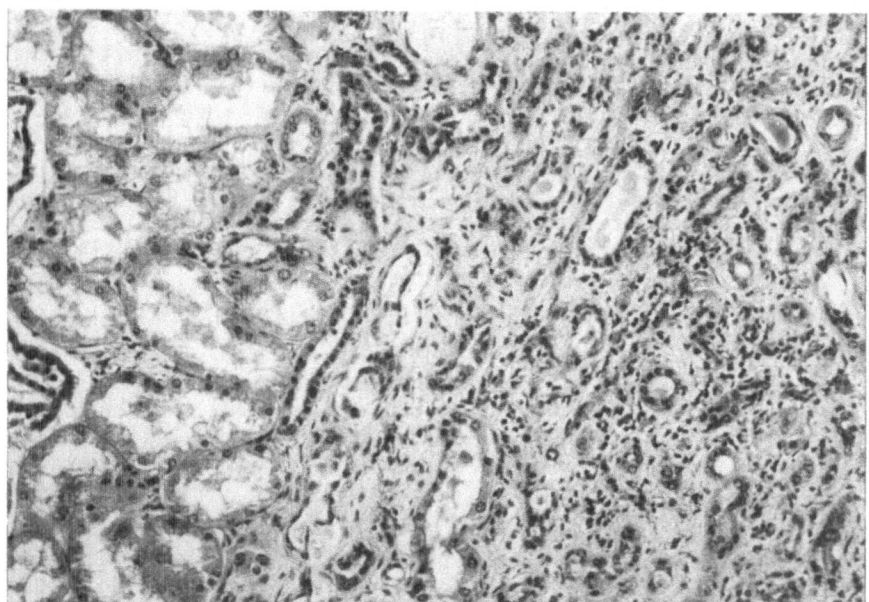

Figure 15.9 Tubulo-interstitial atrophy. Unremarkable proximal tubules packed close together with hardly any intervening interstitium constrasting with area of tubulo-interstitial atrophy. × 134

noted at 1 year post-transplantation in 27 patients[38,39]. The degree of interstitial fibrosis correlated with high cumulative CsA dose during the first 6 months of treatment, as well as with the number of acute CsA nephrotoxic episodes. Nine patients had repeat biopsies 1.5–4 years post-transplant with little evidence of progressive fibrosis. CsA-associated arteriolar lesions were seen very infrequently in this study, and the authors stated it was not easily distinguished from vascular rejection.

The Oxford group[41] compared biopsies from 100 patients who were treated with CsA and prednisolone for 90 days, and subsequently switched to azathioprine and prednisolone, with biopsies from patients treated with azathioprine and prednisolone throughout. Elective biopsies were done on 7, 21, 90 and 365 days post-transplantation as well as when clinically indicated. A total of 107 biopsies in the CsA group was compared with 127 in the azathioprine group. Glomerular changes in both groups were minimal, with capillary thrombosis present only in those with acute rejection. Both groups had evidence of tubular atrophy and interstitial fibrosis. Although there were no specific features of CsA toxicity the incidence of severe interstitial fibrosis was higher in the CsA group but not statistically significant. It was 38% in the CsA group and 18% in the azathioprine group at 90 days and 39% and 29%, respectively, at 365 days. Vascular changes of intimal oedema, cellular infiltration, fibrinoid necrosis and intimal fibrosis were the same in both groups and lesions of 'CsA-associated arteriolopathy', as described by Mihatsch[33], were not found to be increased in the CsA group. The authors reported the increase in fibrosis in the CsA group was probably related to chronic rejection rather than drug toxicity, since it was preceded by diffuse cellular infiltration and accompanied by severe changes in arteries.

Variable amounts of interstitial fibrosis associated with tubular atrophy were seen in a group of 17 patients treated with CsA for sight-threatening uveitis[13]. All patients had normal serum creatinine prior to therapy and elevated levels at time of biospy.

Diffuse interstitial fibrosis is associated with long ischaemia time, and is often accompanied by prolonged oliguria[36]. Morphologically the renal cortical tubules are separated initially by oedema and subsequently by fine fibrosis. The proximal tubules are often irregularly dilated with the lining epithelium exhibiting degenerative changes and individual cell necrosis (Figures 15.10 and 15.11). This abnormality is often present in kidneys of patients with ATN, and is therefore not specifically related to CsA. CsA, of course, may well prolong and enhance the abnormality.

Glomerular and vascular abnormalities associated with CsA are:

    glomerular and vascular platelet – fibrin thrombi;
    arteriolar eosinophilic hyaline sclerosis;
    arteriolar intimal mucoid thickening and fibrosis;
    glomerular segmental-global sclerosis.

Glomerular and vascular thrombi. CsA-associated abnormalities were initially reported in bone marrow transplant patients who had poor renal function

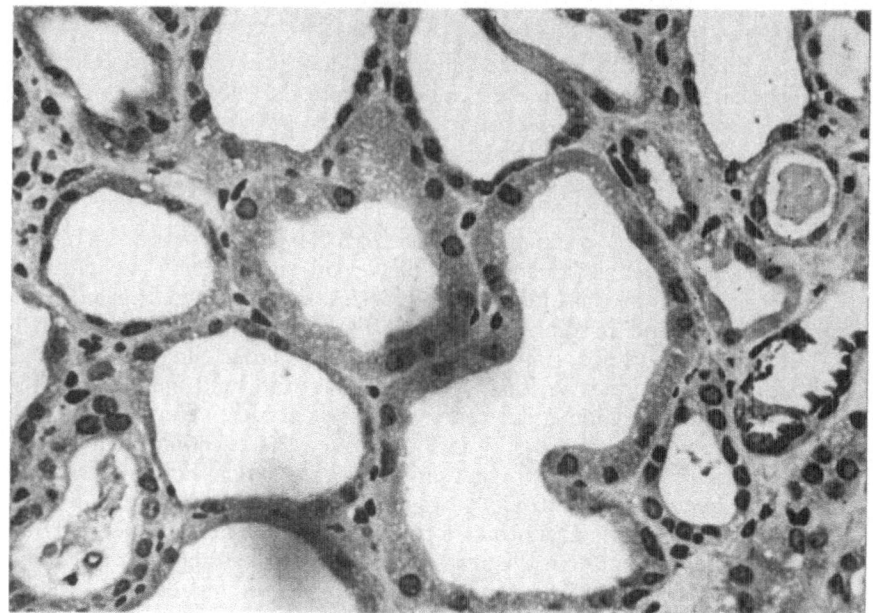

Figure 15.10   Acute tubular necrosis. Irregularly dilated proximal tubules lined by degenerating, attenuated epithelium. × 335

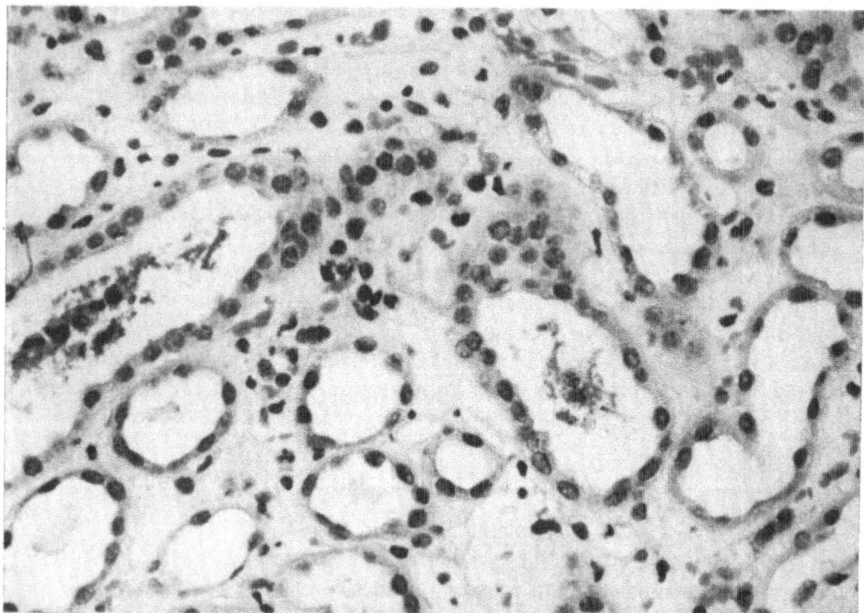

Figure 15.11   Diffuse interstitial oedema and early fibrosis. Widely separated proximal tubules showing evidence of ATN. The separation of tubules is due to interstitial oedema together with delicate fibres of collagen. × 335

and exhibited glomerular necrosis and arteriolar thrombi in the kidneys at postmortem[48]. It was postulated that these patients had a syndrome similar to the haemolytic uraemic syndrome as a consequence of CsA toxicity. The patients also had active graft-versus-host disease (GVHD) and systemic infections. Neild et al.[49] reported glomerular and/or afferent arteriolar platelet-fibrin thrombi in renal biopsy specimens from seven renal allograft recipients treated with CsA and prednisolone. All patients had high plasma CsA levels and none of the patients was considered to be undergoing rejection. Such thrombi were not previously seen by them in biopsy material from patients treated with prednisolone and azathioprine, except rarely associated with acute vascular rejection. In a subsequent report, however, Neild et al.[50] reported glomerular thrombi in CsA-treated renal grafts undergoing rejection, those with nephrotoxicity and those with apparent stable function. In the writer's experience glomerular–arteriolar platelet–fibrin thrombi can be seen in rejection and even in the absence of overt evidence of vascular rejection, can be seen in renal allografts treated with azathioprine and prednisolone as well as in the CsA-treated allografts (Figures 15.12–15.15). The incidence of glomerular platelet thrombi in routine elective biopsies of renal allografts with stable function is no different in CsA-patients compared to those treated with azathioprine and prednisolone (Dunhill, personal communication). A microangiopathic haemolytic anaemia with renal dysfunction has been reported in a hepatic allograft patient treated with CsA and prednisolone[51]. The patient at the same time had a urinary tract infection and hypertensive encephalopathy.

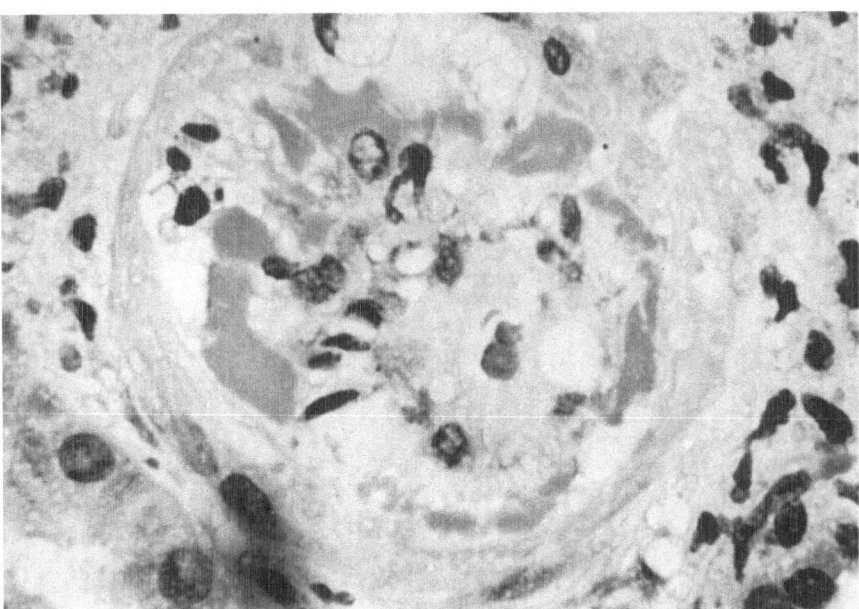

Figure 15.12 Arteriolar platelet – fibrin thrombi. Intimal deposition of fibrin and platelets within an ateriole. Incidental finding in an allograft with normal function and otherwise normal histology. × 335

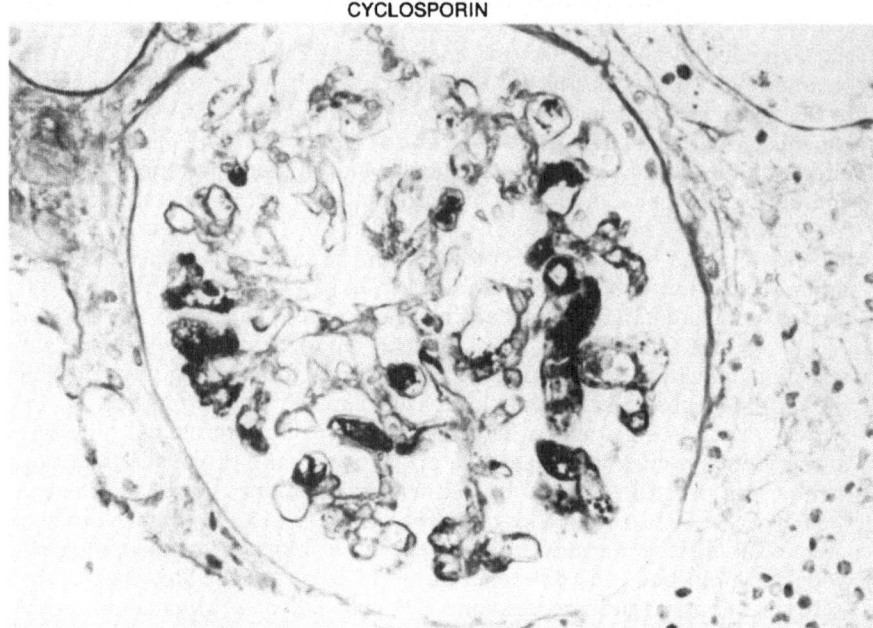

Figure 15.13 Glomerular platelet thrombi. Immunoperoxidase stain showing aggregates of platelets within glomerular capillary loops. Incidental finding in otherwise normal allograft. × 335

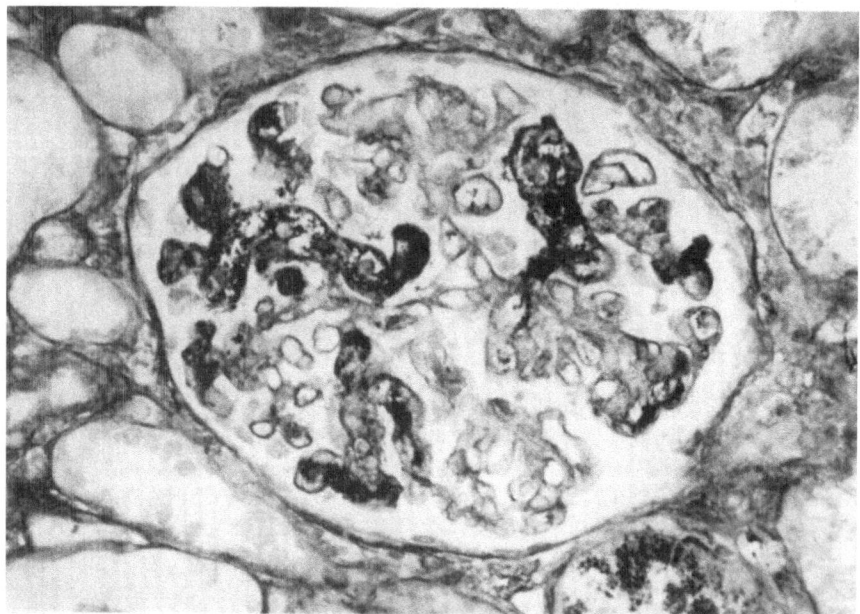

Figure 15.14 Glomerular platelet thrombi. Aggregates of platelets within glomerular capillary loops showing positive staining with monoclonal antibody to platelets. Biopsy from a patient with CsA toxicity. × 335

344

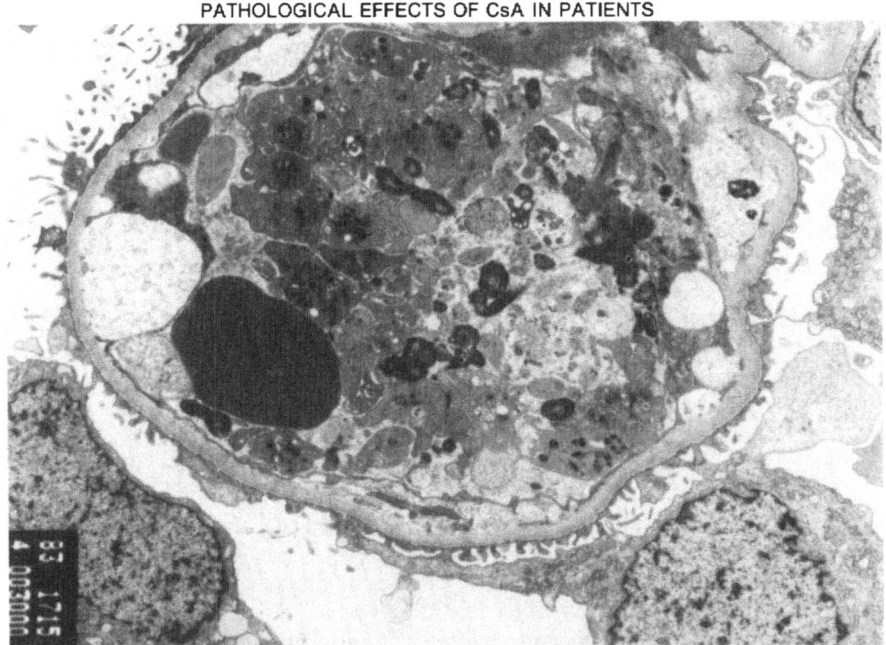

Figure 15.15 Electronmicrograph of platelet thrombi. Same case as Figure 15.14. × 5400

Clinical improvement occurred with withdrawal of CsA and introduction of azathioprine. In another report[52] of a CsA-treated liver transplant patient' there was complicating thrombotic thrombocytopenic purpura and severe microangiopathic haemolytic anaemia with concomitant histological evidence of rejection. This patient was successfully treated with intensive plasma exchange and *continued administration* of CsA.

Leithner *et al.*[53] reported a case of a patient who had a cadaveric renal transplant whose primary disease was haemolytic uraemic syndrome (HUS). The patient developed renal failure with a microangiopathic haemolytic anaemia and thrombocytopenia; renal biospy showed extensive thrombosis of arterioles and glomerular capillaries. Acute rejection was considered unlikely as there was no fever or graft tenderness. Rat aortic rings incubated in patient's plasma revealed lack of prostacyclin-stimulating activity. The graft was eventually removed as there was no response to fresh frozen plasma. It was difficult to be certain if the patient had HUS or acute humoral rejection. Moreover, if it was HUS, was it a spontaneous recurrence of the patient's original disease or was it triggered by CsA? HUS is known to recur in renal allografts of patients who have not been treated with CsA[54]. Hamilton *et al.*[55], on the other hand, reported a case of end-stage HUS who underwent renal transplantation and was treated with CsA as the sole immunosuppressive agent. Three years later the serum creatinine was 118 μmol/l and creatinine clearance 37 ml/min, with no evidence of any haemolytic or thrombotic activity.

Landmann *et al.*[56] described two forms of vaculopathy associated within intravascular coagulation. One was a proliferative arteriopathy of interlobular

345

and arcuate arteries with loss of graft; this was labelled vascular rejection. The other was intravascular coagulation with glomerular and/or arteriolar thrombi *without* arteriopathy and no loss of grafts; this was described as CsA-associated arteriolopathy (see below). In 230 biopsies from non-CsA patients 13 h ıd arterial lesions leading to graft loss. In 200 biopsies from CsA patients, on tıe other hand, 13 had arterial lesions leading to graft loss and seven had the glomerular/arteriolar lesions. As the latter lesion was seen only in the CsA group they concluded it was due to the drug.

Hyaline eosinophilic arteriolar sclerosis. This was first described by Mihatsch *et al.*[33], who observed nodular circumferential, acellular deposits within the media of arterioles associated with loss of myocytes. The lesions are similar to the arteriolar necrosis—sclerosis that is seen in hypertensive and diabetic arteriolopathy. The acellular deposits are intensely eosinophilic, stain bright magenta with the PAS stain and bright red with trichrome stains. With immunofluorescence the deposits stain intensely with IgM and/or C3 (Figures 15.16–15.19). In a study of 61 biopsies from 31 renal transplant patients on CsA alone compared with 104 historical controls treated with azathioprine and prednisolone, Mihatsch *et al.*[33] reported the *arteriolar* lesions to be limited to the former group. In vascular rejection *arterial* lesions were predominant and if arteriolar lesions occurred they were always accompanied by lesions in arteries. They never observed vascular rejection limited to arterioles in the non-CsA group, and therefore concluded the frequent occurrence of arteriolar

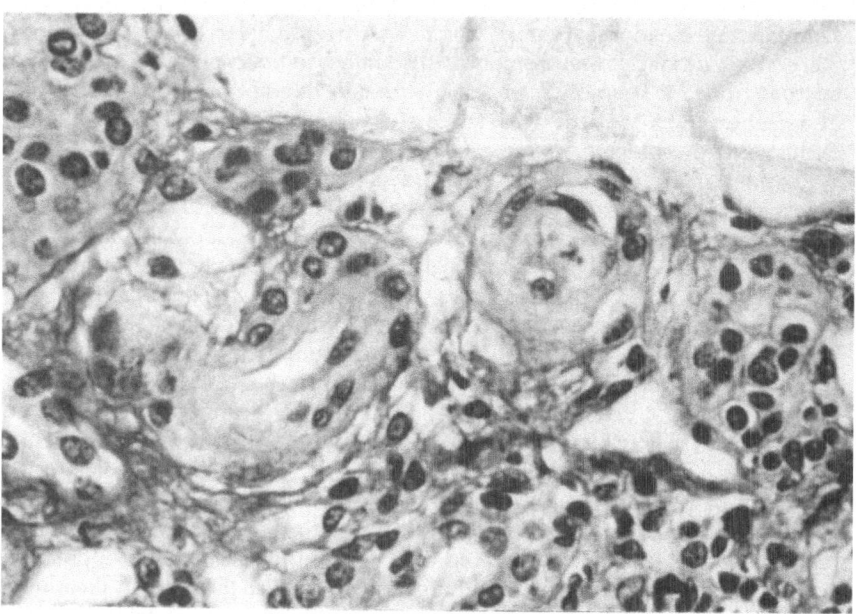

Figure 15.16 Arteriolar sclerosis. (On CsA) Acellular dense hyaline thickening of the wall with loss of myocytes. This change may appear focal and nodular (↑) or circumferential (↑↑). These lesions can be quite difficult to identify especially then there is additional tubular atrophy. × 335

346

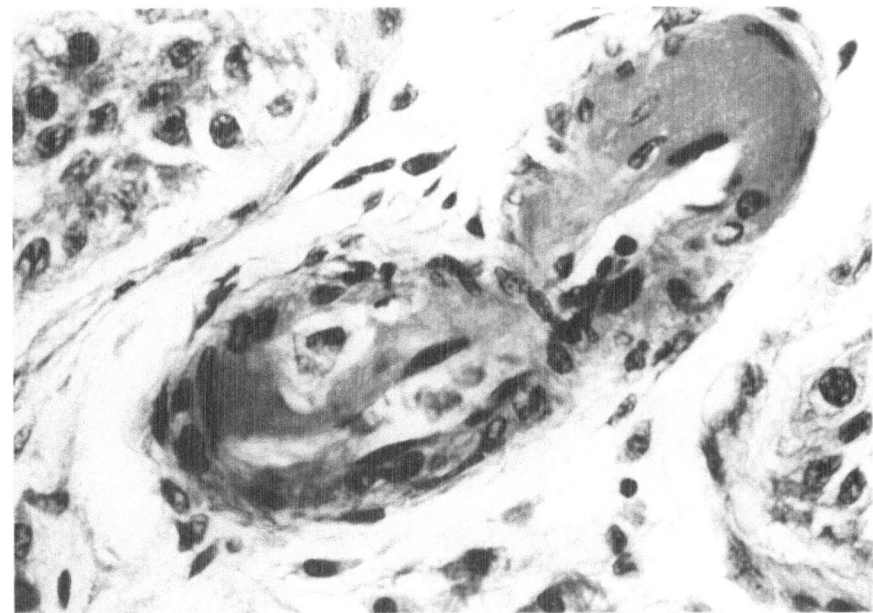

Figure 15.17 Arteriolar sclerosis. (No CsA) Marked hyaline thickening involving part of the wall. Note loss of myocytes in this region (↑). × 335

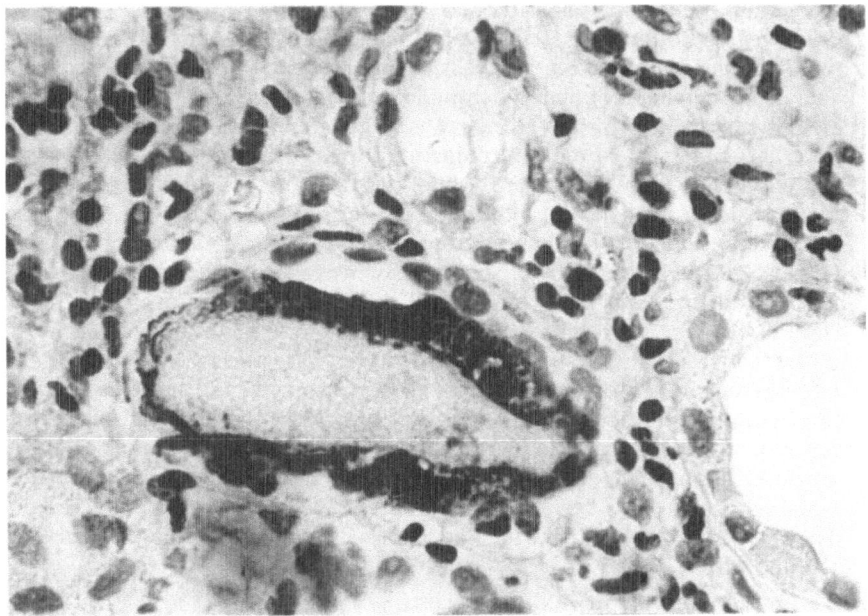

Figure 15.18 Arteriolar sclerosis. Immunoperoxidase stain for IgM. × 335

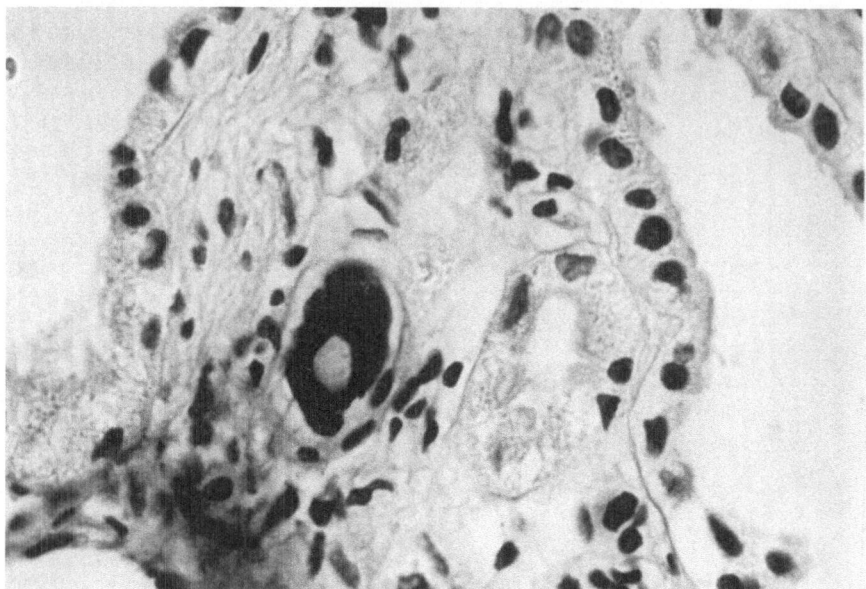

Figure 15.19 Arteriolar sclerosis. Immunoperoxidase stain for IgM. × 335

lesions in CsA patients must be due to CsA toxicity.

However, Porter et al.[57] in 1966, long before CsA was on the scene, reported thickening of arteriolar walls by large subendothelial hyaline deposits containing immunoglobulin and complement. In a series of routine biopsies of grafts after 2 years this change was encountered by him in 48%. There have been a number of reports comparing the histology of CsA-treated renal allografts with non-CsA-treated grafts, and the majority of these have not found a higher incidence of arteriolar changes with CsA[38,39,41,42,50]. Although arteriolar hyaline change was present in renal biopsies of patients treated with CsA for uveitis it was not significantly increased compared to controls[13]. Similar findings were reported in renal biopsies of liver transplant patients treated with CsA[8,9]. In a recent report[24] of long-term CsA nephrotoxicity in cardiac allograft patients, the arteriolar changes were present in 14 of 15 renal biopsies, but there was no control group for comparison. It must be stressed that peroperative biopsies of donor kidneys at the time of transplantation reveal hyaline arteriolar sclerosis in approximately 5–10% of the cases; these are from donors who did not have a known history of hypertension and were between 40 and 60 years of age (personal observation, Figure 15.20). The significance of hyaline arteriolar sclerosis should therefore be interpreted with caution.

Arteriolar intimal mucoid thickening. Significant luminal narrowing has been reported secondary to an oedematous mucoid widening of the intima[33]. The intima, though wide, is relatively hypocellular and may have a few delicate strands of fibrous tissue (Figure 15.21). Similar lesions can be seen in

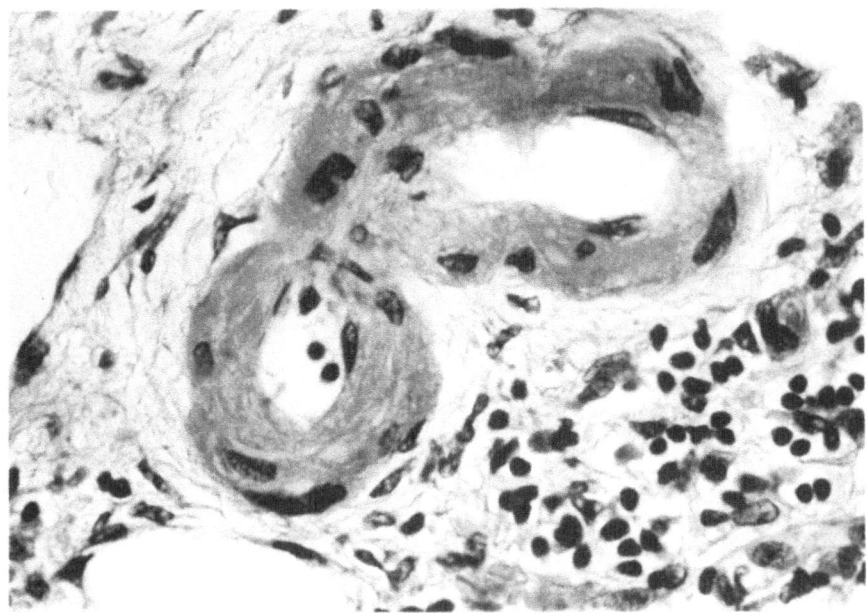

Figure 15.20 Arteriolar sclerosis. Incidental finding in 46-year-old donor who was the victim of a road traffic accident. × 335

hypertension and the haemolytic uraemic syndrome, and also in non-CsA-treated renal allografts.

Glomerular segmental–global sclerosis. Recent reports[8–10], especially on liver and heart transplant patients, have reported a greater incidence of ischaemic glomeruli in CsA-treated recipients when compared to non-CsA controls. The changes consist of thickening and wrinkling of glomerular capillary walls, abnormal widening of Bowman's capsule, segmental and global sclerosis of tufts. These changes were seen most frequently in patients who had been on CsA for longer than 1 year. On the other hand in a report on patients treated with CsA for uveitis, renal biopsies at 1 year showed a variable number of completely sclerosed glomeruli which was not significantly different from controls[13]. In most CsA-treated long-term renal transplants the incidence of glomerular ischaemic changes has not been greater than in non-CsA controls[15,33,36,38,40–42,45].

Pathogenesis of renal lesions associated with CsA therapy

Although a long list of morphological abnormalities have been reported none of these is specific or diagnostic of nephrotoxicity. However, it is apparent that there are some abnormalities which are seen more frequently in CsA-treated patients when compared to non-CsA controls. Admittedly these abnormalities are often not statistically significant and merely indicate a trend.

349

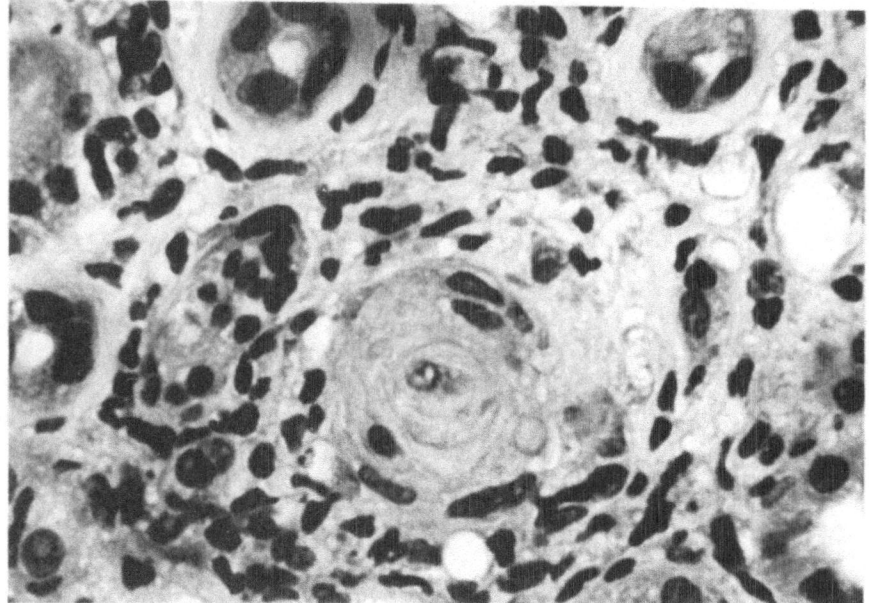

Figure 15.21 Arteriolar mucoid thickening. Marked luminal narrowing secondary to oedematous mucoid widening of the intima. These lesions can be seen in graft rejection (CsA and non-CsA treated), hypertension and the haemolytic uraemic syndrome. × 335

The features that are recurrently observed, especially in patients on long-term CsA and chronic nephrotoxicity, are *tubulo-interstitial scarring, glomerular sclerosis* and *hyaline arteriolar sclerosis* with luminal narrowing. On the other hand it must also be noted that there are well-controlled studies which have not shown any difference in morphological abnormalities between CsA and non-CsA groups. The major reason for this discrepancy may be that most centres have different protocols of immunosuppression, with variable CsA dosage, single-drug or combination therapy, continuous CsA therapy or withdrawal of CsA after a limited period of time and so on. Although all centres admit to functional nephrotoxicity, which can occur even with low-dose regimes, the incidence of structural abnormalities probably depends on the variables mentioned.

What, then, is the pathogenesis of these lesions? Is CsA the sole culprit or is it aided and abetted by other unrelated factors? Are the lesions inevitable; can they be prevented? Is renal damage progressive? Much of the pathogenesis as we know it has been discussed in the preceding sections and some of these questions have been touched upon. An attempt will be made here to correlate the pathogenesis with the morphological lesions.

The evolution of the morphological lesions of CsA toxicity is thought to be due to *direct tubular damage and/or vascular mechanisms* (see above). Thiru *et al.*[15] postulated that although acute tubulo-interstitial changes are not specific for CsA toxicity, such damage could account for the early fall in renal function. With time there is chronic tubular atrophy and interstitial fibrosis. Superimposed on these changes is probably some degree of ongoing acute damage. This may be the reason for the functional improvement that occurs when the dose of CsA is reduced and/or switched to some other drug. It is well established that renal function is more closely related to structural changes observed in the tubules than to those in the glomeruli[58,59]. There is impaired salt reabsorption through damaged proximal tubules, resulting in increased sodium concentration in the tubular fluid at the macular densa: this would lead to a fall in GFR through the tubular-glomerular feedback mechanism[60]. The toxic effects of CsA are most damaging in the early post-transplant period when the graft tissue is made more vulnerable by a variety of insults, such as ischemic damage and rejection. The lack of progressive deterioration in renal function in most cases may be due to the fact that the CsA dose is reduced to maintenance levels, and also the impact of these other insults has been reduced or eliminated. Moreover renal function may be stabilized at the expense of the functional reserve capacity of the allograft. Only when the reserve capacity is exhausted will continued renal damage be reflected by further functional deterioration. The length of time required for the renal reserve capacity to dissipate would presumably depend on a number of variables, including dose of CsA, supplementary steroids, hypertension, infections, evolution of rejection and many other unrecognized factors.

The other mechanism of CsA toxicity is, of course, primary vascular damage with secondary tubulo-interstitial scarring and glomerular sclerosis. Interstitial fibrosis is often focal and linear, suggesting a vascular distribution pattern. On the other hand most studies report no correlation between severity of arteriolar lesions and the extent of fibrosis. As discussed earlier there is substantial experimental and *in vitro* evidence to indicate CsA has an inhibitory effect on the synthesis of PGI2 which causes vasodilatation and prevents platelet aggregation. The vascular lesions of CsA have been described almost exclusively in the kidney and not in other organs, thus implying the inhibitory effect on PGI2 is mainly on the renal vasculature. The lesions similar to HUS are seen either in kidneys grafts[33,49,61,62], or in native kidneys of bone marrow and liver transplant patients[48,51,52] when there is concomitant GVHD and/or infection and septicaemia. In patients with classical HUS it is known that there is a background deficiency of a plasma factor which normally stimulates PGI2 production; an additional factor, e.g. infection, is required in such individuals for HUS to occur[63]. Similarly if CsA does impair mechanisms normally regulating vascular PGI2, as suggested by *in vitro* studies on rabbit aorta[26], it is possible that an additional factor may be required before the clinical picture of HUS is precipitated. This additional factor may be rejection, GVHD, infection, septicaemia, viraemia or any other factors which affect endothelial integrity.

Furthermore the arteriolar hyaline sclerosis described by Mitatsch *et al.*[33] is seen in renal allografts treated with CsA but not to a significant degree in native kidneys of patients receiving CsA for other organ grafts or autoimmune disorders. This may well mean that these lesions in renal allografts could represent vascular rejection, being modified by the inhibitory effect of CsA on PGI2. Finally, vascular lesions cannot be produced experimentally, even

351

by massive doses of CsA, unless the animal models have some additional trigger for endothelial damage such as spontaneous hypertension or chronic serum sickness[25,27]. The same principle seems to apply to the effects of CsA in clinical practice. In the author's opinion the vascular lesions associated with CsA are due not to CsA toxicity on its own, but to CsA triggering, enhancing or acting with other causes of endothelial damage. These other causes of endothelial damage would include ischaemia, infection, rejection in organ transplants, GVHD in bone marrow transplants and an immune insult in autoimmune disorders.

Prevention of nephrotoxicity

It is possible to prevent or suppress CsA-induced nephrotoxicity? The therapeutic window between immunosuppression and toxicity is very narrow, making it difficult to achieve this goal. A number of protocols have been tried by different centres and some of these suggestions are mentioned below.

1. Initiation of CsA therapy delayed until after the onset of adequate renal function in cadaveric renal allografts, so as to avoid potentiating the ischaemic injury to which such grafts are vulnerable.
2. Withdraw CsA 3–6 months after therapy. This covers the period during which the allograft is most susceptible to acute rejection, and at the same time removes the drug before irreversible chronic changes develop. A disadvantage of this protocol is that a significant number of grafts develop 'rebound rejection' when CsA is withdrawn and azathioprine instituted.
3. Low-dose triple therapy to minimize CsA toxicity.
4. Keep CsA trough levels towards the lower end of the recommended therapeutic range of 200–800 ng/ml.
5. Control CsA dosage by serum creatinine levels rather than CsA levels, and aim at keeping the serum creatinine at a clinically acceptable level and not be satisfied with levels of 150–200 μmol/l.

HYPERTENSION

Hypertension is common in renal transplant recipients but its exact pathogenesis is ill-understood. Several factors are thought to predispose to hypertension, including persistence of pre-existing hypertension, allograft rejection, transplant artery stenosis, inappropriate renin secretion from diseased native kidneys and steroid therapy. CsA-treated renal transplant patients can have raised blood pressure, but more significantly CsA therapy is associated with hypertension in recipients of cardiac and bone marrow transplants. The mechanism by which CsA elevates the blood pressure is not known. It is likely that the hypertensive effect is either related to the nephrotoxicity or due to some primary effect of CsA on the systemic vasculature. While there is evidence for stimulation of the renin–angiotensinogen system in rat models of CsA nephrotoxicity[25] renin levels are low or low–normal in the clinical situation[64]. However, recently Myers et al.[24] have shown extreme elevation

352

of plasma-inactive renin with impaired intrarenal conversion to active renin. They also reported that rigorous control of the hypertension in CsA-treated heart transplant patient did not prevent chronic renal injury.

In the Canadian trial[2] of renal transplantation 42 of 103 patients receiving CsA and Prednisolone were hypertensive, compared with 32 of 107 patients receiving classical therapy of azathioprine and prednisolone. In the European multi-centre trial, on the other hand, 27 of 60 patients treated with CsA alone were hypertensive compared with 39 of 59 patients on classical therapy[65]. Recently the Oxford Group[66] have shown the importance of concomitant steroid therapy in the induction of post-transplant hypertension. They compared renal transplant recipients on short-term CsA with conversion to azathioprine and prednisolone at 90 days to patients treated with azathioprine and prednisolone throughout. Blood pressure was similar in the two groups during the first 90 days, but after conversion the CsA group mean blood pressure fell from 155/94 to 142/81 within 7 days. This fall correlated significantly with a fall in serum creatinine levels from $231\,\mu$mol/l to $140\,\mu$mol/l. Blood pressure subsequently remained lower in the converted group compared to those treated with azathioprine and prednisolone throughout. At 6 months 72% of the converted group required hypertensive medication, whereas the figure was 90% in the control group. It therefore seems that concomitant steroid therapy may be important in the incidence of hypertension in CsA-treated patients.

HEPATOTOXICITY

Hepatotoxicity represented by elevated serum bilirubin, alkaline phosphatase and serum transaminase levels was reported in the initial pilot study of CsA[1]. The dose of CsA used was large, 25 mg/kg body weight, but similar toxicity (27–34% incidence) has since been reported in trials using smaller doses of CsA, 17 mg/kg and 14 mg/kg[67,68]. Reduction of CsA dosage resulted in regression of the abnormal liver function in most cases. It must be remembered that liver dysfunction has been recorded in renal transplant recipients prior to the era of CsA, and been attributed to azathioprine and/or other drug therapy. Sutherland et al.[69] reported no significant difference in serum bilirubin or liver enzyme levels between patients treated with CsA and prednisolone compared to those treated with azathioprine, prednisolone and anti-lymphocyte serum. Recently Lorber et al.[70] reported at least one episode of hepatotoxicity in 49% of 466 renal allograft patients treated with CsA and prednisolone. The hepatotoxic episodes generally occurred during the very early post-transplant period, were self-limited and resolved with dose reduction in 41% of the cases. In 7%, however, there were recurrent or persistent liver function abnormalities and in another 2.4% there was evidence of biliary calculous disease. In a control group of 279 renal transplant recipients treated with azathioprine and prednisolone none had evidence of cholelithiasis.

Assessment of possible hepatotoxicity of CsA in hepatic transplant recipients is difficult because of other causes of liver dysfunction – rejection, cholestasis, cholangitis, obstruction and recurrence of original disease. Histologically there is no specific feature of CsA toxicity. Although a fine vacuolar-feathery change is often seen in the cytoplasm of hepatocytes the degree of overlap of this feature in rejection and other non-specific causes of hepatic injury make it an unreliable feature for diagnosis of CsA toxicity, (personal communication, D.G.D. Wight). In all cases hepatotoxic reactions are generally reversible and responsive to CsA dose reduction. It must, however, be remembered that concomitant therapy with other hepatotoxic drugs can potentiate the effects of CsA.

INFECTIONS

In initial clinical usage CsA was prescribed in large doses and combined with other immunosuppressive agents, corticosteroids, azathioprine and cytimun. The patients were consequently over-immunosuppressed with a high incidence of bacterial, viral and fungal infections[1]. Since then multiple reports have appeared comparing the clinical effects of CsA, with or without low-dose prednisolone, to classical immunosuppressive protocols. In the randomized Canadian Multicentre Trial there was significantly less infection, particularly CMV infection and bacterial septicaemia in the CsA–prednisolone group compared to the non-CsA group[2]. Similarly Najarian et al.[71] and Kahan et al.[72] have noted a major decrease in infectious complications in the CsA group when compared to the non-CsA group. In the European Multicentre Trial, however, there was no difference in the incidence of infection, including viral infection, when the CsA-alone group was compared to the conventional therapy group[65]. Similarly, Tilney et al.[73] found no difference between the CsA–prednisolone group as compared with the group receiving azathioprine and prednisolone. The differences in these reports can be explained by the contributions of other components in the immunosuppressive regime. In the European Multicentre Trial acute rejection in both groups was treated with pulse doses of intravenous methylprednisolone, and Tilney et al. used T12 monoclonal antibody for antirejection therapy. In the Canadian Multicentre Trial, on the other hand, the classical group had for maintenance immunosuppression azathioprine and prednisolone, plus a variety of other agents including ALG, cyclophosphamide and plasmapheresis; acute rejection was treated with further steroids and/or ALG. Similarly Najarian et al. used ALG as well as azathioprine and prednisolone in the classical group, but no ALG in the CsA group. It therefore seems that it is the addition of other agents, in particular ALG, that alters the balance between the CsA and non-CsA groups. The advantage of CsA therapy appears to lie in its ability to decrease rejection and thereby increase graft survival without the use of additional immunosuppression by agents such as ALG[74]. It thus causes increased graft survival without a concomitant increase in infection. It has been reported that CMV infections are observed in only 3% of CsA-treated recipients in the first 2 months post-transplant compared to 15% in azathioprine- and prednisolone-treated recipients[75]. There have been a few centres that have reported a high incidence of Pneumocystis carinii pneumonia among CsA recipients[73,76], but the explanation for this is not yet available.

354

There have been no controlled studies to define quantitatively the relative risks of infection at different periods in the post-transplant course. Overall it appears that the incidence of infection in CsA-treated patients is less than in those treated with azathioprine and prednisolone, and in particular much less than in those treated with additional ALG. Finally it must always be kept in mind that interactions between CsA and a variety of antibiotics can complicate therapy and also cause nephrotoxicity.

MALIGNANT NEOPLASMS

One of the long-term consequences of immunosuppression is the evolution of malignant tumours. Soon after the introduction of CsA into clinical transplantation the Cambridge group reported[77,78] three lymphomas in a series of 34 transplant patients who had received the drug. All the patients had been heavily immunosuppressed with CsA and multiple other immunosuppressive agents. After initial fears it was soon realized that the development of lymphomas in CsA patients is by virtue of its powerful immunosuppressive activity rather than through a direct oncogenic action.

According to the records of the Transplant Tumour Registry[79] 141 malignancies had developed in 5550 organ transplant recipients treated with CsA up to May 1986. Only 8% of the patients with tumours had been treated with CsA as the sole immunosuppressive agent. Of the 141 malignancies the commonest was non-Hodgkin's lymphoma, 41%; next in order were skin cancer 15%, and Kaposi's sarcoma 8%. On the other hand, in the 2598 tumours of classically immunosuppressed transplant recipients the distribution was skin cancers 40%, lymphomas 12%, carcinoma of cervix 6% and Kaposi's sarcoma 3%. There were also other important differences between the two groups. The lymphomas appeared much earlier in the CsA group, average of 11 months (range 1–68) post-transplant compared with an average of 42 months (range 1–190) in the alternative group. Furthermore, unlike in the classically immunosuppressed group the lymphomas often involved lymph nodes and multiple organs, but rarely involved the brain and were more likely to regress after reduction of immunosuppressive therapy. This last feature suggests that some of the so-called lymphomas most probably represent extreme lymphoproliferation rather than true neoplasms (see below). The reduced incidence of skin cancers, predominantly squamous cell carcinomas, as well as carcinomas of the cervix, vulva and perineum, may be a reflection of the length of follow-up. It is known that skin cancers in particular show a progressive increase in incidence with the length of follow-up, and therefore the pattern of distribution of tumours in CsA patients may change with time. Another interesting feature of the tumours in the CsA group was the small but significant number of endocrine-related tumours and renal cell carcinomas[79,80]. Nineteen of 141 tumours were of endocrine organs (ovary, testis, thyroid and carcinoid) or of organs that are influenced by hormones (breast, prostate). This occurrence may be a chance event and it is speculative whether CsA has hormonal side-effects which may promote these tumours. (CsA is known to elevate serum prolactin levels.) A further difference between

355

the CsA and non-CsA groups was that in the former a larger number of tumours, 35 of 141 (25%), occurred in recipients of extrarenal organs, whereas in the latter group only 51 of 2422 patients (2%) were recipients of extrarenal organs. Most of the CsA-related tumours that occurred in extrarenal organ recipients (27 of 35; 77%) were lymphomas.

What, then, is the pathogenesis of the lymphomas? In vitro and in vivo studies in dogs, sheep, pigs, rodents and rabbits treated with CsA have not shown the drug to be carcinogenic[81]. However, in a study of non-human primates treated with CsA for heart or heart and lung transplants 12 of 97 animals developed lymphomas[82]. A herpes-like virus with antigens cross-reactive with Epstein–Barr virus (EBV) was found in the tumour cells. The association between Burkitt's lymphoma, malaria and EBV is well known[83]. It has been repeatedly shown that all patients with Burkitt's lymphoma, both the African type and the sporadic cases in temperate climates, have antibodies to EBV, and that the virus genome is expressed in the tumour cells which are also Epstein–Barr nuclear-antigen positive. In malaria there is massive stimulation of B cells with excessive immunoglobulinaemia, and at the same time there is evidence of immunosuppression with a defect in the processing of antigens by macrophages and defective T suppressor cell activity[84]. EBV is known to selectively infect B lymphocytes which possess surface receptors for the virus[85]. This induces a polyclonal B-cell proliferation, both in vitro and in vivo, which in the immunocompetent patient is self-limited and controlled by EBV-specific cytotoxic T cells and antibodies to EBV-specific antigens[86]. This occurs in patients with infectious mononucleosis. After the acute event latent virus will be present in B lymphocytes and will be under the tight control of EBV-specific T cells. In the immunosuppressed patient there is impaired T-cell function which may allow uncontrolled proliferation of the B cells either in a primary infection or activation of the latent infection. Analogous to the malaria scenario chronic antigenic stimulation from the allograft may further stimulate continued B cell proliferation. This proliferation will in the first instance be polyclonal without cytogenetic abnormalities and regress with reduction or cessation of immunosuppression. If immunosuppression is continued, however, a clonal cytogenic abnormality may occur (8 : 14 translocation) and proceed to a monoclonal B-cell proliferation – malignant lymphoma. The higher incidence of lymphomas in recipients of extrarenal organs, especially cardiac transplants, could be because these patients have disorders, e.g. cardiomyopathy, which are in themselves partly due to some form of T cell abnormality.

Morphology of lymphoproliferative lesions

The lesions tend to involve multiple lymph node groups, the gastrointestinal tract, in particular the terminal ileum, tonsils, pharynx, lungs, liver, renal allografts and retroperitoneum. The gastrointestinal tumours are often multicentric and present either as bleeding problems or with peritonitis secondary to perforation. Histologically they all have features of polymorphic B cell proliferations and produce extensive architectural obliteration of the organs involved. Overall the hyperplastic lesions tend to have a plasmacytoid differentiation without much atypia or necrosis. The lymphomas, on the other hand, are composed of cells of varying size, often large, with large vesicular nuclei and prominent nucleoli. The nuclei can be either cleaved or non-cleaved and mitoses are abundant. There is often extensive necrosis. The majority of these tumours are classified as diffuse large cell lymphomas, either cleaved or non-cleaved cell subtype; a few are designated immunoblastic lymphomas. With immunohistochemical stains the hyperplastic proliferative lesions tend to be polyclonal with varying numbers of cells staining for heavy chains alpha, gamma, mu, and light chains kappa and lambda. The malignant lymphomas, on the other hand, tend to be monoclonal with the majority of tumour cells staining for a single heavy chain and light chain. There has been recent evidence, using immunoglobulin gene rearrangement techniques, that some lymphomas may even be bioclonal or multiclonal[87].

GINGIVAL HYPERPLASIA

Gingival hyperplasia, clinically and pathologically similar to that seen with penylhydantoin and nifedipine[88], is rarely evident before 3 months of CsA therapy[32,89]. It appears to be more common in children, and tends to occur in patients with poor oral hygiene. The hyperplasia is occasionally severe enough to require gingivectomy. There has recently been a report of two cases of Kaposi's sarcoma occuring in gingival hyperplasia induced by CsA[90].

DERMATOLOGICAL TOXICITY

One of the most common dermatological side-effects of CsA is dose-dependent hypertrichosis on the face and upper trunk, affecting more than 80% of the patients[32,91]. There are also variable degrees of hirsutism with soft downy hair growth in the male distribution. The cause of this CsA-induced hair growth is unclear. A recent study[9] showed no significant influence of therapeutic doses of CsA on specific sex hormone actions. The authors therefore postulated the mode of action to be at the cellular level in the hair follicles, with transformation of lanugo hair producing follicles into terminal hair follicles, and/or stimulation of dormant follicles. This report also included a renal transplant patient with longstanding alopecia areata universalis, who experienced considerable regrowth of eyebrows and scalp hair during CsA therapy. This effect of CsA in alopecia was considered to reflect not only the stimulating potency of the drug on hair growth but also perhaps the modulating effect on the immune system in a disease which is thought to have autoimmune characteristics. In a recent report[92] 19 children (aged 3.9–18.5 years) given renal allografts and treated with CsA and prednisolone, developed facial changes by 6 months post-transplant. There was pronounced coarsening of the face with thickening of the nares, lips and ears, prominence of the supraorbital ridges and mandibular prognathism. Such changes were not seen in patients receiving prednisolone and azathioprine.

357

NEUROLOGICAL TOXICITY

Tremor was one of the early side-effects to be observed. It appears to be similar to 'essential tremor', is common in the early post-transplant phase, especially when high doses of CsA are employed, and usually resolves with reduction of dose[32]. Such tremor, with or without burning paraesthesiae of palms and soles, is observed in approximately 22% of recipients but is rarely present after 1 year or at doses below 5 mg/kg body weight[94]. Convulsions, either *de novo* or in patients with a previous history, have been reported in children with bone marrow transplants[95,96]. The patients had been given additional high-dose methyl prednisolone for GVHD. Convulsions were not observed in patients who were not given high-dose steroids. It is, however, very difficult to be certain of the contribution made by the drugs in the causation of diffuse neurological dysfunction in patients that have acute GVHD and its attendant complications of vasculitis and haemorrhage. It has been postulated[97] that the rejection process or GVHD might cause vasoactive substances to be released[98], and this could sensitize the cerebral circulation and produce an encephalopathy without having to involve CsA or steroids.

CAPILLARY LEAK SYNDROME

CsA has been associated with the development of pulmonary oedema − capillary leak syndrome − in some bone marrow transplant patients and in two liver transplant patients[95,99,100]. The patients developed dyspnoea, hypoxia and bilateral pulmonary infiltrates on chest radiography. Fluid retention had been postulated to be important for the development of this syndrome. An additional factor was thought to be CsA potentiating pre-existing endothelial cell damage provoked by other processes like GVHD in bone marrow transplant patients, or to high concentrations of CsA reaching the lung via central venous catheters, as in the liver transplant patients. Recently there has been a report of this syndrome in a diabetic patient receiving simultaneous kidney and pancreas transplants[101]. Two periods of pulmonary oedema occurred with intraveous CsA administration, and disappeared when the drug was given orally. The patient did not have fluid retention and intravenous administration of CsA was through a central vein in the first instance and via the Scribner shunt in the second instance. The authors concluded the capillary leak was attributable to the solvent cremaphor (20% w/v) and not to CsA.

MISCELLANEOUS TOXIC EFFECTS

Minor gastrointestinal symptoms have been reported by patients on CsA and include anorexia, nausea and vomiting. Breast tenderness without lumps has been reported in patients given CsA for uveitis[102]. Two renal transplant recipients developed benign breast lumps after CsA treatment[103]. One had previous fibrocystic disease of the breast and developed a benign fibroadenoma with elevated levels of prolactin 1 year post-transplant. The second patient, treated only with CsA, developed a fibroadenoma which was resected 1 year after grafting. Three months later she developed lumps in both breasts, and two fibroadenomata were removed from the right breast as previously. The lump in the left breast was not excised. CsA dose was reduced and she had a severe rejection episode which resolved on changing to conventional therapy. The lump in the left breast resolved after cessation of CsA therapy.

ABO-autoimmune haemolytic anaemia has been documented[104] in a CsA-treated renal transplant patient of blood group B Rh+ given a kidney from an O Rh+ donor. It was thought the autoantibodies developed as a result of the immunosuppression whereby lymphocytes with anti-B specificity normally suppressed by suppressor lymphocytes were released from the suppression. The drug rarely causes dose-related myeloid depression with leukopenia and thrombocytopenia.

CONCLUSION

Although CsA has been shown to have some major and minor problems of toxicity, it has many advantages, both in terms of improved graft survival and in the avoidance of the side-effects of corticosteroids. In the present state of the art the benefits to be gained from the use of CsA in transplantation far outweigh the risks. However, many questions still remain to be answered, and it is hoped the solutions will be revealed not far into the future.

REFERENCES

1. Calne, R. Y., White, D. J. G., Thiru, S., Evans, D. B., McMaster, P., Dunn, D. C., Craddock, G. N., Pentlow, B. D. and Rolles, K. (1978) Cyclosporin A in patients receiving renal allografts from cadaver donors. *Lancet*, **2**, 1323–1327.
2. Canadian Multicentre Transplant Study Group (1983) A randomised clinical trial of cyclosporin in cadaveric renal transplantation. *N. Engl. J. Med.*, **309**, 809–812.
3. Hall, B. M., Tiller, D. J., Duggin, G. G., Horvath, J. S., Farnsworth, A., May, J., Johnson, J. R. and Sheil, A. R. (1985) Post-transplant acute renal failure in cadaver renal recipients treated with cyclosporine. *Kidney Int.*, **28**, 178–186.
4. Merion, R. M., White, D. J. G., Thiru, Sathia, Evans, D. B. and Calne, R. Y. (1984) Cyclosporine: five years experience in cadaveric renal transplantation. *N. Engl. J. Med.*, **310**, 148–154.
5. Calne, R. Y. and Wood, A. J. (1985) Cyclosporine in cadaveric renal transplantation: 3-year follow up of a European multicentre trial. *Lancet*, **2**, 549–552.
6. The Canadian Transplant Study Group (1985) Examination of parameters influencing the benefit : detriment ratio of cyclosporine in renal transplantation. *Am. J. Kidney Dis.*, **5**, 328–332.
7. Morris, P. J., Chapman, J. R., Allen, R. D., Ting, A., Thompson, J. E., Dunnill, N. S. and Wood, R. F. M. (1987) Cyclosporinconversion versus conventional immunosuppression: long-term follow-up and histological evaluation. *Lancet*, **1**, 586–591.
8. Wheatley H. C., Datzman, M., Williams, J. W., Miles, D. E. and Hatch, F. E. (1987) Long-term effects of cyclosporine on renal function in liver transplant recipients. *Transplantation*, **43**, 614–647.
9. Dische F. E., Neuberger, J., Keating, J., Parsons, V., Calne, R. Y. and Williams, R. (1988). Kidney pathology in liver allograft recipients after long-term treatment with cyclosporin A. *Lab. Invest.*, **58**, 395–402.
10. Myers, B. D. (1986) Cyclosporine toxicity. *Kidney Int.*, **30**, 964–974.
11. Myers, B. D., Ross, J., Newton, L., Luetscher, J. and Perlroth, M. (1984) Cyclosporine-associated chronic nephropathy. *N. Engl. J. Med.*, **311**, 699–705.

12. Hesse, C. L., Sutherland, D. E. R., Mauer, S. M. and Najarian, J. S. (1985) Creatinine clearance and serum creatinine levels before and after pancreas transplantation in 11 patients. *N. Engl. J: Med.*, **312**, 48.

13. Palestine, A. G., Austin III, H. A., Barlow, J. E., Antonovyeh, T. T., Sabris, S. G., Preuss, H. G. and Nussenblatt, R. B. (1986) Renal histopathologic alterations in patients treated with cyclosporine for uveitis. *N. Engl. J. Med.*, **314**, 1293–1298.

14. Miescher, P. A., Favre, H., Chatelanat, F. and Mihatsch, M. J. (1987) Combined steroid–cyclosporine treatment of chronic autoimmune disease: clinical results and assessment of nephrotoxicity by renal biopsy. *Klin. Wochenschr.*, **65**, 727–736.

15. Thiru, S., Maher, E. R., Hamilton, D. V., Evans, D. B. and Calne, R. Y. (1983) Tubular changes in renal transplant recipients on cyclosporine. *Trans. Proc.*, **15**, 2846–2850.

16. Whiting, P. H., Thomson, A. W., Blair, J. T. and Simpson, J. G. (1982) Experimental cyclosporine nephrotoxicity. *Br. J. Exp. Pathol.*, **63**, 88–92.

17. Kahan, B. D. (1986) Cyclosporin nephrotoxicity: pathogenesis, prophylaxis, therapy and prognosis. *Am. J. Kidne Dis.*, **5**, 323–331.

18. Baxter, C. R., Duggin, G. G., Willis, N. S., Hall, B. M., Horvath, J. S. and Tiller, D. J. (1982) Cyclosporin A induced increases in renin storage and release. *Res. Commun. Chem. Pathol. Pharmacol.*, **37**, 305–309.

19. Osman, E. A., Barrett, J. J., Bewick, M. and Parsons, V. (1984) Does cyclosporine affect renal blood vessels? *Lancet*, **1**, 1470.

20. Humes, H. D., Jackson, N. M., O'Connor, R. P., Hunt, D. A. and White, M. P. (1985) Pathogenic mechanisms of nephrotoxicity: Insights into cyclosporine nephrotoxicity. *Transplant Proc.*, **17**, 51–54.

21. Paller, M. S. and Murray, B. M. (1985) Renal dysfunction in animal models of cyclosporine toxicity. *Transplant. Proc.*, **17** (Suppl. 1), 155–158.

22. Sullivan, B. A., Hak, L. J. and Finn, W. F. (1985) Cyclosporine nephrotoxicity: studies in laboratory animals. *Transplant. proc.*, **17**, 145–148.

23. Paller, M. S., Murray, B. M. and Ferris, T. F. (1985) Decreased blood flow after cyclosporine infusion. *Kidney Int.*, **27**, 346–349.

24. Myers, M. D., Sibley, R., Newton, L., Tomlanon, S. J., Boshkos, C., Stinson, E., Leutscher, J. A., Wray, D. J., Krasny, D., Coplon, N. S. and Perlroth, M. G. (1988) The long-term course of cyclosporine-associated chronic nephropathy. *Kidney Int.*, **33**, 590–600.

25. Siegl, H., Ryffel, B., Petric, R., Shoemaker, P. and Muller, A. (1983) Cyclosporine, the resin–angiotensin–aldosterone system and renal adverse reactions. *Transplant. Proc.*, **15**, 2719–2721.

26. Neild, G. H., Rocchi, G., Imberti, L., Fumagalli, F. and Brown, Z. (1983) Effect of cyclosporine on prostacyclin synthesis by vascular tissue in rabbits. *Transplant. Proc.*, **15**, 2398–400.

27. Neild, G. H., Ivory, K. and Williams, D. G. (1983) Glomerular thrombi and infarction in rabbits with serum sickness following cyclosporine therapy. *Transplant. Proc.*, **15**, 2782–2786.

28. Rossi, V., Breviaro, F., Ghezzi, P., Dejana, E. and Mantovani, A. (1985) Prostacyclin synthesis induced in vascular cells by interleukin 1. *Science*, **229**, 174–176.

29. Voss, B. L., Hamilton, K. K., Samara, E. N. S. and McKee, P. A. (1988) Cyclosporine suppression of endothelial prostacyclin generation. *Transplantation*, **45**, 793–796.

30. Heikki, H. and Edgington, T. S. (1983) Allogeneic induction of the human T cell instructed monocyte procoagulant response is rapid and is elicited by HLA-DR. *J. Exp. Med.*, **158**, 962–968.

31. Hamilton, D. V., Evans, D. B., Henderson, R. G., Thiru, S., Calne, R. Y. and White D. J. G. (1982) Long-term nephrotoxicity of cyclosporin A in transplantation. *Dialysis Transplant.*, **11**, 146–160.

32. Hamilton, D. V., Evans, D. B. and Thiru, S. (1982) Toxicity of Cyclosporin A in organ grafting. In White, D. J. G. (ed.), *Cyclosporin A* (Amsterdam: Elsevier), pp. 393–409.

33. Mihatsch, M. J., Thiel, G., Spichtin, H. P., Oberholzer, M., Brunner, F. P., Harder, F., Olivieri, V., Bremer, R., Ryffel, B., Stocklin, E., Torhorst, J., Gudat, F., Zollinger, H. U. and Loertscher, R. (1983) Morphological findings in kidney transplants after treatment with cyclosporine. *Transplant. Proc.*, **15**, 2821–2835.

34. Farnsworth, A., Hall, B. M., Bishop, G. A., Duggin, G. C., Goodman, B., Horvath, J., Johnson, J., Ng, A., Sheil, A. G. R. and Tiller, D. J. (1983) Pathology in renal transplant

patients treated with cyclosporine A. *Transplant. Proc.*, **15**, 2852–2854.
35. Sibley, R. K., Rynasiewicz, J., Ferguson, R. M., Fryd, D., Sutherland, D. E. R. (1983) Morphology of cyclosporine nephrotoxicity and acute rejection in patients immunosuppressed with cyclosporine and prednisolone. *Science*, **94**, 225–234.
36. Farnsworth A., Horvath, J., Hall, B. M., Sheil, A. G. R., Ng, A. B. P., Tiller, D. J. and Duggin, G. C. (1984) *Am. J. Surg. Pathol.*, **8**, 243–252.
37. Mihatsch, M. J., Thiel, G., Ryffel, B. B., Von Overbeck, J. and Zollinger, H. U. (1985). Morhological patterns in cyclosporine-treated renal transplant recipients. *Transplant. Proc.*, **17**, 101–115.
38. Klintmalm, G., Bohman, S.-O., Sundelin, B. and Wilczek, H. (1984) Interstitial fibrosis in renal allografts after 12–46 months of cyclosporin treatment. Beneficial effects of low doses in early post-transplant period. *Lancet*, **2**, 950–953.
39. Bohman, S.-O., Klintmalm, G., Ringdn, O., Sundelin, B. and Wilczek, H. (1985) Interstitial fibrosis in human kidney grafts after 12 to 46 months of cyclosporine therapy. *Transplant. Proc.*, **17**, 1168–1171.
40. Bignardi, L., Neild, G. H., Hartley, R. B., Taube, D. H., Cameron, J. S., Rudge, C. J., Williams, D. G. and Ogg, C. S. (1987) Histopathological changes in Cyclosporine treated renal allografts biopsied at 1 and 12 months. *Nephrol. Dial. Transplant.*, **2**, 366–370.
41. d'Ardenne, A. J., Dunnill, M. S., Wood, R. F. M., Thompson, J. F. and Morris, P. J. (1985) Cyclosporine treatment does not cause specific histologic changes in human renal allografts. *Transplant. Proc.*, **17**, 1166–1167.
42. Morris, P. J., Allen, R. D., Thompson, J. F., Chapman, J. R., Ting, A., Dunnill, M. S. and Wood, R. F. M. (1987) Cyclosporin conversion versus conventional immunosuppression. Long term follow up and histological evaluation. *Lancet*, **1**, 586–591.
43. Merion, R. M., White, D. J. G. and Calne, R. Y. (1983) Early renal allograft rejection episodes are less aggressive with Cyclosporine A immunosuppression. *Transplant Proc.*, **15**, 2172–2177.
44. Flechner, S. M., Payne, W. D., Van Buren, C. T., Kerman, R. H. and Kahan, B. D. (1983) The effect of cyclosporine on early graft function in human renal transplantation. *Transplantation*, **36**, 268–272.
45. Bergstrand, A., Bohmann, S. O., Farnsworth, A., Gokel, J. M., Krause, P. H., Lang, W., Mihatsch, M. J. Oppedal, B., Sell, S., Sibley, R. K., Thiru, S., Verani, R., Wallace, A. C., Zollinger, H. U., Ryffel, B., Thiel, G. and Wonigeit, K. (1985) Renal histopathology in kidney transplant recipients immunosuppressed with cyclosporin A. *Clin. Nephrol.*, **24**, 107–119.
46. Thiru, S. and Calne, R. Y. (1981) Giant mitochondria, renal transplant biopsy and cyclosporin A. *Lancet*, **2**, 147.
47. Thomson, A. W., Whiting, P. H., Blair, J. T., Davidson, R. J. L., Simpson, J. G. (1981) Pathological changes developing in the rat during a 3 week course of high dosage cyclosorin A and their reversal following drug withdrawal. *Transplantation*, **32**, 271–227.
48. Shulman, J., Striker, G., Deeg, H. J., Kennedy, M., Storb, R. and Thoams, E. D. (1981) Nephrotoxicity of cyclosporine after allogeneic marrow transplantation. *N. Engl. J. Med.*, **305**, 1392–1395.
49. Neild, G. H., Reuben, R., Hartley, R. B. and Cameron, J. S. (1985) Glomerular thrombi in renal allografts associated with Cyclosporin treatment. *J. Clin. Pathol.*, **38**, 253–258.
50. Neild, G. H., Taube, G. H., Hartley, R. B., Bignardi, L., Cameron, J. S., Williams, D. G., Ogg, C. S. and Rudge, C. J. (1986) Morphological differentiation between rejection and Cyclosporin nephrotoxicity in renal allografts. *J. Clin. Pathol.*, **39**, 152–159.
51. Bonser, R. S., Adu, D., Franklin, I. and McMaster, P. (1984) Cyclosporin induced haemolytic syndrome in liver allograft recipients. *Lancet*, **2**, 1337.
52. Dzik, W. H., Georgi, B. A., Khettry, U. and Jenkins, R. L. (1987) Cyclosporine-associated thrombotic thrombocytopenic purpura following liver transplantation – successful treatment with plasma exchange. *Transplantation*, **44**, 570–572.
53. Leithner, C., Sinzinger, H., Pohanka, E., Schwarz, M. and Kretschmer, G., Syre, C. (1983) Occurrence of haemolytic uremic syndrome under cyclosporine treatment: accident or possible side effect mediated by a lack of prostacyclin-stimulating plasma factor? *Transplant. Proc.*, **15**, 2787–2789.
54. Morzuka, M., Croker, B. P., Seigler, H. F. and Tisher, C. C. (1982) Evaluation of recurrent

glomerulonephritides in kidney allografts. *Am. J. Med.*, **72**, 588–598.
55. Hamilton, D. V., Calne, R. Y. and Evans, D. B. (1982) Haemolytic-uraemic syndrome and cyclosporin A. *Lancet*, **2**, 151–152.
56. Landmann, J., Mihatsch, M. J., Ratschek, M. and Thiel, G. (1987) Cyclosporine A and intravascular coagulation. *Transplant. Proc.*, **19**, 1817–1819.
57 Porter, K. A., Rendal, J. M., Stolinski, C., Terasaki, P. I., Marachioro, T. L. and Starzl, T. E. (1966) Light and electronmicroscopic study of biopsies from 33 human renal allografts and an isograft $1\frac{3}{4}$–$2\frac{1}{2}$ years after transplantation. *Ann. N.Y. Acad. Sci.*, **19**, 615–625.
58. Risdon, R. A., Sloper, J. C. and DeWardener, H. E. (1968) Relationship between renal function and histological changes found in renal biopsy specimens from patients' with persistent glomerulonephritis. *Lancet*, **2**, 363–365.
59. MacKensen-Haen, S., Baden, R., Grund, K. E. and Bohle, A. (1981). Correlations between renal cortical interstitial fibrosis, atrophy of the proximal tubules and impairment of the glomerular filtration rate. *Clin. Nephrol.*, **15**, 167–171.
60. Thurau, K. and Boylan, J. W. (1976) Acute renal success. The unexpected logic of oliguria in acute renal failure. *Am. J. Med.*, **61**, 308–315.
61. Sommer, B. G., Henry, M. L. and Ferguson, R. M. (1986). Cyclosporine-associated renal arteriopathy. *Transplant. Proc.*, **18**, 151–154.
62. Giroux, L., Smeesters, C., Corman, J., Paquin, F., Allaire, G., St-Louis G. and Daloze, P. (1986) Hemolytic uremic syndrome in renal allografted patients treated with cyclosporin. *Can. J. Physiol. Pharmacol.*, **65**, 1125–1131.
63. Wiles, P. G., Solomon, L. R., Lauler, W., Mallick, N. P. and Johnson, M. (1981) Inherited plasma factor deficiency in haemolytic–uraemic syndrome. *Lancet*, **1**, 1105–1106.
64. Adu, D., Turne, J., Michael, J. and McMaster, P. (1983) Hyperkalaemia in cyclosporin treated renal allograft recipients. *Lancet*, **2**, 370–371.
65. European Multicentre Trial Study Group (1983) Cadaveric renal transplantation: One year follow-up of a multicentre trial. *Lancet*, **2**, 986–990.
66. Chapman, J. R., Marcer, R., Arias, M., Raine, A. E. G., Dunnill, M. S. and Morris, P. J. (1987) Hypertension after renal transplantation. *Transplantation*, **43**, 860–864.
67. Klintmalm, G. B. G., Iwatsuki, S. and Starzl, T. E. (1981) Cyclosporin A hepatotoxicity in 66 renal allograft recipients. *Transplantation*, **32**, 488–491.
68. Kahan, B. D., Wideman, C., Reid, M., Gibbons, S., Jarowenko, M., Flechner, S. and Van Buren, C. T. (1984) The value of serial serum trough cyclosporine levels in human renal transplantation. *Transplant. Proc.*, **16**, 1195–1199.
69. Sutherland, D. E. R., Fryd, D. S., Strand, M. H., Canafax, D. M., Ascher, N. L., Payne, W. D., Simmons, R. L. and Najarian, J. S. (1985) Results of the Minnesota randomized prospective trial of Cyclosporine versus azathioprine–antilymphocyte globulin for immunosuppression in renal allograft recipients. *Am. J. Kidney Dis.*, **5**, 318–22.
70. Lorber, M. I., Van Buren, C. T., Flechner, S. M., Williams, C. and Kahan, B. D. (1987) Hepatobiliary and pancreatic complications of Cyclosporine therapy in 466 renal transplant recipients. *Transplantation*, **43**, 35–40.
71. Najarian, J. S., Fryd, D. S., Strand, M., Canafax, D. M., Ascher, N. L., Payne, W. D., Simmons, R. L. and Sutherland, D. E. R. (1985) A single institution, randomized, prospective trial of Cyclosporine versus azathioprine–ALG for immunosuppression in renal allograft recipients. *Ann. Surg.*, **201**, 142–157.
72. Kahan, B. D., Van Buren, C. T., Fechner, S. M., Jarowenka, M., Yasumura, T., Rogers, A. J., Yoshimura, N., LeGrue, S., Drath, D. B. and Kerman, R. H. (1985) Clinical and experimental studies using cyclosporine in renal transplantation. *Surgery*, **97**, 125–140.
73. Tilney, N. L., Milford, E. L., Araujo, J. L., Strom, T. B., Carpenter, C. B. and Kirkman, R. L. (1984) Experiences with cyclosporine and steroids in clinical renal transplantation. *Ann. Surg.*, **200**, 605–613.
74. Tolkoff-Rubin, N. E. and Rubin, R. H. (1986). The impact of cyclosporine therapy on the occurrence of infection in the renal transplant recipient. *Transplant. Proc.*, **18**, 168–73.
75. Ho, M., Gui, X. E. and Atchison, R. W. (1983) The effects of cyclosporine on viruses. *Transplant. Proc.*, **15**, 2917–2919.
76. Dummer, J. S., Hardy, A., Poorsattar, A. and Ho, M. (1983). Early infections in kidney, heart and liver transplant recipients on cyclosporin. *Transplantation*, **36**, 259–267.
77. Calne, R. Y., Rolles, K., White, D. J. G., Thiru, S., Evans, D. B., McMaster, P., Dunn, D.

B., Craddock, G. N., Henderson, R. G., Aziz, S. and Lewis, P. (1979) Cyclosporin A initially as the only immunosuppressant in 34 recipients of cadaveric organs: 32 kidneys, 2 pancreases and 2 livers. *Lancet*, **2**, 1033–1036.

78. Thiru, S., Calne, R. Y. and Nagington, J. (1981) Lymphoma in renal allograft patients treated with Cyclosporin A as one of the immunosuppressive agents. *Transplant. Proc.*, **13**, 359–3⸵3.

79. Penn, I. (1987) Cancers following cyclosporine therapy. *Transplantation*, **43**, 32–34.

80. Penn, I. and First, M. R. (1986) Development and incidence of cancer following cyclosporine therapy. *Transplant. Proc.*, **18**, 210–213.

81. Powles, R. L., Clink, H. M., Spence, D., Morgenstern, G., Watson, J. G., Selby, P. J., Woods, M., Barrett, A., Jameson, B., Sloane, J., Lawler, S. D., Kay, H. E. M., Lawson, D., McElwain, T. J. and Alexander, P. (1980) Cyclosporin A to prevent GVHD in man after allogenic bone-marrow transplantation. *Lancet*, **1**, 327–329.

82. Reitz, B. A. and Bieber, C. P. (1982) Cancer after the use of cyclosporin A in animals. *Cancer Surv.*, **1**, 613–619.

83. O'Conor, G. T. (1970) Persistent immunologic stimulation as a factor in oncogenesis, with special reference to Burkitt's tumour. *Am. J. Med.*, **48**, 279–285.

84. Editorial (1978) Malaria and immunology. *Lancet*, **2**, 974–975.

85. Hanto, D. W., Frizzera, G., Kazimiera, J., Gajl-Peczalska and Simmons, R. L. (1985) Epstein–Barr virus, immunodeficiency and B cell lymphoproliferation. *Transplantation*, **39**, 461–472.

86. Bird, A. G., McLachlan, S. M. and Britton, S. (1981) Cyclosporin A promotes outgrowth *in vitro* of Epstein–Barr virus-induced B-cells lines. *Nature*, **289**, 300–301.

87. Clearly, M. L. and Sklar, J. (1984) Lymphoproliferative disorders in cardiac transplant recipients are multiclonal lymphomas. *Lancet*, **2**, 489–491.

88. Butler, T. T., Kalkwarff, K. L. and Kaldahl, W.B. (1987) Drug-induced gingival hyperplasia: phenytoin, cyclosporine and nifedipine. *J. Am. Drug. Assoc.*, **114**, 56–60.

89. Wysocki, G. P. Gretzinger, H. A., Lacipacis, A., Ulan, R. A., Stiller, C. R. Fibrous hyperplasia of the gingiva: A side effect of cyclosporine A therapy. *Oral Surg.*, **55**, 274–278.

90. Qunibi, W. Y., Akhtar, M., Ginn, E. and Smith, P. (1988) Kaposis sarcoma in cyclosporine-induced gingival hyperplasia. *Am. J. Kidney Dis.*, **11**, 349–352.

91. Harper, J. I., Kendra, J. R., Desai, S., Staughton, R. C. D., Barrett, A. J. and Hobbs, J. R. (1984) Dermatological aspects of the use of CsA for prophylaxis of graft versus host disease. *Br. J. Dermatol.*, **10**, 469–474.

92. Gebhart, W., Schmidt, J. B., Schemper, M., Spona, J., Kopsa, H. and Zazgornik, J. (1986). Cyclosporin-A-induced hair growth in human renal allograft recipients and alopecia areata. *Arch. Dermatol. Res.*, **278**, 238–240.

93. Reznik, V. M., Lyons Jones, K., Durham, B. L. and Medoza, S. A. (1987) Changes in facial appearance during cyclosporin treatment. *Lancet*, **2**, 1405–1406.

94. Kahan, B. D., Flechner, S. M., Lorber, M. I., Jensen Chris, Golden, D. and Van Buren, C. T. (1986) Complications of cyclosporin therapy. *World J. Surg.*, **10**, 348–360.

95. Barrett, A. J., Kendra, J. R., Lucus, C. F., Joss, D. V., Joshi, R., Pendharkar, P. and Hugh-Jones, K. (1982) Cyclosporin A as prophylaxis against graft versus host disease in 36 patients. *Br. Med. J.*, **285**, 162–166.

96. Durrant, S., Chipping, P. M., Palmer, S. and Gordon-Smith, E. C. (1982) Cyclosporine A, methyl prednisolone and convulsions. *Lancet*, **2**, 829–830.

97. Gross, M. L. P., Pearson, R. M., Kennedy, J., Moorhead, J. F. and Sweny, P. (1982). Rejection encephalopathy. *Lancet*, **2**, 1217.

98. Lewis, G. P. and Mangham, B. A. (1979) Pharmacology of graft rejection. *Trends Pharmacol. Sci.*, **1**, 18–21.

99. Powles, R. L., Kay, H. E. M. and Clink, M. M. (1983) Mismatched family donors for bone marrow transplantation as treatment for acute leukaemia. *Lancet*, **1**, 612–615.

100. Powell-Jackson, P. R., Carmichael, F. J. L., Calne, R. Y. and William, R. (1984) Adult respiratory distress syndrome and convulsions associated with administration of cyclosporine in liver transplant recipients. *Transplantation*, **38**, 341–343.

101. Blaauw, A. A. M., Leunissen, K. M. L., Cheriex, E. C., Wolters, J., Kootstra, G. and Van Hooff, J. P. (1987) Disappearance of pulmonary leak syndrome when intravenous cyclosporine is replaced by oral cyclosporine. *Transplantation*, **40**, 758–759.

102. Palestine, A. G., Nussenblatt, R. B. and Chan, C. C. (1984) Side effects of systemic Cyclosporine in patients not undergoing transplantation. *Am. J. Med.*, **77**, 652–656.
103. Calne, R. Y., Rolles, K., White, D. J. G., Thiru, S., Evans, D. B. E., Henderson, R., Hamilton, D. V., Boone, N., McMaster, P., Gibby, O. and Williams, R. (1981) Cyclosporin A in clinical organ grafting. *Transplant. Proc.*, **13**, 349–359.
104. Nyberg, G., Sandberg, L., Rydberg, L., Gabel, H., Persson, H., Wedel, N., Ahlman, J. and Brunger, H. (1984) ABO-autoimmune haemolytic anaemia in a renal transplant patient treated with cyclosporine. *Transplantation*, **37**, 529–530.

Index